Medical Radiology

Diagnostic Imaging

For further volumes:
http://www.springer.com/series/4354

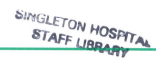

Olle Ekberg
Editor

Dysphagia

Diagnosis and Treatment

Foreword by
Maximilian F. Reiser

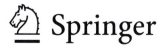 Springer

Editor
Olle Ekberg
Department of Clinical Sciences
Skåne University Hospital
Lund University
Malmö
Sweden

ISSN 0942-5373
ISBN 978-3-642-17886-3   ISBN 978-3-642-17887-0   (eBook)
DOI 10.1007/978-3-642-17887-0
Springer Heidelberg New York Dordrecht London

Library of Congress Control Number: 2012945741

Printed on acid-free paper

Springer is part of Springer Science+Business Media (www.springer.com)

To my wife Guje
with romance, felicity and affection

Olle Ekberg

Foreword

Dysphagia is a symptom of many and diverse diseases causing serious derogation of the quality of life. Diagnosis and treatment of dysphagia requires knowledge and experience of specialists from multiple disciplines, such as ENT specialists, neurologists, gastroenterologists and various other disciplines. For the radiologists involved in interdisciplinary teams, which are devoted to the diagnosis and treatment of dysphagia, knowledge of the anatomy and physiology is fundamental. Familiarity with the clinical background and available treatment options is mandatory.

The curriculum of most postgraduate institutions does not include profound training in specialized examinations of dysphagia. Professor Ekberg and the other authors of this book have great merits by providing comprehensive information covering anatomy, physiology, pathophysiology, pathology and clinical background. This book includes chapters on gastroesophageal reflux disease, globus and dysphagia, pediatric aspects on dysphagia, dysphagia in systemic disease, the geriatric pharynx and esophagus, voice and dysphagia as well as psychiatric aspects of dysphagia. The functional and cross-sectional imaging methods for the assessment of swallowing and its disorders are described in detail.

After the first edition in 2004 this second edition incorporates all newly discovered knowledge in this rapidly advancing field.

On behalf of the series editors of Medical Radiology—Diagnostic Imaging I would like to extend our sincere thanks to Prof. Ekberg and his co-workers for this extraordinary work. We are sure that it will be a great help for those interested in dysphagia and treatment of patients suffering from this symptom.

In addition to radiologists, specialists of various other medical disciplines can obtain most valuable information.

Munich   Maximilian F. Reiser

Preface

In preparing this volume, my aim has been to organize and set down, as concisely as possible, what may be considered the basic facts concerning the diagnosis and treatment of dysphagia. A principal focus is how to analyze the symptom of dysphagia, which is of the utmost importance and forms the basis for selection of any further steps in evaluation. In the clinical work-up, radiology is crucial. This was the topic of the book *Radiology of the Pharynx and Esophagus*, published by Springer in 2004. The continued rapid advances in dysphagology in the intervening period have prompted me to revise and expand that book. Seventeen chapters have been updated and refreshed, while 19 are completely new and place dysphagia in an even broader and deeper context. Particularly the consequences like malnutrition and dehydration are thoroughly described.

The current book therefore contains detailed information on anatomy, physiology, pathophysiology, pathology and clinical background as well as different aspects of nutrition and malnutrition. It bridges the gap between basic anatomy and physiology and the clinical management of patients with dysphagia.

The authors of the individual chapters are experts in their fields and most of them are engaged in hands-on practical work with patients.

The skilful assistance provided by Ms. Eva Prahl has been invaluable in bringing together all the loose ends to create what I hope will be a well-received volume.

I also wish to thank all the contributors to the volume and, particularly, Ms. Corinna Schaefer and Ms. Daniela Brandt of the publisher's staff. Their enthusiasm and skilful guidance have been invaluable.

Olle Ekberg

Contents

Part IV   Treatment

Contributors

Kasim Abul-Kasim Faculty of Medicine, Diagnostic Centre for Imaging and Functional Medicine, Skåne University Hospital, Malmö, Sweden; Lund University, Malmö, Sweden

Karin Aksglæde Division for Gastrointestinal Motility Disorders, Department of Radiology, Aarhus University Hospital, Nørrebrogade 44, 8000 Aarhus C, Denmark, e-mail: kariaksg@rm.dk

Jacqui Allen Department of Otolaryngology, North Shore Hospital, Takapuna, Auckland, New Zealand, e-mail: jeallen@voiceandswallow.co.nz; Jacqueline.Allen@waitematadhb.govt.nz

Samuel Hannes Baldinger University Polyclinic for Endocrinology, Diabetes and Clinical Nutrition, University Clinic for General Medicine, University Hospital, Bern, Switzerland

Filippo Barbiera Unità Operativa di Radiologia "Domenico Noto", Azienda Ospedali Civili Riuniti "Giovanni Paolo II", 92019, Sciacca, Italy

Ahmed Ba-Ssalamah Department of Radiology, Medical University of Vienna, Vienna, Austria, e-mail: ahmed.ba-ssalamah@meduniwien.ac.at

Peter C. Belafsky Center for Voice and Swallowing, University of California, Davis, Sacramento, CA, 95817, USA, Unità Operativa di Radiologia "Domenico Noto", Azienda Ospedali Civili Riuniti "Giovanni Paolo II", 92019 Sciacca, Italy

Jane E. Benson Russell H. Morgan Department of Radiology and Radiological Science, The Johns Hopkins University School of Medicine, 600 North Wolfe Street, Baltimore, MD 21205, USA, e-mail: jbenson@jhmi.edu

Katarina Bodén Department of Diagnostic Radiology, Karolinska University Hospital and Karolinska Institute, Stockholm, Sweden

Edmundo Brito-de la Fuente Innovation and Development Centre Clinical Nutrition and Pharmaceuticals, Science Production and Technology, Fresenius Kabi Deutschland GmbH, 61440, Oberursel, Germany, e-mail: edmundo.brito@fresenius-kabi.com

Margareta Bülow Neurological Department and Diagnostic Centre of Imaging and Functional Medicine, Skåne University Hospital, 205 02 Malmö, Sweden, e-mail: margareta.bulow@med.lu.se

S. Burton Abteilung Neurologie, m&i-Fachklinik Bad Heilbrunn, Wörnerweg 30, 83670 Bad Heilbrunn, Germany

Silvia Carrión Unidad de Exploraciones Funcionales Digestivas, Hospital de Mataró, Universitat Autònoma de Barcelona, Barcelona, Spain, Centro de Investigación Biomédica en red de Enfermedades Hepáticas y Digestivas (Ciberehd), Instituto de Salud Carlos III, Madrid, Spain

Massimo Castagnola Istituto di Biochimica e Biochimica Clinica, Facoltà di Medicina, Università Cattolica and Istituto per la Chimica del Riconoscimento Molecolare, CNR, Rome 00168, Italy

Michael Y. Chen Department of Radiology, Medical Center Boulevard, Wake Forest University School of Medicine, Winston-Salem, NC 27157, USA

Pere Clavé Centro de Investigaeión Biomédica, Universitat Autònoma de Barcelona, Hospital de Mataró, Barcelona, Spain

Jason D. Conway Department of Gastroenterology, Medical Center Boulevard, Wake Forest University School of Medicine, Winston Salem, NC 27157, USA, e-mail: jconway@wakehealth.edu

Doris-Maria Denk-Linnert Section of Phoniatrics, Department of Otorhinolaryngology, Vienna Medical School, Medical University of Vienna, Währinger Gürtel 18-20, 1090 Vienna, Austria, e-mail: doris-maria.denk-linnert@meduniwien.ac.at

Edith Eisenhuber Krankenhaus Goettlicher Heiland, Dornbacher Strasse 20-28, 1170, Vienna, Austria

Olle Ekberg Department of Clinical Sciences/Medical Radiology, Shane University Hospital, Lund University, 205 02 Malmö, Sweden; Diagnostic Centre of Imaging and Functional Medicine, Skåne University Hospital, 205 02 Malmö, Sweden; Department of Diagnostic Radiology, Malmö University Hospital, 205 02 Malmö, Sweden, e-mail: olle.ekberg@med.lu.se

Jörgen Ekström Department of Pharmacology, Institute of Neuroscience and Physiology, Sahlgrenska Academy at the University of Gothenburg, Box 431, SE-405 30, Göteborg, Sweden, e-mail: jorgen.ekstrom@pharm.gu.se

Lars I. Eriksson Department of Anaesthesiology and Intensive Care Medicine, Karolinska University Hospital and Karolinska Institute, Stockholm, Sweden

Daniele Farneti Voice and Swallowing Center, "Infermi" Hospital, Rimini, Italy, e-mail: lele_doc@libero.it

Pascale Fichaux Bourin Unité de la Voix et de la Déglutition, Department of Ear' Nose and Throat, CHU de Toulouse, Hôpital Larrey, 31059 Toulouse Cedex 9, France, e-mail: fichaux-bourin.p@chu-toulouse.fr

Barbara J. Fueger Department of Radiology, Medical University of Vienna, Vienna, Austria

Peter Funch-Jensen Division for Gastrointestinal Motility Disorders, Department of Radiology, Aarhus University Hospital, Nørrebrogade 44, 8000 Aarhus C, Denmark, Aleris-Hamlet Hospital, and Clinical Institute, Aarhus University, Aarhus C, Denmark

Críspulo Gallegos Departamento de Ingeniería Química, Universidad de Huelva, 21071 Huelva, Spain

Shaheen Hamdy Department of Inflammation Sciences, Salford Royal NHS Foundation Trust, University of Manchester, Manchester, M6 8HD, UK; Department of GI Sciences (Clinical Sciences Building), Salford Royal NHS Foundation Trust, Inflammation Sciences Research Group, University of Manchester, Manchester, M6 8HD, UK, e-mail: e-mail: shaheen.hamdy@manchester.ac.uk

Christian Hannig Institut für Röntgendiagnostik des Klinikums rechts der Isar, Technische Universität München, Ismaningerstrasse 22, 82756, Munich, Germany

Anna I. Hårdemark Cedborg Department of Anaesthesiology and Intensive Care Medicine, Karolinska University Hospital and Karolinska Institute, Stockholm, Sweden

Hanne Witt Hedström Department of Neuroradiology, Karolinska University Hospital and Karolinska Institute, Stockholm, Sweden

Bengt Jeppsson Department of Surgery, University Hospital of Skane-Malmö, Institute of Clinical Sciences, Lund University, Malmö, Sweden

Nina Khosravani Department of Pharmacology, Institute of Neuroscience and Physiology, Sahlgrenska Academy at the University of Gothenburg, Box 431, SE-405 30, Göteborg, Sweden

Martijn P. Kos ENT Department, Waterland Hospital, Purmerend, The Netherlands

Christiane Kulinna-Cosentini Department of Radiology, Medical University of Vienna, Währinger Gürtel 18-20, 1090, Vienna, Austria

Richard Kuylenstierna Department of Otorhinolaryngology, Karolinska University Hospital and Karolinska Institute, Stockholm, Sweden

A. Laverty Abteilung Neurologie, m&i-Fachklinik Bad Heilbrunn, Wörnerweg 30, 83670 Bad Heilbrunn, Germany

Alessandro Laviano Department of Clinical Medicine, Sapienza University, Rome, Italy

Johannes Lenglinger Motility Laboratory, Department of Surgery, Medical University of Vienna, Vienna, Austria, e-mail: johannes.lenglinger@meduniwien.ac.at

Marc S. Levine Department of Radiology, Hospital of the University of Pennsylvania, 3400 Spruce Street, Philadelphia, PA 19104, USA, e-mail: marc.levine@uphs.upenn.edu

M. Macleod Abteilung Neurologie, m&i-Fachklinik Bad Heilbrunn, Wörnerweg 30, 83670 Bad Heilbrunn, Germany, e-mail: marjorymacleod1950@yahoo.co.uk

Hans F. Mahieu ENT Department, Meander Medical Center, Amersfoort, The Netherlands, e-mail: hf.mahieu@meandermc.nl

Thomas Mandl Department of Rheumatology, Skåne University Hospital, 205 02 Malmö, Sweden

Bonnie Martin-Harris MUSC Evelyn Trammell Institute for Voice and Swallowing Disorders, Otolaryngology Head and Neck Surgery, Medical University of South Carolina, Charleston, SC, USA

Irene Messana Dipartimento di Scienze Applicate ai Biosistemi, Università di Cagliari, Cittadella Universitaria Monserrato, 09042 Cagliari, Monserrato, Italy

Emilia Michou Department of Inflammation Sciences, Salford Royal NHS Foundation Trust, University of Manchester, Manchester M6 8HD, UK

Satish Mistry Department of Inflammation Sciences, Salford Royal NHS Foundation Trust, University of Manchester, Manchester M6 8HD, UK

Francesco Mozzanica Department of Biomedical and Clinical Sciences "L. Sacco", University of Milan, Via GB Grassi, 74 20157 Milan, Italy

Göran Nylander Diagnostic Centre of Imaging and Functional Medicine, Skåne University Hospital, 205 02 Malmö, Sweden

Rolf Olsson Diagnostic Centre of Imaging and Functional Medicine, Skåne University Hospital, 205 02 Malmö, Sweden, e-mail: rolf.olsson@med.lu.se

David J. Ott Department of Radiology, Medical Center Boulevard, Wake Forest University School of Medicine, Winston-Salem, NC 27157, USA

Peter Pokieser Department of Radiology, University of Vienna, Währinger Gürtel 18-20, 1090 Vienna, Austria, e-mail: peter.pokieser@meduniwien.ac.at

Mario Prosiegel Abteilung Neurologie, m&i-Fachklinik Bad Heilbrunn, Wörnerweg 30, 83670 Bad Heilbrunn, Germany, e-mail: mario.prosiegel@fachklinik-bad-heilbrunn.de

Michèle Puech Unité de la Voix et de la Déglutition, Department of Ear' Nose and Throat, CHU de Toulouse, Hôpital Larrey, 31059 Toulouse Cedex 9, France

Stephen E. Rubesin Department of Radiology, University of Pennsylvania School of Medicine, MRI Building 1-08, University of Pennsylvania Medical Center, 3400 Spruce St., Philadelphia, PA 19104-4283, USA, e-mail: Stephen.Rubesin@uphs.upenn.edu

Martina Scharitzer Department of Radiology, University of Vienna, Währinger Gürtel 18-20, 1090 Vienna, Austria

Wolfgang Schima Department of Radiology, Krankenhaus Goettlicher Heiland, Dornbacher Strasse 20-28, 1170 Vienna, Austria, e-mail: wolfgang. schima@khgh.at; wolfgang.schima@meduniwien.ac.at

Antonio Schindler Department of Biomedical and Clinical Sciences "L. Sacco", University of Milan, Via GB Grassi, 74 20157, Milan, Italy, e-mail: antonio. schindler@unimi.it

Rainer Schöfl 4th Department of Internal Medicine, Hospital of the Elisab-ethinen, Fadingerstraße 1, 4020 Linz, Austria

Renée Speyer Mozartstraat 47, 6521 GB, Nijmegen, The Netherlands, e-mail: r.speyer@online.nl

Zeno Stanga University Polyclinic for Endocrinology, Diabetes and Clinical Nutrition, University Clinic for General Medicine, University Hospital, Bern, Switzerland, e-mail: zeno.stanga@insel.ch

Christina Stene Department of Surgery, Ängelholm Hospital, Institute of Clinical Sciences, Lund University, Malmö, Sweden, e-mail: christina.stene@ med.lu.se

Eva Sundman Department of Anaesthesiology and Intensive Care Medicine, Karolinska University Hospital and Karolinska Institute, Stockholm, Sweden

Per Thommesen Division for Gastrointestinal Motility Disorders, Department of Radiology, Aarhus University Hospital, Nørrebrogade 44, 8000 Aarhus C, Denmark

Dipesh H. Vasant Department of Inflammation Sciences, Salford Royal NHS Foundation Trust, University of Manchester, Manchester M6 8HD, UK

Eric Verin Service de Physiologie, Hôpital Charles Nicolle, CHU de Rouen, Rouen, France,

Arastoo Vossough Department of Radiology, Hospital of the University of Pennsylvania, 3400 Spruce Street, Philadelphia, PA 19104, USA

Virginie Woisard Unité de la Voix et de la Déglutition, Department of Ear· Nose and Throat, CHU de Toulouse, Hôpital Larrey, 31059 Toulouse Cedex 9, France

Anita Wuttge-Hannig Gemeinschaftspraxis für Radiologie, Strahlentherapie und Nuklearmedizin, Dres. Wuttge-Hannig-Rosskopf-Schepp-Sindelar, Karl-splatz 3-5, 80335 Munich, Germany, e-mail: Olle.Ekberg@med.lu.se

Part I

Anatomy and Physiology

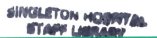

Anatomy and Physiology

Olle Ekberg and Göran Nylander

Contents

O. Ekberg (✉) · G. Nylander
Diagnostic Centre of Imaging and Functional Medicine,
Skåne University Hospital, 205 02 Malmö, Sweden
e-mail: olle.ekberg@med.lu.se

Abstract

The oral cavity, pharynx and esophagus constitute three anatomically and functionally integrated areas that are involved in swallowing. They are made up of muscular tubes surrounded by cartilages and bones. Swallowing in controlled by the brain stem in the central nervous system where the swallowing centre is located.

1   Introduction

The swallowing apparatus is made up of three anatomically and functionally separated, but integrated, areas, namely, the oral cavity, the pharynx, and the esophagus. These are tubular structures with muscular walls, in certain areas containing bone and cartilage. Each compartment functions independently, but for a successful swallowing process a finely tuned coordination between the compartments is necessary. Each compartment acts as a hydrodynamic pump. Between these pumps are interconnected valves.

To interpret the findings of the radiological examination, detailed knowledge of anatomy and physiology in this area is mandatory. In this context it is also important to understand that the larynx, both anatomically and physiologically, is an integrated part of the pharynx during swallowing. The nomenclature used in this chapter corresponds to anglicized Latin commonly in use (Williams et al. 1989). The description below refers to the adult individual. Those interested in newborns and infants are referred to works by Bosma (1973, 1976).

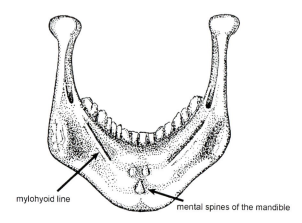

mylohyoid line

mental spines of the mandible

Fig. 1 The mandible seen posteriorly

2 Anatomy of the Pharynx and Larynx

2.1 Cartilages of the Larynx and Pharynx

Several of the important swallowing muscles insert on the inside of the mandible (Fig. 1). On the inside and medial surface of the mandible there is a centimeter-sized crest called the mylohyoid line, where the mylohyoid muscle inserts. Anteriorly in the midline on the posterior surface of the mandible there are a couple of eminences (mental spines) on which the geniohyoid and genioglossus muscles insert. These muscles then also insert within the tongue and on the hyoid bone, respectively. The hyoid bone is made up of a body and four horns, two on each side (Fig. 2). The upper two are called the lesser cornu of the hyoid bone, and the lower ones are called the greater cornu of the hyoid bone. From the lesser cornu there is a ligament that connects the cornu with the styloid process of the skull base. This ligament is called the stylohyoid ligament.

The thyroid cartilage is made up of two quadrilateral laminae, their anterior borders fused inferiorly and with a convexity superiorly and anteriorly. It also has a notch in the midline and superiorly. Posteriorly the cartilage has four horns (cornu). Two of these have a superior direction (superior cornu of the thyroid cartilage) and two have an inferior direction (inferior cornu of the thyroid cartilage; Fig. 3).

The superior cornu is connected via the thyrohyoid ligament with the greater cornu of the hyoid bone. The inferior cornu articulate directly against the cricoid cartilage. The hyoid bone and the thyroid cartilage

are connected, not only with the median and lateral thyrohyoid ligaments but also by the thyrohyoid membrane (Fig. 4). There is a lateral opening in the thyrohyoid membrane through which the laryngeal artery, vein, and nerve pass. There is also a small cartilage in the posterior and lateral part of the thyrohyoid ligament. This is called the triticeal cartilage.

The cricoid cartilage has the shape of a signet ring and is made up of a thin anterior part called the arcus of the cricoid cartilage and a posterior thicker portion called the lamina of the cricoid cartilage (Fig. 5). On its lateral margin the cricoid cartilage has an articulate facet for the inferior cornu of the thyroid cartilages. The lamina continues superiorly and dorsally in an eminence that ends with an articulate facet. Against this surface the arytenoid cartilages articulate. Two inferior horns of the thyroid cartilage articulate as described above against the cricoid cartilage. The thyroid and cricoid cartilages are also connected via the cricothyroid ligament (Fig. 6). Inferiorly to the cricoid cartilage is the trachea.

The core of the epiglottis is made up of cartilage. This thin foliate lamella has the form of a racket with a plate and a shaft. The shaft (petiolus) has a ligament (thyroepiglottic ligament) that connects it to the posterior surface of the thyroid cartilage (Fink and Demarest 1978; Fig. 7a).

The anterior surface of the epiglottis has a fan-shaped ligament connecting it to the hyoid bone (Fig. 7b). This ligament is an extension of the median glossoepiglottic ligament.

The arytenoid cartilages are shaped like small pyramids and are located at the posterior and superior corners of the cricoid cartilage. On top of this pyramid is another small cartilage, namely, the corniculate cartilage (Fig. 8).

Thereby there is a wall of cartilages, ligaments, and membranes extending from the hyoid bone and inferiorly. It reaches all the way to the anterior surface of the trachea. In the following the relation of the musculature and mucous membrane to these stabilizing structures will be described.

2.2 Muscles

The floor of the mouth is made up of several muscles, the positions of which are given in Figs. 9 and 10. The caudal extreme of the floor of the mouth is made up of the geniohyoid muscle and the mylohyoid muscle. The

Fig. 2 The hyoid bone seen superiorly and from the left (**a**) and anteriorly (**b**)

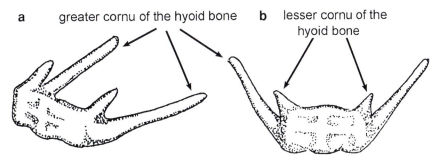

a   greater cornu of the hyoid bone   b   lesser cornu of the hyoid bone

Fig. 3 The thyroid cartilage seen anteriorly (**a**), anteriorly and from the left (**b**), and from the left (**c**)

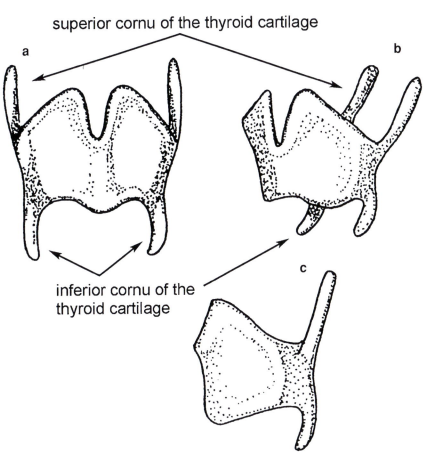

superior cornu of the thyroid cartilage

inferior cornu of the thyroid cartilage

latter inserts on the mylohyoid line on the mandible. It extends to the hyoid bone, where it inserts (Fig. 9). It is made up of a broad muscular diaphragm that covers most of the floor of the mouth. Covering this muscle is the geniohyoid muscle extending from the mental spines in the midline of the mandible to the body of the hyoid bone. The stylohyoid muscles extend from the styloid process to the lesser cornu on both sides (Fig. 10). Inferiorly are the thyrohyoid muscle, the hyoid bone, and the thyroid cartilage (Fig. 9). Inferior to the hyoid bone are the sternohyoid muscles and the omohyoid muscles.

2.2.1   Muscles of the Tongue

The genioglossus muscle is the largest muscle of the tongue and it extends from the mental spines on the mandible. This fan-shaped muscle widens as it extends backwards into the tongue. The superior fibers run to the tip of the tongue, and the middle fibers run to the dorsum of the tongue and a few of the inferior fibers extend to the hyoid bone, where the muscle inserts on the body of the hyoid bone (Fig. 11a). The hyoglossus muscle extends from the body and greater cornu of the hyoid bone and extends

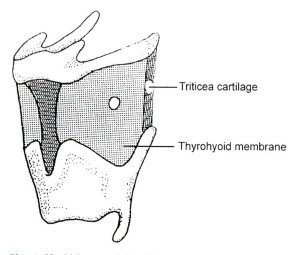

Fig. 4 Hyoid bone and thyroid cartilage seen anteriorly and from the left. *Light hatching* the thyrohyoid membrane, *dark hatching* the lateral and median thyrohyoid ligaments. There is a hole in the membrane for the passage of vessels and nerves

from there superiorly into the lateral portions of the tongue (Fig. 11b). The styloglossus muscle extends from the styloid processes of the skull base and the stylomandibular ligaments. It then extends into the lateral part of the tongue all the way to the tip of the tongue (Fig. 11c).

These three muscles join within the tongue and the muscle bundles fuse (Fig. 11d).

There are also a couple of external tongue muscles that connect the tongue with the skull base, the mandible, and the hyoid bone. Other tongue muscles are separated from these structures and are located solely within the tongue. They can be divided into four muscles: (1) the longitudinal superficial muscle, (2) the longitudinal deep muscle, (3) the transverse lingual muscles, and (4) the vertical lingual muscles. A small portion of the transverse lingual muscles runs up into the soft palate, where it is called the glossopalatine muscle (Fig. 12). Another small portion of this muscle is called the glossopharyngeal muscle and extends into the pharyngeal wall musculature (Fig. 12). In this way the musculature of the tongue inserts on the skull base, mandible, hyoid bone, soft palate, and lateral pharyngeal wall.

2.2.2 Muscles of the Soft Palate

The soft palate has an important function during swallowing. It is made up of a fibrous aponeurosis on which a couple of swallowing muscles insert. The levator veli palatini muscle extends from the inferior and lateral surface of the temporal bone close to the foramen of the internal carotid artery as well as from the inferior aspect of the tubal cartilage (of the auditory tube). The muscle then extends inferiorly, medially, and anteriorly and inserts on the midportion of the aponeurosis of the soft palate (Fig. 13). The tensor veli palatini muscle extends from the skull base and from the pterygoid processes of the sphenoid bone and extends first inferiorly and then turns at a right angle medially over the hamulus of the pterygoid process to spread horizontally in the aponeurosis of the soft palate (Fig. 14).

The palatopharyngeal muscle is the most prominent muscle in the soft palate and constitutes the arch. It extends from the inferior body of the tubal cartilage, pterygoid processes, and aponeurosis of the soft palate. This is the posterior extreme of the soft palate. The muscle then extends further inferiorly and posteriorly and forms part of the posterior wall of the pharynx. It also reaches the posterior surface of the thyroid cartilage (Fig. 15).

2.2.3 Muscles of the Pharynx

All muscles in the oral cavity, larynx, and pharynx are striated. Of the two arches that surround the tonsils, the medial arch is made up of the previously described palatopharyngeal muscle and the lateral arch is made up of the glossopalatine muscle (Fig. 16).

The walls of the pharynx are made up of a fibrous fascia connected to the mucosa on the inside and to the musculature on the outside of the wall. Superiorly towards the skull base there is no proper muscular layer. The only layers here are the mucosa and fascia, called the fibrous layer of the pharynx. This has a width of about 2 cm. Further inferiorly are the constrictor musculatures (Fig. 17). The main part of the wall of the pharynx is made up of constrictor muscles and elevators. The elevators are located on the inside, which is unique in the gastrointestinal tract. The muscles surrounding the oropharyngeal junction area are schematically shown in Fig. 18.

The pharyngeal constrictors are made up of three portions. The superior pharyngeal constrictor extends from above with four portions, namely, from the pterygoid process of the sphenoid bone, from the pterygomandibular raphe, from the mylohyoid line on the mandible, and also from the transverse

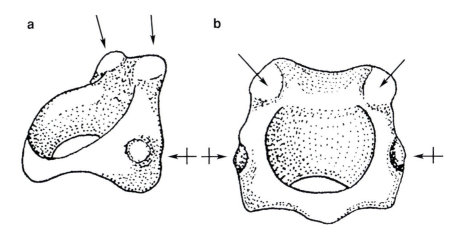

Fig. 5 The cricoid cartilage seen from the left (**a**) and anteriorly (**b**). There are two articulate surfaces for the arytenoid cartilages (*plain arrows*). There are also articulate surfaces for the cricoid cornu of the thyroid cartilage (*crossed arrows*)

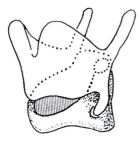

Fig. 6 The thyroid cartilage and cricoid cartilage with the cricothyroid ligament (*shaded*)

musculature of the tongue. These muscle bundles join and extend posteriorly. They make up the wall of the pharynx and meet in the midline dorsally in the pharyngeal raphe (Figs. 17, 18).

The middle pharyngeal constrictor extends from the hyoid processes and from the stylohyoid ligament. This ligament runs from the styloid process in the skull base to the minor processes of the hyoid bone. It then extends as a plate posteriorly and superiorly, joining the muscles from the other side in the posterior midline in the pharyngeal raphe (Figs. 18, 19).

The inferior pharyngeal constrictor extends from the cricoid cartilage, from the thyroid cartilage, and also from the lateral thyrohyoid ligament (Figs. 17, 18, 19, 20). This muscle extends somewhat superiorly and posteriorly surrounding the pharynx and joining the muscle from the other side in a pharyngeal raphe in the posterior midline. Inferiorly the pharyngeal constrictors form a superiorly convex arch.

There are several muscles that elevate the pharynx. The stylopharyngeal muscle extends from the styloid process and its surroundings at the skull base and

extends inferiorly and anteriorly in a gap between the superior and middle pharyngeal constrictors. It partly joins with the contralateral muscles and extends inferiorly to insert on the edges of the epiglottis and also on the posterior margin of the thyroid cartilage (Figs. 21, 22).

The palatopharyngeal muscle is the biggest of the elevators. It inserts on the posterior border of the hard palate and the palatine aponeurosis and on the pterygoid process. It extends inferiorly and inserts on the back of the thyroid cartilage and also within the constrictor musculature (Fig. 15).

2.2.4 The Pharyngoesophageal Segment

The pharyngeal constrictors make up the muscle wall of the pharynx almost from the skull base and down into the esophagus. Inferiorly to the constrictors there is one more muscle, namely, the cricopharyngeal muscle (Zaino et al. 1970; Fig. 20). This muscle is made up of an oblique portion, a transverse portion (which makes up the bulk of the muscle), and a longitudinal portion of muscle bundles inferiorly. The oblique part extends obliquely, superiorly, and posteriorly from the lateral part of the cricoid cartilage. It is close to the inferior constrictor. Like the latter muscle, it is usually considered that the oblique muscles connect in the pharyngeal raphe. This portion of the cricopharyngeal muscle is anatomically and functionally the inferior (small) portion of the pharyngeal constrictors. The transverse or semicircular portion extends posteriorly from the posterior and lateral part of the cricoid cartilage. Where the two muscles merge in the posterior midline there is *no* fibrous raphe. The two longitudinal muscles, also called esophageal elevators, extend from the inferior portion of

Fig. 7 a The thyroid cartilage and epiglottis (seen anteriorly) are connected with the thyroepiglottic ligament. **b** The hyoid bone (*H*) (seen from the *left*) is connected to the epiglottis via the hyoepiglottic ligament (*hl*)

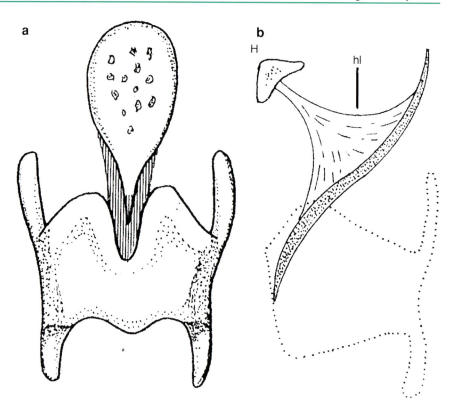

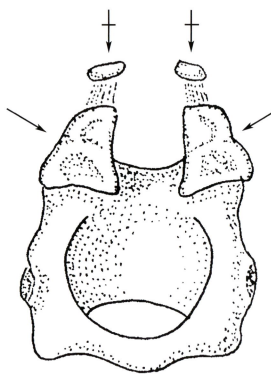

Fig. 8 Cricoid cartilage (seen anteriorly). The arytenoid cartilages (*plain arrows*) and corniculate cartilages (*crossed arrows*) are located on top

the cricoid cartilage and extend on each side of the esophagus, where they join the longitudinal musculature of the esophagus, which in turns comes from the median part of the lamina of the cricoid cartilage. Normally the inferior constrictor muscle overlaps the cricopharyngeal muscle, which in turn overlaps the circular muscle of the esophagus (Ekberg and Lindström 1987). However, between the oblique and transverse part of the crico-pharyngeal muscles there is a small triangular gap which is a weak point called Killian's opening or Laimer's tri-angle. It is through this weak area that the Zenker diverticulum extends. Laterally, there is a similar weak point inferior to the transverse portion and above the insertion of the longitudinal portion of the cricoid mus-cles. Through this gap the Killian–Jamieson diverticula extend (Jamieson 1934).

2.3 The Larynx

During swallowing, the larynx acts like a valve that closes off the airways from the foodway. The closure of the larynx is achieved by the following mecha-nisms. The tilting down of the epiglottis is achieved in a clear-cut two-step fashion. The first movement is

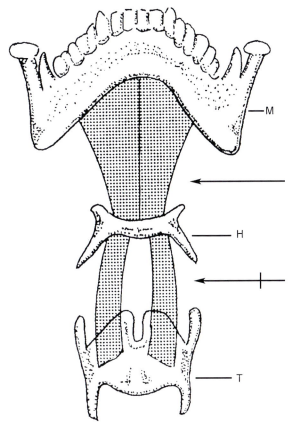

Fig. 9 The mandible (*M*), hyoid bone (*H*), and thyroid cartilage (*T*) seen anteriorly. The mylohyoid (*plain arrow*) and thyrohyoid (*crossed arrow*) muscles are indicated

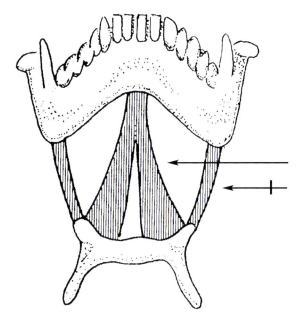

Fig. 10 The mandible and hyoid bone seen from below and anteriorly. The geniohyoid (*plain arrow*) and stylohyoid (*crossed arrow*) muscles are indicated

from the upright resting position of the epiglottis to a transverse position. This movement can be explained as consequential to the elevation of the hyoid bone and the approximation between the thyroid cartilage and the hyoid bone. This movement of the epiglottis is thereby the result of contraction of the muscles that elevate the hyoid bone, namely, the stylohyoid, digastric, mylohyoid, and geniohyoid muscles. In addition, the thyrohyoid muscle approximates the hyoid bone and the thyroid cartilage. The epiglottis is laterally fixed by the pharyngoepiglottic plicae and, during laryngeal elevation and thyroid approximation to the hyoid bone, is tilted to the transverse position with these plicae as turning points. The second movement of the epiglottis has been attributed either to the passing bolus which should push the movable lip of the epiglottis further down into the esophageal inlet or to the peristaltic contraction in the pharyngeal constrictor musculature. It is more probable that the second movement of the

epiglottis is accomplished by one of the muscles that inserts on the epiglottis. These muscles are the stylopharyngeal, thyroepiglottic, and aryepiglottic muscles. None of these muscles have such a direction that they are able to tilt the epiglottis down from its upright resting position. However, when the epiglottis has attained a transverse position, the conditions may have changed. Still, the stylopharyngeal muscle cannot possibly bring about the second movement, and it is more likely that a contraction in this muscle results in a tilting back of the epiglottis to the upright position. It is possible that the aryepiglottic muscle may be able to pull the epiglottis downwards against the "ary" region, but never as far down as into the esophageal inlet. When these two muscles have been excluded, the thyroepiglottic muscle remains as an able candidate to accomplish the tilting down of the epiglottis. With the epiglottis in the transverse position this muscle has a favorable direction in relation to the epiglottis. A contraction of the thyroepiglottic muscle is therefore very likely to pull the epiglottis down over the ary region. Furthermore, it will change the form of the epiglottis from a downward convex form to an upward convex form. A contraction of the aryepiglottic muscle in this new position of the epiglottis with its tip in the esophageal inlet will tighten the laryngeal inlet in the same manner as the string in a

Fig. 11 The tongue musculature, hyoid bone (*H*), and styloid process (*SP*). **a** Genioglossus muscle, **b** hyoglossus muscle, **c** styloglossus muscle, **d** composite drawing of the three muscles shown in **a–c**

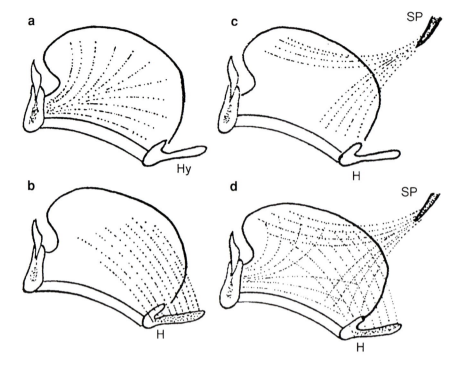

tobacco pouch. It is possible to distinguish two different steps in the closure of the vestibule, both of which are clearly separated from the closure of the rima glottidis. In the first step the supraglottic space of the vestibule is closed by the apposition of the lateral walls. This closure of the supraglottic space is caused by contraction and thickening of the superior portion of the thyroarytenoid muscle. The compressed supraglottic space has an orientation in the sagittal plane.

In the second step the closure of the vestibule is effected by a compression of the subepiglottic space from below. This is caused by the posterior aspect of the epiglottis with its superimposed fat cushion that is gradually pressed against the prominence of the ary region. The compressed subepiglottic space has an orientation nearly in the horizontal plane, with its anterior part more caudally than the posterior part. The tilting down of the epiglottis is probably due to a contraction of the thyroepiglottic muscles. A backward bulging of the superior–anterior wall of the vestibule is achieved by a folding of the median soft tissue linking the thyroid cartilage to the hyoid bone. This tissue comprises the epiglottic cartilage, the preepiglottic fat cushion, and its bounding ligaments, namely, the thyroepiglottic, the median thyrohyoid, and the hyoepiglottic ligaments. In analogy with other folds in this

region the above structures have been designated "the median thyrohyoid fold" (Fink 1976).

The described sequence of events in the closure of the vestibule by a compression from below—the supraglottic followed by the subepiglottic space—is important as it implies a peristaltic-like mechanism that can clear the vestibule of bolus material. After a swallowing act, the vestibule is free from foreign particles when it opens again.

The thyroepiglottic muscle and the aryepiglottic muscles pull the epiglottis downwards over the laryngeal inlet (Fig. 22). The aryepiglottic muscle runs within the aryepiglottic folds from the ary cartilage in a superior and anterior direction and inserts on the lateral border of the epiglottis (Fig. 22). Within the larynx there are several muscles, namely, the dorsal cricoarytenoid muscles, the lateral cricoarytenoid muscles, and the arytenoid muscle (Figs. 23, 24). The dorsal cricoarytenoid muscle runs from the posterior surface of the cricoid cartilage superiorly and laterally to insert on the lateral and inferior corner of the arytenoid cartilage. The lateral arytenoid muscle runs from the lateral part on the cricoid cartilage superiorly and posteriorly to insert in the same area as the prior described muscle. The arytenoid muscle runs between the two arytenoid cartilages and has a pars recta and

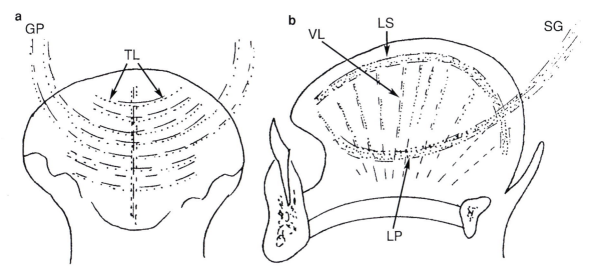

Fig. 12 Internal tongue musculature. The tongue seen **a** anteriorly and **b** from the left. *TL* transverse lingual muscles, *VL* vertical lingual muscles, *LS* longitudinal superficial muscle, *LP* longitudinal deep muscle, *GP* glossopharyngeal muscle, *SG* styloglossus muscle

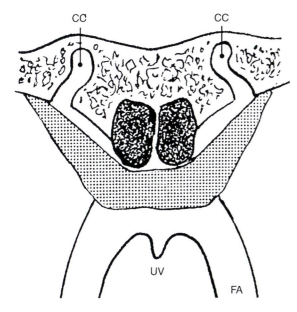

Fig. 13 Levator veli palatini muscle (*shaded*). The picture shows the skull base with choanae (*dark*) as well as the carotid canal (*CC*). The uvula (*UV*) and the faucial arcs (*FA*) are indicated

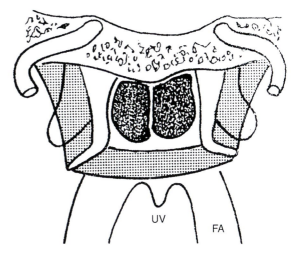

Fig. 14 Tensor veli palatini muscle (*shaded*). The picture shows the skull base with choanae (*dark*) as well as the carotid canal. The pterygoid process (*P*) and the hamulus of the pterygoid process (*H*) are indicated, as are the uvula (*UV*) and the faucial arcs (*FA*)

also a pars obliqua (Fig. 24). The thyroarytenoid muscle runs from the inside of the lamina of the thyroid cartilage and runs dorsally and laterally to insert on the arytenoid cartilage (Fig. 25a). It creates a muscle plate that laterally covers the larynx and the inlet to the larynx. The inferior portion is more bulky and it is made up of a lateral part and a vocal part. This latter is often

called the vocalis muscle within the vocal folds. The somewhat weaker and superior portion of the thyroarytenoid muscle is sometimes called the ventricularis muscle because it forms the ventricular fold. The thyroarytenoid muscle closes the rima glottidis and at the same time compresses the inferior portion of the laryngeal vestibule which we call the supraglottic space.

The cricothyroid muscle is a strong muscle that runs between the cricoid and thyroid cartilages. The pars

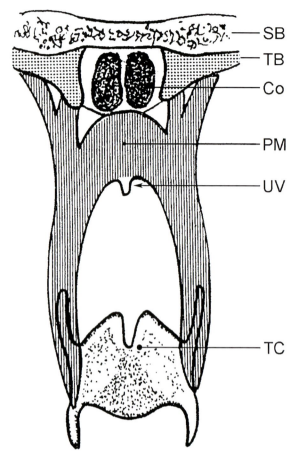

Fig. 15 The palatopharyngeal muscle seen posteriorly. *SB* skull base, *TB* tubal cartilage, *CO* choanae, *SP* soft palate, *UV* uvula, *TC* thyroid cartilage

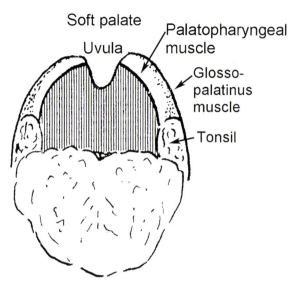

Fig. 16 The pharyngeal arches seen anteriorly. The locations of the palatopharyngeal and glossopharyngeal muscles are indicated

recta of this muscle runs superiorly and posteriorly from the cricoid cartilage and inserts on the thyroid cartilage. The pars obliqua of the muscle runs from the cricoid cartilage superiorly and posteriorly to insert on the inferior cornu of the thyroid cartilage (Fig. 25b).

2.4   The Mucosal Surface

The previous sections have described a framework of bones, cartilages, ligaments, and muscles, constituting the oral cavity, larynx, and pharynx. Inside this framework is the mucous membrane (Figs. 26, 27).

The posterior part of the tongue reaches all the way to the vallecula. This corresponds to the level of the hyoid bone. There is a pocket on each side of the midline, the vallecula. Posteriorly and laterally the valleculae are bordered by a mucosal fold above the stylopharyngeal

muscle. This fold is called the pharyngoepiglottic fold. The two valleculae are separated in the midline by a mucosal fold, the median glossoepiglottic fold (Figs. 26, 27). The tongue base and valleculae contain a rich network of lymphatic tissue. The vallecula may also contain vessels in the submucosa, which causes a weblike appearance (Ekberg et al. 1986). Further inferiorly (Fig. 27) there is a fold reaching from the lateral border of the epiglottis to the ary region. The folds surround the inlet of the laryngeal vestibule. This is the aryepiglottic fold which harbors the aryepiglottic muscle. There are two small protuberances caudally/inferiorly due to the cuneiform tubercle superiorly and the corniculate tubercle inferiorly. Between the two corniculate tubercles there is a cleft called the interarytenoid incisure. The aryepiglottic fold is made up of the aryepiglottic muscle posteriorly and the thyroepiglottic muscle anteriorly. The lamina of the cricoid cartilage causes an impression of the pharyngeal lumen. On both sides of these impressions there are two recesses called the piriform sinuses.

3   Anatomy of the Esophagus

The esophagus can be divided into different parts according to the surrounding anatomical structures (Fig. 28). The superior part, the pharyngoesophageal segment (functional term), also called the upper

Fig. 17 The pharyngeal musculature seen posteriorly. **a** Palatopharyngeal muscles and elevator of the pharynx. **b** Constrictor muscles. (Drawing by Sigurdur V. Sigurjonsson)

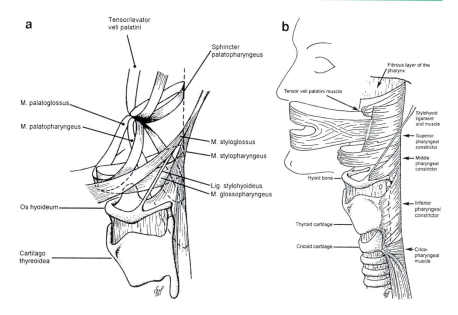

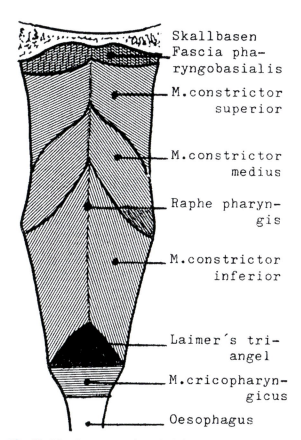

Fig. 18 The pharynx seen from the left. (Drawing by Sigurdur V. Sigurjonsson)

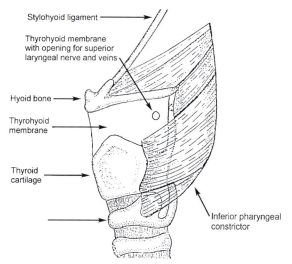

Fig. 19 The hyoid bone, thyroid cartilage, and cricoid cartilage with muscles and membranes seen from the left

esophageal segment (anatomical term), corresponds to the cricopharyngeal muscle and surrounding pharynx and cervical esophagus. This is also called introitus esophagi or Killian's mouth. From here to the impression of the aorta is the paratracheal esophagus (Fig. 28). This is located close to the membranous part of the trachea. The aorta makes a short impression from the left into the aortic lumen.

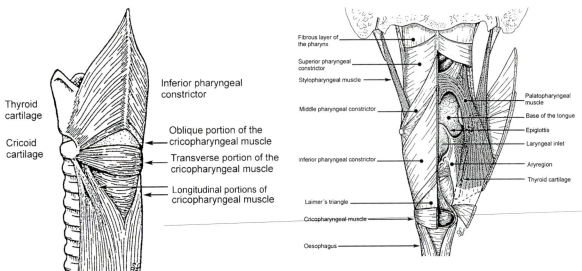

Fig. 20 The cricopharyngeal muscle seen from posteriorly and from left. (Drawing by Sigurdur V. Sigurjonsson. From Ekberg and Nylander 1982)

Fig. 21 The pharyngeal musculature seen posteriorly and with the right side of the pharynx cut open so that it can be seen from inside. The three constrictor muscles are overlapping. The stylopharyngeal muscle runs from the styloid process inferiorly to insert on the epiglottis, thyroid cartilage, and pharyngeal wall through a gap between the superior and middle constrictors. (Drawing by Sigurdur V. Sigurjonsson)

Inferiorly to this and above the left main bronchus is the aortobronchial portion, which is a short, relatively wide segment. The left main bronchus makes a short impression in the esophagus from the left. The cardial portion is that segment of the esophagus which is located close to the left atrium of the heart. A schematic drawing of the gastroesophageal region is given in Fig. 29.

The esophagus is made up of three layers, the mucosa, the submucosa, and the muscularis (Fig. 30). The mucosa is made of squamous cell epithelium. Under the epithelium there is a submucosal layer of musculature as everywhere else in the alimentary canal. The mucosa also contains glands and vessels. The mucosa has a tendency to create longitudinal mucosal folds.

The esophagus has two layers of muscles, an inner circular and an outer longitudinal muscle layer. The longitudinal muscles insert on the posterior aspect of the lamina of the cricoid cartilage. The upper third of the esophagus is made up of striated musculature, whereas the lower two thirds is smooth muscles. The transitional zone, however, has a varying position. The circular muscle layer is thinner cranially and increases in thickness distally. Between the two muscle layers there are a multitude of neurons in a plexus formation (Auerbach's plexus). In this there

are both sympathetic and parasympathetic nerves. There is a close proximity between the vagus nerve and the esophagus, especially inferiorly.

4 Neuroanatomy and Physiology of Swallowing

There are several reviews on the neuroanatomy and neurophysiology of swallowing, the most contemporary by Miller (1999). Several of the cranial nerves are involved in the control of swallowing (Perlman and Christensen 1997). Oral sensation is transmitted in the trigeminal nerve. Efferent information in the trigeminal nerve goes to the mylohyoid muscle, the anterior belly of the digastric muscle, and the four muscles of mastication: the masseter, temporalis, and pterygoid muscles.

Taste sensation is mediated in the facial nerve. Efferent control from the facial nerve goes to the salivary glands and to muscles of facial expression, the stylohyoid and platysma muscles, as well as the posterior belly of the digastric muscle.

The glossopharyngeal nerve conveys taste information from the posterior part of the tongue. It also conveys sensation from the pharynx. It innervates only the stylopharyngeal muscle efferently.

Fig. 22 The stylopharyngeal muscle and epiglottic musculature seen posteriorly (a), posteriorly and from the right (b), and from the right (c). (Drawing by Sigurdur V. Sigurjonsson. From Ekberg and Sigurjonsson 1982)

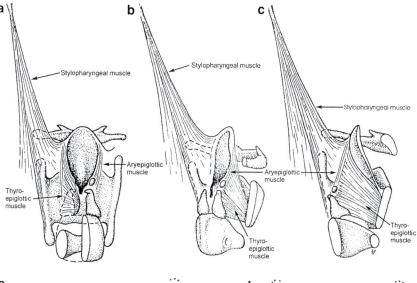

Fig. 23 The cricoid cartilage, arytenoid cartilage, and muscles seen from the left (a) and posteriorly (b)

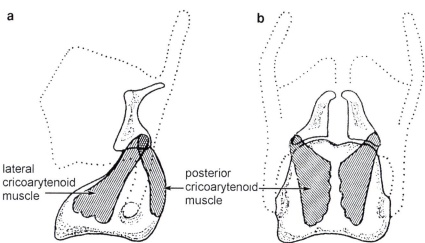

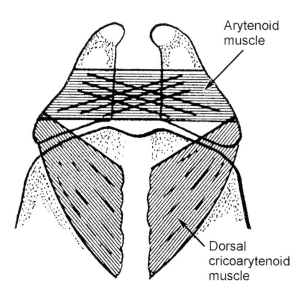

Fig. 24 The cranial portion of the cricoid cartilage, the arytenoid cartilage, and muscles seen posteriorly

The vagus nerve is the most important nerve for swallowing. It innervates the pharyngeal and laryngeal mucosa. The recurrent laryngeal nerve conveys sensation from below the vocal folds and also the esophagus. Efferent control in the vagus nerve comes from the ambiguus nucleus (striated muscle) and the posterior nucleus of the vagus nerve (smooth muscles and glands).

The hypoglossal nerve provides efferent control of all the intrinsic and some of the extrinsic muscles of the tongue.

The locations of the central swallowing pathways include several cortical and subcortical regions. One such area is located immediately in front of the precentral sulcus cortex. Stimulation in this area evokes mastication followed by swallowing. It is likely that the cortical and subcortical areas merely modify swallowing as pharyngeal and esophageal swallowing can be evoked also in the absence of these areas. This

Fig. 25 **a** The larynx cut open in the midline and seen from the left. **b** The larynx seen anteriorly and from the left

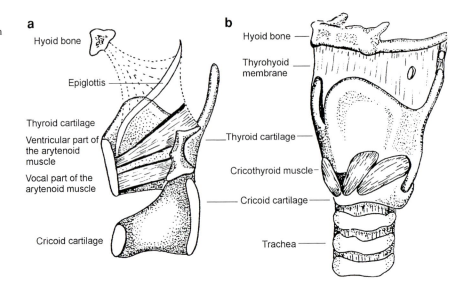

Fig. 26 The pharynx seen from the left

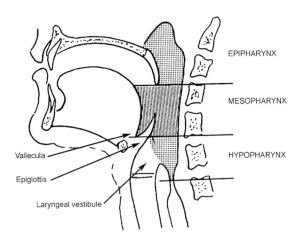

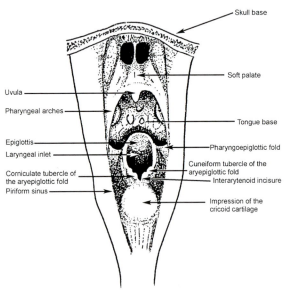

Fig. 27 The pharynx cut open in the posterior midline and seen from behind

indicates that the brainstem is the primary swallowing area.

Afferent information from the oral cavity and pharynx is mediated via the vagus nerve and other nerves to the nucleus of the solitary tract in the brainstem. Close to the nucleus of the solitary tract is an afferent swallowing center that interprets the information. If it is found appropriate for swallowing, information goes to a swallowing center close to the ambiguus nucleus. Control of the pharynx is managed from that swallowing center. Information also goes to a dorsal swallowing center close to the posterior nucleus of the vagus nerve. The oral stage of

swallowing is completely voluntary, whereas the pharyngeal stage of swallowing is automatic. This automatism means that there is a none-or-all situation. Once the pharyngeal swallow has been elicited, it is always completed. It is not modified during the pharyngeal swallowing process and it cannot be interrupted. Swallowing has priority over other activities controlled from the ambiguus nucleus such as breathing, speech, and positioning. The esophageal stage of

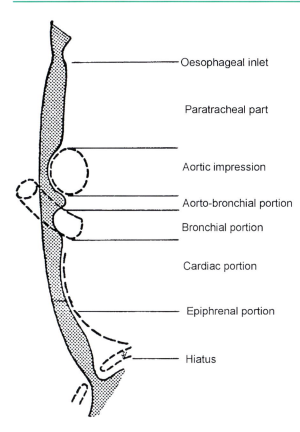

Oesophageal inlet

Paratracheal part

Aortic impression

Aorto-bronchial portion

Bronchial portion

Cardiac portion

Epiphrenal portion

Hiatus

Fig. 28 The different parts of the esophagus

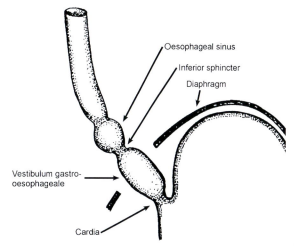

Oesophageal sinus

Inferior sphincter

Diaphragm

Vestibulum gastro-oesophageale

Cardia

Fig. 29 The gastroesophageal region

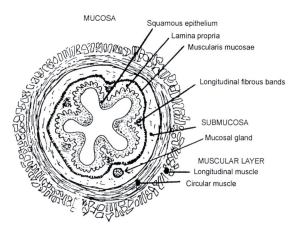

MUCOSA

Squamous epithelium

Lamina propria

Muscularis mucosae

Longitudinal fibrous bands

SUBMUCOSA

Mucosal gland

MUSCULAR LAYER

Longitudinal muscle

Circular muscle

Fig. 30 Cross section of the esophagus

swallowing is autonomic, which means that it may occur also without control from the brainstem. It is also self-regulatory, i.e., a second swallow interrupts the first, and a secondary peristaltic wave can be elicited. This is achieved by the enteric nervous system.

The oral stage of swallowing includes ingestion, which is a complex act. It also involves blending, mixing, and mincing of ingested material. When the ingested material is found to be appropriate for swallowing (by analyzing information from the nucleus of the solitary tract), the tongue usually scoops up a suitable amount of ingested material, which is from now on called a "bolus," onto the top of the tongue. From there it is propelled by a sweeping movement of the tongue into the pharynx. The pharyngeal stage of swallowing includes sealing off the nasopharynx with the soft palate opposing the posterior pharyngeal wall and also the closing of the airways by elevation and closure of the larynx and tilting down of the epiglottis. Opening of the pharyngoesophageal segment is also mandatory.

The pharyngeal constrictors achieve the final rinsing of the pharynx. An important item is the elevation of the pharynx and larynx. When the bolus reaches the upper part of the esophagus, peristaltic activity occurs. This means that esophageal tonicity is abolished and the bolus is propelled downwards by a combination of gravity and contraction in the circular musculature. When this occurs in connection with pharyngeal swallowing, it is called primary peristalsis. If it occurs by local distension, for instance, by retained material or regurgitated/reflux material, it is called secondary peristalsis. If contraction is non-propulsive, it is called simultaneous contraction. In the elderly patient this has also been called tertiary contraction.

References

Bosma JF (ed) (1973) Fourth symposium on oral sensation and perception: development in the fetus and infant. DHEW publication no. (NIH) 73-546. US Department of Health, Education, and Welfare, Bethesda

Bosma JF (ed) (1976) Symposium on development of the basicranium. DHEW publication no. (NIH) 76-989. US Department of Health, Education, and Welfare, Bethesda

Ekberg O, Lindström C (1987) The upper esophageal sphincter area. Acta Radiol 28:173–176

Ekberg O, Nylander G (1982) Dysfunction of the cricopharyngeal muscle: a cineradiographic study of patients with dysphagia. Radiology 143:481–486

Ekberg O, Sigurjonsson SV (1982) Movement of the epiglottis during deglutition: a cineradiographic study. Gastrointest Radiol 7:101–107

Ekberg O, Birch-Iensen M, Lindström C (1986) Mucosal folds in the valleculae. Dysphagia 1:68–72

Fink BR (1976) The median thyrohyoid "fold": A nomenclature suggestion. J Anat 122:697–699

Fink BR, Demarest RJ (1978) Laryngeal biomechanics. Harvard University Press, Cambridge

Jamieson JB (1934) Illustrations of regional anatomy. Livingstone, Edinburgh, Sect 2:44

Miller AJ (1999) The neuroscientific principles of swallowing and dysphagia. Singular Publishing Group, San Diego

Perlman AL, Christensen J (1997) Topography and functional anatomy of the swallowing structures. In: Perlman AL, Schulze-Delrieu K (eds) Deglutition and its disorders: anatomy, physiology, clinical diagnosis, and management. Singular Publishing Group, San Diego, pp 15–42

Williams PL, Warwich R, Dyson M, Bannister LH (eds) (1989) Gray's anatomy, 37th edn. Churchill Livingstone, Edinburgh

Zaino C, Jacobson HG, Lepow H, Ozturk CH (1970) The pharyngoesophageal sphincter. Thomas, Springfield

Saliva and the Control of Its Secretion

Jörgen Ekström, Nina Khosravani, Massimo Castagnola, and Irene Messana

Contents

J. Ekström (✉) · N. Khosravani
Department of Pharmacology,
Institute of Neuroscience and Physiology,
Sahlgrenska Academy at the University of Gothenburg,
Box 431, SE-405 30 Göteborg, Sweden
e-mail: jorgen.ekstrom@pharm.gu.se

M. Castagnola
Istituto di Biochimica e Biochimica Clinica,
Facoltà di Medicina, Università Cattolica
and Istituto per la Chimica del Riconoscimento
Molecolare, CNR, 00168 Rome, Italy

I. Messana
Dipartimento di Scienze Applicate ai Biosistemi,
Università di Cagliari, Cittadella Universitaria
Monserrato, 09042 Monserrato, Cagliari, Italy

Abstract

The various functions of saliva—among them digestive, protective and trophic ones—not just limited to the mouth, and the relative contribution of the different types of gland to the total volume secreted as well as to various secretory rhythms over time are discussed. Salivary reflexes, afferent and efferent pathways, as well as the action of classical and non-classical transmission mechanisms regulating the activity of the secretory elements and blood

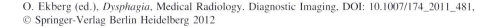
O. Ekberg (ed.), *Dysphagia*, Medical Radiology. Diagnostic Imaging, DOI: 10.1007/174_2011_481,

vessels are in focus. Sensory nerves of glandular origin and an involvement in gland inflammation are discussed. Although, the glandular activities are principally regulated by nerves, recent findings of an "acute" influence of gastro-intestinal hormones on saliva composition and metabolism, are paid attention to, suggesting, in addition to the cephalic nervous phase, both a regulatory gastric and intestinal phase. The influence of nerves and hormones in the long-term perspective as well as old age, diseases and consumption of pharmaceutical drugs on the glands and their secretion are discussed with focus on xerostomia and salivary gland hypofunction. Treatment options of dry mouth are presented as well as an explanation to the troublesome clozapine-induced sialorrhea. Final sections of this chapter describe the families of secretory salivary proteins and highlight the most recent results obtained in the study of the human salivary proteome. Particular emphasis is given to the post-translational modifications occurring to salivary proteins before and after secretion, to the polymorphisms observed in the different protein families and to the physiological variations, with a major concern to those detected in the pediatric age. Functions exerted by the different families of salivary proteins and the potential use of human saliva for prognostic and diagnostic purposes are finally discussed.

1   Functions of Saliva: An Overview

Saliva exerts digestive and protective functions and a number of other functions, depending on the species, usually grouped under the heading "additional functions." *Digestive functions* include the mechanical handling of food such as chewing, bolus formation, and swallowing. The chemical degradation of food is by amylase and lipase—these enzymes continue to exert their activities in the stomach, amylase exerting its activity until the acid penetrates the bolus. The group of digestive functions also includes the process of dissolving the tastants, and thus allowing them to interact with the taste buds. If pleasant, taste sets up a secretory reflex of gastric acid as part of the cephalic regulation of gastric secretion. To the *protective functions* belong the lubrication of the oral structures by mucins, the dilution of hot or cold food, and spicy food, the ability of the buffer

(by bicarbonate, phosphates, and protein) to maintain salivary pH around 7.0 (note that in many laboratory animals, the pH is higher, 8.5–9.0), the remineralization of enamel by calcium, the antimicrobial defense action by immunoglobulin A, α-defensins, and β-defensins, and wound healing by growth-stimulating factors such as epidermal growth hormone, statherines, and histatines. Additionally, saliva is necessary for articulate speech, for excretion (as discussed below), and for social interactions (such as kissing). Moreover, saliva exerts trophic effects. It maintains the number of taste buds. Further, it has recently become apparent that the composition of saliva secreted during fetal life may be of importance for the development of oral structures (Jenkins 1978; Tenouvo 1998; Mese and Matsuo 2007; Inzitari et al. 2009; Castagnola et al. 2011a). It has already been mentioned that the salivary enzymes accompanying the bolus are still active in the stomach. There are further examples of the fact that the action of saliva is not restricted to the mouth. Swallowed saliva protects the esophageal wall from being damaged by regurgitating gastric acid as is the case with a lowered tone of the lower esophageal sphincter (Shafik et al. 2005). The defense mechanisms of saliva protect the upper as well as the lower respiratory tract from infectious agents (Fig. 1).

Although the exocrine function of the salivary glands is in focus, it is worth noting that salivary glands have, in addition, excretory and possibly endocrine functions. Circulating non-protein-bound fractions of hormones, such as of melatonin, cortisol, and sex steroids, passively move into the saliva, as do a number of pharmaceutical drugs (Gröschl 2009). Interestingly, melatonin, when in the oral cavity, exerts antioxidative, immunomodulatory, and anticancerogenic effects (Cutando et al. 2007). Iodide is actively taken up by the glands by the same transport system as in the thyroid gland, a situation that may be deleterious for the salivary glands if the iodide is radioactive and is used in the treatment of thyroid tumors (Mandel and Mandel 2003). Salivary substances may appear in the blood as indicated by amylase and epidermal growth factor, which suggests endocrine functions of the glands (Isenman et al. 1999).

In animals, saliva may be secreted to lower the body temperature by evaporative cooling (panting of dogs and spreading of saliva on the scrotum and the fur by rats), for grooming (rats and cats) and, by salivary pheromones, to mark territory or to attract mates (mice and pigs); particularly, sex steroids of the saliva serve as olfactory signals (Gregersen 1931; Hainsworth 1967; Gröschl 2009).

Fig. 1 Functions of saliva

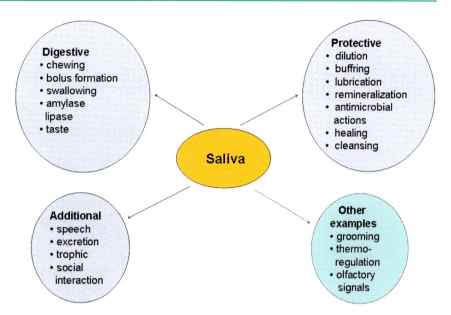

Digestive
- chewing
- bolus formation
- swallowing
- amylase lipase
- taste

Protective
- dilution
- buffring
- lubrication
- remineralization
- antimicrobial actions
- healing
- cleansing

Saliva

Additional
- speech
- excretion
- trophic
- social interaction

Other examples
- grooming
- thermo-regulation
- olfactory signals

Fig. 2 Parotid gland and accessory gland. (With permission from Elsevier)

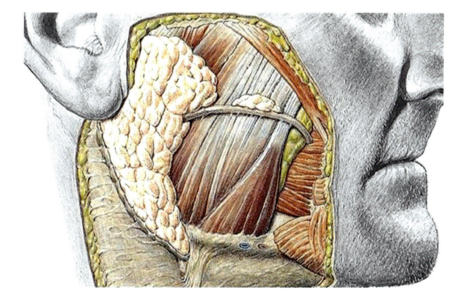

2 Major and Minor Salivary Glands and Mixed Saliva

Saliva is produced by three pairs of major glands, the parotids, the submandibulars, and the sublinguals, located outside the mouth, and hundreds of minor glands—each the size of a pinhead and located just below the oral epithelium (Figs. 2 and 3). As judged by magnetic resonance imaging, the volume of the parotid gland is about 2.5 times that of the submandibular gland and eight times that of the sublingual gland (Ono et al. 2006). Similar relationships are obtained when the comparisons are based on gland

Fig. 3 Submandibular and sublingual glands. Note the many small ducts from the sublingual gland. (With permission from Elsevier)

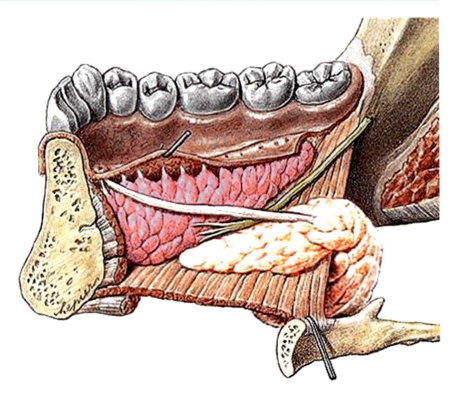

weights, the parotid gland weighing 15–30 g (Gray 1988). The saliva from the parotid and submandibular glands reaches the oral cavity via long excretory ducts (7 and 5 cm, respectively), the parotid duct (also called Stensen's duct) opening at the level of the second upper molar, and the submandibular duct (Wharton's duct) opening on the sublingual papilla. In about 20% of the population, the parotid duct is surrounded by a small accessory gland. Sublingual saliva empties into the submandibular duct via the major sublingual duct (Bartholin's duct) or directly into the mouth via a number of small excretory ducts opening on the sublingual folder. Likewise, the saliva of minor glands, such as of the buccal, palatine (located just in the soft palate), labial, lingual, and molar glands, empties into the mouth directly via small, separate ducts just traversing the epithelium (Tandler and Riva 1986). Unless saliva is collected directly from the cannulated duct, the saliva in the mouth will be contaminated by the gingival crevicular fluid, blood cells, microbes, antimicrobes, cell and food debris, and nasopharyngeal secretion. Consequently, mixed saliva ("whole saliva") collected by spitting or drooling is not pure saliva, although the term "saliva" is usually used.

3   Spontaneous, Resting, and Stimulated Secretion

Some salivary glands have an inherent capability to secrete saliva (Emmelin 1967). The type of gland differs among different species. In humans, only the minor glands secrete saliva spontaneously. Although these glands are innervated and may increase their secretory rate in response to nervous activity, they secrete saliva at a low rate, without exogenous influence during the night. In daytime and at rest, a nervous reflex drive—set up by low-grade mechanical stimuli due to movements of the tongue and lips, and mucosal dryness—acts on the secretory cells, particularly engaging the submandibular gland (Fig. 4). In the clinic, the saliva secreted at rest is often called "unstimulated secretion," despite the involvement of nervous activity. With respect to stimulated secretion, the parotid contribution becomes more dominant: in response to strong stimuli, such as citric acid, the flow rate is about equal to that from the submandibular gland, whereas in response to chewing, the flow rate is twice as high as that from the submandibular gland. The total volume of saliva secreted amounts to 1–2 L per 24 h. The flow rate

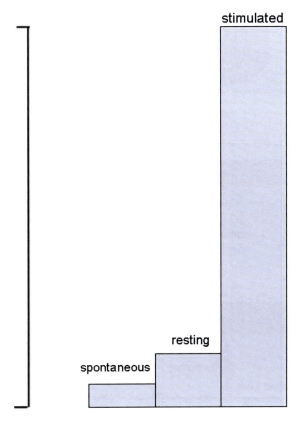

Fig. 4 Different rates of salivary flow

characterized as mucous glands. The deep posterior lingual glands (von Ebner's glands), found in circumvallate and foliate papillae close to most of the taste buds, are, however, of the serous type. Though, the contribution of the minor glands is small, they continuously, during day and night, provide the surface of the oral structures with a protective layer of mucin-rich saliva that prevents the feeling of mouth dryness from occurring. Together with the sublingual glands, they are responsible for 80% of the total mucin secretion per 24 h.

4 The Salivary Response Displays Circadian and Circannual Rhythms

On the whole, the flow rate of resting as well as of stimulated saliva is higher in the afternoon than in the morning (Ferguson and Botchway 1980; Dawes 1975), the peak occurring in the middle of the afternoon. Also the salivary protein concentration follows this diurnal pattern. In addition, the flow of the resting saliva is higher during winter than during summer, indicating a circannual rhythm (Elishoov et al. 2008). Just a small change in the ambient temperature (by 2 °C) in a warm climate is enough to inversely affect the flow rate (Kariyawasam and Dawes 2005).

correlates with gland size, and is higher in males than in females (Heintze et al. 1983). The relative contributions of each type of gland to the total volume secreted are as follows: roughly 30% for the parotid glands, 60% for the submandibular glands, 5% for the sublingual glands, and 5% for the minor glands (Dawes and Wood 1973). Different types of glands produce different types of secretion. Depending on the reaction to the histochemical staining of the acinar cells for light-microscopy examination, the cells are classified as (basophilic) serous or (eosinophilic) mucous cells. The serous cells are filled with protein-storing granules and are associated with the secretion of water and enzymes, whereas the mucous cells are associated with the secretion of the viscous mucins stored in vacuoles. The parotid gland is characterized as a serous gland, the submandibular gland is characterized as a seromucous gland (10% mucous cells and 90% serous cells), and the sublingual gland and most of the minor glands are

5 The Diversity of the Salivary Response

Pavlov drew attention to the fact that the volume of saliva secreted and its composition vary in a seemingly purposeful way in response to the physical and chemical nature of the stimulus (see Babkin 1950). Not only does the secretion adapt "acutely" to the stimulus, but also long-term demands may induce changes in gland size and secretory capacity. The variety in the salivary response is attained by the involvement of different types of glands, different types of cells within a gland, different types of reflexes displaying variations in intensity, duration, and engagement of the two divisions of the autonomic innervation, different types of transmitter and varying transmitter ratios, different types of receptors, and various intracellular pathways either running in parallel or interacting synergistically (Fig. 5).

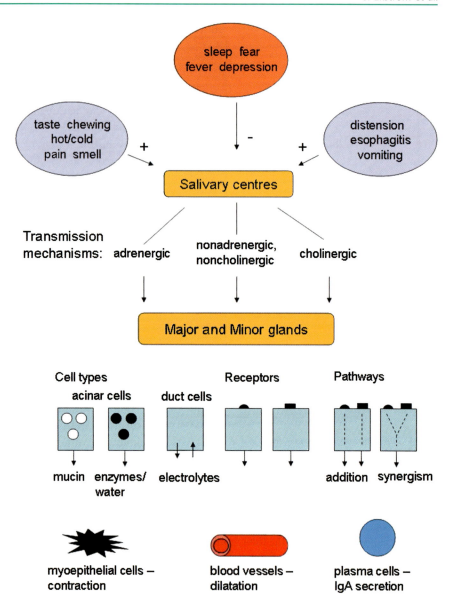

Fig. 5 Afferent and efferent nerves, and various elements of salivary glands

6 Afferent Stimuli for Secretion

Eating is a strong stimulus for the secretion of saliva (Hector and Linden 1999). A number of sensory receptors are activated in response to food intake: gustatory receptors, mechanoreceptors, nociceptors, and olfactory receptors (Fig. 5). All four modes of taste (sour, salt, sweet, and bitter) elicit secretion ("gustatory salivary reflex") but sour, followed by salt, is the most effective stimulus. Taste buds reside in the papillae of the tongue. The sensation of salt is particularly experienced at the tip of the tongue and that of bitter at the dorsum of the tongue, whereas the sensations of sweet and sour are experienced in between. Regions other than the tongue, in particular the soft palate, but also the epiglottis, the esophagus, the nasopharynx, and the buccal wall, also contain areas of taste buds. Chewing causes the teeth to move sideways, thereby stimulating mechanoreceptors of the periodontal ligaments ("masticatory salivary reflex"). In addition, gingival mucosal tissue mechanoreceptors are activated during chewing. Olfactory receptors are located at the cribriform plate,

i.e., at the roof of the nasal cavity, and they respond to volatile molecules of the nasal and the retronasal airflow (the latter arising from the oral cavity or the pharynx). Sniffing increases the airflow and thereby the access of stimuli to the receptor area. The epithelium containing the olfactory receptors has a rich blood supply. Interestingly, blood-borne odorants may pass through the vessel walls and stimulate these receptors. The submandibular glands, but not the parotid glands, are regulated by an "olfactory salivary reflex." Irritating odors, do, however, mobilize the parotid gland, in addition to the submandibular gland, in this case in response to the stimulation of epithelial trigeminal "irritant receptors." The nociceptors may also be activated in response to spicy food (e.g., chilli pepper). Thermal stimuli also influence the rate of secretion. Ice-cold drinks cause a greater volume of saliva to be produced than do hot drinks (Dawes et al. 2000). Dryness of the mucosa acts as yet another stimulus for secretion ("dry mouth reflex"; Cannon 1937). Salivary secretion as a consequence of pain is a well-known phenomenon, and both pain receptors and mechanoreceptors may cause secretion elicited by esophageal distension due to swallowing dysfunctions (Sarosiek et al. 1994). When applied unilaterally, the stimulus may evoke secretion from the glands of both sides. However, the secretory response is more pronounced on the stimulated side. Afferent signals arising from the anterior part of the tongue preferentially engage the submandibular gland, whereas signals arising from the lateral and posterior parts preferentially engage the parotid gland (Emmelin 1967). Patients suffering from chronic gastroesophageal reflux of acid may experience salivation in response to
acid directly hitting the muscle layers of a damaged esophageal wall ("esophageal salivary reflex"; Helm et al. 1987). This reflex is also elicited in healthy subjects (Shafik et al. 2005). Salivation is part of the vomiting reflex set up by a number of stimuli, including distension of the stomach and duodenum as well as of chemical stimuli acting locally or centrally. The phenomenon of conditioned reflexes has been tightly associated with salivary secretion since the pioneering work by Pavlov on dogs. In humans, however, it is difficult to establish conditioned salivary reflexes to sight, sound, or anticipation of food. The feeling of "mouth watering" at the sight of an appetizing meal is attributed to anticipatory tongue

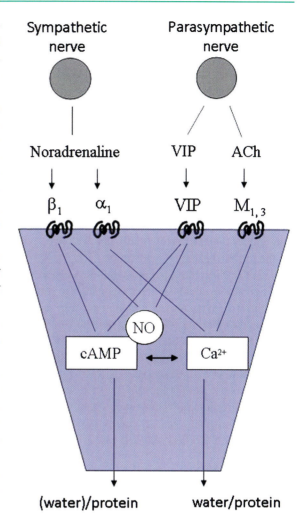

Fig. 6 Acinar cells: transmitters, receptors, and intracellular pathways

and lip movements as well as to an awareness of preexisting saliva in the mouth (Hector and Linden 1999).

7   Efferent Stimuli for Secretion

Since the days of the ninetieth century pioneers of experimental medicine who were exploring the action of nerves, the secretion of saliva has been thought to be solely under nervous control (Garrett 1998). Recent studies, however, imply an "acute" role for hormones in the regulation of saliva composition (see below). The secretory elements (acinar, duct, and myoepithelial cells) of the gland are invariable richly supplied with parasympathetic nerves. The sympathetic innervation differs in intensity between the glands, however. In humans, the secretory elements of the parotid glands are reported to be supplied with fewer sympathetic nerves than the submandibular glands, and the labial glands are thought to lack a sympathetic secretory innervation (Rossoni et al. 1979). The parasympathetic innervation is responsible for the secretion of large volumes of saliva, whereas, in the event of a sympathetic secretory innervation, the sympathetically nerve-evoked flow of saliva is usually sparse. Both the parasympathetic and the sympathetic innervations cause the secretion of proteins. Whereas gustatory reflexes activate both types of autonomic nerves, masticatory reflexes preferentially involve the activity of the parasympathetic innervation (Jensen Kjeilen et al. 1987). Since the accompanying flow of saliva is much greater in response to parasympathetic stimulation than to sympathetic stimulation, the salivary protein concentration is lower in parasympathetic saliva than in sympathetic saliva. In case of a double innervation of the secretory cells, parasympathetic and sympathetic nerves interact synergistically with respect to the response (Emmelin 1987). The secretion of saliva requires a large water supply from the circulation. Parasympathetic activity causes vasodilation, and the glandular blood flow may increase 20-fold.

8   Autonomic Transmitters and Receptors

Traditionally, acetylcholine is the parasympathetic postganglionic transmitter and noradrenaline the sympathetic postganglionic transmitter that act on the secretory elements of the glands (Fig. 6). Noradrenaline acts on α_1-adrenoceptors and β_1-adrenoceptors, whereas acetylcholine acts on muscarinic M1 and M3 receptors. The parasympathetic nerve of the salivary glands has been found to use other transmission mechanisms besides the cholinergic one, i.e., peptidergic (vasoactive intestinal peptide, calcitonin-gene-related peptide, substance P, neurokinin A, neuropeptide Y) and nitrergic (nitric oxide, NO) mechanisms (Ekström 1999a). The cotransmitters to acetylcholine may, on their own, evoke secretory effects and potentiate the acetylcholine-evoked responses (Ekström 1987). For instance, vasoactive intestinal peptide causes the secretion of proteins with no (or little) fluid. However, in concert with

acetylcholine, both the protein and the fluid secretion are enhanced by vasoactive intestinal peptide. Although the parasympathetic innervation of the salivary glands contains the NO synthesizing enzyme NO synthase, NO of parasympathetic origin does not seem to take part in the regulation of the secretory activity. Instead, NO of intracellular origin is mobilized, and particularly upon sympathetic nerve activity (Ekström et al. 2007). With respect to the parasympathetic-evoked vasodilator response, both vasoactive intestinal peptide and NO, besides acetylcholine, are involved.

9   Secretory Units

The glands are divided into lobules, each lobule consisting of a number of secretory units composed of acini and ducts. The acini, the lumen of which is surrounded by the secretory cells, form a blind end, and the saliva produced passes through intercalated, intralobular, and excretory ducts before finally emptying into a main excretory duct; on its way through the duct system, the primary saliva is modified.

10   Fluid and Protein Secretion

Fluid and protein secretion is an active, energy-dependent process. The acinar cells are responsible for the secretion of fluid. They are also responsible for most of the protein secretion, whereas the duct cells contribute to a minor proportion of the total protein output. Large volumes of water are transported from the interstitium to the lumen by paracellular and transcellular passages in response to the osmotic force exercised by intraluminal NaCl. An intracellular rise in calcium concentration opens basolateral channels for potassium and apical channels for chloride. Potassium leaves the cell for the interstitium and chloride leaves the cell for the lumen. Next, the luminal increase in chloride concentration drags sodium, via paracellular transport, from the interstitium to the lumen and, as a result, water will move along the osmotic gradient produced by NaCl (Poulsen 1998; Melvin et al. 2005) (Fig. 7a and b).

The primary isotonic saliva formed in the acini undergoes changes during its passage through the duct system. The water permeability of the ducts is

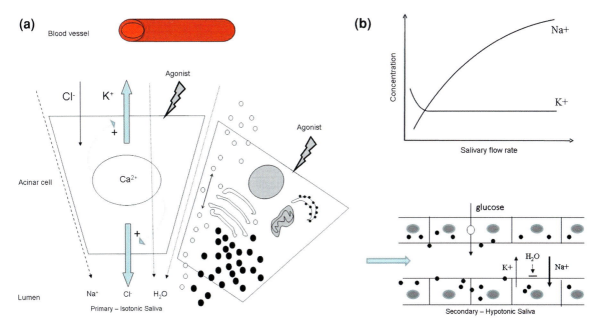

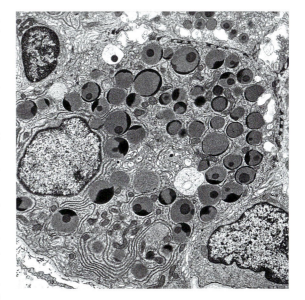

Fig. 7 a Acinar cells: water and protein secretion via vesicular and granular pathways—primary secretion. **b** Duct cells: modifications of saliva—secondary secretion

extremely small. Sodium and chloride are reabsorbed without accompanying water. A certain secretion of potassium and bicarbonate occurs at a lower rate than the rate of reabsorption of sodium and chloride. Consequently, the so-called secondary saliva that enters the mouth is hypotonic. The low salivary sodium concentration, one fifth of that of the primary saliva, makes it possible for the taste buds to detect salt at low concentrations.

The permeability of the duct system may increase under conditions that elevate the blood level of circulating catecholamines, released from the adrenal medulla, as illustrated by the appearance of glucose in the saliva in response to cold stress, mental stress, and physical exercise (Borg-Anderson et al. 1992; Teesalu and Roosalu 1993).

Immunoglobulins, in particular immunoglobulin A, are transported across the epithelial cells of acini and ducts. They are formed by plasma cells within the gland. After release to the interstitium, they form a complex with polymeric immunoglobulin receptor, which serves as transporter (Brandtzaeg 2009), a complex that splits in the saliva.

The secretion of proteins is of two types (Gorr et al. 2005). The constitutive (vesicular) secretion is a direct release of proteins as soon as they are

Fig. 8 Serous acinus of a human submandibular gland filled with secretory granules. Osmium maceration method. Magnification ×2,500. (Courtesy of Alessandro Riva, Cagliari University)

synthesized by the Golgi vesicles. The constitutive secretion is responsible for a continuous secretion of several proteins without any ongoing external stimuli. The constitutive secretion is, however, also influenced

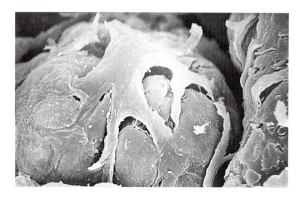

Fig. 9 Myoepithelial cells on the surface of, and embracing, a human parotid acinus. NaOH maceration method. Scanning electron microscope image, magnification ×2,000. (Courtesy of Alessandro Riva, Cagliari University)

by the nervous activity and, upon intense and prolonged stimulation, the importance of this pathway will increase concomitantly with the depletion of granules, as demonstrated experimentally (Garrett and Thulin 1975). Granular secretion is the regulated type of secretion. After synthesis, the proteins are stored in granules (Fig. 8). Upon stimulation, the granules empty their content of proteins into the lumen, i.e., the secretion occurs by exocytosis. The various routes for secretion may allow variations in the composition of the secretions (Ekström et al. 2009). Mobilization of the intracellular messenger adenosine $3',5'$-cyclic monophosphate (cAMP) by stimulation of β_1-adrenergic receptors and vasoactive intestinal peptide receptors is associated with protein secretion by exocytosis and a small volume response. Mobilization of the intracellular messenger Ca^{2+} by stimulation of muscarinic receptors (M1, M3) and α_1-adrenergic receptors is associated with fluid secretion—and particularly large volumes in response to muscarinic agonists—and protein secretion via vesicular secretion and, with intense stimulation, also via exocytosis (Ekström 2002). In acinar cells, agonists using cAMP may activate NO synthase of neuronal type but of nonneuronal origin to generate NO, which catalyzes the formation of guanosine $3',5'$-cyclic monophosphate (cGMP) (Sayardoust and Ekström 2003). The NO/cGMP pathway may contribute to the protein secretion partly by prolonging the action of cAMP (Imai et al. 1995), partly by catalyzing the generation of cyclic adenosine diphosphate ribose, which triggers the release of Ca^{2+} by its action on ryanodine-

sensitive receptors of intracellular Ca^{2+} stores (Gallacher and Smith 1999) (Fig. 7).

The combined mobilization of Ca^{2+} and cAMP results in synergistic interactions with respect to both fluid and protein secretion (Ekström 1999a). Moreover, the two sets of autonomic innervations are also involved in protein synthesis. The nonadrenergic, noncholinergic mechanisms play a major role in parasympathetically nerve-induced protein synthesis (Ekström et al. 2000). The sympathetically nerve-induced protein synthesis is exerted via the two types of adrenergic receptors with a predominance for β-adrenergic receptors (Sayardoust and Ekström 2004). Importantly, the parasympathetic nonadrenergic, noncholinergic mechanisms have been shown to take part in the regulation of salivary gland activities under reflex activation due to taste and chewing (Ekström 1998, 2001; Ekström and Reinhold 2001).

11   Myoepithelial Cell Contraction

Myoepithelial cells display characteristics in common with both smooth muscle cells and epithelial cells. They embrace acini and ducts (Fig. 9). They receive a dual innervation, and both muscarinic receptors and α_1-adrenergic receptors cause the cells to contract; in some species, tachykinins also cause contraction (Garrett and Emmelin 1979). Myoepithelial cell contraction increases the ductal pressure, which may be of importance for the flow of high-viscosity mucin-rich saliva and for overcoming various obstacles to the flow. Moreover, the contraction of the myoepithelial cells may play a supportive role for the underlying parenchyma, particularly at a high rate of secretion.

12   Blood Flow

Salivary glands are supplied with a dense capillary network comparable with that of the heart (Edwards 1988; Smaje 1998). The capillaries are extremely permeable to water and solutes but not to macromolecules such as albumin. Parasympathetically induced vasodilatation may generate a 20-fold increase in gland blood flow, which ensures the secretory cells produce large volumes of saliva over a long period of time. The parasympathetic transmitter vasoactive intestinal peptide, besides acetylcholine, plays a major role in the vasodilator response, which also involves the action of NO. Stimulation of the sympathetic innervation causes vasoconstriction by α_1-adrenergic receptors and neuropeptide Y receptors. However, the sympathetic innervation of the blood vessels of the gland is activated not in response to a meal but in response to a profound fall in systemic blood pressure in order to restore the blood pressure. The sympathetic vasoconstrictor nerve fibers originate from the vasomotor center and are separated from the sympathetic secretomotor nerve fibers taking part in alimentary reflexes (Emmelin and Engström 1960). Interestingly, the sympathetic nerve fibers innervating the blood vessels contain the potent constrictor transmitter neuropeptide Y, whereas the sympathetic secretomotor fibers lack this peptide (Ekström et al. 1996; Ekström 1999a, b).

13   Salivary Centers

The parasympathetic salivary center is located in the medulla oblongata and is divided into a superior and an inferior salivatory nucleus, and, in addition, an intermediate zone. The superior nucleus connects (the facial nerve) with the submandibular and the sublingual glands, whereas the inferior nucleus connects (the glossopharyngeal nerve) with the parotid gland (Emmelin 1967; Matsuo 1999). The intermediate zone makes connections with both the submandibular gland and the parotid gland. The sympathetic salivary center resides in the upper thoracic segments of the spinal cord. Higher centers of the brain exert both excitatory (glutamate) and inhibitory (γ- aminobutyric acid and glycine) influences on the salivary centers. The inhibitory influence is illustrated by the reduced flow of saliva associated with depression, fever, sleep, and emotional stress. Mouth dryness in response to stress is *not* a consequence of sympathetic activity: there are no inhibitory sympathetic fibers innervating the secretory cells (Garrett 1988).

14   Efferent Nerves

The parasympathetic preganglionic nerve fibers of the submandibular and sublingual glands leave the facial nerve and join, via the chorda tympani nerve, the lingual nerve to form the chorda-lingual nerve to reach the submandibular ganglion. The postganglionic nerve fibers of the submandibular ganglion innervate the submandibular and sublingual parenchyma (Rho and Deschler 2005). In humans, this ganglion is located outside the parenchyma of the two glands, which is in contrast to the intraglandular localization in many laboratory animals. The parasympathetic preganglionic nerve fibers of the parotid gland travel via the tympanic branch of the glossopharyngeal nerve (Jacobson's nerve), the tympanic plexus, and the lesser superficial petrosal nerve and, after relaying in the otic ganglion, the postganglionic nerve fibers are usually thought to reach the gland via the auriculotemporal nerve. With respect to the preganglionic innervation of the parotid gland, reflex studies suggest that not only fibers of the glossopharyngeal nerve but also fibers of the facial nerve (chorda tympani nerve) contribute, since cutting the chorda tympani nerve in the tympanic membrane reduces the response (Reicher and Poth 1933; Diamant and Wiberg 1965). The routes of the postganglionic cholinergic nerve fibers may differ as judged by extensive animal studies. Cholinergic nerve fibers may detach at an early stage from the auriculotemporal nerve, to reach the gland via the internal maxillary artery. Moreover, and in contrast to the general textbook view, the facial nerve passing through the parotid gland parenchyma, with its twigs, supplies the secretory cells with a cholinergic innervation that takes part in the reflex secretion (Ekström and Holmberg 1972; Khosravani et al. 2006; Khosravani and Ekström 2006). The facial nerve is therefore a potential contributor to the development of Frey syndrome (Dunbar et al. 2002). Frey syndrome is characterized by sweating, redness, flushing, and warming over the parotid region when eating. It develops over a period of months following parotid gland surgery, neck dissection, blunt trauma to the cheek, and chronic infection of the parotid area. It is considered to be due to aberrant regeneration of postganglionic parasympathetic cholinergic nerve fibers of the auriculotemporal nerve that innervate sweat glands and skin vessels following loss of the sympathetic postganglionic cholinergic innervation but may, in the light of a secretory role for the facial nerve, also involve regenerating parasympathetic postganglionic cholinergic nerve fibers of the facial nerve. Since botulinus toxin, preventing transmitter exocytosis, is more effective than the muscarinic receptor antagonist atropine in the treatment of the syndrome, a cotransmitter or cotransmitters to acetycholine is/are likely to contribute to the symptoms; vasoactive intestinal peptide is such a cotransmitter (Drummond 2002).

The routes of the parasympathetic nerves of the minor glands (Tandler and Riva 1986) are via the buccal branch of the mandibular nerve with respect to the molar, buccal, and labial glands (postganglionic nerves originate from the otic ganglion), via the lingual nerve with respect to the lingual glands (Remak's ganglia, intralingually located), and via the palatine nerve with respect to palatine glands (sphenoplatine ganglion).

The sympathetic preganglionic nerve fibers ascend in the paravertebral sympathetic trunk to synapse with their postganglionic nerve fibers in the superior cervical ganglion, which then reach the glands via the arteries. However, their actual anatomical pathways are not completely defined, e.g., the parotid gland may be reached both via the external carotid artery and via intracranial routes (Garrett 1988).

15   Sensory Nerves of Glandular Origin

Pain in the salivary gland region is a well-known phenomenon in response to gland swelling upon inflammation or sialolithiasis. Although the pain is usually attributed to an increase in the intercapsular tension and activation of afferent nerves of the glandular fascia (Shapiro 1973; Leipzig and Obert 1979), sensory nerves occur in the glands and are therefore likely to be involved in the response. Nerve fibers showing colocalization of substance P and calcitonin-gene-related peptide are of sensory origin, and in the glands, these fibers are present in close connection with ducts and blood vessels (Ekström et al. 1988). The facial nerve and the great auricular nerve are pathways for nerves of this type of the parotid gland, originating from the trigeminal ganglion and dorsal root ganglia, respectively (Khosravani et al. 2006, 2008); in addition, the great auricular nerve innervates the parotid fascia (Zohar et al. 2002). The lingual nerve is thought to supply the submandibular and sublingual glands with sensory fibers of trigeminal origin. The periductal sensory nerves may serve protective functions. They may release defense substances from the duct cells (such as β-defensins)

and by causing the myoepithelal cells to contract, noxious substances may be expelled and ductal distension may be overcome. Both substance P and calcitonin-gene-related peptide evoke protein extravasation and periglandular edema. Therefore, the perivascular sensory nerve fibers may be involved in gland swelling and gland inflammation. A role for sensory nerves in chronic inflammation has been pointed out, for instance, in asthma. In analogy, there might be a role for these nerves in chronic salivary gland inflammation. The levels of both substance P and calcitonin-gene-related peptide increase following extirpation of the superior cervical ganglion (Ekström and Ekman 2005), a phenomenon that may be associated with the clinical condition of parotid postsympathectomy pain upon eating (Schon 1985).

16   Hormones

Animal experiments demonstrate a long-term influence of sex steroids, growth hormone, and thyroid hormones on salivary gland metabolism, morphology, and secretory capacity (Johnson 1988). In humans, the development of postmenopausal hyposalivation illustrates the consequence of the loss of the continuous influence of estrogen and progesterone (Meurman et al. 2009). The opposite, i.e., excessive salivation, has been reported during pregnancy (Jenkins 1978). Apart from the effect of circulating catecholamines from the adrenal medulla in response to sympathetic activity, little attention has been paid to a short-term hormonal influence on the glands and their secretion. Aldosterone-induced ductal uptake of sodium (without water), lowering the sodium concentration of the saliva, is a well-known phenomenon in the parotid gland of the sheep, but in humans the effect of aldosterone is small (Blair-West et al. 1967). Recent animal investigations on the effect of some gastrointestinal hormones—gastrin, cholecystokinin, and melatonin, the latter found in large amounts in the intestines—do, however, imply that the secretory activity of salivary glands, like other exocrine glands of the digestive tract, are under the control of both nerves and hormones, and that the secretion from the salivary glands can be divided into three separate phases depending on the location from where the stimulus for secretion arises during a meal (Cevik Aras and Ekström 2006, 2008; Ekström and Cevik

Fig. 10 Physiological changes at old age contributing to hyposalivation

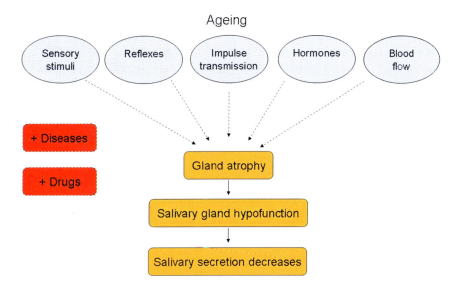

Aras 2008; Cevik Aras et al. 2011). Thus, in addition to the well-known cephalic phase (nerves), a gastric phase (gastrin) and an intestinal phase (cholecystokinin and melatonin) may regulate salivary gland secretion. The hormones cause the secretion of proteins and stimulate the synthesis of secretory proteins but have little effect on the volume response. Ongoing studies show that human glands, like animal glands, are supplied with receptors for the three hormones and further, in vitro, release proteins from pieces of human gland tissues upon administration of the hormones (Riva et al. 2010).

Gastrointestinal hormones such as cholecystokinin, gastrin, and melatonin exert anti-inflammatory actions on salivary glands (Cevik Aras and Ekström 2010).

17 Trophic Effects of Nerves: Gland Sensitivity to Chemical Stimuli and Gland Size

When the amount of a drug required to elicit a certain submaximal biological response diminishes, the tissue is referred to as being supersensitive (Emmelin 1965; Ekström 1999b). Salivary glands, in particular, have been used as model organs to explore the phenomenon of supersensitivity. Depriving the glands of their receptor stimulation by trauma, surgery, or the pharmacological action of drugs results in the gradual development of denervation supersensitivity. The

sensitization is most pronounced in response to the loss of influence of the postganglionic parasympathetic nerve. Restoration of a functional innervation normalizes the sensitivity. Experimentally, variations in the gland sensitivity can be brought about in animals supplied with functionally intact reflex arcs by varying the intensity of the reflex stimulation, the gland subjected to disuse (liquid diet) being more sensitive to stimuli than the gland subjected to overuse (chewing-demanding pelleted diet)—thus illustrating that the state of "normal sensitivity" is indeed a relative phenomenon (Ekström and Templeton 1977). Supersensitivity is attributed to intracellular events rather than to a change in the number of receptors on the cell membrane. The phenomenon is usually regarded as nonspecific but it seems, in fact, possible to demonstrate agonist-specific patterns associated with the degree of disuse of the various intracellular pathways (Ekström 1999b).

As might be expected, under physiological conditions the gland size is of primary importance for the volume response of the gland. Preclinical studies show that when the chewing-demanding diet is changed to a liquid diet in rats, the parotid gland loses about 50% of its dry weight, the amount of saliva secreted as a response to submaximal muscarinic stimulus is reduced by 40%, and the maximally evoked muscarinic volume response is reduced by 25% (Ekström and Templeton 1977). Parasympathetic postganglionic denervation causes a profound decrease in gland weight (by 30–40%). However, loss of the action of acetylcholine on the gland is probably not the cause: prolonged treatment with the muscarinic antagonist atropine results in no decrease in weight. Instead parasympathetic nonadrenergic, noncholinergic transmission mechanisms maintain the gland weight, and induce mitotic activity in the glands (Ekström et al. 2007). The nature of the transmitter or transmitters involved is unknown.

As previously pointed out, salivary glands are supplied with β_1-adrenergic receptors (Ekström 1969); however, the sympathetic system seems to play a minor role in the regulation of gland size under physiological conditions. Although the β-adrenergic agonist isoprenaline is known to cause gland swelling after prolonged treatment of asthma and isoprenaline in preclinical studies is known to increase gland weights severalfold (Barka 1965), sympathetic denervation only slightly, if at all, reduces gland weight. In agreement, treatment with the β_1-adrenergic receptor antagonist metoprolol causes only a small decrease in gland weight (Ekström and Malmberg 1984). It should be noted that the severalfold gain in weight caused by isoprenaline does not correspond to a similar increase in secretory capacity (Ohlin 1966).

18   Ageing

The secretory capacity is usually thought to decline with age; however, functional data do not support such an assumption (Vissink et al. 1996; Nagler 2004; Österberg et al. 1992). No doubt, the proportion of fat and fibrovascular tissue gradually increases with time and consequently, the proportion of functional parenchyma decreases. However, despite these morphological changes, the secretory volumes of unstimulated and stimulated saliva are only slightly affected, if at all. With respect to the composition of saliva, the individuality of the glands comes to light since the parotid saliva composition is considered unchanged whereas the mucin secretion of the mucous/seromucous glands as well as the immunoglobulin A secretion of the labial glands is thought to decrease (Fig. 10).

A number of events associated with ageing will make salivary gland functions particularly vulnerable, and in concert, these events may eventually have implications for the production of the saliva. For instance, the intensity of the reflex activity diminishes owing to reduction in the number of olfactory and taste receptors as well as loss of teeth; the neuroglandular junction widens, diminishing the concentration of transmitters acting on the receptors; the blood levels of the sex steroids decrease; and the blood perfusion of the glands is reduced. To this list of changes, diseases and pharmaceutical drugs are added. In 70-year-olds, 64% of women and 55% of men were found to be receiving medication in a recent Swedish study; the average number of drugs was 4.0 for women and 3.3 for men (Johanson 2011).

19   Xerostomia, Salivary Gland Hypofunction, and Dry Mouth

Usually, the salivary secretion is estimated after an overnight fast or 2 h after a meal (Birkhed and Heintze 1989; Navazesh and Kumar 2008). To collect whole unstimulated/resting saliva, the subject, sitting in a chair, is instructed to swallow and then to lean the body forward, allowing the saliva to drip passively through a funnel into an (ice-chilled) graduated (or preweighed) cylinder for 15 min. The stimulated whole saliva is usually collected over 5 min: by chewing paraffin wax, usually at a fixed frequency (e.g., 40 or 70 strokes per min); by citric acid applied either on the dorsum of the tongue for 30 s or as a solution (2.5%) held in the mouth for 1 min; or by sucking a lemon-flavored candy. The saliva pouring into the mouth is spat into a cylinder, preferentially at fixed intervals. The secretion is expressed per milliliters per minute or per milligrams per minute (the density of saliva is assumed to be 1.0 g/ml).

In humans, salivary ducts are not usually cannulated to measure the flow of saliva from individual glands. However, by applying the Lashley–Crittenden "cup" over the orifice of the parotid duct, one can record the flow of parotid saliva. Devices of various types have been constructed for the collection of submandibular/sublingual secretion—but here, saliva from the two types of gland is mixed. By the so-called Periotron method, saliva from the minor glands can be estimated (Eliasson and Carlén 2010). A filter paper is placed over a small area of the oral epithelium, and the fluid collected on the filter paper is measured using the change in conductance to indicate fluid.

An unstimulated flow rate of whole saliva less than 0.1 ml/min and a stimulated flow rate of whole saliva less than 0.7 ml/min are considered to indicate *salivary gland hypofunction* (Ericsson and Hardwick 1978). *Xerostomia* is the subjective sensation of dryness of the oral mucosa. Importantly, xerostomia and salivary gland hypofunction may or may not be related phenomena—only about 55% of those complaining of xerostomia show, by objective measurement, a decrease in saliva volume (Field et al. 1997; Longman et al. 1995). The term "dry mouth" refers to the oral sensation of dryness with or without the demonstration of salivary gland hypofunction.

The thickness of the fluid layer covering the oral mucosa varies markedly, being 70 μm at the posterior dorsum of the tongue and 10 μm at the hard palate (DiSabato-Mordaski and Kleinberg 1996; Wolff and Kleinberg 1998). The volume of saliva in the mouth is dependent not only on the secretion of saliva but also on evaporation, absorption of fluid through the oral mucosa, and swallowing. Mouth breathing and speaking are the main causes of the fluid loss by evaporation; the hard palate with its thin fluid layer is directly exposed to the flow of inspired air (Thelin et al. 2008). An excess of saliva in the mouth elicits a swallowing reflex. Usually, the volume of saliva that enters the mouth at rest exceeds the volume lost by evaporation and swallowing. Despite wide differences in the rate of unstimulated secretion, a decrease by about 50% of this secretion in an individual will give rise to the sensation of oral dryness (Dawes 1987; Wolff and Kleinberg 1999). In this case, the thickness of the saliva film of the anterior dorsum of the tongue and the hard palate is less than 10 μm. It is also from these locations that the subject experiences the most pronounced symptoms of xerostomia (Wolff and Kleinberg 1999). A decrease in the labial secretion by only 20% is correlated to the feeling of oral dryness (Eliasson et al. 1996).

20 Causes of Dry Mouth

The prevalence of dry mouth is 15–40%. The condition is more common among women and increases with age (Österberg et al. 1984; Nederfors et al. 1997). Dry mouth dramatically impairs the quality of life (Ship et al. 2002; Wärnberg et al. 2005), and is both a physical and a social handicap. It is associated with difficulties in chewing, swallowing, and speaking. The lips are cracked and dry. Taste acuity weakens and oral mucosal infections, dental caries and halitosis develop. Among known causes of dry mouth are chronic gland inflammation as Sjögren syndrome, diabetes, depression, head and neck radiotherapy, radioiodide therapy, HIV/AIDS, orofacial trauma, surgery, and use of medications (Grisius and Fox 1988). Drugs presently in use may interfere with the reflexly elicited secretion at the level of the central nervous system and/or at the level of the neuroglandular junction. In this connection, it should be remembered that the salivary glands are effectors of the autonomic nervous system and that they are supplied with the same set of receptor types as other effector organs of this system. Consequently, when a dysfunction of an effector within this system is treated by interfering with the transmission mechanisms, e.g., overactive urinary bladder (by muscarinic receptor antagonists) or hypertension (see below), the functions of the salivary glands are invariably influenced. Drugs with antimuscarinic actions cause a marked reduction in the volume of saliva produced. Although the volume is not always changed to any great extent, the composition of the saliva may have undergone changes resulting in the subjective feeling of oral dryness. The use of drugs belonging to the cardiovascular category or the psychotropic category is particularly correlated with a decreased rate of secretion as a side effect. Antihypertensive drugs may block α_1- adrenergic receptors and β_1-adrenergic receptors, and stimulate prejunctional (neuronal) α_2-adrenergic receptors (which inhibits the transmitter release). Although diuretics in in vitro experiments influence various electrolyte exchange processes in the glands and dry mouth is a common complaint in response to the treatment with diuretics, the salivary flow rate in humans is only slightly affected, if at all (Atkinson et al. 1989; Nederfors et al. 1989). Oral mucosal tissue dehydration has been suggested as cause of the dry mouth feeling. Antiarythmics block β_1-adrenergic receptors and exert anticholinergic effects. Apart from the central action of antidepressants, this group of drugs blocks peripherally the muscarinic receptors. Antipsychotics have not only antimuscarinic actions but also have anti-α_1-adrenergic actions. Importantly, when one set of receptor type is blocked, not only is the response mediated by this particular receptor abolished, but the synergistic interaction provided by the receptor is also abolished.

Several hundred drugs are said to be xerogenic, and dry mouth is the third most common side effect of drug treatment. It is important to realize that reference guides to drugs causing dry mouth are usually put together on the basis of the sensation of oral dryness rather than on the basis of the actual measurement of the saliva output. There is a correlation between the total intake of the number of drugs and dry mouth (with or without hyposalivation). The use of four drugs or more increases the probability that the phenomenon of dry mouth will occur. If the number of drugs is increased, the chance of consuming a drug producing dry mouth by itself or by its interaction with other drugs is likely to increase.

21 Treatment of Dry Mouth

The options to treat dry mouth are, unfortunately, limited and focused on maintaining the salivary reflexes by flavored gums or lozenges, or by the use of salivary substitutes such as artificial saliva, oral rinses, and oral gels. These treatments are of short duration. In addition, scrutiny of the medication list may make it possible to achieve a reduction in the number of drugs taken by the patients or in the dose of individual drugs and, in addition, replacement with drugs with less xerogenic effects may be effected. A number of drugs for systemic use have been introduced, such as parasympathomimetics, cholinesterase inhibitors, the bile stimulating agent anethole trithione, the mycolytic agents bromhexine and guafensin, the immune-enhancing substance interferon-α, the cytoprotective amifostine, and the antimalarial drug hydroxychloroquine. In many cases, the clinical effects are questionable, and moreover some of these drugs are associated with serious side effects. The parasympathomimetics pilocarpine (Salagen®) and cevimeline (Evoxac®) stimulate the flow of saliva but may also cause nausea, sweating, gastrointestinal discomfort, respiratory distress, urges to empty the bladder, and hypotension. Recent clinical trials using topical application of the cholinesterase physostigmine on the oral mucosa have demonstrated local treatment of dry mouth as an alternative approach to systemic treatment (Khosravani

et al. 2009). After diffusion of the drug through the mucosal barrier, the underlying mucin-producing minor glands are stimulated to secrete saliva, while at the same time the systemic effects are minimized. The patient suffering from dry mouth should maintain meticulous oral hygiene, including the use of a fluoride-rich gel, frequent visits to the dental hygienist, and in addition, avoiding food and beverages that are sweet, acidic, or carbonated.

22 Sialorrhea

Neuromuscular dysfunctions associated with cerebral palsy, Parkinson disease, amyotrophic lateral sclerosis, and stroke are examples of conditions that cause drooling. Under these conditions, saliva pools in the mouth owing to lack of swallowing rather than to an increased rate of secretion of saliva (Young et al. 2011). An increase in the rate of secretion may occur in the treatment of Alzheimer disease and myasthenia gravis owing to the medication with reversible cholinesterases (Freudenreich 2005; Ecobichon 1995). Sialorrhea is reported as a side effect of clozapine in about one third of patients under treatment for schizophrenia (Praharaj et al. 2010). Clozapine is an atypical antipsychotic drug used when traditional antipsychotics fail to treat schizophrenia. During the night, patients are troubled with choking sensations and the aspiration of saliva. The situation may be so bothersome that the drug regimen is discontinued. The phenomenon has been largely unexplained, and some authors have referred it to a weakened swallowing reflex. A number of various categories of drugs have been suggested for the treatment of clozapine-induced hypersalivation, usually with limited success and with side effects of their own (Sockalingam et al. 2007). Recent preclinical studies have shown that both clozapine and its main metabolite N-desmethylclozapine exert mixed actions on the salivation (Ekström et al. 2010a, b; Godoy et al. 2011). Upon reflex secretion, the two drugs decrease the flow of saliva by antagonistic actions on muscarinic M3 receptors and α_1-adrenergic receptors. During sleep and at rest, an agonistic action by the drugs on muscarinic M1 receptors maintains a low-grade, continuous flow of saliva.

Fig. 11 Approximate percentages (w/w) of the different protein families present in human adult whole saliva, assuming a comparable contribution of parotid and submandibular/sublingual glands. (Modified from Messana et al. 2008b)

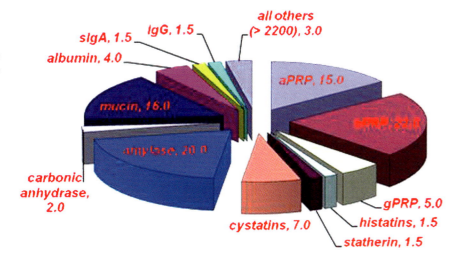

23 Protein Components of Human Saliva and Posttranslational Modifications

The recent availability of mass spectrometry (MS)-based techniques applicable to the study of complex protein mixtures has stimulated the effort to obtain a qualitative and quantitative comprehensive understanding of the protein composition of saliva.

Indeed, MS techniques are capable of identifying and quantifying thousands of protein components in complex samples. The mass spectrometer makes it possible to obtain precise mass values through the measure of the mass-to-charge ratio (m/z) of the ions generated from peptides and proteins at the source. Selected ions may also be submitted to a fragmentation process (this technique is called MS/MS), and the determination of the m/z ratio of the fragments allows the peptide structure to be investigated. Thus, the power of MS rests in the possibility to obtain information on not only the exact mass of a given peptide/protein, but also on its sequence. Two main strategies may be used to investigate protein mixtures: the top-down and the bottom-up approaches. In the bottom-up approach, the nonfractionated sample is submitted to digestion, typically by trypsin, and the resulting digestion mixture is fractionated and analyzed by MS. Thus, presence and quantification of the proteins in the sample are inferred from the ensemble of identified digestion peptides, supposing that any peptide identified derives from a unique protein. Even though this approach is of high throughput, the digestion step introduces a limitation, since relevant naturally occurring cleavages may obviously not be disclosed. The top-down approach overcomes this problem, since peptide and protein separation followed by MS analysis is performed with undigested samples. However, top-down platforms often cannot cover the entire proteome, because some proteins can escape from the analysis (e.g., proteins insoluble in acidic milieu). High-performance liquid chromatography (HPLC) is more suitable than gel electrophoresis as a separation step technique for the analysis of the salivary proteome, since it is mainly represented by peptides and small/medium-sized proteins. Moreover, with respect to gel electrophoresis, HPLC offers the advantage that MS analysis can be performed online, i.e., peptides and proteins are submitted directly to the ion source of the MS apparatus.

24 The Salivary Proteome

Most of the about 2,400 different proteins of whole saliva characterized in recent years by proteomic studies are not of glandular origin but probably originate from exfoliating epithelial cells and oral microflora. Proteins of gland secretion origin should not be more than 200–300 in number, and they represent more than 85% by weight of the salivary proteome (Fig. 11). They belong to the following major families: α-amylases, carbonic anhydrase, histatins, mucins, proline-rich proteins (PRPs), further divided in acidic, basic, and basic glycosylated PRPs, statherin, P–B peptide, and salivary-type (S-type) cystatins.

Table 1 Families of major salivary proteins: function, origin, genes, name of mature proteins, and main posttranslational modifications (*PTMs*)

Family	Function	Origin	Gene	Mature proteins	Other PTMs
α-Amylases	Antibacterial, digestion, tissue coating	Pr Sm/Sl	*AMY1A*	α-Amylase 1	Disulfide bond, N-glycosylation, phosphorylation, proteolytic cleavages
Acidic PRPs	Lubrication, mineralization, tissue coating	Pr Sm/Sl	*PRH1, PRH2*	Db-s, Pa, PIF-s, Pa 2-mer, Db-f, PIF-f, PRP-1, PRP-2, PRP-3, PRP-4, P–C peptide	Disulfide bond, further proteolytic cleavages, phosphorylation, protein network
Basic PRPs	Binding of tannins, tissue coating	Pr	*PRB1, PRB2, PRB3, PRB4*	II-1, II-2, CD-IIg, IB-1, IB-6, IB-7, IB-8a (Con1−/+), P–D, P–E, P–F, P–J, P–H, PRP Gl 1–8, protein N1, salivary PRP Po	Disulfide bond (Gl 8), further proteolytic cleavages, N- and O-glycosylation, phosphorylation, protein network
Glycosylated PRPs	Antiviral, lubrication				
Carbonic anydrase VI	Buffering, taste	Pr Sm	*CA6*	Carbonic anhydrase 6	Disulfide bond, glycosylation
Cystatins	Antibacterial, antiviral, mineralization, tissue coating	Pr Sm/Sl	*CST1, CST2, CST3, CST4, CST5*	Cystatin SN, cystatin SA, cystatin C, cystatin S, cystatin D	Disulfide bond, O-glycosylation, phosphorylation, sulfoxide, truncated forms
Histatins	Antifungal, antibacterial, mineralization, wound-healing	Pr Sm/Sl	*HTN1, HTN3*	Histatin 1, histatin 2, histatin 3, histatin 5, histatin 6	Further proteolytic cleavages, phosphorylation, sulfation
Lactoferrin	Antibacterial, antifungal, antiviral, innate immune response	All salivary glands	*LTF*	Lactoferrin	Disulfide bond, glycosylation, phosphorylation
Lysozyme	Antibacterial	Pr Sm	*LYZ*	Lysozyme C	Disulfide bond
Mucins	Antibacterial, antiviral, digestion, lubrication, tissue coating	All salivary glands	*MUC5B, MUC19, MUC7*	Mucin-5B, mucin-19, mucin-7	Disulfide bond, N- and O-glycosylation, phosphorylation
Peptide P–B	Not defined	Pr Sm/Sl	*SMR3B (PROL3)*	Proline-rich peptide P–B	Proteolytic cleavages
Statherins	Inhibits crystal formation, lubrication, mineralization, tissue coating	Pr Sm/Sl	*STATH*	Statherin, statherin SV2	Phosphorylation, proteolytic cleavages, protein network

Modified from Castagnola et al. (2011b)

PRP proline-rich protein, *Pr* parotid, *Sm* submandibular, *Sl* sublingual, *GCF* gingival crevicular fluid

The function, origin, and encoding genes of the major salivary proteins are reported in Table 1, together with the name of mature proteins and the main posttranslational modifications occurring before, during, and after secretion.

Histatins are a family of small peptides, the name referring to the high number of histidine residues in their structure. All the members of this family arise from histatin 1 and histatin 3, which share very similar sequences and are encoded by two genes

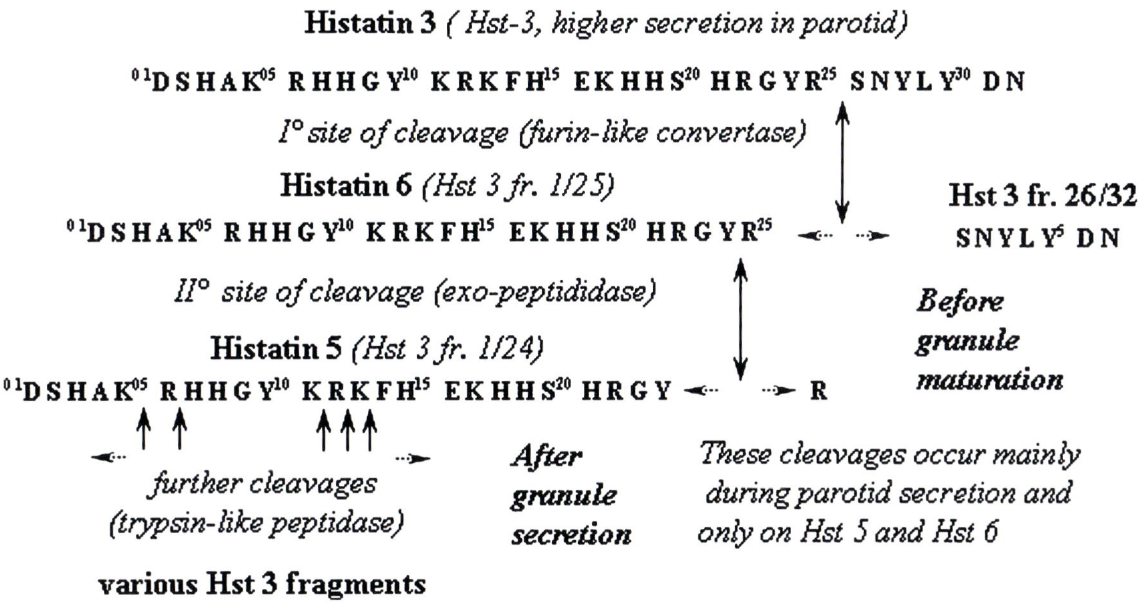

Histatin 3 *(Hst-3, higher secretion in parotid)*

^{01}D S H A K^{05} R H H G Y^{10} K R K F H^{15} E K H H S^{20} H R G Y R^{25} S N Y L Y^{30} D N

I° site of cleavage (furin-like convertase)

Histatin 6 *(Hst 3 fr. 1/25)*

Hst 3 fr. 26/32

^{01}D S H A K^{05} R H H G Y^{10} K R K F H^{15} E K H H S^{20} H R G Y R^{25}

S N Y L Y^{5} D N

II° site of cleavage (exo-peptididase)

Before granule maturation

Histatin 5 *(Hst 3 fr. 1/24)*

^{01}D S H A K^{05} R H H G Y^{10} K R K F H^{15} E K H H S^{20} H R G Y R

further cleavages (trypsin-like peptidase)

After granule secretion

These cleavages occur mainly during parotid secretion and only on Hst 5 and Hst 6

various Hst 3 fragments

Fig. 12 The sequential proteolytic cleavage of histatin 3, which generates histatin 6 and histatin 5, before granule maturation, and a multitude of other fragments after granule secretion. (From data reported in Castagnola et al. 2004; Messana et al. 2008a)

(*HTN1* and *HTN3*) located on chromosome band 4q13 (Sabatini and Azen 1989). Statherin is an unusual tyrosine-rich 43-residue phosphorylated peptide involved in oral cavity calcium ion homeostasis and tooth mineralization (Schwartz et al. 1992). Its gene (*STATH*) is localized on chromosome band 4q13.3 (Sabatini et al. 1987), near the histatin genes. Usually P–B peptide is included in the basic PRP family. However, it is the product of *PROL3* gene localized on chromosome band 4q13.3, very close to the statherin gene, and several characteristics of P–B peptide suggest a functional relationship with statherin (Inzitari et al. 2006). Cystatin S, SN, and SA are salivary cystatins; they are inhibitors of cysteine proteinases and this property suggests its role in the protection of the oral cavity from pathogens and in the control of lysosomal cathepsins (Bobek and Levine 1992). Cystatin S1 and cystatin S2 correspond to monophosphorylated and diphosphorylated cystatin S, respectively. The loci expressing all the S-type cystatins (*CST1–CST5*) are clustered on chromosome band 20p11.21 together with the loci of cystatins C and D. Whereas cystatin SA seems to be specifically expressed in the oral cavity, cystatin S and SN have also been detected in other bodily fluids and organs, such as tears, urine, and seminal fluid (Dickinson 2002; Ryan et al. 2010). Human salivary

acidic PRPs consist of five principal isoforms codified by two distinct loci called *PRH1* and *PRH2* localized on chromosome band12p13.2. They show acidic character in the first 30 amino acid residues of the N-terminal region; the remaining part is basic and, similarly to basic PRPs, shows repeated sequences rich in proline and glutamine. Basic and glycosylated (basic) PRPs are the most complex group of salivary peptides, encoded by four different genes named *PRB1–PRB4* clustered on chromosome band 12p13.2. Numerous homologous and unequal crossing-overs are present within the tandem repeats of the third exon, producing frequent length polymorphisms.

Salivary amylases consist of two families of isoenzymes, called A and B, each family comprising three isoforms whose differences are connected to different posttranslational modifications (Scannapieco et al. 1993).

Salivary mucins are divided in two distinct classes: the large gel-forming mucins (MG1) and the small soluble mucins (MG2). MG1 represents a heterogeneous family of 20×10^6–40×10^6 Da glycoproteins expressed by *MUC5B*, *MUC4*, and *MUC19* genes (Offner and Troxler 2000; Thomsson et al. 2002). MG2, a much smaller mucin of 130–180 kDa, is the product of the *MUC7* gene mapped to chromosome bands 4q13–4q21 (Bobek et al. 1996). Mucins are composed of approximately 15–20% protein and up to 80% carbohydrate, present largely in the form of serine and threonine O-linked glycans (Strous and Dekker 1992; Gendler and Spicer 1995). The polypeptide backbone can be divided into three regions. The central region contains tandemly repeated sequences of eight 169 amino acids. This domain serves as the attachment site for the O-glycans, and each mucin has a unique, specific tandem-repeat sequence. Many mucins with monomeric molecular masses greater than 2×10^6 Da form multimers more than ten times bigger than that size.

25 Polymorphism of the Salivary Proteome

The human salivary proteome shows high interindividual variability. The different isoforms of salivary proteins may be genetic in origin (different alleles codifying acidic PRPs, basic PRPs, mucins, cystatins; differential splicing), but may also derive from several posttranslational modifications which occur during the trafficking of the proteins through the secretory pathway and after secretion.

One of the better known examples of polymorphism and modifications occurring before, during, and after secretion concerns acidic PRPs. The two loci which encode acidic PRPs have different alleles. The *PRH2* locus is biallelic, and the expression products are PRP-1 and PRP-2. There are three alleles of the *PRH1* locus and they express Pif-s (parotid isoelectric-focusing variant, slow), Db-s (double band, slow), and Pa (parotid acidic protein) proteins (Inzitari et al. 2005). All the isoforms are N-terminally modified (pyroglutamic moiety) and are subjected to phosphorylation before granule storage. The major derivatives are diphosphorylated, but low levels of monophosphorylated and triphosphorylated forms are also detected in saliva. Another important modification is the cleavage. Before granule storage PRP-1, PRP-2, Pif-s, and Db-s are in part cleaved at the Arg-106 residue by a specific enzyme of the convertase family. Cleavage generates four truncated derivatives, called PRP-3, PRP-4, Pif-f, and Db-f, and a common C-terminal peptide of 44 amino acids, called P–C peptide (Messana et al. 2008a). The Pa isoform is not cleaved, since the Arg-106 → Cys substitution eliminates the consensus sequence

recognized by the proteinase. However, the cysteine residue generates a disulfide bridge and only the Pa dimeric form may be detected in whole saliva.

Also histatins, statherin, P–B peptide, and principally basic PRPs undergo proteolytic cleavage before granule storage and during secretion, but the entire forms of basic PRPs, differently from the other salivary proteins, are not detected in saliva (Messana et al. 2008a). Following proteolytic cleavage, many salivary peptides are also subjected to the removal of C-terminal residues by the action of specific carboxypeptidases, and this modification is considered an event common to all the secretory processes (Steiner 1998). An important example concerns the formation of histatin 5 from histatin 6. The two histatins derive from the parent peptide of 32 amino acid residues called histatin 3. Histatin 3, from the presence of the RGYR↓ convertase consensus sequence recognized by an unknown, but specific, proteinase acting before granule storage, generates histatin 6 (histatin 3 fr 1/25). Subsequently, an unknown carboxypeptidase removes the C-terminal arginine residue, generating histatin 5 (histatin 3 fr 1/24). Sequentially, histatins 5 and 6 are subjected to further proteolytic cleavages after granule secretion as shown in Fig. 12 (Castagnola et al. 2004; Messana et al. 2008a).

Before granule storage salivary proteins are also subjected to phosphorylation, glycosylation, and sulfation. MG1, MG2, glycosylated PRPs, and amylase are salivary glycosylated proteins (Ramachandran et al. 2006). The glycomoiety may be N- and/or O-linked and the sugars show the same architectures demonstrated for other glycoproteins (Guile et al. 1998). In the same way, the tyrosylprotein sulfotransferase involved in the polysulfation of histatin 1 seems to be the same enzyme acting in other tissues (Cabras et al. 2007).

The salivary proteome changes dynamically also after secretion under the action of endogenous and exogenous enzymes, the latter derived from microorganisms resident in the oral cavity. For instance, it has been demonstrated that a glutamine endoproteinase localized in dental plaque—likely of microbial origin—generates in the oral cavity a lot of small fragments (from seven to 20 amino acid residues) from different basic PRPs (Helmerhorst et al. 2008). Another important modification occurring in the oral cavity is the formation of cross-linked derivatives of salivary proteins, generating a protective

Table 2 Different contributions to salivary peptides and proteins

Peptide or family	Parotid glands	Sm/Sl glands	Plasma exudate	GCF
Acidic PRP (all the isoforms)	●●●●	●●●		
Basic PRP	●●●●			
Basic glycosylated PRP	●●●			
Histatin 3	●●●●	●●●		
Histatin 1	●●●	●●●		
Statherin	●●●●	●●●●		●
P–B peptide	●●	●●●●		●
"S-type" cystatins	●	●●●●		
Amylase	●●●●	●		
MG1		●●●●		
MG2		●●●		
Albumin (HSA)			●●	●●
Thymosins β_4 and β_{10}			?	●●
α-Defensins 1–4			●	●●

Modified from Messana et al. (2008b)

GCF gingival crevicular fluid, *HSA* human serum albumin, *Four circles* high contribution, *three circles* medium contribution, *two circles* low contribution, *one circle* very low contribution, *question mark* unknown

proteinaceous network on tooth surfaces (enamel pellicle) and oral mucosa. This protein film is important for the integrity of tooth enamel, because it acts as a boundary lubricant on the enamel surface (Douglas et al. 1991). Moreover, interactions between pellicle proteins and bacterial surfaces are responsible for specificity of the bacterial colonization during the earliest stage of plaque formation (Gibbons and Hay 1988). This protein network could also interact with the oral epithelial cell plasma membrane and its associate cytoskeleton and might contribute to the mucosal epithelial flexibility and turnover. Histatins, statherin, and acidic PRPs are among the proteins involved. It has been indeed demonstrated that acidic PRPs, statherin, and the major histatins are substrates of oral transglutaminase 2 and they participate in cross-linking reactions (Yao et al. 1999).

26 Physiological Variability

The composition of oral fluid varies depending on various factors. It has already been reported that the contribution of the different salivary glands to whole saliva in resting and stimulated conditions is different, and parotid saliva is the prevalent contributor to stimulated saliva. It has been also demonstrated that the protein composition of mixed submandibular/sublingual saliva is different from that of parotid saliva (Table 2). For instance, the levels of acidic PRPs, histatin 1, and α-amylases are higher in parotid saliva than in submandibular/sublingual saliva. Conversely, S-type cystatins are more concentrated in submandibular/sublingual saliva. Furthermore, the secretion of some peptides is gland-specific: basic PRPs are secreted only by the parotid glands. Finally, among the other proteins detected in whole saliva, α-defensins 1–4 and β-thymosins 4 and 10 originate mainly from gingival crevicular fluid (Pisano et al. 2005).

As a consequence, the salivary output is characterized by variations not only of the flow rate but also of the protein concentration and composition.

Age is another important factor affecting protein saliva composition. A recent study performed on human preterm newborns demonstrated the profound difference in the protein composition of their saliva with respect to that of adults (Castagnola et al. 2011a). Indeed, in saliva from preterm human newborns, more than 40 protein masses usually undetected in adult saliva were revealed. Among them, stefin A and stefin B (three isoforms), S100A7 (two isoforms), S100A8, S100A9 (eight isoforms), S100A11, S100A12, small PRP-3 (two isoforms), lysozyme C, thymosins β_4 and

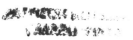

β_{10}, antileukoproteinase, histone H1c, and α- and β-globins were identified. The salivary concentration of these proteins decreased as a function of postconceptional age, reaching the values observed in full-term newborns at about 270 days of postconceptional age, and the values observed in adult whole saliva later in development. Interestingly, the shape of decrease for many proteins was different, suggesting that the variations were connected to coordinate and hierarchical actions of these proteins. Many of the identified proteins are candidates as tumor markers in the adult. This observation led to the suggestion that during fetal development, the interplay between these proteins contributes to the molecular events that regulate cell growth and death. A preliminary study showed that salivary glands are responsible for the high levels of oral thymosin β_4 detected in preterm newborn saliva, whereas in adult saliva this peptide is primarily derived from crevicular fluid (Inzitari et al. 2009; Nemolato et al. 2009). These studies suggest that salivary glands switch their secretion to adult salivary proteins only after the normal term of delivery.

Whereas basic PRPs in whole saliva do not reach their mature concentrations until the age of adolescence (Cabras et al. 2009), other proteins show mature levels as early as an age of 3 years or show variable concentrations as a function of age, i.e., acidic PRPs, histatin 5, histatin 6, histatin 1, and cystatin S. For instance, acidic PRPs show a minimum of concentration around 6–9 years of age, probably in connection with events occurring in the mouth during the replacement of the deciduous dentition. A process called "exfoliation" might cause a decrease in the concentration of specific salivary protein and peptides, owing to their recruitment to dental and gingival surfaces. The higher concentration of histatin 1 around 3–5-years of age is of particular interest, since it may be associated with its recently demonstrated wound-closing properties (Oudhoff et al. 2008).

27 Function of Salivary Proteins

No doubt exists about the fundamental role of saliva and its protein content in the protection of oral mucosa and teeth. It is enough to consider the devastating macroscopic effects detectable in the oral cavity of patients affected by severe Sjögren syndrome. The mucosal epithelium is subjected to wounds and infections. The dental arc is compromised by recurrent periodontitis and caries. It is, however, very difficult to establish, at the molecular level, not only the specific role played by each salivary protein in oral protection but also the interactions between the different salivary proteins in their protection of the mouth and, since saliva is swallowed, of the entire digestive tract. Some roles seem evident, such as the lubricating and protecting role of mucins, and the buffering properties of carbonic anhydrase, as reported in Table 1. The high concentration of salivary amylase is traditionally associated with starch predigestion. However, owing to the low enzymatic activity of the enzyme, some researchers are convinced that oral amylase plays a presently not specified role in the protection of the mouth.

The information obtained by recent proteomic studies are a clue and a stimulus for the understanding of the roles of the different families of salivary proteins in the oral cavity. For instance, it is challenging to decipher the significant qualitative and quantitative differences in gland secretions, which suggest specific molecular requirements for different oral districts. Other suggestions could emerge from the variations observed in protein composition during the pediatric age which could offer valuable information on possible functions. Except for their tannin-binding properties (Lu and Bennick 1998), the function of basic PRPs is still almost completely obscure. Recent studies demonstrated that an unidentified component of the basic PRP family displays antiviral activity against HIV (Robinovitch et al. 2001), and a peptide fragment of ten amino acid residues considerably inhibits *Propionibacterium acnes* growth (Huang et al. 2008), revealing interesting antiviral properties for peptide fragments related to basic PRPs.

Acidic PRPs are responsible for the modulation of the salivary calcium ion concentration and are involved in the formation of acquired enamel pellicle and oral mucosal pellicle, networks originating from cross-linking of the proteins caused by the action of transglutaminase 2. However, no information is available on the functional differences exerted by the entire and truncated isoforms or on the possible role of P–C peptide, the C-terminal peptide deriving from the cleavage of all the isoforms of acidic PRPs.

Most salivary peptides and proteins are directly or indirectly involved in innate immunity and in the modulation of the oral microflora (Gorr 2009). In this respect, the antifungal activity shown by histatin 3 and its fragments on *Candida albicans* species is particularly interesting. Recently, it was demonstrated that histatin 3 binds to heat shock cognate protein 70 (HSC70) during the G1/S transition in human gingival fibroblasts (Imamura et al. 2009); it prevents ATP-dependent dissociation of the HSC70–p27 complex, and it induces DNA synthesis. These findings suggest that histatin 3 may also be involved in oral cell proliferation.

Recently, it was shown that histatin 1 displays wound-healing activity (Oudhoff et al. 2008). Interestingly, histatin 1 induced cell spreading and migration in a full-skin human wound model; however, the peptide did not stimulate cell proliferation. N- to C-cyclization potentiated peptide activity 1,000-fold, indicating that a specific peptide conformation was responsible for the effect (Oudhoff et al. 2009a). The minimally active domain was found to be fragment 20–32 of the parent histatin peptide. The wound-healing effect was strongly inhibited by mucin-5B, probably by blocking reepithelialization. Interestingly, histatin 1 stimulated wound closure of primary cells of both oral and nonoral origin (Oudhoff et al. 2009b), which suggests a therapeutic application of histatin 1 derived peptides in the treatment of skin wounds.

Statherin is a singular salivary phosphopeptide of 43 amino acid residues involved in the inhibition of calcium phosphate precipitation and in the formation of acquired enamel pellicle (Schüpbach et al. 2001). However, statherin may have other relevant oral functions implicated in the formation of the oral epithelial protein pellicle, and it probably has a functional connection with the P–B peptide, whose function is still completely obscure (Messana et al. 2008b).

28 Pathological Modifications

Saliva is a very attractive bodily fluid for the diagnosis of diseases for several reasons: (1) collection of saliva is usually economical, "safe," "easy," and can be performed without the help of health care workers, allowing home-based sampling; (2) collection of saliva is considered an acceptable and noninvasive process by patients because it does not provoke any pain (and so saliva can be easily collected for patients

in the pediatric age range) (Tabak 2001). Nowadays, saliva is used effectively for the detection of specific antibodies (i.e., HIV, hepatitis C), hormones, and pharmaceuticals (i.e., drugs of abuse). However, the widespread use of saliva for diagnostics is complicated by the above-reported dynamism and polymorphism that characterizes the salivary proteome. The present and future analytical ability of proteomic techniques to contemporaneously quantify the great variety of possible translational salivary states will inevitably lead to defining "individual salivary profiles." The challenges are to establish the differences between particular polymorphisms or posttranslational modifications connected with diseases and further, to determine whether these differences inhibit or promote the development of specific diseases.

The salivary proteome presents several unique proteins; thus saliva-based diagnostics may provide information complementary to that from blood- and urine-based diagnostics. Since about one quarter of the salivary proteome overlaps with the plasma proteome (Loo et al. 2010), it will be important to establish if disease-linked plasma modifications are reflected in the saliva secreted in order to rely upon noninvasive tests for disease screening, detection, and monitoring.

Indeed, several studies have shown that systemic diseases may affect the human salivary proteome. The salivary biomarkers characterized so far show satisfactory clinical sensitivity and specificity (i.e., good prediction of the patients with the disease and normal values in healthy subjects). An interesting example concerns the detection of low phosphorylation levels of three salivary peptides (statherin, histatin 1, acidic PRPs) in a subset (about 60%) of patients with autism spectrum disorder (Castagnola et al. 2008). A set of salivary proteins has been shown to display a different concentration in children affected by type 1 diabetes compared with healthy subjects (Cabras et al. 2010), i.e., a significant increase of amounts of the short form of S100A9, α-defensins 1–3, and various fragments deriving from P–C peptide paralleled by a decrease of the amounts of P–C peptide, statherin, P–B peptide, and histatins 3, 5, and 6.

Many studies have addressed the early detection of different oral tumors such as oral squamous cell carcinoma (Jou et al. 2010; Shintani et al. 2010; Hu et al. 2008) and head and neck squamous cell carcinoma (Dowling et al. 2008; Ohshiro et al. 2007; de Jong et al. 2010; Chen et al. 2002). Because the research groups used different proteomic platforms, it is not surprising that the results may differ. Jou et al. (2010), using 2D electrophoresis followed by matrix-assisted laser desorption/ionization (MALDI) time-of-flight (TOF) MS, found the level of salivary transferrin to be increased in patients with oral squamous cell carcinoma. Shintani et al. (2010), using surface-enhanced laser desorption/ionization TOF analyses, showed an increase in the level of a truncated form of cystatin SN. Hu et al. (2008), using both liquid chromatography–MS/MS and 2D electrophoresis, found increased amounts of protectin, catalase, profilin, and S100A9 for oral squamous cell carcinoma. The salivary proteome of patients affected by primary Sjögren syndrome has also been extensively investigated (Giusti et al. 2007; Ryu et al. 2006; Peluso et al. 2007; Fleissig et al. 2009). The principal platform utilized was based on 2D electrophoresis followed either by MALDI-TOF MS or by electrospray ionization MS/MS analyses of the tryptic protein digests. Some controversial results were, however, obtained. For instance, whereas Giusti et al. (2007) found the level of salivary α-amylase decreased, Fleissig et al. (2009) found it increased, suggesting that the search of new biomarkers has to be performed in a large number of patients and validation of most of the results reported is necessary.

Even though it is a demanding task, for widespread introduction of saliva-based diagnostics it is mandatory to define proper reference proteomes and further, to standardize analytical procedures. As for blood and urine samples, the time and site of specimen collection, as well as the definition of specific treatments for sample stabilization, need to be established. Thus, high-throughput proteomic approaches, applied under standardized conditions, will result in the introduction of simple, sensitive, and specific analytical procedures to demonstrate salivary biomarkers in clinical practice.

References

Atkinson JC, Shiroky JB, Macynski A, Fox PC (1989) Effects of furosemide on the oral cavity. Gerodontology 8:23–26

Bobek LA, Levine MJ (1992) Cystatins–inhibitors of cysteine proteinases. Crit Rev Oral Biol Med 3:307–332

Bobek LA, Liu J, Sait SN, Shows TB, Bobek YA, Levine MJ (1996) Structure and chromosomal localization of the human salivary mucin gene, MUC7. Genomics 31:277–282

Babkin BP (1950) Secretory mechanism of the digestive glands, 2nd edn. Hoeber, New York

Barka T (1965) Induced cell proliferation: the effect of isoproterenol. Exp Cell Res 37:662–679

Birkhed D, Heintze U (1989) Salivary secretion rate, buffer capacity, and pH. In: Tenovuo J (ed) Human saliva. Clinical chemistry and microbiology, vol 11. CRC, Boca Raton

Blair-West JR, Coghlan JP, Denton DA, Wright RDI (1967) Alimentary canal II. In: Code CF (ed) Handbook of physiology, 6th edn. American Physiological Society, Bethesda

Borg-Andersson A, Ekström J, Birkhed D (1992) Glucose in human parotid saliva in response to cold stress. Acta Physiol Scand 146:283–284

Brandtzaeg P (2009) Mucosal immunity: induction, dissemination and effector functions. Scand J Immunol 70:505–515

Cabras T, Fanali C, Monteiro JA, Amado F, Inzitari R, Desiderio C, Scarano E, Giardina B, Castagnola M, Messana I (2007) Tyrosine polysulfation of human salivary histatin 1. A post-translational modification specific of the submandibular gland. J Proteome Res 6:2472–2480

Cabras T, Pisano E, Boi R, Olianas A, Manconi B, Inzitari R, Fanali C, Giardina B, Castagnola M, Messana I (2009) Age-dependent modifications of the human salivary secretory protein complex. J Proteome Res 8:4126–4134

Cabras T, Pisano E, Mastinu A, Denotti G, Pusceddu PP, Inzitari R, Fanali C, Nemolato S, Castagnola M, Messana I (2010) Alterations of the salivary secretory peptidome profile in children affected by type 1 diabetes. Mol Cell Proteomics 9:2099–2108

Cannon WB (1937) Digestion and health. Secker and Warburg, London

Castagnola M, Inzitari R, Rossetti DV, Olmi C, Cabras T, Piras V, Nicolussi P, Sanna MT, Pellegrini M, Giardina B, Messana I (2004) A cascade of 24 histatins (histatin 3 fragments) in human saliva. Suggestions for a pre-secretory sequential cleavage pathway. J Biol Chem 279:41436–41443

Castagnola M, Messana I, Inzitari R, Fanali C, Cabras T, Morelli A, Pecoraro AM, Neri G, Torrioli MG, Gurrieri F (2008) Hypo-phosphorylation of salivary peptidome as a clue to the molecular pathogenesis of autism spectrum disorders. J Proteome Res 7:5327–5332

Castagnola M, Inzitari R, Fanali C, Iavarone F, Vitali A, Desiderio C, Vento G, Tirone C, Romagnoli C, Cabras T, Manconi B, Sanna MT, Boi R, Pisano E, Olianas A, Pellegrini M, Nemolato S, Heizmann CW, Faa G, Messana I (2011a) The surprising composition of the salivary proteome of preterm human newborn. Mol Cell Proteomics 10:M110.003467

Castagnola M, Cabras T, Vitali A, Sanna MT, Messana I (2011b) Biotechnological implication of the salivary proteome. Trends Biotechnol 29:409–418

Çevik-Aras H, Ekström J (2006) Cholecystokinin- and gastrin-induced protein and amylase secretion from the parotid gland of the anaesthetized rat. Reg Pept 134:89–96

Çevik-Aras H, Ekström J (2008) Melatonin-evoked in vivo secretion of protein and amylase from the parotid gland of the anaesthetized rat. J Pineal Res 45:413–421

Çevik-Aras H, Ekström J (2010) Anti-inflammatory action of cholecystokinin and melatonin in the rat parotid gland. Oral Dis 16:661–667

Çevik-Aras H, Godoy T, Ekström J (2011) Melatonin-induced protein synthesis in the rat parotid gland. J Physiol Pharmacol 62:95–99

Chen YC, Li TY, Tsai MF (2002) Analysis of the saliva from patients with oral cancer by matrix-assisted laser desorption/ionization time-of-flight mass spectrometry. Rapid Commun Mass Spectrom 16:364–369

Cutando A, Gómez-Moreno G, Arana C, Acuña-Castroviejo D, Reiter RJ (2007) Melatonin: potential functions in the oral cavity. J Periodontol 78:1094–1194

Dawes C (1975) Circadian rhythms in the flow rate and composition of unstimulated and stimulated human submandibular saliva. J Physiol 244:535–548

Dawes C (1987) Physiological factors affecting salivary flow rate, oral sugar clearance, and the sensation of dry mouth. J Dent Res 66:648–653

Dawes C, Wood CM (1973) The contribution of oral minor mucous gland secretions to the volume of whole saliva in man. Arch Oral Biol 18:337–342

Dawes C, O'Connor AM, Aspen JM (2000) The effect on human salivary flow rate of the temperature of a gustatory stimulus. Arch Oral Biol 45:957–961

de Jong EP, Xie H, Onsongo G, Stone MD, Chen XB, Kooren JA, Refsland EW, Griffin RJ, Ondrey FG, Wu B, Le CT, Rhodus NL, Carlis JV, Griffin TJ (2010) Quantitative proteomics reveals myosin and actin as promising saliva biomarkers for distinguishing pre-malignant and malignant oral lesions. PLoS One 5:e11148

Diamant H, Wiberg A (1965) Does the chorda tympani in man contain secretory fibres for the parotid gland? Acta Otolaryngol 60:255–264

Dickinson DP (2002) Cysteine peptidases of mammals: their biological roles and potential effects in the oral cavity and other tissues in health and disease. Crit Rev Oral Biol Med 13:238–275

DiSabato-Mordaski T, Kleinberg I (1996) Measurement and comparison of the residual saliva on various oral mucosal and dentition surfaces in humans. Arch Oral Biol 41:655–665

Douglas WH, Reeh ES, Ramasubbu N, Raj PA, Bhandary KK, Levine MJ (1991) Statherin: a major boundary lubricant of human saliva. Biochem Biophys Res Commun 180:91–97

Dowling P, Wormald R, Meleady P, Henry M, Curran A, Clynes M (2008) Analysis of the saliva proteome from patients with head and neck squamous cell carcinoma reveals differences in abundance levels of proteins associated with tumour progression and metastasis. J Proteomics 71:168–175

Drummond PD (2002) Mechanisms of gustatory flushing in Frey's syndrome. Clin Auton Res 12:179–184

Dunbar EM, Singer TW, Singer K, Knight H, Lanska D, Okun MS (2002) Understanding gustatory sweating. What have we learned from Lucja Frey and her predecessors? Clin Auton Res 12:179–184

Ecobichon DJ (1995) Toxic effects of pesticides. In: Klassen CD (ed) Casarett and Doulll's toxicology. The basic science of poisons, 5th edn. McGraw- Hill, New York

Edwards AV (1988) Autonomic control of salivary blood flow. In: Garrett JR, Ekström J, Anderson LC (eds) Glandular mechanisms of salivary secretion. Frontiers of oral biology, vol 10. Karger, Basel

Ekström J (1969) 4(2-hydroxy-3-isopropylaminopropoxy) acetanilide as a beta-receptor blocking agent. Experientia 25:372

Ekström J (1987) Neuropeptides and secretion. J Dent Res 66:524–530

Ekström J (1998) Non-adrenergic, non-cholinergic reflex secretion of parotid saliva in rats elicited by mastication and acid applied on the tongue. Exp Physiol 83:697–700

Ekström J (1999a) Role of non-adrenergic, non-cholinergic autonomic transmitters in salivary glandular activities in vivo. In: Garrett JR, Ekström J, Anderson LC (eds) Neural mechanisms of salivary gland secretion. Frontiers of oral biology, vol 11. Karger, Basel

Ekström J (1999b) Degeneration secretion and supersensitivity in salivary glands following denervations, and the effects on choline acetyltransferase activity. In: Garrett JR, Ekström J, Anderson LC (eds) Neural mechanisms of salivary gland secretion. Frontiers of oral biology, vol 11. Karger, Basel

Ekström J (2001) Gustatory-salivary reflexes induce non-adrenergic, non-cholinergic acinar degranulation in the rat parotid gland. Exp Physiol 86:475–480

Ekström J (2002) Muscarinic agonist-induced non-granular and granular secretion of amylase in the parotid gland of the anaesthetized rat. Exp Physiol 87:147–152

Ekström J, Çevik-Aras H, Sayardoust S (2007) Neural- and hormonal-induced protein synthesis and mitotic activity in the rat parotid gland and the dependence on NO-generation. J Oral Biosci 49:31–38

Ekström J, Çevik Aras H (2008) Parasympathetic non-adrenergic, non-cholinergic transmission in rat parotid glands: effects of cholecystokinin-A and -B receptor antagonists on the secretory response. Reg Pept 146:278–284

Ekström J, Ekman R (2005) Sympathectomy-induced increases in calcitonin gene-related peptide (CGRP)-, substance P- and vasoactive intestinal peptide (VIP)-levels in parotid and submandibular glands of the rat. Arch Oral Biol 50:909–917

Ekström J, Ekman R, Håkanson R, Sjögren S, Sundler F (1988) Calcitonin gene-related peptide in rat salivary glands: neuronal localization, depletion upon nerve stimulation, and effects on salivation in relation to substance P. Neuroscience 26:933–949

Ekström J, Ekman R, Luts A, Sundler F, Tobin G (1996) Neuropeptide Y in salivary glands of the rat: origin, release and secretory effects. Regul Pept 61:125–134

Ekström J, Godoy T, Riva A (2010a) Clozapine: agonistic and antagonistic salivary secretory actions. J Dent Res 89:276–280

Ekström J, Godoy T, Riva A (2010b) N-Desmethylclozapine exerts dual and opposite effects on salivary secretion in the rat. Eur J Oral Sci 118:1–8

Ekström J, Havel GE, Reinhold A (2000) Parasympathetic non-adrenergic, non-cholinergic-induced protein synthesis and mitogenic activity in rat parotid glands. Exp Physiol 85:171–176

Ekström J, Holmberg J (1972) Choline acetyltransferase in the normal and parasympathetically denervated parotid gland of the dog. Acta Physiol Scand 86:353–358

Ekström J, Malmberg L (1984) Beta 1-adrenoceptor mediated salivary gland enlargement in the rat. Experientia 40:862–863

Ekström J, Murakami M, Inzitari R, Khosravani N, Fanali C, Cabras T, Fujita-Yoshigaki J, Sugiya H, Messana I, Castagnol M (2009) RP-HPLC-ESI-MS characterization of novel peptide fragments related to rat parotid secretory protein in parasympathetic induced saliva. J Sep Sci 32:2944–2952

Ekström J, Reinhold AC (2001) Reflex-elicited increases in female rat parotid protein synthesis involving parasympathetic non-adrenergic, non-cholinergic mechanisms. Exp Physiol 86:605–610

Ekström J, Templeton D (1977) Difference in sensitivity of parotid glands brought about by disuse and overuse. Acta Physiol Scand 101:329–335

Eliasson L, Birkhed D, Heyden G, Strömberg N (1996) Studies on human minor salivary gland secretion using the Periotron method. Arch Oral Biol 41:1179–1182

Eliasson L, Carlén A (2010) An update on minor salivary gland secretions. Eur J Oral Sci 118:435–442

Elishoov H, Wolff A, Kravel LS, Shiperman A, Gorsky M (2008) Association between season and temperature and unstimulated parotid and submandibular/sublingual secretion rates. Arch Oral Biol 53:75–78

Emmelin N (1965) Action of transmitters on the responsiveness of effector cells. Experientia 15:57–65

Emmelin N (1967) Nervous control of salivary glands. In: Code CF (ed) Handbook of physiology alimentary canal II, 6th edn. American Physiological Society, Bethesda

Emmelin N (1987) Nerve interactions in salivary glands. J Dent Res 66:509–517

Emmelin N, Engström J (1960) On the existence of specific secretory sympathetic fibres for the cat's submaxillary gland. J Physiol 153:1–8

Ericsson Y, Hardwick L (1978) Individual diagnosis, prognosis and counseling for caries prevention. Caries Res 12:94–102

Ferguson DB, Botchway CA (1980) A comparison of circadian variation in the flow rate and composition of stimulated human parotid, submandibular and whole salivas from the same individuals. Arch Oral Biol 25:559–568

Field EA, Longman LP, Bucknall R, Kaye SB, Higham SM, Edgar WM (1997) The establishment of a xerostomia clinic: a prospective study. Br J Oral Maxiofac Surg 35:96–103

Fleissig Y, Deutsch O, Reichenberg E, Redlich M, Zaks B, Palmon A, Aframian DJ (2009) Different proteomic protein patterns in saliva of Sjögren's syndrome patients. Oral Dis 15:61–68

Freudenreich O (2005) Drug-induced sialorrhea. Drugs Today (Barc) 41:411–418

Gallacher DV, Smith PM (1999) Autonomic transmitters and Ca $^{2+}$ -activated cellular responses in salivary glands in vitro. In: Garrett JR, Ekström J, Anderson LC (eds) Neural mechanisms of salivary gland secretion. Frontiers of oral biology, vol 11. Karger, Basel

Garrett JR (1988) Innervation of salivary glands: neurohistological and functional aspects. In: Sreebny LM (ed) In the salivary system. CRC, Boca Raton

Garrett JR (1998) Historical introduction to salivary secretion. In: Garrett JR, Ekström J, Anderson LC (eds) Glandular mechanisms of salivary secretion. Frontiers of oral biology, vol 10. Karger, Basel

Garrett JR, Emmelin N (1979) Activities of salivary myoepithelial cells: a review. Med Biol 57:1–28

Garret JR, Thulin A (1975) Changes in parotid acinar cells accompanying salivary secretion in rats on sympathetic or parasympathetic nerve stimulation. Cell Tissue Res 159:179–193

Gendler SJ, Spicer AP (1995) Epithelial mucin genes. Ann Rev Physiol 57:607–634

Gibbons RJ, Hay DI (1988) Human salivary acidic proline-rich proteins and statherin promote the attachment of Actinomyces viscosus LY7 to apatitic surfaces. Infect Immun 56:439–445

Gorr S-U (2009) Antimicrobial peptides of the oral cavity. Periodontol 2000 51:152–180

Giusti L, Baldini C, Bazzichi L, Ciregia F, Tonazzini I, Mascia G, Giannaccini G, Bombardieri S, Lucacchini A (2007) Proteome analysis of whole saliva: a new tool for rheumatic diseases—the example of Sjögren's syndrome. Proteomics 7:1634–1643

Godoy T, Riva A, Ekström J (2011) Clozapine-induced salivation: interaction with N-desmethylclozapine and amisulpride in an experimental rat model. Eur J Oral Sci 119:275–281

Gorr SU, Venkatesh SG, Darling DS (2005) Parotid secretory granules: crossroads of secretory pathways and protein storage. J Dent Res 84:500–509

Gray H (1988) Gray's anatomy: the classical collector's edition. Bounty Books, New York

Gregersen MI (1931) A method for uniform stimulation of the salivary glands in the unaesthetized dog by exposure to a warm environment, with some observations on the quantitative changes in salivary flow during dehydration. Am J Physiol 97:107–116

Grisius MM, Fox PC (1988) Salivary gland dysfunction and xerostomia. In: Linden RWA (ed) The scientific basis of eating. Frontiers of oral biology, vol 9. Karger, Basel

Gröschl M (2009) The physiological role of hormones in saliva. Bioessays 31:843–852

Guile GR, Harvey DJ, O'Donnell N, Powell AK, Hunter AP, Zamze S, Fernandes DL, Dwek RA, Wing DR (1998) Identification of highly fucosylated N-linked oligosaccharides from the human parotid gland. Eur J Biochem 258:623–656

Hainsworth RF (1967) Saliva spreading, activity, and body temperature regulation in the rat. Am J Physiol 212:1288–1292

Hector MP, Linden RWA (1999) Reflexes of salivary secretion. In: Garrett JR, Ekström J, Andersson LC (eds) Neural mechanisms of salivary glands. Frontiers of oral biology, vol 11. Karger, Basel

Heintze U, Birkhed D, Björn H (1983) Secretion rate and buffer effect of resting and stimulated whole saliva as a function of age and sex. Swed Dent J 7:227–238

Helm JF, Dodds WJ, Hogan WJ (1987) Salivary response to esophageal acid in normal subjects and patients with reflux esophagitis. Gastroenterology 93:1393–1397

Helmerhorst EJ, Sun X, Salih E, Oppenheim FG (2008) Identification of Lys-Pro-Gln as a novel cleavage site specificity of saliva-associated proteases. J Biol Chem 283: 19957–19966

Hu S, Arellano M, Boontheung P, Wang J, Zhou H, Jiang J, Elashoff D, Wei R, Loo JA, Wong DT (2008) Salivary proteomics for oral cancer biomarker discovery. Clin Cancer Res 14:6246–6252

Huang CM, Torpey JW, Liu YT, Chen YR, Williams KE, Komives EA, Gallo RL (2008) A peptide with a ProGln C terminus in the human saliva peptidome exerts bactericidal activity against Propionibacterium acnes. Antimicrob Agents Chemother 52:1834–1836

Imai A, Nashida T, Shimomura H (1995) Regulation of cAMP phosphodiesterases by cyclic nucleotids in rat parotid gland. Biochem Mol Biol Int 37:1029–1036

Imamura Y, Fujigaki Y, Oomori Y, Usui S, Wang PL (2009) Cooperation of salivary protein histatin 3 with heat shock cognate protein 70 relative to the G1/S transition in human gingival fibroblasts. J Biol Chem 284:14316–14325

Inzitari R, Cabras T, Onnis G, Olmi C, Mastinu A, Sanna MT, Pellegrini MG, Castagnola M, Messana I (2005) Different isoforms and post-translational modifications of human salivary acidic proline-rich proteins. Proteomics 5:805–815

Inzitari R, Cabras T, Rossetti DV, Fanali C, Vitali A, Pellegrini M, Paludetti G, Manni A, Giardina B, Messana I, Castagnola M (2006) Detection in human saliva of different statherin and P-B fragments and derivatives. Proteomics 6:6370–6379

Inzitari R, Cabras T, Pisano E, Fanali C, Manconi B, Scarano E, Fiorita A, Paludetti G, Manni A, Nemolato S, Faa G, Castagnola M, Messana I (2009) HPLC-ESI-MS analysis of oral human fluids reveals that gingival crevicular fluid is the main source of oral thymosins beta(4) and beta(10). J Sep Sci 32:57–63

Isenman L, Liebow C, Rothman S (1999) The endocrine secretion of mammalian digestive enzymes by exocrine glands. Am J Physiol 276:E223–E232

Jenkins GN (1978) The physiology and biochemistry of the mouth. Blackwell, Oxford

Jensen Kjeilen JC, Brodin P, Aars H, Berg T (1987) Parotid salivary flow in response to mechanical and gustatory stimulation in man. Acta Physiol Scand 131:169–175

Johanson CN (2011) Cariological and salivary studies in 70-year-old cohorts. Dissertation, University of Gothenburg

Johnson DA (1988) Regulation of salivary glands and their secretion by masticatory, nutritional and hormonal factors. In: Sreebny LM (ed) The salivary system. CRC, Boca Raton

Jou YJ, Lin CD, Lai CH, Chen CH, Kao JY, Chen SY, Tsai MH, Huang SH, Lin CW (2010) Proteomic identification of salivary transferrin as a biomarker for early detection of oral cancer. Anal Chim Acta 681:41–48

Kariyawasam AP, Dawes C (2005) A circannual rhythm in unstimulated salivary flow rate when the ambient temperature varies by only about 2 degrees C. Arch Oral Biol 50: 919–922

Khosravani N, Ekman R, Ekström J (2008) The peptidergic innervations of the rat parotid gland. Effects of section of the auriculo-temporal nerve and/or otic ganglionectomy. Arch Oral Biol 53:238–242

Khosravani N, Birkhed D, Ekström J (2009) The cholinesterase inhibitor physostigmine for the local treatment of dry mouth: a randomized study. Eur J Oral Sci 117:209–217

Khosravani N, Sandberg M, Ekström J (2006) The otic ganglion in rats and its parotid connection: cholinergic pathways, reflex secretion and a secretory role for the facial nerve. Exp Physiol 91:239–247 (Erratum in: Exp Physiol 91:481, 2006)

Khosravani N, Ekström J (2006) Facial nerve section induces transient changes in sensitivity to methacholine and in acetylcholine synthesis in the rat parotid gland. Arch Oral Biol 51:736–739

Leipzig B, Obert P (1979) Parotid gland swelling. J Fam Pract 9:1085–1093

Loo JA, Yan W, Ramachandran P, Wong DT (2010) Comparative human salivary and plasma proteomes. J Dent Res 89:1016–1023

Longman LP, Higham SM, Rai K, Edgar WM, Field EA (1995) Salivary gland hypofunction in elderly patients attending a xerostomic clinic. Gerodontology 12:67–72

Lu Y, Bennick A (1998) Interaction of tannin with human salivary proline-rich proteins. Arch Oral Biol 43:717–728

Mandel SJ, Mandel L (2003) Radioactive iodine and the salivary glands. Thyroid 13:265–271

Matsuo R (1999) Central connections for salivary innervations and efferent impulse formation. In: Garrett JR, Ekström J, Anderson LC (eds) Neural mechanisms of salivary gland secretion. Frontiers of oral biology, , vol 11. Karger, Basel

Melvin JE, Yule D, Shuttleworth T, Begenisich T (2005) Regulation offluid and electrolyte secretion in salivary gland acinar cells. Annu Rev Physiol 67:445–469

Messana I, Cabras T, Pisano E, Sanna MT, Olianas A, Manconi B, Pellegrini M, Paludetti G, Scarano A, Fiorita A, Agostino S, Contucci AM, Calò L, Picciotti PM, Manni A, Bennick A, Vitali A, Fanali C, Inzitari R, Castagnola M (2008a) Trafficking and postsecretory events responsible for the formation of secreted human salivary peptides: a proteomics approach. Mol Cell Proteomics 7:911–926

Messana I, Inzitari R, Fanali C, Cabras T, Castagnola M (2008b) Facts and artifacts in proteomics of body fluids. What proteomics of saliva is telling us? J Sep Sci 31:1948–1963

Mese H, Matsuo R (2007) Salivary secretion, taste and hyposalivation. Oral Rehabil 34:711–723

Meurman JH, Tarkkila L, Tiitinen A (2009) The menopause and oral health. Maturitas 63:56–62

Nagler RM (2004) salivary glands and the aging process: mechanistic aspects, health-status and medicinal-efficacy monitoring. Biogerontology 5:223–233

Navazesh M, Kumar SKS (2008) Measuring salivary flow: challenges and opportunities. J Am Dent Assoc 139: 35S–40S

Nederfors T, Isaksson R, Mörnstad H, Dahlöf C (1997) Prevalence of perceived symptoms of dry mouth in an adult Swedish population—relation to age, sex and pharmacotherapy. Community Dent Oral Epidemiol 25:211–216

Nederfors T, Twetman S, Dahlöf C (1989) Effects of the thiazide diuretic bendroflumethiazide on salivary flow rate and composition. Scand J Dent Res 97:520–527

Nemolato S, Messana I, Cabras T, Manconi B, Inzitari R, Fanali C, Vento G, Tirone C, Romagnoli C, Riva A, Fanni D, Di Felice E, Faa G, Castagnola M (2009) Thymosin beta(4) and beta(10) levels in pre-term newborn oral cavity and foetal salivary glands evidence a switch of secretion during foetal development. PLoS One 4:e5109

Offner GD, Troxler RF (2000) Heterogeneity of high-molecular-weight human salivary mucins. Adv Dent Res 14:69–75

Ohlin P (1966) Effects of isoprenaline treatment of secretory responses and respiratory enzymes of the submaxillary gland of the rat. J Oral Ther Pharmacol 3:190–193

Ohshiro K, Rosenthal DI, Koomen JM, Streckfus CF, Chambers M, Kobayashi R, El-Naggar AK (2007) Pre-analytic saliva processing affect proteomic results and biomarker screening of head and neck squamous carcinoma. Int J Oncol 30:743–749

Ono K, Morimoto Y, Inoue H, Masuda W, Tanaka T, Inenaga K (2006) Relationship of the unstimulated whole saliva flow rate and salivary gland size estimated by magnetic resonance image in healthy young humans. Arch Oral Biol 51:345–349

Österberg T, Landahl S, Heidegård B (1984) Salivary flow, saliva pH and buffering capacity in 70-year-old men and women. J Oral Rehab 11:157–170

Österberg T, Birkhed D, Johanson CN, Svanborg A (1992) Longitudinal study of stimulated whole saliva in an elderly population. Scand J Dent Res 100:340–345

Oudhoff MJ, Bolscher JG, Nazmi K, Kalay H, van 't Hof W, Amerongen AV, Veerman EC (2008) Histatins are the major wound-closure stimulating factors in human saliva as identified in a cell culture assay. FASEB J 22:3805–3812

Oudhoff MJ, Kroeze KL, Nazmi K, van den Keijbus PA, van 't Hof W, Fernandez-Borja M, Hordijk PL, Gibbs S, Bolscher JG, Veerman EC (2009a) Structure-activity analysis of histatin, a potent wound healing peptide from human saliva: cyclization of histatin potentiates molar activity 1,000-fold. FASEB J 23:3928–3935

Oudhoff MJ, van den Keijbus PA, Kroeze KL, Nazmi K, Gibbs S, Bolscher JG, Veerman EC (2009b) Histatins enhance wound closure with oral and non-oral cells. J Dent Res 88:846–850

Peluso G, De Santis M, Inzitari R, Fanali C, Cabras T, Messana I, Castagnola M, Ferraccioli GF (2007) Proteomic study of salivary peptides and proteins in patients with Sjögren's syndrome before and after pilocarpine treatment. Arthritis Rheum 56:2216–2222

Pisano E, Cabras T, Montaldo C, Piras V, Inzitari R, Olmi C, Castagnola M, Messana I (2005) Peptides of human gingival crevicular fluid determined by HPLC-ESI-MS. Eur J Oral Sci 113:462–468

Poulsen JH (1998) Secretion of electrolytes and water by salivary glands. In: Garrett JR, Ekström J, Anderson LC (eds) Glandular mechanisms of salivary secretion. Frontiers of oral biology, vol 10. Karger, Basel, pp 55–72

Praharaj SK, Jana AK, Goswami K, Das PR, Goyal N, Sinha VK (2010) Salivary flow rate in patients with schizophrenia on clozapine. Clin Neuropharmacol 33:176–178

Ramachandran P, Boontheung P, Xie Y, Sondej M, Wong DT, Loo JA (2006) Identification of N-linked glycoproteins in human saliva by glycoprotein capture and mass spectrometry. J Proteome Res 5:1493–1503

Reichert FL, Poth EJ (1933) Pathways for the secretory fibres of salivary glands in man. Proc Soc Exp Biol Med 30: 973–977

Rho MB, Deschler DG (2005) Salivary gland anatomy. In: Witt RL (ed) Salivary gland diseases. Surgical and medical management. Thieme, New York

Riva A, Loy F, Diana M, Isola R, Lantini MS, Ekström J (2010) Secretory effects of pentagastrin and melatonin on human parotid gland in vitro. An HRSEM study. In: XXI international symposium on morphological sciences. Taormina - Messina, 18/22 September - 2010, p 60

Robinovitch MR, Ashley RL, Iversen JM, Vigoren EM, Oppenheim FG, Lamkin M (2001) Parotid salivary basic proline-rich proteins inhibit HIV-I infectivity. Oral Dis 7:86–93

Rossoni RB, Machado AB, Machado CRS (1979) A histochemical study of catecholamines and cholinesterases in the autonomic nerves of human minor salivary glands. Histochem J 11:661–688

Ryan CM, Souda P, Halgand F, Wong DT, Loo JA, Faull KF, Whitelegge JP (2010) Confident assignment of intact mass tags to human salivary cystatins using top-down Fourier-transform ion cyclotron resonance mass spectrometry. J Am Soc Mass Spectrom 21:908–917

Ryu OH, Atkinson JC, Hoehn GT, Illei GG, Hart TC (2006) Identification of parotid salivary biomarkers in Sjogren's syndrome by surface-enhanced laser desorption/ionization time-of-flight mass spectrometry and two-dimensional difference gel electrophoresis. Rheumatology (Oxford) 45: 1077–1086

Sarosiek J, Rourk RM, Piascik R, Namiot Z, Hetzel DP, McCallum RW (1994) The effect of esophageal mechanical and chemical stimuli on salivary mucin secretion in healthy individuals. Am J Med Sci 308:23–31

Sabatini LM, Carlock LR, Johnson GW, Azen EA (1987) cDNA cloning and chromosomal localization (4q11–13) of a gene for statherin, a regulator of calcium in saliva. Am J Hum Genet 41:1048–1060

Sabatini LM, Azen EA (1989) Histatins, a family of salivary histidine-rich proteins, are encoded by at least two loci (HIS1 and HIS2). Biochem Biophys Res Commun 160: 495–502

Sayardoust S, Ekström J (2003) Nitric oxide-dependent in vitro secretion of amylase from innervated or chronically denervated parotid glands of the rat in response to isoprenaline and vasoactive intestinal peptide. Exp Physiol 88:381–387

Sayardoust S, Ekström J (2004) Nitric oxide-dependent protein synthesis in parotid and submandibular glands of anaesthetized rats upon sympathetic stimulation or isoprenaline administration. Exp Physiol 89:219–227

Scannapieco FA, Torres G, Levine MJ (1993) Salivary alpha-amylase: role in dental plaque and caries formation. Crit Rev Oral Biol Med 4:301–307

Schon F (1985) Postsympathectomy pain and changes in sensory neuropeptides: towards an animal model. Lancet 2:1158–1160

Schüpbach P, Oppenheim FG, Lendenmann U, Lamkin MS, Yao Y, Guggenheim B (2001) Electron-microscopic demonstration of proline-rich proteins, statherin, and histatins in acquired enamel pellicles in vitro. Eur J Oral Sci 109:60–68

Schwartz SS, Hay DI, Schluckebier SK (1992) Inhibition of calcium phosphate precipitation by human salivary statherin: structure-activity relationships. Calcif Tissue Int 50:511–517

Shafik A, El-Sibai O, Shafik AA, Mostafa R (2005) Effect of topical esophageal acidification on salivary secretion:

identification of the mechanism of action. J Gastroenterol Hepatol 20:1935–1939

Shapiro SL (1973) Recurrent parotid gland swelling. Eye Ear Nose Throat 52:147–150

Shintani S, Hamakawa H, Ueyama Y, Hatori M, Toyoshima T (2010) Identification of a truncated cystatin SA-I as a saliva biomarker for oral squamous cell carcinoma using the SELDI ProteinChip platform. Int J Oral Maxillofac Surg 39:68–74

Ship J, Pillemer SR, Baum BJ (2002) Xerostomia and the geriatric patient. J Am Geriatr Soc 50:535–543

Smaje LH (1998) Capillary dynamics in salivary glands. In: Garrett JR, Ekström J, Anderson LC (eds) Glandular mechanisms of salivary secretion. Frontiers of oral biology, vol 10. Karger, Basel

Sockalingam S, Shammi C, Remington G (2007) Clozapine-induced hypersalivation: a review of treatment strategies. Can J Psychiatry 52:377–384

Steiner DF (1998) The proprotein convertases. Curr Opin Chem Biol 2:31–39

Strous GJ, Dekker J (1992) Mucin-like glycoproteins. Crit Rev Biochem Mol Biol 27:57–92

Tabak LA (2001) A revolution in biomedical assessment: the development of salivary diagnostics. J Dent Educ 65:1335–1339

Tandler B, Riva A (1986) Salivary glands. In: Mjör IA, Fejerskov O (eds) Human oral embryology and histology. Munksgaard, Copenhagen

Teesalu S, Roosalu M (1993) Mixed salivary glucose and other carbohydrate leverls and their changes in emotional stress and in physical activity. Acta Physiol Scand 149:P57

Tenouvo J (1998) Antimicrobial functions of human saliva—how important is it for oral health? Acta Odontol Scand 58:250–256

Thelin WR, Brennan MT, Lockhart PG, Singh ML, Foc PC, Papas AS, Boucher RC (2008) The oral mucosa as a therapeutic target for xerostomia. Oral Dis 14:683–689

Thomsson KA, Prakobphol A, Leffler H, Reddy MS, Levine MJ, Fisher SJ, Hansson GC (2002) The salivary mucin MG1 (MUC5B) carries a repertoire of unique oligosaccharides that is large and diverse. Glycobiology 12:1–14

Vissink A, Spijkervet F, Amerongen A (1996) Aging and saliva: a review of the literature. Spec Care Dent 16:95–103

Wärnberg GE, Einarson S, Jonsson M, Aronsson JI (2005) Impact of dry mouth on oral health-related quality of life in older people. Gerodontology 22:219–226

Wolff MS, Kleinberg I (1999) The effect of ammonium glycopyrrolate (Robinul)-induced xerostomia on oral mucosal wetness and flow of gingival crevicular fluid in humans. Arch Oral Biol 44:97–102

Wolff MS, Kleinberg I (1998) Oral mucosal wetness in hypo- and normosalivators. Arch Oral Biol 43:455–462

Yao Y, Lamkin MS, Oppenheim FG (1999) Pellicle precursor proteins: acidic proline-rich proteins, statherin, and histatins, and their crosslinking reaction by oral transglutaminase. J Dent Res 78:1696–1703

Young CA, Ellis C, Johnson J, Sathasivam S, Pih N (2011) Treatment for sialorrhea (excessive saliva) in people with motor neuron disease/amyotrophic lateral sclerosis. Cochrane Database Syst Rev 11(5):CD006981

Zohar Y, Siegal A, Siegal G, Halpern B, Levy M, Gal R (2002) The great auricular nerve: does it penetrate the parotid gland? An anatomical and microscopical study. J Craniomaxillofac Surg 30:318–321

Feeding and Respiration

Olle Ekberg, Anna I. Hårdemark Cedborg, Katarina Bodén,
Hanne Witt Hedström, Richard Kuylenstierna, Lars I. Eriksson,
and Eva Sundman

Contents

O. Ekberg (✉)
Department of Diagnostic Radiology,
Skåne University Hospital, 205 02 Malmö, Sweden
e-mail: olle.ekberg@med.lu.se

A. I. Hårdemark Cedborg · L. I. Eriksson · E. Sundman
Department of Anaesthesiology and Intensive Care
Medicine, Karolinska University Hospital and Karolinska
Institute, Stockholm, Sweden

K. Bodén
Department of Diagnostic Radiology,
Karolinska University Hospital and Karolinska Institute,
Stockholm, Sweden

H. W. Hedström
Department of Neuroradiology, Karolinska University
Hospital and Karolinska Institute, Stockholm, Sweden

R. Kuylenstierna
Department of Otorhinolaryngology, Karolinska
University Hospital and Karolinska Institute,
Stockholm, Sweden

Abstract

Coordination of breathing and swallowing is
essential for normal bolus transportation through
the pharynx and for protection of the airways.
During passage of the bolus through the pharynx,
respiration is interrupted. Normal swallowing
occurs during the expiratory phase of breathing.
Incoordination of the feeding respiratory pattern
may lead to penetration of the bolus into the
airways. This may cause choking, death, aspiration
pneumonia, or chronic laryngitis.

1 Introduction

Swallowing and breathing are closely controlled by
specialized neuronal groups colocalized to the brainstem. Interaction occurs between neuronal groups
controlling breathing and those controlling swallowing (Dick et al. 1993; Saito et al. 2002; Ertekin and
Aydogdu 2003). Such central neuronal control, together with local anatomic conditions and sensory input
from the larynx and pharynx, allows safe and direct
passage of air, liquids, and solids. Moreover, factors
primarily thought to influence breathing (e.g., arterial
partial pressure of CO_2) affect swallowing (Nishino
et al. 1998; Sai et al. 2004), and other factors controlling pharyngeal function affect breathing pattern
(Nilsson et al. 1997; Hadjikoutis et al. 2000; Butler
et al. 2007; Terzi et al. 2007). Posture and positioning
are such factors.

Miller (1999), in his neurophysiological investigations of swallowing, concluded that brainstem
neuronal control is involved in the central inhibition

O. Ekberg (ed.), *Dysphagia*, Medical Radiology. Diagnostic Imaging, DOI: 10.1007/174_2012_587,
© Springer-Verlag Berlin Heidelberg 2012

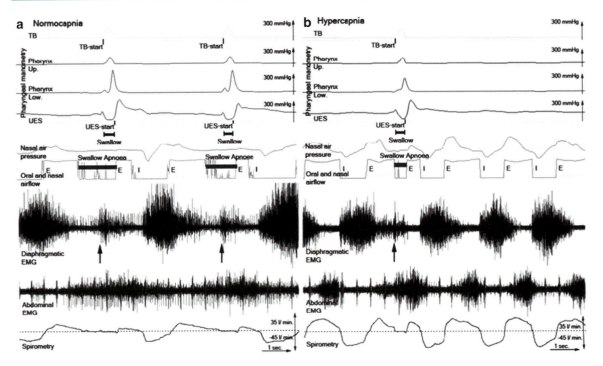

Fig. 1 Registrations of pharyngeal manometry, nasal air pressure, and oral and nasal respiratory airflow by the bidirectional gas flow discriminator, diaphragmatic and abdominal EMG, and spirometry. Recordings of two swallows at normocapnia (**a**) and one swallow at hypercapnia (**b**). The swallows presented show the respiratory phase pattern E–E (inspiration–expiration–swallow–expiration). The start of pharyngeal swallowing was defined as the start of pressure rise at the tongue base (*TB-start*) and the end was defined as the point in time when the upper esophageal sphincter started to contract

(*UES-start*). The duration of pharyngeal swallowing is marked with a *horizontal bar* (swallow). Swallowing apnea was detected by the respiratory airflow discriminator as an oscillating signal, representing zero airflow. Diaphragmatic activity during swallowing apnea is marked with *arrows*. Pharyngeal manometry was recorded at the tongue base (*TB*), upper/lower level of the pharynx (*Pharynx Up./Pharynx Low.*) and upper esophageal sphincter (*UES*). *I* inspiration, *E* expiration. (Reprinted from Hårdemark Cedborg et al. 2009)

of respiration during swallowing. Therefore, swallowing apnea is not an effect of closure of the vocal folds even though, together with laryngeal closure, it often occurs at the same time as apnea.

Swallowing apnea has also been registered in patients after laryngectomy (Hiss et al. 2003). The presence of swallowing apnea also remains 10 years after laryngectomy. Therefore, swallowing apnea is a central phenomenon and not the result of obstructive forces of closed airways during swallowing. On the other hand, closure of the laryngeal vestibule, including vocal folds, is an important part of the protective mechanism that hinders the bolus from reaching the airways. Swallowing apnea may start long before vocal fold closure; however, it ends when the vocal folds begin to reopen.

2   Feeding Respiratory Pattern

In a recent study, Hårdemark Cedborg et al. (2009) explored breathing during spontaneous swallowing using a bidirectional gas flow discriminator. They used a complex experimental setting in volunteers including manometry for registration of pressure at the level of the tongue base, midpharynx, and upper esophageal sphincter and including nasal and oral airflow. A diaphragmatic and abdominal EMG was used as well. Spirometry was used for quantitative registration of airflow in liters per minute. They studied spontaneous swallowing during normocapnia and hypercapnia. The latter was achieved by subjects breathing air with the addition of 5% CO_2. The term

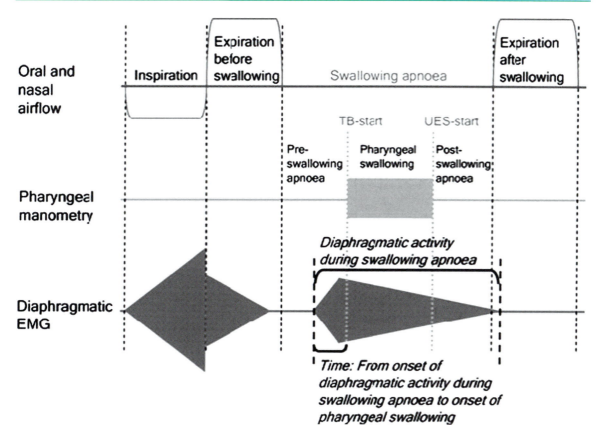

Fig. 2 A swallow preceded and followed by expiration (E–E pattern) and the diaphragmatic activity during swallowing apnea. The time from the onset of diaphragmatic activity during swallowing apnea to the onset of pharyngeal swallowing was measured and is marked in the figure. The start of pharyngeal swallowing is defined as the start of the pressure rise at the tongue base (*TB-start*) and the end of pharyngeal swallowing is defined as the start of the pressure rise at the upper esophageal sphincter (*UES-start*). (Reprinted from Hårdemark Cedborg et al. 2009)

"spontaneous swallowing" refers to the fact that the subjects were allowed to swallow saliva spontaneously and were not given any instruction for how to swallow. Hypercapnia was used to evaluate how an increased respiratory drive and higher breathing frequency interfered with spontaneous swallowing (Fig. 1).

Hårdemark Cedborg et al. (2009) found that all swallows occur during expiration. The normal sequence is that expiration is interrupted by a period of apnea, during which time the bolus passes through the pharynx. Then the expiration is resumed. The expiration before swallowing may be as short as 30 ms. Expiration before swallowing lasts about 1.3 s and expiration after swallowing lasts about 1.5 s. The preswallowing expiration time could be very short but could always be discerned. They speculated that swallowing is in fact controlled by the respiratory

neurons, in that sense that swallowing was only allowed to occur during an expiratory phase. By studying the EMG pattern, they confirmed the phrenic nerve activity described by Saito et al. (2002). This EMG pattern is distinctly different from that of an inspiration and was not followed by airflow. They called this "active breath holding." This central control of breathing ensures that respiration is stopped before pharyngeal swallowing and that a significant proportion (approximately 200 ml) of the tidal volume is "put on hold" by the activated diaphragm, only to be expired at the end of swallowing apnea. Expiratory airflow after swallowing clears the laryngeal inlet from misdirected bolus material, and thereby aspiration is prevented (Fig. 2).

In an experimental prospective study, Gross et al. (2003) showed that during a standardized pudding-like consistency swallow at three randomized lung

Fig. 3 Temporal
coordination of swallowing
and respiratory events in **a** the
upright and left decubitus
positions with normocapnia
and **b** the left decubitus
position with normocapnia
and with hypercapnia. All
values are in milliseconds and
are mean values ± the 95%
confidence interval. *TB*
tongue base, *UES* upper
esophageal sphincter, *PhCM*
middle pharyngeal
constrictor, *PhCL* lower
pharyngeal constrictor.
(Reprinted from Bodén et al.
2009)

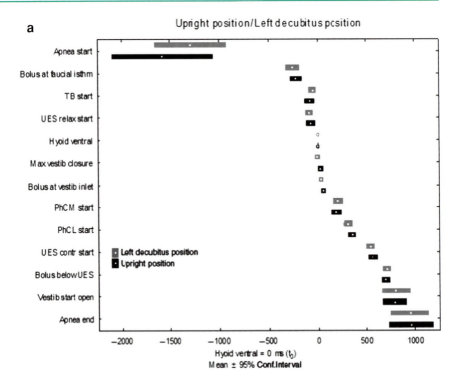

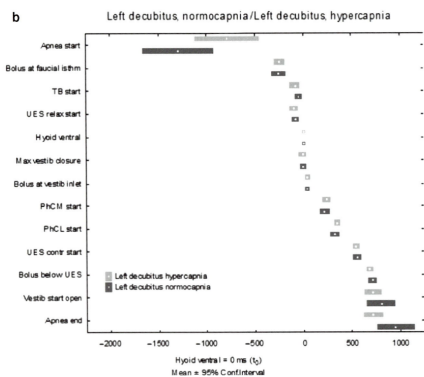

volumes (total lung capacity, functional residual capacity, and residual volume), the pharyngeal activity duration of deglutition for swallows produced at residual volume was significantly longer than that for swallows occurring at total lung capacity or at functional residual capacity. No significant differences were found for the bolus transit time or intramuscular electromyography of the superior constrictor. This supports the hypothesis that the respiratory system may have a regulatory function related to swallowing and that positive subglottic air pressure may be important for swallowing integrity.

Hårdemark Cedborg et al. (2009) also studied the length of preswallowing and postswallowing apnea. The duration of swallowing apnea decreased considerably at hypercapnia. Interestingly, they found that the duration of preswallowing apnea shortened, whereas the duration of postswallowing apnea did not change during hypercapnia. Hence, the temporal positioning of pharyngeal swallowing is asymmetrical, occurring in the late part of swallowing apnea at normocapnia but not at hypercapnia. This means that when breathing at a high frequency the preswallowing apnea period shortens considerably and that may put the patient at risk of misdirected swallowing. This may be a considerable problem in patients with chronic obstructive pulmonary disease who have a high respiration frequency (Martin et al. 1994; Martin-Harris et al. 2003, 2005). Chronic aspiration may then aggravate the patient's pulmonary condition, introducing a vicious cycle (Gross et al. 2009).

Respiration and swallowing coordination is not affected by changes in body position, bolus types, and respiratory drive (Hårdemark Cedborg et al. 2010). However, during water swallows, the duration of preswallowing apnea is significantly longer than that of spontaneous saliva swallow (Hårdemark Cedborg et al. 2010). During water swallow, the duration of the postswallowing apnea is also very constant.

Elderly adults have been shown to have a longer swallowing apnea duration than young and middle-aged adults (Hiss et al. 2001). That study also showed that women have a longer swallowing apnea duration than men and that the swallowing apnea duration increases as the bolus volume increases.

Martin-Harris et al. (2005) showed a higher occurrence of inhalation with swallowing apnea, with increased occurrence in individuals older than 65 years. Although it was not shown, the hypothesis is that this predisposes the elderly to aspiration pneumonia. However, they also found that the elderly have a prolonged swallowing apnea duration. Particularly, the onset of apnea could occur rather early compared with the onset in young individuals.

The coordination of respiration and swallow rhythms has also been studied in preterm and term infants (Gewolb and Vice 2006). The initial feeding efforts at 32–34 weeks (postmenstrual age) are characterized by periods of apneic suckle-feeding that alternate with tidal respiration. With further development, respiration is interposed into spaces partitioned by the swallows and the breathing efforts are integrated into an oral suck–swallow–breathing rhythm.

It has also been shown that an increase in respiratory drive by inhalation of 7% CO_2 in preterm infants is accompanied by a decrease in the rate of both sucking and swallowing during nutritive feeding. Increased ventilatory drive may directly inhibit nutritive feeding behavior in premature infants. Also, this speaks in favor of respiratory neurons in the brainstem that have superior control of swallowing and not vice versa (Timms et al. 1993).

Temporal coordination of swallowing and respiratory events has also been studied in a more global perspective (Bodén et al. 2009; Fig. 3). This confirms several of the studies forming the basis for the concept of a fixed pattern generator that controls muscular activity in the swallowing apparatus (Miller 1999).

References

Bodén K, Hårdemark Cedborg AI, Eriksson LI, Witt Hedström H, Kuylenstierna R, Sundman E, Ekberg O (2009) Swallowing and respiratory pattern in young healthy individuals recorded with high temporal resolution. Neurogastroenterol Motil 21:1163–e101

Butler SG, Stuart A, Pressman H, Poage G, Roche WJ (2007) Preliminary investigation of swallowing apnea duration and swallow/respiratory phase relationships in individuals with cerebral vascular accident. Dysphagia 22:215–224

Dick TE, Oku Y, Romaniuk JR, Cherniack NS (1993) Interaction between central pattern generators for breathing and swallowing in the cat. J Physiol 465:34–44

Ertekin C, Aydogdu I (2003) Neurophysiology of swallowing. Clin Neurophysiol 114:2226–2244

Gewolb IH, Vice FL (2006) Maturational changes in the rhythms, patterning, and coordination of respiration and swallow during feeding in preterm and term infants. Develop Med Child Neurol 48:589–594

Gross RD, Atwood CW Jr, Grayhack JP, Shaiman S (2003) Lung volume effects on pharyngeal swallowing physiology. J Appl Physiol 95:2211–2217

Gross RD, Atwood CW Jr, Ross SB, Olszewski JW, Eichhorn KA (2009) The coordination of breathing and swallowing in chronic obstructive pulmonary disease. Am J Respir Crit Care Med 179:559–565

Hadjikoutis S, Pickersgill TP, Dawson K, Wiles CM (2000) Abnormal patterns of breathing during swallowing in neurological disorders. Brain 123:1863–1873

Hiss SG, Treole K, Stuart A (2001) Effects of age, gender, bolus volume, and trial on swallowing apnea duration and swallow/respiratory phase relationships of normal adults. Dysphagia 16:128–135

Hiss SG, Strauss M, Treole K, Stuart A, Boutilier S (2003) Swallowing apnea as a function of airway closure. Dysphagia 18:293–300

Hårdemark Cedborg AI, Sundman E, Bodén K, Witt Hedström H, Kuylenstierna R, Ekberg O, Eriksson LI (2009) Coordination of spontaneous swallowing with respiratory airflow and diaphragmatic and abdominal muscle activity in healthy adult humans. Exp Physiol 94:459–468

Hårdemark Cedborg AI, Bodén K, Witt Hedström H, Kuylenstierna R, Ekberg O, Eriksson LI, Sundman E (2010) Breathing and swallowing in normal man—effects of changes in body position, bolus types, and respiratory drive. Neurogastroenterol Motil 22:1201–e316

Martin BJ, Logemann JA, Shaker R, Dodds WJ (1994) Coordination between respiration and swallowing: respiratory phase relationships and temporal integration. J Appl Physiol 76:714–723

Martin-Harris B, Brodsky MB, Michel Y, Ford CL, Walters B, Heffner J (2005) Breathing and swallowing dynamics across the adult lifespan. Arch Otolaryngol Head Neck Surg 131:762–770

Martin-Harris B, Brodsky MB, Price CC, Michel Y, Walters B (2003) Temporal coordination of pharyngeal and laryngeal dynamics with breathing during swallowing: single liquid swallows. J Appl Physiol 94:1735–1743

Miller AJ (1999) The neuroscientific principles of swallowing and dysphagia. Singular Publishing Group, San Diego, pp 73–92

Nilsson H, Ekberg O, Bülow M, Hindfelt B (1997) Assessment of respiration during video fluoroscopy of dysphagic patients. Acad Radiol 4:503–507

Nishino T, Hasegawa R, Ide T, Isono S (1998) Hypercapnia enhances the development of coughing during continuous infusion of water into the pharynx. Am J Respir Crit Care Med 157:815–821

Sai T, Isono S, Nishino T (2004) Effects of withdrawal of phasic lung inflation during normocapnia and hypercapnia on the swallowing reflex in humans. J Anesth 18:82–88

Saito Y, Ezure K, Tanaka I (2002) Swallowing-related activities of respiratory and non-respiratory neurons in the nucleus of solitary tract in the rat. J Physiol 540:1047–1060

Terzi N, Orlikowski D, Aegerter P, Lejaille M, Ruquet M, Zalcman G, Fermanian C, Raphael JC, Lofaso F (2007) Breathing–swallowing interaction in neuromuscular patients: a physiological evaluation. Am J Respir Crit Care Med 175:269–276

Timms BJM, DiFiore JM, Martin RJ, Miller MJ (1993) Increased respiratory drive as an inhibitor of oral feeding of preterm infants. J Pediatr 123:127–131

Oral and Pharyngeal Function and Dysfunction

Olle Ekberg

Contents

O. Ekberg (✉)
Diagnostic Centre of Imaging and Functional Medicine,
Skåne University Hospital,
205 02 Malmö, Sweden
e-mail: olle.ekberg@med.lu.se

Abstract

Normal pharyngeal swallow is coordinated in a precise and exact manner. It is controlled from a swallowing centre in the brain stem. Normal swallowing is adjusted to bolus volume temperature and viscosity. Abnormal pharyngeal swallow may lead to misdirected swallowing that challenges the airways. Inefficient transportation into the esophagus, stomach and bowel may lead to dehydration and malnutrition.

1   Introduction

Normal pharyngeal swallow is precisely scheduled and symmetric. It is finely tuned and coordinated in a precise and exact manner to establish a safe swallow (Miller 1986; Dodds 1989). The swallowing process is regulated by a command center in the brainstem, a central program generator which receives input from the cerebral cortex and peripheral muscle and directs the sequence of swallowing. This process is both voluntary and involuntary and incorporates motor activity from the oral cavity, pharynx, and esophagus. It involves both motor and sensory activity. There is an evolving amount of knowledge concerning normal and abnormal swallowing (Jones and Donner 1991; Ekberg and Wahlgren 1985; Hannig and Hannig 1987; Brühlmann 1985; Pokieser et al. 1995; Dodds 1989).

O. Ekberg (ed.), *Dysphagia*, Medical Radiology. Diagnostic Imaging, DOI: 10.1007/174_2011_391,

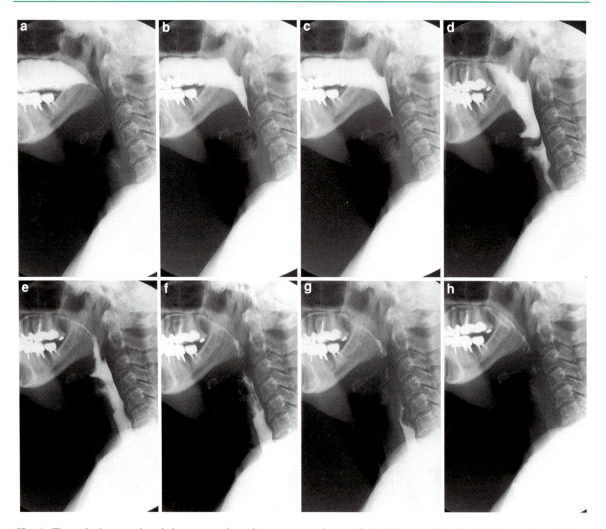

Fig. 1 The oral, pharyngeal, and pharyngoesophageal segment (PES) stages are readily appreciated radiographically. This is a sequence of a barium swallow (**a**–**h**) in lateral projection. The bolus is gathered in the oral cavity (**a**–**c**) and is propelled into the pharynx by an upward and backward movement of the back of the tongue (**d**) (*arrow*). The tilting down to a horizontal position of the epiglottis is seen in **d**. The airways are closed and none of the barium reaches into the laryngeal vestibule or trachea. The PES opens. The upward and forward movements of the larynx including the hyoid superiorly and the PES inferiorly are extremely important for the normal execution of pharyngeal transit. There are no, or only minimal, remnants of barium in the pharynx after swallowing

2 The Normal Swallow

2.1 The Oral Stage

The oral, pharyngeal, pharyngoesophageal segment (PES), and esophageal stages of swallowing are readily appreciated radiographically (Fig. 1). The oral stage of swallowing is bolus-specific, i.e., the patient handles different boluses differently, i.e., a strawberry is handled differently from a cup of tea. Therefore, the oral stage is notoriously more difficult to evaluate radiologically than the rest of the swallowing apparatus. However, the oral stage should be included in the radiologic evaluation. The recording should start with the ingestion. During oral processing there is superior and inferior and some anterior–posterior movement of the hyoid bone. However, liquid barium should not be processed or modified in the oral cavity. Therefore, oral preparation for swallowing is tested with a solid or semisolid bolus. When the ingested material is ready to be swallowed, the material is brought onto the back of the tongue, which obtains the shape of a groove (Hamlet et al. 1988). This is the preparatory position for swallowing.

No part of the bolus is allowed to leak anteriorly from the mouth through the lips. Even more important radiologically is to observe if posterior leak occurs. The patient should be able to control the sealing of the tongue base to the soft palate and posterior pharyngeal wall.

2.2 The Pharyngeal Stage

The pharyngeal swallow is initiated voluntarily and the material to be swallowed is usually called a bolus from this point. Initiation of the pharyngeal swallow coincides with the beginning of the anterior movement of the hyoid bone from an elevated position. Pharyngeal constriction is probably cued by the bolus interfering with sensory innervation at the faucial isthmus. Radiologically it is convenient to use the beginning of the anterior hyoid movement as the starting point of pharyngeal swallow. The tongue then propels the bolus posteriorly into the pharynx and further down into the PES and cervical esophagus. If the pharyngeal constrictor wall has normal compliance, only minor dilatation of the pharynx occurs (Fig. 2).

The palatopharyngeal isthmus is closed by elevation of the muscular palate and constrictor convergence, which is most medial of the lateral walls. Normally, no regurgitation of barium into the nasopharynx occurs.

In a patient with severe oral impairment, the pharyngeal phase may be elicited by injecting a small barium bolus directly into the pharynx through a soft tube. This may be placed into the pharynx via either the mouth or the nose. Such techniques, however, are used only for examination and not for feeding. Patients with uncoordinated, weak, or jerky tongue movements commonly cannot correctly position the bolus on the tongue. Accordingly, the tongue cannot displace the bolus posteriorly. There is a strong correlation between an abnormal anterior movement of the hyoid bone and overall abnormal oral and pharyngeal function, as well as defective opening of the PES.

Protection of the airways occurs at four separable anatomically and functionally different sites, i.e., the vocal folds, the supraglottic portion of the laryngeal vestibule, the subepiglottic portion of the laryngeal vestibule, and the epiglottis (Curtis and Hudson 1983; Curtis and Sepulveda 1983; Ekberg 1982). The most crucial of these levels is the supraglottic portion of the

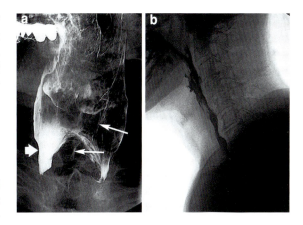

Fig. 2 An 80-year-old man with cerebrovascular disease. There is paresis in the right side of the pharynx. This is not seen in lateral projection (**b**) and is only seen in frontal projection (**a**). There is pooling of contrast medium in the right piriform sinus (*broad arrow*). Small amounts of barium are also seen coating the inside of the laryngeal vestibule down to the false vocal cords

laryngeal vestibule. Barium in the vestibule commonly extends into the trachea, as the vocal folds offer poor protection of the lower airway (Ekberg and Hilderfors 1985). Radiographic observation of barium penetration into the larynx and trachea is strategic in dysphagia evaluation. Bedside evaluation for aspiration has a low sensitivity. This is partly because many of these patients have sensory impairment in the larynx and/or trachea and fail to cough (Splaingard et al. 1988).

Of even more fundamental importance, and basically a prerequisite for airway closure and constrictor activity, is the elevation of the pharynx and larynx. The airways are also protected by a movement of the thyroid cartilage toward the hyoid, and by closure of the laryngeal vestibule. Additional protection is offered by the epiglottis and the vocal folds. Closure of the larynx starts at the vocal folds and progresses in a superior direction in a peristaltic-like manner.

The constrictors have a minor role in the conveyance of a bolus through the pharynx. The tongue base pressure does not differ significantly between those individuals with and those individuals without retention (Olsson et al. 1997). This finding is important because many research groups advocate normal tongue-base and constrictor activity as a prerequisite for a successful outcome of cricopharyngeal myotomy (Buchholz 1995). Tongue-base pressure has been appreciated as the driving force of the bolus, and the tongue base has been associated with a compensatory function, namely, overcoming weak pharyngeal constrictors by increasing tongue-base activity. This tongue driving force propels the bolus and the pharyngeal constrictors stabilize the pharyngeal tube; the tongue then closes the lumen behind the bolus to prevent retrograde escape (McConnel et al. 1988; Cerenko et al. 1989; McConnel 1988).

In patients with pharyngeal retention, the PES does not open as much as in patients without such retention. This reduced opening of the PES is not associated with an increased intrabolus pressure, but is seen together with decreased laryngeal elevation. This is in agreement with a study in which traction on the PES was found to be the main force leading to the PES opening (Hsieh et al. 1995). The suprahyoid muscles are therefore much more important than other muscles in the pharynx. Also, tongue-base pressure, which is reflected by the intrabolus pressure, was the same in patients with and in patients without retention. Thus, pharyngeal shortening could be the most important mechanism in pharyngeal bolus transport (Ergun et al. 1993a, b).

Such intrabolus pressure was shown to be the same for the two groups in this study.

The pharyngeal phase of swallowing is complex because of the intricate anatomic relationships and the close temporal activation of the more than two dozen muscles that are required to function together to effectively transport the bolus from the mouth to the esophagus. In a classic electromyographic study by Doty and Bosma (1956), temporal activation of the muscles of deglutition was shown. Activation begins in the mylohyoid muscle, and the muscle action is then propelled inferiorly. Early events during the pharyngeal phase of swallowing include activation and sealing of the nasopharynx and contraction of the mylohyoid, hyoglossus, and geniohyoid muscles (i.e., the suprahyoid pharyngeal shorteners). A number of other muscles also contract early, namely, those that effect airway protection, such as the intrinsic and extrinsic muscles of the larynx. Contraction of the superior pharyngeal constrictor, styloglossus, palatoglossus, pterygopharyngeal, palatopharyngeal, stylopharyngeal, salpingopharyngeal, stylohyoid, and posterior digastric muscles then occurs. In terms of bolus transportation, this early stage represents the conveyance of the bolus from the oral cavity into the pharynx. This activity is often described as being achieved by the tongue thrust, although a multitude of muscles are involved (McConnel et al. 1988; Cerenko et al. 1989; McConnel 1988). The pharyngeal constrictors give only stability to the gullet—they do not contribute to bolus transportation in other ways (Dodds 1989). In contrast, the late part of the pharyngeal stage consists of contraction of the thyrohyoid, sternohyoid, sternothyroid, and omohyoid muscles (i.e., the strap muscles), and also the middle and inferior pharyngeal constrictors. This latter activity is thought to clear the bolus from the pharynx. The late pharyngeal constrictor activity for clearance of the pharynx is seen as a contracting wave traversing inferiorly from the superior pharyngeal constrictor level. This wave is usually best appreciated on the anteroposterior view as an inverted V-shape to the tail of liquid or semisolid bolus (Dodds 1989). It is impairment of such clearance that is recognized as retention in the valleculae, piriform sinus, or both.

The exact reason why laryngeal elevation leads to retention in patients with manometrically normal pharyngeal constrictor activity is not clear. It is possible that reduced elevation is caused by impaired function of the suprahyoid muscles and other elevators. Such impaired function might lead to abnormal compliance of the wall, against which the constrictors may then act. As retention was not seen in a location immediately cranial to the cricopharyngeal muscle, it is more likely that a defective opening reflects a more profound and widespread dysfunction in the pharynx. Defective opening may be the sole result of impaired elevation of the pharynx.

2.3   The Pharyngoesophageal Segment

The PES is the transition between the pharynx and the esophagus. Between swallows it is kept closed as a sphincter of circular striated muscles. Anatomically it consists of the cricopharyngeal muscle and the inferior portion of the pharyngeal constrictors and the superior portion of the cervical esophagus. The length of the segment is about 3–4 cm, where the cricopharyngeal muscle makes up 1–1.5 cm. Closure is the effect of muscle tonicity and the pressure from surrounding tissues (Kahrilas et al. 1988). Normal opening, which is crucial for bolus transport, is achieved by relaxation of muscle tone. However, this probably only accounts for 10–20% of the total sphincter tone. More important is the movement of the PES superiorly and anteriorly together with the larynx and the hyoid bone. In addition, intrabolus pressure created mainly by the tongue-base and constrictor activity also helps to open the PES.

2.4   The Esophageal Stage

This is comprehensively presented in Sect. 5.1.

3   The Abnormal Swallow

In terms of what abnormalities can be expected on the four different anatomic levels, a rule of thumb is that dysfunction is by far the principal abnormality in the oral cavity and pharynx. In the PES, dysfunction and structural abnormalities may coexist. In the esophagus, structural abnormalities predominate.

3.1   The Oral Stage

Leaking of barium anteriorly through the lips, laterally into the buccal pouches, or posteriorly into the pharynx is abnormal. An overly large ingestion in a patient with impaired pharyngeal function and misdirected swallowing is also abnormal. This may indicate impairment of bolus sizing. Impaired lingual movement or jerky uncoordinated movements of the tongue during the preparatory phase of swallowing are also abnormal.

In patients with neurologic diseases, oral dysfunction regularly predominates over pharyngeal dysfunction. Radiographically, this can be appreciated as defective containment, i.e., leakage of barium anteriorly through the lips, laterally into the buccal pouches, or posteriorly into the pharynx, where it potentially may reach the airways if the laryngeal vestibule is not closed. If the patient swallows an abnormally large bolus, this may indicate impairment of bolus sizing. Abnormalities in the oral phase of swallowing, i.e., impaired lingual movement or a soft tissue defect, generally lead to delayed oral transit and clearance of the oral bolus with retention of barium. Premature spill of barium into the pharynx may be accompanied by

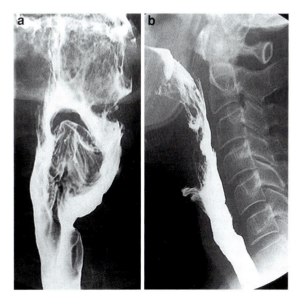

Fig. 3 A 49-year-old man with sudden onset of dysphagia. There is a left-sided weakness of the pharynx. The left side of the pharynx bulges laterally. There is also abnormal opening of the PES, probably due to impaired constrictor strength cranially. The pharyngeal constrictor abnormality is not appreciated in the lateral projection (**a**) and is only appreciated in the frontal projection (**b**)

failed initiation of swallowing, aspiration, or both. Impaired oral function is often associated with abnormal pharyngeal swallow (Fig. 3). Normally, the oral phase of swallowing undergoes a smooth transition into the pharyngeal phase with vigorous transport of the swallowed bolus into and through the pharynx. In some patients, however, the pharyngeal phase is delayed but otherwise normal.

3.2   The Pharyngeal Stage

Abnormal initiation of the pharyngeal stage of swallowing is easily appreciated when the bolus is conveyed into the pharynx without the pharynx being elevated and without occurrence of constrictor activity. Again, lack of anterior displacement of the hyoid bone is a conspicuous indicator of a serious abnormality. Demonstration of dissociation between the oral and pharyngeal stages depends upon observation of structural displacement. Except for this failure of voluntary elicitation of pharyngeal swallow, the oral as well as the pharyngeal stages of swallowing basically appear radiologically normal. In borderline cases, in which the bolus is retained in the valleculae or in the piriform sinuses for 2–5 s, the assessment of normalcy is based upon observation of the bolus.

The ultimate consequences of this dissociation is that the bolus reaches the pharynx when the larynx is still open. Even if the barium does not penetrate into the larynx, the delayed initiation is a potential threat to safe swallowing. Even the slightest amount of barium in the vestibule indicates an abnormality (Fig. 4). The wide range of normalcy can be observed during chewing and swallowing of a mixture of solids and liquid, especially during talking etc. when the barium and/or solids are brought into the pharynx while chewing continues without tongue propulsion being elicited. Again, what happens to the bolus is more important than observing wall displacement in this circumstance. It is even more important to recognize that if pharyngeal swallow is not triggered at the faucial isthmus either by the bolus or by the tongue, swallowing may be elicited from the vallecula or from the posterior pharyngeal wall.

Defective closure of the velopharynx is due to either soft palate dysfunction or defective function in the superior pharyngeal constrictor. Medial movement of the lateral wall is more extensive than the anterior movement of the posterior constrictor wall. Compensation may be in the form of a Passavant's ridge, a protrusion similar to that seen as a compensatory maneuver in speech in individuals with a cleft palate.

The pharyngeal constrictors play a crucial role in swallowing (Ardran and Kemp 1956). If the constrictor muscles are paretic, the pharynx is flaccid and allows an abnormal expansion of the chamber during the compression phase of swallowing (Figs. 3, 4). Such lack of distensibility may result in impaired transit of bolus from the oral cavity into the esophagus even if the tongue acts normally (Thulin and Welin 1954; Ekberg et al. 1986). This can be seen as a dilated and wide flaccid pharynx, but this is a nonspecific finding. Action of the pharyngeal constrictors is also crucial for clearing barium from the pharynx. However, there are pitfalls (Fig. 5). This constrictor activity is best evaluated in the posteroanterior view (Fig. 2). The consequence of defective constrictor activity is residual barium in the pharynx after swallowing. As the middle pharyngeal constrictor is the pharyngeal constrictor most commonly involved, retention occurs at the level of the laryngeal inlet and may lead to aspiration after swallowing.

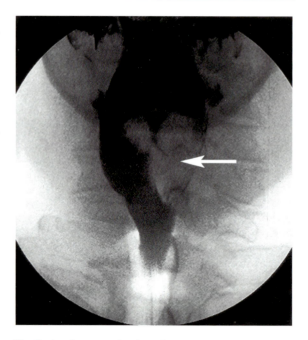

Fig. 4 Another example of a unilateral pharyngeal constrictor paresis, this time on the right side. The deviation of contrast medium into the right side may erroneously give the impression of a tumor on the normal left side (*arrow*). This pseudotumor appearance has led to numerous unnecessary endoscopic examinations

In the pharynx, retention of contrast medium may occur and indicate abnormalities in the tongue-base and/or in the pharyngeal constrictors. The finding of any contrast medium that reaches into the laryngeal vestibule and trachea is abnormal (Figs. 1, 2, 3). This is especially true if the patient does not cough during this event. This indicates desensitization and is seen in patients with impairment lasting for more than about 2 months. Defective tilting down of the epiglottis is also abnormal and is generally seen together with impaired movement of the hyoid bone and larynx. More fundamental abnormalities are impaired elevation of the larynx and pharynx together with the hyoid bone at the initiation of pharyngeal swallow. This is seen in patients who do not elicit the pharyngeal stage of swallowing. We have used the beginning of the anterior movement of the hyoid bone as a key event. During the preparatory stage the hyoid bone and larynx are moving up and down, but at the initiation of the pharyngeal swallow the hyoid bone starts to move anteriorly (from an elevated position). If that movement is missing, the patient does not elicit pharyngeal swallow and is thereby at great risk if fed orally.

Fig. 5 **a**, **b** Barium swallow, single-contrast full column films. **c**, **d** Double-contrast films. In this 30-year-old woman there are extremely large tonsils (*arrow*). This finding was seen in both frontal and lateral projection. They may simulate normal or exaggerated function in the constrictor musculature, but they are in fact caused by a morphologic abnormality. Such hypertrophic tonsils may cause dysphagia

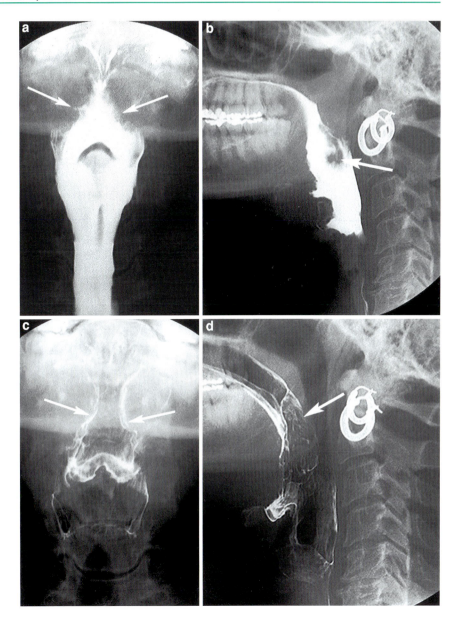

3.2.1 Misdirected Swallowing

Confusion exists regarding the terminology confined to barium reaching into the airways. "Penetration" has been used either to describe barium reaching into the airways *during* swallowing or merely to describe barium reaching only into the laryngeal vestibule and not beyond the vocal folds. "Aspiration" has been used either to describe barium reaching into the airways *after* swallowing and usually due to residue in the pharynx or to describe barium reaching beyond the vocal folds. Different use of the terminology has created unnecessary confusion. It is much more rational to describe

(1) when the barium reaches into the airways, namely, *before*, *during*, or *after* elicitation of pharyngeal swallow, and (2) how far into the airways the barium reaches, namely, *into the subepiglottic, supraglottic portion* of the laryngeal vestibule or *beyond the vocal folds*. There is no consensus regarding the terminology and therefore it is warranted to be precise as the implicit meaning of "penetration" and "aspiration" is not widely accepted.

Of crucial importance is the coordination between the oral and pharyngeal stages of swallowing. The most common cause of misdirected swallowing is

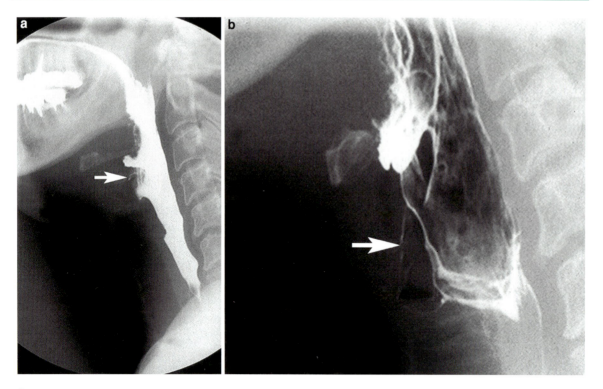

Fig. 6 This patient complained of an occasional sensation of having a foreign body in the neck. She pointed to the lateral part of her neck. Several swallows were normal. However, small amounts of barium eventually reached into the laryngeal vestibule. This was due to a slight dissociation (1.7 s) between the oral and pharyngeal stages of swallowing. This was enough to cause misdirected swallowing into the laryngeal vestibule. The patient then indicated that she had the foreign body sensation in the neck. This was seen both on single-contrast full column films (**a**) (*arrow*) and on double-contrast films (**b**) (*arrow*)

dissociation between the oral and pharyngeal stages of swallowing. This means that those two compartments are acting normally but the synchronization between them is impaired. The oral stage includes propulsion of the bolus into the pharynx. The pharyngeal stage of swallowing includes elevation of the hyoid bone, the larynx, and the pharynx. It is crucial to observe a conspicuous anterior movement of the hyoid bone as this is an indicator of elicitation of pharyngeal swallow. Any patient who does not show such hyoid bone movement potentially has a severe pharyngeal dysfunction. There should also be an approximation between the larynx and the hyoid bone due to contraction of the thyrohyoid muscles. In normal individuals the timing of the oral and pharyngeal stages is tightly coordinated and there is usually a time lag of not more than 0.5 s between when the apex of the bolus passes the faucial isthmus and start of the anterior movement of the hyoid bone. In patients with such a tight coordination, misdirected swallowing is seldom seen. However, the longer the

delay, the more likely misdirected swallowing is to occur. Such incoordination between the oral and pharyngeal stages of swallowing is particularly common in the elderly. It is often the sole cause of misdirected swallowing (Fig. 6).

Airway closure and constrictor activity are both important elements of swallowing. Absence of elevation of the pharynx and larynx as well as failure of anterior movement of the hyoid bone are crucial elements of abnormal function. These are seen not only in the neurologically impaired patient but also after extensive surgery and/or radiotherapy. During barium swallow, the quality of the cough reflex is readily appreciated and can be defined as to the level where it is elicited, as well as roughly how much and for how long the barium must be in contact with the laryngeal and/or tracheal mucosa. However, for proper quantification of misdirected swallowing to the trachea, scintigraphy is more accurate than barium swallow (Muz et al. 1987).

Discovery of misdirection of the barium into the larynx and/or trachea should not lead to the interruption of the study. On the other hand, there are patients with massive penetration into the trachea in whom a very limited study is sufficient for answering the clinician's immediate questions concerning possible oral feeding. It is important to elucidate the underlying pathophysiologic processes in these patients and a few swallows should be observed in lateral projection. However, the risk of acquiring bronchopneumonia secondary to misdirected bolus is probably much less than many would expect (Ekberg and Hilderfors 1985).

According to Kun et al. (1987), elderly patients have misdirected swallowing due to dysfunction in the oral stage or a combination of oral and pharyngeal stage dysfunction. Oral stage dysfunction was due to ingestion of a large volume or rapid acquisition. However, dissociation between the oral and pharyngeal stages was the main finding. It has been shown that thermal stimulation of the faucial isthmus reduces such a dissociation (Logemann 1983; Logemann and Kahrilas 1990). For many years such tactile and thermal stimulation of the faucial isthmus has been a widely used technique for treatment of these patients.

Misdirected swallowing has been considered a major cause of aspiration pneumonia. If major aspiration occurs during barium swallow, it is common for the patient to be fed nonorally. The rationale for such treatment has been questioned (Siebens and Linden 1985). It was shown that patients who were fed nonorally showed more frequent aspiration pneumonia than those who were fed orally. Their explanation was that saliva contaminated with bacteria in the oral cavity caused the pneumonia. The oral hygiene in these patients is usually low. It was concluded that artificial feeding does not seem to be a satisfactory solution for preventing pneumonia in elderly patients with prandial aspiration.

Patients who have defective protection of the airways during swallowing are also at risk of fatal choking episodes. Prandial aspiration most often results in reflexive coughing, gagging, and forced exploration. This is often referred to by the patient as "choking." It is usually uncomfortable but brief and usually familiar in nature to the patient. This is in contrast to airway obstruction during oral intake, which may be fatal unless the occluding material is removed or displaced. Such food asphyxia is an important cause of accidental death in children (Editorial 1981; Lima 1989). It is estimated that 8,000–10,000 adults choke to death each year (Donner and Jones 1985). The development of the Heimlich maneuver and its inclusion as part of basic cardiopulmonary resuscitation training has increased public awareness of the problem in the USA (Heimlich 1985). The cause of near-fatal choking episodes has been studied in 58 individuals (Feinberg and Ekberg 1990). Most of these patients who had survived a Heimlich maneuver applied because of food impaction showed abnormalities during the barium swallow. Most of them aspirated liquid bolus. This was due to bolus leak or dissociation. Some patients also showed defective closure of the laryngeal vestibule. However, a subset of patients (14 of 58) were able to vocalize during the near-fatal choking episode and they demonstrated structural abnormalities of the PES and the esophagus. Therefore, patients who have had a near-fatal choking episode should undergo an elective radiologic barium study in order to reveal an underlying cause and prevent new episodes that may otherwise prove to be fatal.

4 Dysfunction of the Pharyngoesophageal Segment

Defective opening of the PES is a common finding. This may be seen as a posterior indentation of the cricopharyngeal muscle. However, it has been shown that the indentation per se does not impinge on the lumen diameter (Olsson and Ekberg 1995). In fact, the diameter of the PES at the level of the cricopharyngeal muscle is the same in patients with and without that posterior cricopharyngeal bar. Instead the pharynx is dilated above and the cervical esophagus is dilated below the cricopharyngeal bar, thereby giving the false impression of lumen narrowing. Manometrically, the cricopharyngeal muscle in these patients has been shown to act normally, and there are decreased peak amplitudes in the pharynx above. There is also a small subset of patients who have fibrosis of the PES and the cricopharyngeal muscle, but this is rare. Most patients who appear to have an abnormal opening of the PES do have normal morphology and function in that particular segment, and the impairment in fact is defective elevation of the PES and weakness of the pharyngeal constrictors (Olsson and Ekberg 1995). The most common cause of this, in turn, is lack of initiation of the pharyngeal stage of swallowing. Therefore, any surgical

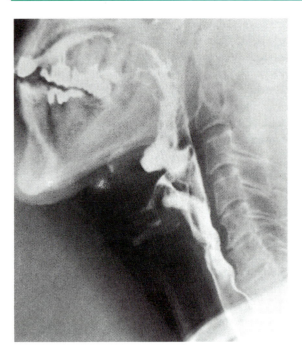

Fig. 7 A 76-year-old woman 2 weeks after a stroke. Lateral radiogram of the pharynx during swallowing. Contrast medium has reached into the pharynx, through the PES, and into the cervical esophagus. The epiglottis is in a horizontal position. The hyoid bone is elevated and brought slightly forward. However, contrast medium has reached into the laryngeal vestibule to the level of the sinus of Morgagni. No contrast medium is seen in the trachea. The patient did not subjectively experience this misdirected swallowing. There was no cough. This indicates chronic aspiration (see also Fig. 8)

procedure on the PES is not likely to be beneficial, the main reason being that only a small fraction of the closure of the PES is due to muscle tonicity.

Failure of the PES to open may be seen in neurologic disease but is generally not accompanied by abnormal pharyngeal bolus transport (Curtis et al. 1984; Ekberg 1986a). Failure of the cricopharyngeal muscle to open or elongate may be due to (1) defective muscle relaxation, (2) defective extensibility, and (3) hypertrophy or hyperplasia. The posterior bar intruding into the barium and created by the cricopharyngeal muscle is seldom an isolated dysfunction. It is commonly associated with abnormal motor function in the segment above (i.e., the inferior pharyngeal constrictor) and/or in the segment below (i.e., the cervical esophageal muscles). Therefore, the cricopharyngeal indentation, though the most conspicuous, is only one aspect of severe motor

dysfunction in the adjacent PES (Ekberg 1986a). Cervical esophageal webs are also common in dysphagic patients (Figs. 5, 7).

Adapted and compensated swallowing basically have the same radiologic appearance and, in most patients, they are notoriously difficult to demonstrate. Therefore, a normal radiologic study does not rule out pharyngeal abnormality.

5   Radiologic Evaluation in Specific Disease Entities

Radiologic evaluation of oral and pharyngeal function during swallowing has a high sensitivity but is non-specific in terms of the type and extent of the underlying abnormality (Figs. 7, 8, 9). Specific disease is seen to cause pharyngeal dysfunction and dysphagia with varying frequency and the cause of dysphagia during the disease varies. This has been studied radiologically in cerebrovascular disease (Veis and Logemann 1985; Donner and Silbiger 1966), poliomyelitis (Silbiger et al. 1967; Ardran et al. 1957), amyotrophic lateral sclerosis (Bosma and Brodie 1969a), myasthenia gravis (Murray 1962), myotonic dystrophy (Bosma and Brodie 1969b), Parkinson's disease (Calne et al. 1970; Robbins et al. 1986), brainstem tumor (Kun et al. 1987), and multiple sclerosis (Daly et al. 1962). Even the distinction between upper and lower motor neuron disease, e.g., cortical bulbar tract dysfunction (pseudobulbar palsy), and lower motor neuron disease, i.e., pontomedullary dysfunction (bulbar palsy), is ambiguous. However, the latter patients usually have more widespread pharyngeal paresis and they also lack initiation of pharyngeal swallow. Basically, all neurologic impairments lead to the same dysfunction. This is especially so for the "end-stage" dysfunction, which tends to lead all types of disease entities down a common pathway with impaired elevation of the larynx and pharynx and impaired anterior movement of the hyoid bone.

The cause of dysphagia in terms of symptoms and functions often does not match. Deterioration or progression of dysphagia is as a rule compensated. So, if we could decompensate swallowing, this would reveal progression. The radiologist may intentionally elicit the decompensation by extension of the neck by provision of a large bolus and other stresses (Ekberg 1986b; Buchholz et al. 1985).

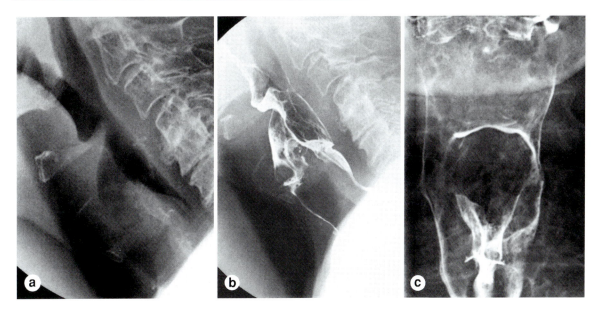

Fig. 8 A 74-year-old man who had undergone radiotherapy to the neck for laryngeal carcinoma 3 years previously. There was no sign of recurrence but the patient now had difficultly swallowing. He had sustained several choking episodes. **a** Lateral radiogram of the pharynx. There is thickening of the prevertebral soft tissue and of the epiglottis. **b** After barium swallow, there is contrast medium in the laryngeal vestibule and in the trachea, but only minor retention in the piriform sinuses. **c** Anteroposterior view of the pharynx. There is minor retention in the effaced valleculae and shallow piriform sinuses. Contrast medium is also seen in the laryngeal vestibule and sinus of Morgagni (see also Fig. 7)

5.1   Cerebrovascular Diseases

Most patients with pharyngeal dysfunction are patients who suffer from stroke. The prevalence of stroke in the USA has been estimated to be approximately 1.6 million persons, with 250,000 new cases of stroke each year. Of these stroke patients, 30–50% will develop dysphagia. Strokes that are multiple (Veis and Logemann 1985; Rosenbek et al. 1991; Horner et al. 1991; Splainard et al. 1988), bilateral (Logemann 1983), or localized in the brainstem (Veis and Logemann 1985; Horner et al. 1991; Logemann and Kahrilas 1990; Linden and Siebens 1983) are considered to cause severe swallowing impairment. However, even unilateral cortical or subcortical strokes (Veis and Logemann 1985; Robbins and Levine 1988; Robbins et al. 1993; Gordon et al. 1987; Meadows 1973) can cause swallowing problems. Dysphagia in the stroke population may last for weeks or months, but occasionally much longer. Although dysphagia is a subjective symptom, dysfunction of the pharyngeal stage of swallowing can be objectively registered using barium swallow and video recording. This technique is now the gold standard for evaluation of normal and abnormal swallowing.

Oropharyngeal impairment is recognized as a frequent cause of morbidity, disability, and costly dependence in stroke patients (Veis and Logemann 1985). Bolus misdirection into the larynx and trachea is perhaps the most significant abnormality that we routinely observe during barium swallow. Especially in the elderly, swallowing dysfunction is prevalent, particularly in those who are hospitalized, institutionalized, or well advanced in years. These patients represent some of the most challenging cases that clinicians must deal with on a routine basis. The diagnosis is difficult and so is management. However, this is not because of unique abnormalities in swallowing behavior or morphodynamics, but is because of the patients themselves (Veis and Logemann 1985). In fact, swallowing problems may go undetected in these patients because the signs and symptoms are vague, subtle, or unreported by the patients' caregivers. Critical management decisions regarding dietary alterations, degree of oral intake, and institution of artificial feeding often depend on the radiologic assessment of such misdirected swallowing.

Radiologists are important members of multidisciplinary teams that address swallowing disorders.

Fig. 9 A 65-year-old woman with no prior history of stroke. She had developed dysphagia 2 years previously. The dysphagia progressed over a couple of weeks. She had difficulty with all kinds of textures and had a very prolonged eating time. **a** The contrast medium is brought into the pharynx. **b** Pronounced dilatation of the pharynx indicating high compliance secondary to weakness of pharyngeal constrictor musculature. **c** Eventually contrast medium reached into the laryngeal vestibule but not further down into the airways. **d** Only very tiny streaks of barium reach through the PES during each swallowing attempt. There was minor anterior movement of the hyoid bone that could indicate that pharyngeal swallow had been elicited. However, there was no constrictor activity. The patient spontaneously learned to compensate for the absence of contractility in the constrictors. (From Ekberg and Olsson 1997)

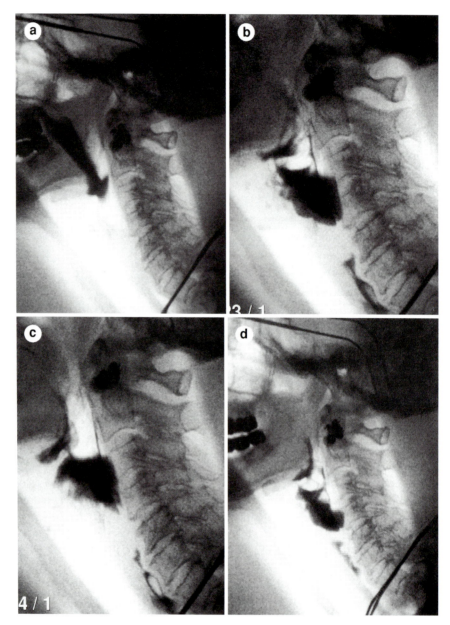

Diagnosis and treatment of dysphagia depend on videofluorographic deglutition examinations during barium swallow. Patients with cerebrovascular disease, Parkinson's disease, and other neurologic conditions, including elderly patients with dementia, need to undergo videofluorographic examination in order to correctly describe functional status and thereby provide a platform for rational therapy. Treatment strategies must be founded on objective grounds (see Sect. 5).

6   The Role of the Radiologist in the Design of Therapy

Treatment of oral and pharyngeal dysfunction strives to correct or compensate for damage to specific neuro-muscular components of the oral and pharyngeal swallow, such as reduced tongue movement, delay in triggering the pharyngeal swallow, pharyngeal constrictor paralysis, and defective closure of the laryngeal vestibule. For evaluation of such therapy, successive radiologic evaluations are necessary (see Sect. 5). The radiologic examination must (1) reveal the anatomic and/or physiologic abnormalities causing the patient's dysphagia, and (2) identify those compensatory strategies or therapy techniques which are most effective in improving the efficiency of the patient's oral and pharyngeal swallow. The radiologic examination should start with ingestion and include also the passage of the bolus into the stomach. Following liquid swallows, the patient should be given other food consistencies, particularly pudding consistency materials and food requiring chewing, such as cookies. A variety of foods mixed with barium can be introduced in the radiologic study. The volume of each food or liquid should be measured because the dynamics of normal pharyngeal swallow vary as the volume of the bolus increases.

Two types of therapy techniques are used for reeducation for oral and pharyngeal dysphagia: (1) "direct" swallowing therapy procedures which passively facilitate swallowing by use of particular foods and liquids; and (2) "indirect" therapy techniques designed to compensate for dysfunction by increasing muscle strength, range of motion, or coordination independent of swallowing. The effectiveness of either of these techniques is assessed by observing the transport of the swallowed bolus during radiography.

References

Ardran GM, Kemp FM (1956) Radiologic investigation of pharyngeal and laryngeal palsy. Acta Radiol Diagn 46:446–457

Ardran GM, Kemp FM, Wegelius C (1957) Swallowing defects after poliomyelitis. Br J Radiol 30:169–189

Bosma JF, Brodie DR (1969a) Disabilities of the pharynx in amyotrophic lateral sclerosis as demonstrated by cineradiography. Radiology 92:97–103

Bosma JF, Brodie DR (1969b) Cineradiographic demonstration of pharyngeal area myotonia in myotonic dystrophy patients. Radiology 92:104–109

Brühlmann WF (1985) Die röntgenkinematographische Untersuchung von Störungen des Schluckaktes. Huber, Bern

Buchholz DW (1995) Cricopharyngeal myotomy may be effective treatment for selected patients with neurogenic oropharyngeal dysphagia. Dysphagia 10:255–258

Buchholz DW, Bosma JF, Donner MW (1985) Adaptation, compensation, and decompensation of the pharyngeal swallow. Gastrointest Radiol 10:235–239

Calne DB, Shaw DG, Spiers AS, Stern GM (1970) Swallowing in parkinsonism. Br J Radiol 43:456–457

Cerenko D, McConnel FMS, Jackson RT (1989) Quantitative assessment of pharyngeal bolus driving forces. Otolaryngol Head Neck Surg 100:57–63

Curtis DJ, Hudson T (1983) Laryngotracheal aspiration: analysis of specific neurmuscular factors. Radiology 149:517–522

Curtis DJ, Sepulveda GV (1983) Epiglottic motion: video recording of muscular dysfunction. Radiology 148:473–477

Curtis DJ, Cruess DF, Berg T (1984) The cricopharyngeal muscle. A video-recording. Am J Roentgenol 146:497–500

Daly DD, Code CF, Andersson HA (1962) Disturbances of swallowing and esophageal motility in patients with multiple sclerosis. Neurology 59:250–256

Dodds WJ (1989) The physiology of swallowing. Dysphagia 3:171–178

Donner MW, Jones B (1985) Editorial. Gastrointest Radiol 10:194–195

Donner MW, Silbiger ML (1966) Cinefluorographic analysis of pharyngeal swallowing in neuromuscular disorders. Am J Med Sci 251:600–616

Doty RW, Bosma JB (1956) An electromyographic analysis of reflux deglutition. J Neurophysiol 19:44–60

Editorial (1981) Inhaled foreign bodies. Br Med J 282: 1649–1650

Ekberg O (1982) Defective closure of the laryngeal vestibule during deglutition. Acta Otolaryngol 93:309–317

Ekberg O (1986a) The cricopharyngeus revisited. Br J Radiol 59:875–879

Ekberg O (1986b) Posture of the head and pharyngeal swallow. Acta Radiol Diagn 27:691–696

Ekberg O, Hilderfors H (1985) Defective closure of the laryngeal vestibule: frequency of pulmonary complications. Am J Roentgenol 145:1159–1164

Ekberg O, Olsson R (1997) Operative techniques in otolaryngology. Head Neck Surg 8:153–162

Ekberg O, Wahlgren L (1985) Dysfunction of pharyngeal swallowing: a cineradiographic investigation in 854 dysphagial patients. Acta Radiol Diagn 26:389–395

Ekberg O, Lindgren S, Schultz T (1986) Pharyngeal swallowing in patients with paresis of the recurrent nerve. Acta Radiol Diagn 27:697–700

Ergun GA, Kahrilas PJ, Lin S, Logemann JA, Harig JM (1993a) Shape, volume, and content of the deglutitive pharyngeal chamber imaged by ultrafast computerized tomography. Gastroenterology 105:1396–1403

Ergun GA, Kahrilas PJ, Logemann JA (1993b) Interpretation of pharyngeal manometric recordings: limitations and variability. Dis Esophagus 6:11–16

Feinberg MJ, Ekberg O (1990) Deglutition in near fatal choking episodes: radiologic evaluation. Radiology 176:637–640

Gordon C, Hewer RL, Wade DT (1987) Dysphagia in acute stroke. Br Med J 295:411–414

Hamlet SL, Stone M, Shawker TH (1988) Posterior tongue grooving in deglutition and speech: preliminary observations. Dysphagia 3:65–68

Hannig C, Hannig A (1987) Stellenwert der Hochfrequenzröntgenkinematographie in der Diagnostik des Pharynx und Ösophagus. Röntgenpraxis 40:358–377

Heimlich JH (1985) A life-saving maneuver to prevent food choking. JAMA 234:398–401

Horner J, Bouyer FG, Alberts MJ, Helms MJ (1991) Dysphagia following brain-stem stroke: clinical correlates and outcome. Arch Neurol 48:1170–1173

Hsieh PY, Brasseur JG, Shaker R, Kern MK, Kahrilas PJ, Ren J (1995) Modeling and timing of UES opening events. Paper presented at the Dysphagia Research Society meeting, Tysons Corner, 26–28 October 1995

Jones B, Donner MW (1991) Normal and abnormal swallowing, imaging in diagnosis and therapy. Springer, Berlin

Kahrilas PJ, Dodds WJ, Dent J, Logemann JA, Shaker R (1988) Upper esophageal sphincter function during deglutition. Gastroenterology 95:52–62

Kun WS, Buchholz D, Kuman AJ, Donner MW, Rosenbaum AE (1987) Magnetic resonance imaging for evaluating neurogenic dysphagia. Dysphagia 2:40–45

Lima JH (1989) Laryngeal foreign bodies in children: a persistent, life-threatening problem. Laryngoscope 99: 415–420

Linden P, Siebens A (1983) Dysphagia: predicting laryngeal penetration. Arch Phys Med Rehab 69:637–640

Logemann JA (1983) Evaluation and treatment of swallowing disorders. College-Hill Press, San Diego

Logemann JA, Kahrilas PJ (1990) Relearning to swallow after stroke-application of maneuvers and indirect biofeedback: a case study. Neurology 40:1136–1138

McConnel FMC (1988) Analysis of pressure generation and bolus transit during pharyngeal swallowing. Laryngoscope 98:71–78

McConnel FMS, Cerenko D, Jackson RT, Guffin TN Jr (1988) Timing of major events of pharyngeal swallowing. Arch Otolaryngol Head Neck Surg 114:1413–1418

Meadows JC (1973) Dysphagia in unilateral cerebral lesions. J Neurol Neurosurg Phychiatry 36:853–860

Miller AJ (1986) Neurophysiological basis of swallowing. Dysphagia 1:91–100

Murray JF (1962) Deglutition in myasthenia gravis. Br J Radiol 35:43–52

Muz J, Mathog RM, Miller PR, Rosen R, Borrero G (1987) Detection and quantification of laryngotracheopulmonary aspiration with scintigraphy. Laryngoscope 97:1180–1185

Olsson R, Ekberg O (1995) Videomanometry of the pharynx in dysphagic patients with a posterior cricopharyngeal indentation. Acad Radiol 2:597–601

Olsson R, Castell J, Johnston B, Ekberg O, Castell DO (1997) Combined videomanometric identification of abnormalities related to pharyngeal retention. Acad Radiol 4:349–354

Pokieser P, Schober W, Schima W (1995) Videokinematographie des Schluckaktes–Indikation, Methodik und Befundung. Radiologe 35:703–711

Robbins J, Levine RL (1988) Swallowing after unilateral stroke of the cerebral cortex: preliminary experience. Dysphagia 3:11–17

Robbins JA, Logemann JA, Kirshner HS (1986) Swallowing and speech production in Parkinson's disease. Ann Neurol 19:283–287

Robbins J, Levine RL, Maser A, Rosenbek JC, Kempster GB (1993) Swallowing after unilateral stroke of the cerebral cortex. Arch Phys Med Rehab 74:1295–1300

Rosenbek JC, Robbins J, Fishback B, Levine RL (1991) The effects of thermal application on dysphagia after stroke. J Speech Hear Res 34:1257–1268

Siebens AA, Linden P (1985) Dynamic imaging for swallowing re-education. Gastrointest Radiol 10:251–253

Silbiger M, Pikielney R, Donner MW (1967) Neuromuscular disorders affecting the pharynx. Invest Radiol 2:442–448

Splainard ML, Hutchins B, Sulton LD, Chaudhuri G (1988) Aspiration in rehabilitation patients: videofluoroscopic versus bedside clinical assessment. Arch Phys Med Rehab 69:637–640

Thulin A, Welin S (1954) Radiographic findings in unilateral hypopharyngeal paralysis. Acta Otolaryngol Suppl 116: 288–293

Veis SL, Logemann JA (1985) Swallowing disorders in persons with cerebrovascular accident. Arch Phys Med Rehabil 66:372–375

Part II

Clinical Evaluation

Evaluation of Symptoms

Doris-Maria Denk-Linnert

Contents

Abstract

Symptoms of pharyngeal/esophageal diseases are mainly related to swallowing function, e.g., dysphagia, aspiration, globus sensation or heartburn. Dysphagia and aspiration may lead to malnutrition, potentially life-threatening pulmonary complications (e.g., aspiration pneumonia) and impairment of life-quality. The most important dysphagia related symptom is aspiration. Other components of dysphagia are drooling, leaking, delayed triggering of the swallowing reflex, retentions, nasal penetration or pharyngeal regurgitation. The etiologies of oropharyngeal dysphagia may be divided into three groups: diseases of the upper aerodigestive tract, neurological diseases and psychogenic disorders. Possible hints to suspect dysphagia and aspiration are indirect and direct symptoms. They necessitate an interdisciplinary diagnostic work-up for revealing etiology and pathophysiology. For the proof or exclusion of aspiration its direct visualization by videoendoscopy and videofluoroscopy remains indispensable and cannot be replaced by screening procedures.

1 Introduction

Symptoms of pharyngeal/esophageal diseases are related to swallowing function, such as dysphagia, odynophagia, globus sensation or heartburn. Patients often do not differentiate between these symptoms and report "swallowing problems." The crossing of airway and digestive tract in the hypopharynx is a critical region for swallowing and respiration: if protection of

D.-M. Denk-Linnert (✉)
Department of Otorhinolaryngology,
Section of Phoniatrics, Medical University of Vienna,
Vienna Medical School, Währinger Gürtel 18–20,
1090 Vienna, Austria
e-mail: doris-maria.denk-linnert@meduniwien.ac.at

the airway during swallowing is not secured, aspiration occurs. Moreover, the pharynx is not only part of the upper digestive tract, but also of the vocal tract and therefore influences resonance and articulation.

Swallowing is one of the most frequent activities of the human body: the human being swallows between 580–2,000 times a day (Garliner 1974; Logemann 1983, 1998). However, swallowing is not only a vital primary function to ensure adequate nutrition and hydration, but also decisively contributes to quality of life and social integration. Dysphagia may lead to malnutrition and, in the case of aspiration, to potentially life-threatening pulmonary complications such as aspiration pneumonia. Furthermore, life-quality of dysphagic patients is impaired (Ekberg et al. 2002). Dysphagia represents a frequent and severe medical problem. It's prevalence is higher among the elderly and is often associated with dementia. For life expectancy, nutritional status, independent oral feeding and prevention of aspiration-related pulmonary complications is of utmost prognostic relevance. In acute-care hospitals, 13–14 % of patients are believed to suffer from dysphagia; in nursing homes, the percentage of dysphagic patients reaches 50 % (Logemann 1995). Moreover, among patients over age 65, aspiration pneumonia is the fourth most frequent cause of death (Sasaki 1991). Every year, about 50,000 Americans die from pulmonary complications of aspiration (Jones and Donner 1991). Therefore, in modern, function-orientated medicine, the management of the dysphagic patient has become of great clinical importance and a focus of scientific interest.

Dysphagia and other swallowing complaints necessitate a thorough diagnostic procedure. Only the knowledge of the underlying cause and of the individual swallowing pathophysiology enable appropriate treatment of the patient.

2   Terminology of Dysphagia

The symptom *dysphagia* is defined as a disturbance of the intake or transport of food from the mouth to the stomach. Furthermore, it includes behavioral, sensory and motor disorders in preparation for the swallow, e.g., disorders of cognitive awareness, visual and olfactory recognition of food, and the physiologic responses to the smell and presence of food (Leopold and Kagel 1996). In the case of *oropharyngeal*

dysphagia, the oral preparatory, oral and/or pharyngeal phases of swallowing are afflicted. If the esophageal phase is disturbed, *esophageal dysphagia* is present. Both types of dysphagia may influence the other; therefore, dysphagia makes the comprehensive evaluation of the aerodigestive tract from the oral cavity to the stomach necessary.

2.1   Components of the Impaired Swallow

To address the pathophysiological aspects, dysphagia has to be regarded as a syndrome. The most important dysphagia-related symptom is *aspiration*, which is defined as the entry of saliva, food or gastric secretion into the airway under the level of the vocal folds. Other components of dysphagia are drooling, leaking, nasal penetration, laryngeal penetration, retention, or pharyngeal regurgitation. The swallowing pathophysiology is analyzed in relation to the phases of swallowing.

Drooling describes complaints of oral spill, i.e., the falling of food, liquid, or saliva from the mouth anteriorly when lip closure is incomplete. *Leaking* is defined as premature loss of the bolus over the tongue base into the pharynx before the swallowing reflex is triggered; consequently, there is a risk of aspiration. A *delayed triggering of the swallowing reflex* occurs in neurological diseases (e.g., stroke) or after extensive surgical resection of the trigger points for the pharyngeal swallow.

Retention (pooling) of saliva or food may be localized in the oral cavity, valleculae or hypopharynx (Fig. 1). Retentions in the anterior or lateral sulcus are due to reduced muscle tone in the labial or buccal musculature. Disturbed lingual function may result in retentions on the floor of the mouth and the valleculae. Weakness, paresis, or scarring of pharyngeal muscles gives rise to pharyngeal retentions.

Nasal penetration (regurgitation) describes the entry of food into the nose and may be caused by incomplete velopharyngeal closure or pharyngeal/esophageal stop of the bolus passage with subsequent overflow into the nasal cavity. In case of *laryngeal penetration*, food or saliva reaches the endolarynx as for as the level of the vocal folds.

Pharyngeal regurgitation is characterized by (parts of) the already swallowed bolus flowing back into the pharynx due to a Zenker's diverticulum or a disturbed esophageal bolus transport.

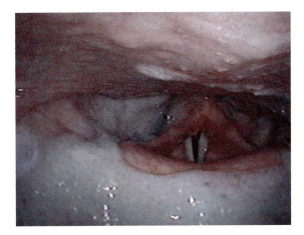

Fig. 1 Retentions of saliva bilaterally in the vallecullae and the right pyriform sinus

2.2 Dysphagia and Other Swallowing Complaints

Dysphagia has to be distinguished from other swallowing complaints, such as globus sensation or odynophagia. *Odynophagia* describes the painful swallow, as occurs in inflammatory or tumorous diseases of the upper aerodigestive tract (e.g., acute tonsillitis, peritonsillar abscess, epiglottitis, hypopharyngeal carcinoma, etc.).

Globus sensation (*globus pharyngis*) is a feeling of a lump or fullness in the throat and discomfort when swallowing saliva. In contrast to dysphagia, swallowing of food is not disturbed. The symptom mainly occurs during swallowing of saliva and decreases or vanishes while swallowing food. In many patients, an underlying cause can be found, e.g., gastroesophageal reflux disease, esophageal motility disorders, hypertensive upper esophageal sphincter (cricopharyngeal achalasia), thyroid gland disease, and cervical spine syndrome or hyperfunctional voice disorder. Therefore, the obsolete term "globus hystericus" should not be used any more. Only if an exact morphological and functional analysis of larynx, pharynx, esophagus and neck does not show any medical entity, a psychogenic etiology can be suspected. Above all, globus sensation and dysphagia may occur in combination.

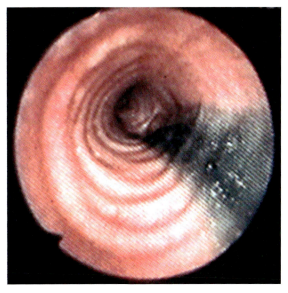

Fig. 2 Aspiration (videoendoscopic view): *blue*-colored aspirated food in the trachea [from Bigenzahn and Denk (1999)]

3 Aspiration

The antero- or retrograde entry of saliva, food or gastric secretion into the airway under the level of the vocal folds is defined as *aspiration* (Fig. 2). To reveal or exclude aspiration is the main goal of the diagnostic procedure in dysphagic patients. The presence/absence of aspiration determines further patient management. In the case of absent or reduced cough reflex, aspiration does not induce cough, but remains "silent" (*silent aspiration*) and is not immediately noticed. About 40 % of aspirating patients are so-called silent aspirators.

Aspiration can be classified in relation to the triggering of the swallow reflex. It may occur before (predeglutitive), during (intradeglutitive), after the swallow (postdeglutitive) or in combined forms (Logemann 1983). *Aspiration before the swallow* may be present when the triggering of the swallow reflex is absent or disturbed, e.g., after stroke. Incomplete laryngeal closure and/or reduced laryngeal elevation may give rise to *aspiration during the swallow*, as is the case, for example, in vocal fold paralysis or in laryngeal defects after partial

Fig. 3 Aspiration after the swallow (videoendoscopic view): overflow aspiration due to retentions in the hypopharynx. **a** *blue*-colored water [from Bigenzahn and Denk (1999)], **b** jelly

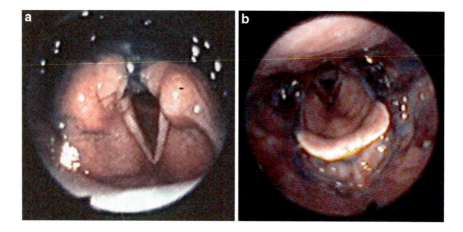

laryngectomy. Reduced pharyngeal peristalsis, reduced laryngeal elevation and disturbed opening of the pharyngo-esophageal sphincter can possibly result in *aspiration after the swallow* (Fig. 3 a, b), e.g., in fibrosis with "frozen" (immobile) larynx after radiation therapy or cricopharyngeal achalasia after stroke.

The severity of aspiration is not only influenced by the amount and type of the aspirated material, but also by the presence of cough reflex and the possibility of voluntary coughing and throat-clearing. Several severity scales are used for the grading of aspiration (Table 1). The clinical aspiration scale (Miller and Eliachar 1994) considers possible pulmonary consequences. In the videoendoscopic aspiration scale (Schröter-Morasch 1996), attention is paid to the cough reflex and voluntary coughing. The videofluoroscopic aspiration scale (Hannig et al. 1995) is based on the amount of aspirated material and the presence/absence of the cough reflex. The penetration-aspiration scale by Rosenbek et al. (1996) describes an eight-point scale. The severity of aspiration is determined by the level of entered material in the airway and if this material can be expelled.

The individual tolerance of aspiration varies widely. Some patients tolerate aspiration of more than 10 % of the bolus, whereas other patients develop aspiration pneumonia even after aspiration of their saliva. Therefore, not only aspiration, but other additional risk factors play an important role. Langmore et al. (1998) found the following predictors for the development of aspiration pneumonia: dependent for feeding, dependent for oral care, number of decayed teeth, tube feeding, more than one medical diagnosis, number of medications, and smoking.

4 Etiology of Dysphagia

The etiologies of dysphagia may be divided into the following groups:

- Diseases of the upper aerodigestive tract (*peripheral "mechanical" dysphagia*)
- Neurological diseases (*neurogenic dysphagia*), and
- *Psychogenic dysphagia*.

Only if after thorough diagnostics, peripheral or neurogenic dysphagia is excluded, psychogenic factors have to be considered. In some cases, the distinction from eating disorders is difficult.

4.1 Mechanical Dysphagia

Diseases of the upper swallowing and respiratory tract or surrounding structures may give rise to dysphagia and aspiration (Table 2). The symptom dysphagia necessitates the exclusion of malignant tumors in the aerodigestive tract. Moreover, not only a tumorous disease of the oral cavity, pharynx or larynx itself, but also the sequelae of therapy—surgical resection, radiation, or chemotherapy—can interfere with bolus transfer or airway protection with consecutive dysphagia and aspiration that requires functional swallowing therapy to regain swallowing function. The various tumor resections in the head and neck are known to create patterns of swallowing disorders, but the same resections need not necessarily result in the same form and degree of dysphagia and aspiration. The extent and localization of the resections carried out are regarded as determining factors for the severity

Table 1 Aspiration scales

Clinical Scale (Miller and Eliachar 1994)

I	Incidental aspiration without complications
II	Intermittent aspiration of liquids; saliva and solid boluses can be swallowed
III	No oral feeding possible, intermittent pneumonias
IV	Life-threatening aspiration; chronic pneumonia/hypoxia

Videoendoscopic Scale (Schröter-Morasch 1996)

I	Incidental aspiration, intact cough reflex
II	Incidental aspiration, no cough reflex, voluntary coughing possible or permanent aspiration, intact cough reflex
III	Permanent aspiration, no cough reflex, voluntary coughing possible
IV	Permanent aspiration, no cough reflex, no voluntary coughing

Videofluoroscopic Scale (Hannig et al. 1995)

I	Aspiration of material that has penetrated into the laryngeal vestibule or ventricle, intact cough reflex
II	Constant aspiration of less than 10 % of the bolus, intact cough reflex
III	Constant aspiration of less than 10 % of the bolus, reduced cough reflex or Constant aspiration of more than 10 % of the bolus, intact cough reflex
IV	Constant aspiration of more than 10 % of the bolus, reduced cough reflex

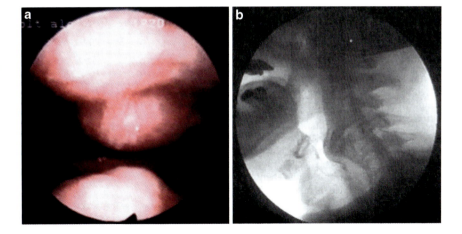

Fig. 4 Diffuse idiopathic skeletal hyperostosis (DISH), **a** Endoscopic view, **b** Radiologic view [from Bigenzahn and Denk (1999)]

of dysphagia. Beside these local factors, also general factors, e.g., patients' general condition or therapy onset postoperatively, influence the outcome of swallowing rehabilitation (Denk and Kaider 1997).

Not only tumors in the pharynx or esophagus, but also thyroid gland disease or cervical osteophyte compression due to diffuse idiopathic skeletal hyperostosis (DISH) (Marks et al. 1998) may be responsible for obstructive dysphagic symptoms that are typically worse for solid than liquid bolus. Patients suffering from DISH (Fig. 4a, b) become especially symptomatic when an additional disease or illness afflicting swallowing function (e.g., stroke) impairs the patient's functional compensatory capability.

4.2 Neurogenic Dysphagia

Nearly all neurological diseases have the potential to disturb the four levels of sensomotoric control of the swallow (central, peripheral nervous system, neuromuscular junction, muscles) and may cause dysphagia and aspiration (Table 2). For the management of the patients (functional therapy, type of nutrition), it is of utmost importance to distinguish between neurologic lesions with recovery potential (e.g., stroke, head trauma, cervical spine cord injury, etc.) and progressive diseases.

Stroke represents the most frequent cause of dysphagia (25 %, Groher and Bukatman 1986). The percentage of dysphagic stroke patients differs with

Table 2 Examples of dysphagia etiologies [modified from Denk and Bigenzahn (1999)]

Type of dysphagia	Aetiology
Mechanical peripheral dysphagia	
Oropharyngeal	Inflammatory diseases
	Malignant tumors in the upper aerodigestive tract/sequelae after tumor therapy (surgery, radiation, chemotherapy)
	Diseases/surgery of the cervical spine
	Long-term intubation
	Cheilognathopalatoschisis
	Tracheo-esophageal fistula
	Diverticula (Zenker's diverticulum)
	Goiter
	Systemic diseases (scleroderma, amyloidosis)
	Graft-versus-host disease
Esophageal	Obstructive esophageal diseases (peptic, tumorous stenosis)
	Motility disorders (gastro-esophageal reflux disease, non-propulsive contractions)
Neurogenic dysphagia	
Central nervous system	
	Stroke
	Degenerative processes: amyotrophic lateral sclerosis, Parkinson's disease, multiple sclerosis
	Cerebral palsy
	Dementia, Alzheimer's disease
	Post-polio syndrome
	Encephalitis
	AIDS
	Posterior fossa tumors
	Head trauma, cervical spine cord injury
	Intoxications
	Drug effects (sedatives, neuroleptics)
	Arnold Chiari malformation
Peripheral nervous system	
	Skull base tumours (chordoma, meningioma)
	Meningitis
	Guillain-Barré syndrome
	Neuropathy (alcoholic, diabetic)
Neuromuscular junction	
	Myasthenia gravis
	Botulism
	Lambert-Eaton syndrome
Muscles	
	Dermatomyositis, polymyositis
	Myopathy (endocrine/metabolic)
	Myotonia, muscular dystrophy
Psychogenic dysphagia	
	Phagophobia

Table 3 Symptoms of dysphagia/aspiration [from Schröter-Morasch (1993)]

Indirect symptoms
Weight loss
Frequent fevers
Coughing
Bronchitis/pneumonia
Changes of voice, articulation/speech and language
\Globus sensation
Heartburn
Non-cardiac chest pain

Direct symptoms
Prolonged duration of swallowing
Pain
Fear of swallowing
Changes in posture
Avoidance of certain consistencies
Drooling
Obstruction
Choking, coughing
Spitting of food
Regurgitation

the time from the onset of stroke: in the first 2 weeks after stroke 41 %, and in the chronic phase 16 % of patients suffer from dysphagia (Kuhlemeier 1994). Finally, within the first year after stroke, 3% (Masiero et al. 2008)—20 % (Brown and Glassenberg 1973) die from aspiration pneumonia.

Beside the swallowing disturbance, neurologic patients can show additional symptoms that have to be considered. Disturbances in the motor system bring about impaired posture and head control, and cognitive deficits lead to a lacking awareness of disease. Severely impaired speech and language (e.g., dysarthria, aphasia) impair communication with the patient.

5 Clinical Symptoms of the Dysphagic Patient

Aspiration is well known as the most threatening symptom of dysphagia. Due to disturbed laryngeal sensibility and absent cough reflex, aspiration often occurs silently. Therefore, the fact that the patient does not cough/choke while eating cannot be regarded as a reliable "clue" symptom to exclude aspiration. *Indirect and direct symptoms of dysphagia/aspiration* (Table 3) are possible hints to suspect dysphagia and aspiration. Direct symptoms occur during the swallowing of food and liquids, whereas indirect symptoms

are not directly associated with the swallow as such, but are due to dysphagia.

Among the *indirect symptoms*, weight loss is regarded as a reliable hint to judge the effects of swallowing impairment, because weight is usually directly related to nutritional state. Frequent fevers, coughing, bronchitis, or pneumonia may be clinical consequences of aspiration. Changes in voice (dysphonia), speech (dysarthria), and language (aphasia) should not be neglected, as they may be related to neurologic diseases. Moreover, anatomical and functional deficits in the upper aerodigestive tract can also lead to dysphonia, altered resonance (e.g., hyperrhinophonia = too much nasal resonance) or impaired articulation (e.g., dysglossia = disturbed articulation due to changes in the peripheral organs of speech). Globus sensation, heartburn and/or non-cardiac chest pain often are present in gastroesophageal reflux disease or esophageal motility disorders. Alterations of taste or mucosal dryness impair swallowing function and the pleasures of oral intake.

Choking or coughing during or immediately after the swallow due to aspiration, prolonged duration of swallowing, pain (odynophagia), or fear of swallowing belong to the *direct symptoms of dysphagia and aspiration*. Furthermore, changes in posture during oral food intake and changes in eating habits (e.g., avoidance of a particular food consistency) merit clinical awareness. Other direct symptoms the patient may report are drooling, nasal regurgitation, spitting of food or regurgitation. The feeling of obstruction may occur not only in patients with tumors, strictures, Zenker's diverticulum, webs, or cervical osteophytes (DISH), but also in neurologic diseases because of pharyngeal muscle weakness, lack of coordination of the swallow, or esophageal motility disorder.

6 Screening Procedures

Various screening protocols try to select the patients who need a thorough swallowing diagnostic work-up. No gold standard exists, and the various studies often cannot be compared because of different protocols, missing validation, and small samplings.

There is no common consent regarding who should perform the screening (the health care team or speech language pathologists) and how it should be carried out. Is a water swallow sufficient (3-ounce water swallow, Suiter and Leder 2008) or should not only water, but

Table 4 Diagnostic procedure [from Denk and Bigenzahn (1999); Denk and Bigenzahn (2005)]

History
Basic Diagnostics (compulsory)
I   ENT/phoniatric examination with clinical observation and videoendoscopic swallowing study (= flexible endoscopic evaluation of swallowing (with sensory testing), FEES (ST))
I   Videofluoroscopic swallowing study
I   If indicated, esophagoscopy
I   In the case of aspiration, chest X-ray
Further diagnostics (optional)
I   Esophagoscopy, gastroscopy
I   Ultrasound of the oral phases of swallowing
Cranial MRI
Scintigraphy
I   Manometry (impedance), pH-metry
I   Electrophysiological methods (electromyography)

also thicker consistencies be tested. The Gugging Swallowing Screen (Trapl et al. 2007) uses semisolid, liquid and solid textures in direct swallowing test. Moreover, an indirect swallowing test as the first step observes a saliva swallow, vigilance, voluntary cough and throat-clearing. Also, the Toronto Bedside Swallowing Screening Test (Martino et al. 2009) considers indirect aspects, such as mobility of the tongue and voice quality, before and after the water swallows.

To increase the sensitivity and specificity, the combination of two tests is recommended, but the discussion remains controversial. Whereas Lim et al. (2001) believes that a water test in combination with pulse oximetry is an apt tool to detect aspiration, Leder (2000) states that the use of changes in $SpO(2)$, heart rate, or blood pressure values as indirect objective markers of aspiration are not suitable.

Due to silent aspiration, the dynamic instrumental methods of videoendoscopy and videofluoroscopy can never be replaced by any screening tool to detect or exclude aspiration.

7   Diagnostic Procedure

For adequate management of patient complaints about swallowing problems, a thorough morphological and functional diagnostic procedure is needed to evaluate the swallow from the oral cavity to the stomach and to reveal the etiology and individual swallow profile. The diagnostic procedure is summarized in Table 4. To address the complexity of swallowing disorders, an interdisciplinary approach is necessary. Very often, the dysphagic patient first presents to the otorhinolaryngologist/phoniatrician who—after taking a thorough history—performs a videoendoscopy of the upper aerodigestive tract and videoendoscopic swallowing study (fiberoptic endoscopic evaluation of swallowing (FEES), (Langmore et al. 1988; Bastian 1991, Fiberoptic evaluation of swallowing with sensory testing (FEESST), Aviv et al. 1998), and, if necessary, refers the patient for a videofluoroscopic swallowing study. Depending on the patient's needs and findings, further examinations have to be performed and further medical disciplines need to become involved, such as gastroenterology, pulmonology, neurology, surgery, maxillofacial surgery, etc.

The diagnostic procedure aims at revealing the components of dysphagia, especially proving or excluding aspiration. Moreover, a classification and quantification of aspiration, as well as a prognostic estimate, have to be performed. Further diagnostic goals are recommendations for therapy and type of feeding, as well as indications for emergency therapies (such as tracheostomy) in the case of intractable aspiration.

7.1   Patient History

Patient history provides valuable information that helps to optimize the diagnostic work-up. The patient is asked to characterize his complaints and to describe their beginning, time characteristics (intermittent or constant occurrence), and influencing factors. However, it is important to know about the influence of bolus consistency on swallowing. In neurologic patients with impaired swallowing reflex and uncoordinated swallow, swallowing liquids is more difficult than semisolids, because they cannot be controlled well. Patients with obstructive diseases (tumors, strictures, webs) often report sticking of solid food, whereas patients suffering from esophageal motility disorders complain about swallowing problems with both liquids and solid food. To estimate the patient's oral intake, a description of his meals and weight during the last weeks may be valuable.

Furthermore, information regarding previous illnesses and therapies (surgery, radiation—often years before), as well as medication, needs to be obtained. The side effects of many drugs can impair swallowing: psychopharmacological drugs possibly interfere with the swallow reflex or induce xerostomia, antipsychotic drugs can cause extrapyramidal symptoms, and spasmolytics may weaken muscles. It has to be pointed out that changes in voice, speech and language should be carefully noted. Above all, the examiner should also take into consideration the patient's general condition, his nutritional status (body weight), and posture, and cognitive and emotional state. Due to the epidemiological changes, dementia will become a challenging problem in our society, and dysphagia may be an early or accompanying symptom. Depending on the patient's needs, a holistic approach, including the mini mental status (Folstein et al. 1975) or the mini nutritional assessment MNA^{TM} (Nestlé Nutrition Services), can help to judge the patient's clinical condition.

Questionnaires may help describe the impaired quality of life due to dysphagia (e.g., The MD Anderson dysphagia inventory, Chen et al. 2001, the dysphagia handicap index, Silbergleit et al. 2012).

7.2 Basic Diagnostic Procedure

The ENT examination plays an important "key" role in the diagnostic work-up because it allows a direct morphological and functional analysis of the upper aerodigestive tract. Since clinical observation and palpation of the swallow alone do not meet the diagnostic demands, a videoendoscopic swallowing study, (FEES (ST), fiberoptic endoscopic evaluation of swallowing

(with sensory testing), see also Sect. 6.2.4) has to be performed. It is a non-invasive dynamic procedure that delivers an immediate evaluation of pharyngeal swallowing function and directly visualizes the upper aerodigestive tract. However, it has the following limitations: no direct visualization of the bolus on it's entire way from the oral cavity to the stomach, no visualization during the swallow, no visualization of the oral and esophageal phases and pharyngo-esophageal segment. Therefore, a videofluoroscopic swallowing study (Ekberg 1992; Logemann 1993, 1998) has to be carried out routinely in many cases as a complementary dynamic diagnostic procedure.

7.3 Further Examinations

If necessary, further diagnostic methods are used (Table 4). Depending on the results of videoendoscopic and videofluoroscopic swallowing studies, esophago-gastroscopy can eventually be performed as a first-line diagnostic method to exclude tumorous lesions or reveal disturbances in the esophageal phase (see also Sect. 6.3). Scintigraphy enables the quantification of bolus transit and aspiration. For an evaluation of neurogenic dysphagia, cranial magnetic resonance imaging (MRI) may detect intracranial lesions responsible for dysphagia. Impedance pH-metry represents the gold standard for diagnostics of suspected gastroesophageal (-pharyngeal) reflux disease. To measure the pressure in the pharynx (especially before surgery of the pharyngo-esophageal segment) impedance manometry, which allows measurement of the intrabolus pressures and pharyngeal contraction, is recommended. Cervical auscultation of the pharyngeal swallow did not gain wide acceptance.

8 Conclusion

Swallowing disorder symptoms necessitate an interdisciplinary, holistic, and thorough diagnostic work-up that reveals etiologic factors and pathophysiological components. The patient should be asked precise questions relating to symptoms, and valuable information should be obtained, allowing suitable diagnostic and therapeutic measures to be taken. Above all, the adequacy of oral nutrition and the presence or absence of aspiration is within the focus of diagnostic and therapeutic interests. Due to an absent cough reflex, aspiration may occur silently. Therefore, diagnostic methods must enable direct visualization of aspiration by videoendoscopy and videofluoroscopy. Aspiration cannot be diagnosed or excluded by patient history or clinical observation alone. However, for appropriate management, the patient's symptoms should be carefully evaluated.

References

Aviv JE, Kim T, Sacco RL, Kaplan S, Goodhart K, Diamond B, Close LG (1998) FEESST: a new bedside endoscopic test of the motor and sensory components of swallowing. Ann Otol Rhinol Laryngol 107(5 Pt 1):378–387

Bastian RW (1991) Videoendoscopic evaluation of patients with dysphagia: an adjunct to the modified barium swallow. Otol HNS 104:339–350

Bigenzahn W, Denk D-M (1999) Oropharyngeale Dysphagien (Oropharyngeal Dysphagia). Ätiologie, Klinik, Diagnostik und Therapie von Schluckstörungen, Thieme, Stuttgart

Brown M, Glassenberg M (1973) Mortality factors in patients with acute stroke. JAMA 224:1493–1495

Chen AY, Frankowski R, Bishop-Leone J, Hebert T, Leyk S, Lewin J, Goepfert H (2001) The development and validation of a dysphagia-specific quality-of-life questionnaire for patients with head and neck cancer: the MD Anderson dysphagia inventory. Arch Otolaryngol Head Neck Surg 127:870–876

Denk D-M, Bigenzahn W (1999) Diagnostik oropharyngealer Dysphagien (Diagnostics of oropharyngeal dysphagia). In: Bigenzahn W, Denk D-M (eds) Oropharyngeale Dysphagien. Ätiologie, Klinik, Diagnostik und Therapie von Schluckstörungen, Thieme, Stuttgart, pp 33–65

Denk D-M, Kaider A (1997) Videoendoscopic biofeedback: a simple method to improve the efficacy of swallowing rehabilitation of patients after head and neck surgery. ORL 59:100–105

Denk DM, Bigenzahn W (2005) Management oropharyngealer Dysphagien. Eine standortbestimmmung [Management of oropharyngeal dysphagia. Current status] HNO 53(7): 661–72

Ekberg O, Hamdy S, Woisard V, Wuttge-Hannig A, Ortega P (2002) Social and psychological burden of dysphagia: its impact on diagnosis and treatment. Dysphagia 17:139–146

Ekberg O (1992) Radiologic evaluation of swallowing. In: Groher ME (ed) Dysphagia. Diagnosis and Management. Butterworth-Heinemann, Stoneham, pp 163–195

Folstein MF, Folstein SE, McHugh PR (1975) Mini-mental state (a practical method for grading the state of patients for the clinician). J Psychiatr Res 12:189–198

Garliner D (1974) Myofunctional therapy in dental practice. Bartel, New York

Groher ME, Bukatman R (1986) The prevalence of swallowing disorders in two teaching hospitals. Dysphagia 1:1–3

Hannig C, Wuttge-Hannig A, Hess U (1995) Analyse und radiologisches staging des typs und schweregrades einer aspiration (analysis and radiological staging of type and grade of aspiration). Radiologe 358:741–746

Jones B, Donner MW (eds) (1991) Normal and abnormal swallowing. Springer, New York

Kuhlemeier KV (1994) Epidemiology and dysphagia. Dysphagia 9:209–217

Langmore S, Schatz K, Olsen N (1988) Fiberoptic examination of swallowing safety: a new procedure. Dysphagia 2: 216–219

Langmore SE, Terpenning MS, Schork A, Chen Y, Murray JT, Lopatin D, Loesche WJ (1998) Predictors of aspiration pneumonia: how important is dysphagia? Dysphagia 13: 69–81

Leder SB (2000) Use of arterial oxygen saturation, heart rate, and blood pressure as indirect objective physiologic markers to predict aspiration. Dysphagia 15(4):201–205

Leopold NA, Kagel MA (1996) Prepharyngeal dysphagia in Parkinson's disease. Dysphagia 11:14–22

Lim SH, Lieu PK, Phua SY, Seshadri R, Venketasubramanian N, Lee SH, Choo PW (2001) Accuracy of bedside clinical methods compared with fiberoptic endoscopic examination of swallowing (FEES) in determining the risk of aspiration in acute stroke patients. Dysphagia 16(1):1–6

Logemann JA (1983) Evaluation and treatment of swallowing disorders. Pro-ed, Austin

Logemann JA (1998) Evaluation and treatment of swallowing disorders. Pro-ed, Austin

Logemann JA (1993) Manual for the videofluorographic study of swallowing, 2nd edn. Pro-ed, Austin

Logemann JA (1995) Dysphagia: evaluation and treatment. Folia Phoniatr Logop 47:140–164

Marks B, Schober E, Swoboda H (1998) Diffuse idiopathic skeletal hyperostosis causing obstructive laryngeal edema. Eur Arch Otolaryngol 255:256–258

Martino R, Silver F, Teasell R, Bayley M, Nicholson G, Streiner DL, Diamant NE (2009) The toronto bedside swallowing screening test (TOR-BSST): development and validation of a dysphagia screening tool for patients with stroke. Stroke 40(2):555–561

Masiero S, Pierobon R, Previato C, Gomiero E (2008) Pneumania in stroke patients with oropharyngeal dysphagia: a six-month folloe-up study. Neurol Sci 29(3):139–145. [Epub 2008 Jul 9]

Miller FR, Eliachar J (1994) Managing the aspirating patient. Am J Otolaryngol 15:1–17

Rosenbek JC, Robbins JA, Roecker EB, Coyle JL, Wood JL (1996) A penetration-aspiration scale. Dysphagia 11(2): 93–98

Sasaki H (1991) Management of respiratory diseases in the elderly. Nippon-Kyobu-Shikkan-Gakkai-Zasshi 29: 1227–1233

Schröter-Morasch H (1993) Klinische untersuchung der am schluckvorgang beteiligten organe (clinical examination). In: Bartolome G et al (eds) Diagnostik und therapie neurologisch bedingter schluckstörungen. Gustav Fischer, Stuttgart, pp 73–108

Schröter-Morasch H (1996) Schweregradeinteilung der aspiration bei patienten mit schluckstörung (Severity of aspiration in dysphagic patients). In: Gross VM (ed) Aktuelle phoniatrisch-pädaudiologische aspekte. R. Gross Verlag, Berlin, pp 145–146

Silbergleit AK, Schultz L, Jacobson BH, Beardsley T, Johnson AF (2012) The dysphagia handicap index: development and validation. Dysphagia 27:46–52

Suiter DM, Leder SB (2008) Clinical utility of the 3-ounce water swallow test. Dysphagia 23(3):244–250

Trapl M, Enderle P, Nowotny M, Teuschl Y, Matz K, Dachenhausen A, Brainin M (2007) Dysphagia bedside screening for acute-stroke patients: the Gugging Swallowing Screen. Stroke 38(11):2948–2952

Neurology of Swallowing and Dysphagia

Mario Prosiegel

Contents

Abstract

Neurogenic dysphagia is difficulty swallowing due to neurological diseases and compromises especially the oral and/or pharyngeal stage. The first section of this chapter deals with the neuroanatomy and neurophysiology of swallowing as a basis for a better understanding of neurogenic dysphagia. Then, diagnostic approaches are described comprising history taking, screening examinations, clinical swallowing examination, and instrumental methods. The third section focuses on those neurological diseases which are frequently associated with dysphagia and ends with the description of the problem that only a few pharmacological and invasive therapeutic interventions against neurogenic dysphagia exist. This expressly underlines the need for swallowing therapy and the development of new therapeutic approaches such as electrical pharyngeal or repetitive transcranial magnetic stimulations.

1 Neuroanatomy and Neurophysiology

This section deals with neuroanatomical and neurophysiological basics of normal and abnormal swallowing: What role do the cerebral hemispheres and the brainstem play in deglutition? How can the pathogenesis of pseudobulbar as well as of bulbar palsy be explained?

Besides such topics, one focus lies also on the upper esophageal sphincter (UES), because opening deficits of the UES are very frequent in neurogenic

M. Prosiegel (✉)
Abteilung Neurologie, m&i-Fachklinik Bad Heilbrunn,
Wörnerweg 30, 83670 Bad Heilbrunn, Germany
e-mail: mario.prosiegel@fachklinik-bad-heilbrunn.de

O. Ekberg (ed.), *Dysphagia*, Medical Radiology. Diagnostic Imaging, DOI: 10.1007/174_2011_339,
© Springer-Verlag Berlin Heidelberg 2012

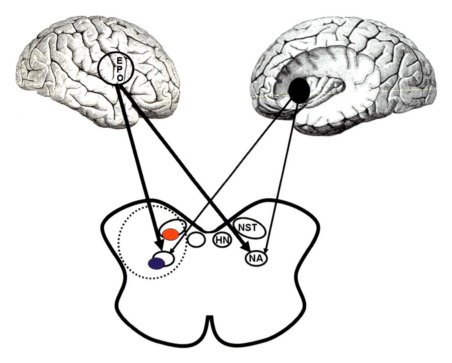

Fig. 1 Swallowing cortex, corticobulbar fibers, and lower brainstem. *Top left*: Right cerebral hemisphere with the frontoparietal operculum (*closed circle*) and the representational areas of the esophagus (*E*), pharynx (*P*) and oral region (*O*). In this example, the right hemisphere is swallowing-dominant, with more corticobulbar fibers (*long thick arrows*) projecting to the ipsilateral and contralateral medulla. *Top right*: Left hemisphere after removal of the operculum; the insula with its anterior swallowing-relevant part (*black area*) can therefore bee seen. *Bottom*: Axial view of the lower brainstem (medulla; lower part=anterior; upper part=posterior). On the *right side* (left side of the medulla) the nucleus of the solitary tract (NST), the nucleus ambiguus (NA), and the hypoglossal nucleus (HN) are shown. On the *left side* (right side of the medulla) the dorsomedial and ventrolateral central pattern generators for swallowing are shown (*red area* and *blue area*, respectively). The *horizontally lined area* corresponds to the site of a dorsolateral medullary infarction with consecutive Wallenberg's syndrome. For details, see the text

dysphagia (for other swallowing muscles see the chapter "Anatomy and Physiology" by O. Ekberg and G. Nylander, this volume).

1.1   Cerebral Hemispheres

In their pioneering work, Penfield and Boldrey (1937) from the Montreal Neurological Institute in Canada performed intraoperative electrical stimulations of the cerebral cortex in awake patients. Thereby, they found certain sensorimotor representational areas with the net result of the well-known sensorimotor homunculus (the "little man inside the brain"). With regard to swallowing, they elicited deglutition by stimulation of the frontoparietal operculum, i.e., the lower portion of the precentral gyrus (primary motor area), of the premotor cortex, and of the postcentral gyrus (primary sensory area)—corresponding to Brodmann's areas (BA) 4 (motor), 6 (premotor), and 3, 2, and 1 (sensory), respectively.

Magnetic resonance imaging (MRI) and functional imaging of the brain, including functional MRI, positron emission tomography, and magnetoencephalography, confirmed these earlier findings and showed that also the anterior insula (BA 14–16) is involved in volitional swallowing (Barritt and Smithard 2009; Hamdy et al. 1999; Humbert and Robbins 2007; Riecker et al. 2009). Furthermore, by use of transcranial magnetic stimulation it was found that the esophageal, pharyngeal, and oral muscles are discretely represented within the motor cortex in a rostrocaudal direction, with esophageal muscles being situated more rostrally than the pharyngeal muscles, which in turn are more rostral than the oral muscles (Hamdy et al. 1996) (Fig. 1).

Functional brain imaging studies also showed that the swallowing cortex is represented bilaterally, but asymmetrically, i.e., it is (in most people) bigger on one side than on the other. The bigger swallowing cortex is called the dominant one. *Swallowing dominance* is independent of the language-dominant side or of handedness (Barrit and Smithard 2009; Hamdy et al. 1999).

The fibers which project from the motoneurons of the swallowing cortex to both sides of the brainstem are called *corticobulbar fibers* and constitute the *corticobulbar (corticonuclear) tract*. When the dominant swallowing cortex and/or its corticobulbar fibers are affected, a significant hemispheric dysphagia occurs (hemispheric dysphagia means swallowing problems caused by cortical and/or subcortical lesions of the left and/or the right cerebral hemisphere, i.e., supratentorial lesions) (Fig. 1). Additionally, right-sided cortical lesions are often associated with "neglect of swallowing," "food stuffing," and consecutive problems in the pharyngeal phase (Robbins and Levin 1988), whereas left-sided lesions may cause swallowing apraxia with corresponding problems in the oral phase (Daniels 2000). Independent of these behavioral/neuropsychological problems, left-sided and right-sided areas of the swallowing cortex seem to play different roles during the early and later phase of swallowing, respectively (Teismann et al. 2009).

Besides the abovementioned swallowing areas, other cortical and subcortical regions are involved in swallowing function, such as the supplementary motor area (SMA) corresponding to the medial part of BA 6, the basal ganglia, and many others. The SMA is responsible for the generation of the readiness potential (*Bereitschaftspotential*), which arises about 1 s before a volitional motor action. It was shown that also a swallowing potential (*Schluckpotential*) exists, which is generated in the SMA too, but spreads to both primary motor areas (whereas the readiness potential spreads to the motor area which is contralateral to the innervated extremity) (Huckabee et al. 2003).

According to Mosier and Bereznaya (2001) one can distinguish two swallowing networks: (1) an "insular loop" including the insula, the primary sensorimotor motor cortex, premotor cortex, posterior

parietal cortex, and the SMA/cingulate gyrus; (2) a "cerebellar loop" comprising the cerebellum, the SMA/cingulate gyrus, the inferior frontal gyrus, the secondary sensory cortex, the corpus callosum, and the basal ganglia as well as the thalamus. The influence of the insula within the "insular loop" might be necessary to synchronize the kinematics of the swallowing movements, whereas the "cerebellar loop" might optimize and modulate movements using feedback information.

As shown by Power et al. (2007), the swallow response time is prolonged in dysphagic patients as compared with healthy volunteers owing to unilateral hemispheric stroke. Interestingly enough, in these stroke patients a sensory deficit of the faucial pillars was found bilaterally in 66% and the duration of laryngeal delay and the degree of the sensory deficit were associated with the severity of predeglutitive aspiration. Very similar results were found in a recent study by Oommen et al. (2010): the stage transition time duration was significantly longer in 52 post-stroke patients—19 aspirators and 33 nonaspirators—than in 12 healthy controls.

Since the cortical swallowing network comprises many sensorimotor areas, one can speculate that sensory input is very critical for an intact swallowing. This view was confirmed by a recent study in decerebrate pigs: the sensory threshold for the swallowing response was increased, since the facilitatory pathways descending from cerebral structures to the brainstem had been lost (Thexton et al. 2007). Therefore, important roles of the cerebral cortex in deglutition seem to be initiation of swallowing, ensuring a normal coupling of the oral and pharyngeal phase (stage transition time) as well as normal sensory properties of the oropharyngeal region, direct modulation of swallowing, and modification of brainstem swallowing responses—in each case mainly dependent on sensory inputs (see also Sect. 1.2).

1.2 Brainstem

Doty and Bosma (1956) conducted a pioneering study on the role of the brainstem in swallowing. By electrical stimulation of the superior laryngeal nerve with 30 Hz in different animals, including monkeys, they could elicit the complete sequential pattern of activation or inhibition of swallowing muscles of the pharyngeal phase. Therefore, they postulated the existence of a swallowing center in the medulla oblongata; this view was confirmed later (for a review, see Jean 2001). There are four swallowing centers—two on each side of the brainstem— for which the term *"central pattern generators"* (*CPGs*) for swallowing was coined. The dorsomedial CPGs (dmCPGs) are situated close beside the nucleus of the solitary tract (NST) and the adjacent reticular formation; they contain so-called master neurons/programming interneurons which generate the temporal–spatial sequence of pharyngeal swallowing muscle activation or inhibition. This information is transmitted to ventrolateral CPGs situated near the nucleus ambiguus (NA); switching neurons/command interneurons of the ventrolateral CPGs distribute the timed output to the cranial nerve nuclei V and VII in the pons as well as to the cranial nerve nuclei IX, X, and XII in the medulla oblongata (Fig. 1). The functioning of the brainstem central network can be influenced by peripheral inputs—e.g., from oropharyngeal mucosal receptors and muscle spindles of the tongue—as well as by central inputs from the cortex; both inputs converge at the NST and serve in particular to adapt the swallowing drive to properties of the bolus to be swallowed. The brainstem is also important for coordinating interactions between respiration and swallowing (Jean 2001; Miller 1993).

Owing to the role of the brainstem in swallowing, unilateral lesions of the medullary region—such as in Wallenberg's syndrome caused by unilateral infarctions in the supply area of the posterior inferior cerebellar artery (Fig. 1)—affecting both ipsilateral CPGs and the NA and the NST, cause complex swallowing disturbances, including unilateral pharyngeal paresis (NA), impaired pharyngeal peristalsis (NA and dmCPG), sensory deficits in the oropharyngeal region (sensory trigeminal nucleus and NST), and secondary UES opening deficit due to impaired hyolaryngeal excursion and/or primary UES opening disturbance due to impaired sphincter relaxation (dmCPG) (Prosiegel et al. 2005a). Dysphagia may be the sole symptom in dorsolateral medullary infarctions but is—owing to ipsilateral vagal paresis—often associated with hoarseness due to unilateral vocal cord paresis. Other symptoms belonging to Wallenberg's syndrome are rotatory nystagmus,

ipsilateral Horner's syndrome, numbness of the face, and ataxia as well as contralateral hypalgesia and thermhypesthesia.

1.3   Pseudobulbar and Bulbar Palsy

Two frequently occurring syndromes associated with dysphagia are pseudobulbar palsy and bulbar palsy. Pseudobulbar palsy is caused by bilateral lesions of the cerebral cortex and/or its corresponding corticobulbar fibers, including those passing through the brainstem. In contrast, bulbar palsy ("bulbus" is an outdated term formerly used for the lower brainstem) is due to bilateral lesions of pontine and medullary cranial nerve nuclei or their axons or is due to bilateral lesions of the cranial nerves themselves.

1.3.1   Pseudobulbar Palsy

The motoneurons of the swallowing cortex are called first motoneurons or upper motoneurons (UMNs). When the swallowing cortex itself and/or and its axons, i.e., the corticobulbar fibers, are lesioned bilaterally, there is diminished input to the brainstem. The consequence is severe dysphagia which affects predominantly the volitional oral phase. Owing to impaired cortical input, the membrane of the motoneurons in the brainstem lower their electrical threshold with consecutive hyperreflexia (e.g., enhanced masseter reflex) and muscle stiffness in terms of spasticity. There are no muscle atrophies, since the second motoneurons/lower motoneurons (LMNs) in the brainstem are intact and, therefore, able to supply the corresponding muscles with the transmitter acetylcholine. This syndrome is called pseudobulbar palsy and occurs in UMN diseases (UMNDs); examples are amyotrophic lateral sclerosis (ALS) due to bilateral degeneration of the UMNs or bilateral subcortical infarctions affecting the corticobulbar tracts. In most cases of pseudobulbar palsy, besides dysphagia also dysarthria and chewing problems occur; pathological crying or laughing is often associated with pseudobulbar palsy too. Bilateral lesions of the corticobulbar tract in the brainstem (e.g., in bilateral anterior mesencephalic infarctions) may also cause pseudobulbar palsy. Very typical for pseudobulbar palsy is *automatic–voluntary dissociation*: emotional or reflex responses are intact or enhanced, whereas volitional activities are disturbed e.g., enhanced palatal reflex, but no elevation of the soft palate during phonation of /A/ or videofluoroscopic study of swallowing (VFSS) is also spasm of the cricopharyngeal muscle.

1.3.2 Bulbar Palsy

In contrast to pseudobulbar palsy, muscle atrophy occurs when the cranial nerve nuclei in the brainstem (or the motoneurons in the spinal cord)—i.e., the LMNs—are affected. Because of diminished input to the corresponding muscles, the muscular membrane develops a decreased electrical threshold with consecutive pathological spontaneous activity. This can be assessed electromyographically or seen clinically in the form of fibrillations of the atrophic tongue (jerks of muscle fibers) or fasciculations of the face or body musculature (jerks of groups of muscle fibers). Other features are weakness of the orofaciopharyngeal muscles and decreased muscle tone in terms of hypotonia with diminished reflexes as well as bulbar (slurred) speech. This syndrome, which is caused by affection of the LMNs, is called bulbar palsy and occurs in LMN diseases (LMNDs) such as ALS (ALS is an example of a combined UMND and LMND). Bulbar palsy may also be caused by lesions of the fibers of the cranial nerve nuclei or of the cranial nerves themselves.

1.4 Upper Esophageal Sphincter

The UES is defined as a high-pressure zone with a rostrocaudal extension of 2–6 cm, which maintains a closed pharyngoesophageal junction and opens phasically during various physiological states (Lang and Shaker 1997). It consists of striated muscles comprising the inferior pharyngeal constrictor, the cricopharyngeal muscle and the upper esophageal musculature. In contrast to the other swallowing muscles, the UES forms a network together with connective tissue (approximately 40%) and consists of more than 70% of slow twitch (tonic, type I) fibers. The number of these tonic fibers is especially high in the horizontal part of the cricopharyngeal muscle as compared with its oblique part as well as in the slow inner layer as compared with the fast outer layer of the UES. Acetylcholine is the transmitter which binds to the nicotinic motor end plates of the muscle fibers,

but many other transmitters (mainly found in blood vessels, glands, and the mucosa) occur in the UES, including neuropeptide Y, calcitonin-gene-related peptide, tyrosine hydroxylase, substance P, and vasoactive intestinal polypeptide. The slow inner layer is innervated by cranial nerve IX (glossopharyngeal nerve), whereas the fast outer layer is supplied by different branches of cranial nerve X (vagus nerve) in the following manner: (1) inferior pharyngeal constrictor —pharyngoesophageal nerve forming the pharyngeal plexus; external superior laryngeal nerve; (2) cricopharyngeal muscle—pharyngeal plexus; external superior laryngeal nerve; recurrent laryngeal nerve (RLN); (3) upper esophageal musculature—recurrent laryngeal nerve (for a review, see Mu and Sanders 2007).

UES opening is a very complex event. Firstly, relaxation of the UES muscles occurs (as can be shown electromyographically). Secondly, about 100 ms later, there is a reduction of UES pressure (as can be shown by use of manometry). Thirdly, again about 100 ms later, UES opening occurs caused by two forces which have to overcome the resistance (R) of the sphincter: (1) traction forces, exerted by the suprahyoid muscles during anterior–superior hyolaryngeal excursion, widen the cricopharyngeal muscle, since the cricopharyngeal muscle originates from the arch of the cricoid cartilage; (2) tongue base retraction with approximation of the base of the tongue to the posterior pharyngeal wall generates the force responsible for the primary pressure on the descending bolus (shortening of the pharynx helps the bolus meet the UES). These forces (F)/pressures (P) can be described mathematically as follows: $F_{\mathrm{Traction}} + P_{\mathrm{Intrabolus}} > R_{\mathrm{UES}}$ (for a review, see Lang et al. 1991). Pharyngeal peristalsis is also important, but its predominant role is to clear pharyngeal bolus residuals.

Defective opening of the UES due to increased tonicity occurs frequently in patients with dysphagia due to medullary lesion (such as in Wallenberg's syndrome or Parkinson's disease (Williams et al. 2002) and is sometimes called cervical achalasia.

Defective tonicity of the UES between swallows (cervical chalasia) may occur in motonic dystrophy, myasthenia gravis, during "off" periods of Parkinson's disease, and after radiotherapy of the neck; it is often asymptomatic, but may cause aerophagia, belching, and/or regurgitation of refluxed material (Ekberg and Olsson 1995).

2 Examinations

Diagnostics in (suspected) neurogenic dysphagia comprise history taking, clinical swallowing examination, and instrumental methods. Bedside screening tests are only necessary in certain cases, which are described in Sect. 2.1.2.

Special diagnostic approaches such as laboratory examination and MRI are dealt with in Sect. 3.6.

2.1 Clinical Examinations

2.1.1 History Taking: Signs and Symptoms in Neurogenic Dysphagia

In many textbooks or articles one can find the statement that dysphagia for liquids is typical for neurogenic dysphagia. Although it often occurs, it is, however, not a pathognomonic symptom for dysphagia of neurogenic origin. In reality, there is a broad range of different signs and symptoms occurring in patients with neurogenic dysphagia. During history taking it is helpful to use a checklist of questions and to ask the patient and his/her relatives to try to answer them as accurately as possible. Interestingly enough, in many cases the relatives may observe, e.g., disturbances of feeding behavior or postural changes which are not or not to the same extent realized by the patients themselves.

Some of the most *important signs and symptoms* are listed in the following: abrupt or gradual beginning of swallowing problems; difficulty with control of saliva; problems with liquids and/or thick consistencies; problems with warm, hot, or cold liquids and/or food; involuntary weight loss; eating and/or drinking more slowly than in the time before symptom onset; eating and/or drinking smaller portions than in the time before symptom onset; unexplained fever and/or pneumonia; coughing and/or choking and/or voice change (e.g., wet, hoarse, nasal) after eating and/or drinking; drooling and/or sialorrhea; increase of secretions; dry mouth; articulation problems (e.g., slurred speech); feeling of a "lump in the throat"; fear of swallowing; pain during swallowing (where?); change of head or trunk posture during swallowing; chewing problems; problems to propel the bolus from the mouth backwards into the pharynx; problems to hold the bolus in the mouth during chewing or swallowing; residuals of food in the mouth after swallowing; nasal regurgitation of food or liquids; feeling of "food sticking" (where?); need for repetitive swallowing in order to remove all residuals; breathing problems; prior or current disease such as chronic pulmonary obstructive disease; prior surgery/medical therapy such as anterior cervical surgery, carotid endarterectomy, or radiochemotherapy for head and neck cancer; current status such as dependence on a percutaneous endoscopic gastrostomy (PEG) tube, nasogastric tube or tracheal cannula; prior and current medication.

2.1.2 Bedside Screening Examinations

Bedside screening examinations should predict the presence or absence of dysphagia or aspiration with sufficient sensitivity and specificity (more than 70%) (Doggett et al. 2002). A bedside screening examination seems to be especially helpful in acute illnesses such as stroke; rapid therapeutic decisions have to be made in those situations with regard to oral administration of food and water versus nil by mouth, because there is often not enough time to perform a clinical swallowing examination or instrumental methods within 72 h. Bedside screening examinations can, however, never replace an accurate clinical swallowing examination or an instrumental method such as flexible endoscopic evaluation of swallowing (FEES) or VFSS (see Sect. 2.2), since the latter ones are necessary for the assessment of the individual swallowing disturbance patterns and thus for applying the corresponding therapeutic interventions.

With regard to acute stroke, Hinchey et al. (2005) convincingly demonstrated the importance of an early screening procedure, which is reflected by the title of their article: "Formal dysphagia screening protocols prevent pneumonia." Indeed, the most dangerous complication of dysphagia is aspiration pneumonia; but also malnutrition—defined as a body mass index of less than 18.5 kg/m^2 (or less than 20 kg/m^2 in elderly persons)—is an important variable, since its occurrence during the acute stroke phase correlates with a poor clinical outcome and with a prolonged length of stay in the hospital (Finestone et al. 1996; Gariballa et al. 1998).

The *Standardized Swallowing Assessment* was developed for use by nurses within the first 24 h after stroke; the sensitivity and specificity for detection of dysphagia were 97% and 90%, respectively; a kappa value of 0.88 indicated good agreement with summative clinical judgment of swallow function (Perry 2001a, b). The Standardized Swallowing Assessment consists of a preswallow screening checklist comprising seven questions/symptoms concerning level of consciousness, ability to sit upright, volitional cough, control of saliva, licking of the lips, breathing, and voice; thereafter, a swallow screen consisting of a water test is performed with consecutive recommendations for interventions (e.g., in the case of problems such as coughing or choking after administration of a teaspoonful of water, the recommendation is "patient nil by mouth," "refer to speech and language therapist").

A well-known instrument for assessing the risk of aspiration in the acute stroke phase was developed by Daniels et al. (1997), often referred to as the *Daniels test*. In their study on 59 patients (within 5 days of admission), the authors determined whether risk factors detected in the clinical examination approximated the VFSS in identification of dysphagia severity. They found that occurrence of two or more of the following variables predicted aspiration with a sensitivity of 92.3% and a specificity of 66.7%, respectively: dysarthria, dysphonia, abnormal (decreased or absent) gag reflex, abnormal volitional cough, cough after swallow, and voice change after swallow. The last two items were assessed by use of a water test in the following manner: patient in sitting position; 5-ml liquid bolus administered from a cup or straw, progressed to 10- and 20-ml volumes; phonation of /Ah/ (change in vocal quality?); all volumes administered twice, i.e., a total of 70 ml; termination of the test in the case of cough or voice change immediately after swallowing or within 1 min after ingestion of the liquid.

With regard to aspiration risk and feeding recommendations, the clinical utility of the *3-oz water swallow test* was examined by Suiter and Leder (2008) in 3,000 patients. The diagnostic categories comprised 850 neurological disorders (most frequently stroke) and 232 neurosurgical disorders. The patients were required to drink 3 oz (90 ml) of water without interruption; the criteria for referral for further assessment of swallowing included inability to complete the task, coughing, choking, or a wet-hoarse vocal quality exhibited either during or within 1 min of test completion. The sensitivity and specificity for assessing the risk of aspiration were 96.5% and

48.7%, respectively. Owing to a high negative predictive value of 98.3%, passing the 3-oz water swallow test was a good predictor for the ability to tolerate oral diet without further dysphagia testing. Failing the test is, however, not a good predictor for unsuccessful swallowing of water, since the false-positive rate is very high. Because of the large amount of water, this test should not be used in patients with compromised medical status, e.g., in frail elderly persons, patients in the acute stroke phase, or persons with severe bulbar type of ALS.

2.1.3 Clinical Swallowing Examination

The clinical swallowing examination aims at detecting disturbances of specific swallowing components as a basis for adequate therapeutic interventions. It comprises—in descending order of cranial nerves—the following examinations: decreased strength of chewing muscles, asymmetry of the mandible, and sensory impairment of the facial and oral region—cranial nerve V; decreased strength and/or motility of facial muscles, fasciculations of the facial musculature, and hypogeusia of the anterior two thirds of the tongue—cranial nerve VII; decreased or absent palatal and pharyngeal reflex, unilateral pharyngeal wall paresis (paralyzed side moving towards the healthy side, also called "Vernet's mouvement de rideau"), sensory impairment of the pharyngeal mucosa, impaired phonation (e.g., wet, hoarse, nasal), disturbed breathing, e.g., stridor, impaired volitional cough, and hypogeusia of the posterior third of the tongue—cranial nerves IX and X; fibrillations and/or atrophy of the tongue, decreased strength and/or motility, and asymmetry of the tongue during rest (to the healthy side) and protrusion (to the affected side)—cranial nerve XII.

Other findings may include dyskinesia or dystonia of the face, jaw, head, and neck; dysarthria; buccofacial apraxia; neglect; attention or memory deficits; and impaired vigilance. Of special importance are pseudobulbar and bulbar signs (see Sect. 1.3).

2.2 Instrumented Methods

The two most important instrumental methods are FEES and VFSS. FEES is dealt with in the chapter "Endoscopy of the Pharynx and Esophagus" by D.-M. Denk and R. Schöfl (this volume). Therefore, only its special role in neurogenic dysphagia is briefly described here.

During *FEES*, the pharyngeal stage is the center of attention with regard to (1) structural abnormalities and sensory deficits (by touching the pharyngeal wall, the epiglottis, or the aryepiglottic fold or by use of FEES with sensory testing), (2) disturbances of control of saliva and/or the ability to swallow real food and liquids, and (3) response to therapeutic interventions such as postural changes. Additionally, showing the video images to the patient and/or to the relatives makes FEES an ideal biofeedback method. In neurological patients with dysphagia, patient outcome with respect to development of pneumonia seems to be similar whether dietary or behavioral management is guided by FEES or VFSS (Aviv et al. 2000). Since with FEES there is no time constraint (because of lacking radiation exposure), FEES can be performed as long as or repeated as often as necessary.

VFSS has many advantages as compared with FEES, among which the most important ones are (1) evaluation of the oral, the pharyngeal, and the esophageal stage, (2) direct visualization of UES opening deficits, (3) accurate measurement of the swallowing reflex/oropharyngeal transition time/swallow response time—usually defined as the interval (in millisesconds) between the first frame showing the apex of the bolus passing the faucial isthmus and the first frame showing anterior movement of the hyoid bone (an interval of more than 500 ms is usually interpreted as oropharyngeal dissociation, which is an important cause of leaking), and (4) visualization of the approximation of the base of the tongue to the posterior pharyngeal wall, which is an important event in the generation of the bolus pressure (see Sect. 1.4).

Manometry of the esophagus and pharynx is dealt with in Chapter. In neurogenic dysphagia, pharyngeal manometry/videomanometry is of special value in patients with opening deficits of the UES. By use of pharyngeal manometry, one can differentiate between primary UES dysfunction (impaired or absent relaxation) and secondary UES opening deficits due to reduced hyolaryngeal excursion and/or impaired bolus pressure. On the basis of certain manometric findings, the indication for cricopharyngeal myotomy (or botulinum toxin injection into the cricopharyngeal muscle) can be made in primary UES dysfunction (see Sect. 3.7.1).

3 Diseases Associated with Neurogenic Dysphagia

This section deals mainly with diseases which are frequently associated with neurogenic dysphagia. For rare causes of dysphagia, *Dysphagia in Rare Conditions* edited by Jones and Rosenbek (2010) is recommended.

3.1 Diseases of the Central Nervous System

3.1.1 Stroke

Stroke is the most frequent cause of dysphagia. The incidence of stroke—comprising brain infarction (80%), intracerebral hemorrhage (15%), and subarachnoidal hemorrhage (5%)—is over 200/100,000 persons per year in industrial countries of the western hemisphere (Hankey and Warlow 1999). According to Mann et al. (2000), dysphagia and aspirations occur in 64% and 22%, respectively, of acute stroke patients as shown videofluoroscopically. About half of these dysphagic patients recover or die within 2 weeks; therefore, about 30% of stroke survivors suffer from chronic dysphagia (Bath et al. 2000). The prognosis is worse in brainstem stroke than in hemispheric stroke: Among dysphagic patients with Wallenberg's syndrome due to dorsolateral medullary infarction who need enteral feeding at the onset, about 30% remain dependent on enteral feeding tubes (Prosiegel et al. 2005b). Whereas in supratentorial stroke leaking of liquids (due to a delayed swallow reflex) is the predominant finding, in medullary stroke various disturbances occur, including unilateral pharyngeal paresis, decreased hyolaryngeal excursion with subsequent secondary opening deficits of the UES, and primary UES dysfunction caused by insufficient relaxation.

A very severe dysphagia develops in bilateral infarctions of the frontoparietal operculum (*bilateral anterior opercular syndrome or Foix–Chavany–Marie syndrome*) with predominant problems in the oral phase (Fig. 2).

Subcortical arteriosclerotic encephalopathy (SAE)—formerly called Binswanger's disease—refers to a combination of periventricular white matter lesions (leukoaraiosis) and lacunar infarction (less than 2 cm in diameter). It is most frequently caused by high

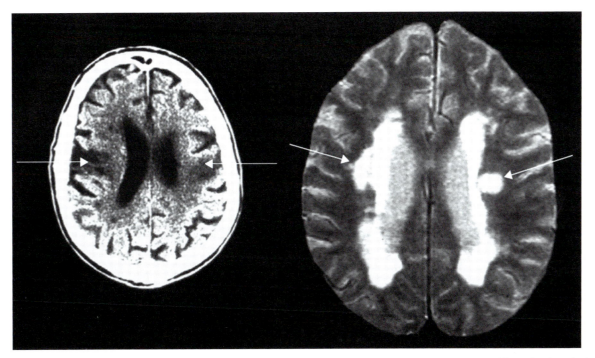

Fig. 2 *Left*: Cranial computed tomography showing bilateral infarctions (*arrows*) in the supply area of the middle cerebral artery affecting the frontoparietal operculum bilaterally causing the so-called bilateral anterior frontoparietal opercular syndrome (Foix-Chavany-Marie syndrome). *Right*: T2-weighted magnetic resonance imaging showing bilateral subcortical infarctions (*arrows*) in a patient with cerebral autosomal dominant arteriopathy with subcortical infarcts and leukoencephalopathy and severy dysphagia; for details, see the text

blood pressure and/or diabetes mellitus; in the case of dementia, it is called subcortical ischemic vascular dementia (SIVD). The severity of subcortical arteriosclerotic encephalopathy/subcortical ischemic vascular dementia is positively correlated with an increase in bolus transit times (Levine et al. 1992) and may, therefore, aggravate or cause swallowing disturbances.

Cerebral autosomal dominant arteriopathy with subcortical infarcts and leukoencephalopathy (CADA-SIL) is a genetic variant of subcortical ischemic vascular dementia and a rare cause of stroke, and occurs mainly in younger persons with a history of migraine. This autosomal dominant genetic disease is associated with mutations in the *NOTCH3* gene on chromosome 19. When the subcortical infarctions are bilaterally situated in the region of the corticobulbar fibers, a severe pseudobulbar palsy may be the consequence (Fig. 2). The diagnosis is made by molecular genetic examination and/or skin biopsy (granular osmiophilic material in dermal arteries as shown by transmission electron microscopy).

Vasculitides are a group of diseases in which inflammatory destruction of vessel walls occurs with consecutive thrombosis or stenosis of (large or small) vessels of the central nervous system (CNS) (and in some types also of the peripheral nervous system). Primary vasculitides comprise giant cell arteritis (temporal arteritis; see below), Takayasu's arteritis (granulomatous arteritis of the aortic arch and its branches, also called "pulseless disease"), polyarteritis nodosa, Wegener's disease/Wegener's granulomatosis (granulomas affecting the kidneys, lungs, and upper respiratory tract, skull base, etc.), Churg–Strauss syndrome (allergic granulomatosis with a history of asthma or allergy), Behçet's disease (uveitis, aphtous ulcers of the mouth and genitals), and isolated or primary CNS vasculitis (see below). In giant cell arteritis/temporal arteritis, besides headache and visual loss, also jaw claudication (pain in the jaw when chewing) as well as tongue claudication (pain in the tongue when chewing) and tongue necrosis may occur. Primary CNS vasculitis/primary angiitis of the CNS is a rare vascular inflammatory disease restricted to the brain and spinal cord of unknown cause; the mean age is 42.48 years at onset of symptoms; the diagnosis of primary CNS vasculitis/

primary angiitis of the CNS is made clinically (head-ache, cerebral infarctions, cognitive dysfunction), by positive leptomeningeal or CNS tissue histopathology and/or cerebral angiography (alternating dilatations and narrowings—also called "beading"—, aneurysms and other irregularities within blood vessels) (for a review, see Kraemer and Berlit 2010). When the infarctions of primary CNS vasculitis/primary angiitis of the CNS affect the dominant swallowing cortex and/or cortico-bulbar fibers, dysphagia may occur. Secondary vascu-litides may complicate other diseases such as connective tissue diseases (see Sect. 3.4.2). For laboratory testing of vasculitides, see Table 1.

When there is a need for *enteral feeding in the acute stroke phase*, a PEG tube should not be inserted to early, i.e., not before about 2 weeks after disease onset: A multicenter randomized controlled trial (Dennis et al. 2005) found that early PEG tube insertion is associated with an increased risk of death or poor outcome (as measured after 6 months with the modified Rankin scale) of 7.8% as compared with early nasogastric feeding. A single-center randomized controlled trial showed that early beginning of high-intensity swallow-ing therapy after stroke (within 7 days) is associated with an increased proportion of patients who returned to a normal diet ($p = 0.04$) and recovered swallowing ($p = 0.02$) by 6 months as compared with "usual care" or low-intensity therapy (Carnaby et al. 2006).

3.1.2 Idiopathic Parkinson Syndrome

The morphologic substrates found in idiopathic Parkinson syndrome (IPS)/Parkinson's disease are intracellular *Lewy bodies* consisting mainly of the protein α-synuclein (therefore IPS belongs to the alpha-synucleinopathies). These inclusion bodies affect not only neurons of the dopaminergic substantia nigra, but also nondopaminergic cells in other brainstem regions such as the pedunculopontine nucleus and the locus ceruleus as well as parasympathic cells of Auerbach's plexus of the esophagus. Therefore, dopaminergic drugs are not very effective with regard to swallowing disturbances in IPS. Deep brain stimulation of the subthalamic nucleus alleviates many symptoms of persons with IPS, but does not influence dysphagic symptoms at all. Deep brain stimulation of the internal pallidum may even cause or aggravate swallowing symptoms. The frequency of dysphagia in IPS increa-ses with the duration of the disease and amounts to over 50%; about half of those affected are (silent) aspirators.

The spontaneous swallowing frequency is decreased and mainly responsible for drooling. Oral and pha-ryngeal symptoms often occur in combination, comprising oral residuals, repetitive pumping motions of the tongue, leaking, piecemeal degluti-tion, residuals in the piriform sinuses, prolonged triggering of the swallow reflex, and UES opening deficits. Aspiration pneumonia is one of the most frequent causes of death in IPS. Manometric studies have shown various esophageal motility disorders in 61–73% of persons with IPS, including decreased peristalsis and diffuse esophageal spasm. The symptoms due to these esophageal disturbances may resemble oropharyngeal problems and should always be kept in mind. As a rule, the diagnosis of IPS is improbable when oropharyngeal dysphagia occurs within the first year after the first symptoms; in those cases, atypical Parkinson syndromes (APS) are the probable cause (for a review, see Pfeiffer 2003).

3.1.3 Atypical Parkinson Syndromes

APS comprise progressive supranuclear palsy (PSP), multiple system atrophy (MSA), dementia with Lewy bodies (DLB), and the rare corticobasal degeneration. DLB and MSA belong to the so-called alpha-synuc-leinopathies such as IPS, but in contrast to IPS, pharmacological interventions against APS symptoms are not very effective.

PSP (*Steele–Richardson–Olszewski syndrome*) is characterized by axial rigidity, dementia, vertical gaze paralysis, postural instability with falls, and dysarthria. Dysphagia occurs initially in about 16% and during the course of the disease in about 83% of persons with PSP (Litvan et al. 1996).

MSA comprises two types. In MSA-P ("P" for "Parkinson"; about 80%)—formerly called striatoni-gral degeneration—parkinsonian symptoms predomi-nate, whereas in MSA-C ("C" for "cerebellar"; about 20%)—formerly called olivopontocerebellar atro-phy—cerebellar symptoms such as gait ataxia are typical. In both types, autonomic disturbances occur, e.g., orthostatic hypotonia and bladder dysfunction. In MSA, neurogenic dysphagia occurs in over 70% of persons (Müller et al. 2001; Higo et al. 2005; O'Sullivan et al. 2008) and laryngeal stridor occurs in over 30% or persons (Yamaguchi et al. 2003).

DLB comprises motor features of parkinsonism, dementia, visual hallucinations, fluctuating course, and hypersensitivity to certain drugs such as

Table 1 Checklist for dysphagia of unknown causes

CIP/CIM/CIPNM, myotonia, myasthenia gravis, LEMS, GBS	Electromyography, repetitive nerve stimulation, motor and sensory nerve conduction studies
MS, neuroborreliosis, CPM/EPM, skull base tumors, Chiari malformations	Cranial CT or MRI
Eagle's syndrome, ventral osteophytes, and/or complications after anterior cervical spine surgery	Lateral cervical radiography, (3D) CT
Diseases of the neuromuscular junction	
Myasthenia gravis	Anti-AChR abs, anti-MuSK abs
LEMS	Anti-VGCC abs
Myositides	Myositis-associated abs such as
PM, DM	Anti-Mi-2 abs, anti-SRP abs, antisynthetase (anti-Jo-1) abs
IBM	Anti-ADDL monoclonal abs
Connective tissue diseases	Antinuclear abs
Sjögren's syndrome	Anti-SS-A/Ro abs, anti-SS-B/La abs
Systemic sclerosis	Anti-scl70/antitopoisomerase abs; anti-PM-Scl abs
MCTD/Sharp's syndrome	Anti-U_1-RNP abs
SLE	Anti-dsDNA abs
Vasculitides	ANCA
Wegener's granulomatosis	Cytoplasmic ANCA (antigen, proteinase 3)
Microscopic polyangiitis	Perinuclear ANCA (antigen, myeloperoxidase)
Churg–Strauss syndrome	Perinuclear ANCA (antigen, myeloperoxidase)
Polyarteritis nodosa	HBsAg (in about 60%)
Polyneuritis cranialis, Miller–Fisher syndrome	Antiganglioside abs against GQ1b or GT1a
Paraneoplastic syndromes	
LEMS	Anti-VGCC abs
Brainstem encephalitis	Anti-Hu, anti-Ri, anti-Ma2 abs
Stiff-person syndrome	Antiamphiphysin, antigephyrin, anti-Ri abs
Idiopathic stiff-person syndrome	Anti-GAD abs
Cerebrospinal fluid examination	Neuroborreliosis, MS, meningitis
CADASIL	Skin biopsy: granular osmiophilic material in dermal arteries (transmission electron microscopy)
Myositides, rare myopathies	Muscle biopsy
CADASIL, SBMA/Kennedy's disease, OPMD	Molecular genetic examination
PCNSV/PACNS	Brain biopsy

CIP critical-illness polyneuropathy, *CIM* critical-illness myopathy, *CIPNM* critical-illness polyneuromyopathy, *LEMS* Lambert–Eaton myasthenic syndrome, *GBS* Guillain–Barré syndrome, *MS* multiple sclerosis, *CPM* central pontine myelinolysis, *EPM* extrapontine myelinolysis , *PM* polymyositis, *DM* dermatomyositis, *IBM* inclusion body myositis, *MCTD* mixed connective tissue disease, *SLE* systemic lupus erythematosus , *CADASIL* cerebral autosomal dominant arteriopathy with subcortical infarcts and leukoencephalopathy, *SBMA* spinobulbar muscular atrophy, *OPMD* oculopharyngeal muscular dystrophy, *PCNSV* primary central nervous system vasculitis, *PACNS* primary angiitis of the central nervous system, *CT* computed tomography, *MRI* magnetic resonance imaging, *AChR* acetylcholine receptor, *abs* antibodies, *MuSK* muscle-specific tyrosine kinase, *dsDNA* double-stranded DNA, *ANCA* antineutrophil cytoplasmic antibodies, *HBsAg* hepatitis B surface antigen, *VGCC* voltage-gated calcium channels, *ADDL* amyloid-β-derived diffusible ligands, *GAD* glutamic acid decarboxylase neuroleptics. Neurogenic dysphagia occurs in over 20% of persons with DLB (Müller et al. 2001).

As compared with IPS, where dysphagia occurs on average after 130 months, swallowing problems develop earlier in APS (PSP, 42 months; MSA, 67 months; DLB, 43 months). After onset of dysphagia, however, the survival time is very similar in IPS, MSA, and PSP (15–24 months) (for a review, see Müller et al. 2001).

3.1.4 Huntington's Disease

Huntington's disease is an autosomal dominant genetic neurodegenerative disease with a prevalence of 2–7/100,000 and disease onset in most cases between the ages of 30–45 years. Beside choreatic movements, personality changes and cognitive decline, and neurogenic dysphagia occur frequently (in over 80%; Edmonds 1966). Tachyphagia and problems with chewing and bolus transfer may be found in the oral phase, but pharyngeal and esophageal disturbances also occur. A differential diagnosis is choreoacanthocytosis. In this autosomal recessive genetic disease including chorea, epilepsy, cognitive decline, and thorny erythrocytes, swallowing problems are characterized by an action-induced tongue protrusion dystonia with widened jaw. Therefore, eating and drinking are very effortful and patients try to compensate for the problem, e.g., by pressing the lips strongly together (for details, see Bader et al. 2010). Pharmacologic therapy against choreic movements includes typical and atypical neuroleptics, benzodiazepines, and the monoamine-depleting agent tetrabenazine.

3.1.5 Dystonia

Among the various types of dystonia, torticollis (cervical dystonia or spasmodic torticollis) is one of the most frequent causes of dysphagia; according to Ertekin et al. (2002) dysphagia occurs in about 70% of patients. In torticollis, the muscles controlling the neck cause sustained twisting. The treatment of choice is botulinum toxin injection.

The combination of oromandibular dystonia and blepharospasmus is called *Meige's or Brueghel's syndrome*, which is often associated with dysphagia. The therapy of choice for the abovementioned dystonias are botulinum toxin injections in the corresponding muscles (neck, masseter muscle and temporalis muscle, lateral pterygoid muscle).

3.1.6 Morbus Wilson

Wilson's disease is a rare (prevalence 1–3/100,000) autosomal recessive genetic disorder with accumulation of copper in various tissues such as liver, cornea, and brain. Clinical symptoms and signs comprise psychiatric problems, cognitive decline, personality changes, symptoms of parkinsonism including a typical hand tremor or dystonia. According to Machado et al. (2006), among 119 patients the following figures for symptoms can be found: dysarthria in 91%, gait disturbances in 75%, dystonia in 69%, rigor in 66%, tremor in 60%, and dysphagia in 50%. The oral, pharyngeal, and esophageal phases may be affected in isolation or in combination. An early diagnosis (low serum copper concentration, high urine copper concentration, liver biopsy, genetic testing) is important, since pharmacological interventions are available with the main aim of removing copper from the body.

3.1.7 Amyotrophic Lateral Sclerosis

ALS is the most common degenerative motoneuron disease of adulthood, with a prevalence of about 7/100,000. It is a disease of unknown cause with combined degeneration of the UMN and the LMN, which occurs in most cases between 50 and 70 years of age; about 90% of cases are sporadic and 10% are genetic (mainly autosomal dominant). UMND causes supranuclear symptoms, also termed "pseudobulbar palsy." LMND affects the cranial nerve nuclei in the pons and medulla oblongata innervating the muscles of the jaw, face, tongue, pharynx, and larynx with subsequent bulbar symptoms of chewing, swallowing, speech, and voice. LMND of the spinal cord may lead to dysphagia as a result of progressive respiratory dysfunction. The survival time ranges on average between 3 and 5 years; in about 25% of cases, the onset is bulbar (bulbar type of ALS; progressive bulbar palsy), with an even worse prognosis. Causal therapy does not exist, but the glutamate antagonist riluzole increases the survival time by about 3 months. Neurogenic dysphagia is very frequent in the course of the disease and occurs in all patients with the bulbar type of ALS. Dysphagic symptoms include problems of the oral phase (with tongue paresis), disturbed pharyngeal peristalsis, and primary or secondary opening deficits of the UES. Swallowing therapy must take into account that too many or long-lasting exercises may exhaust the weakened muscles.

Many ALS patients need thickening of liquids, especially in the case of severely impaired oral control; it has, however, to be considered that thickening may sometimes enhance the swallow effort. When UES dysfunction is a significant problem, thickening may even be dangerous. Since the insertion of a PEG tube is associated with increased morbidity and mortality in patients with a forced vital capacity of less than 60%, patients and relatives have to be informed not too late of the necessity to insert a PEG tube (Kühnlein et al. 2008).

Since type I Chiari malformation, syringobulbia, tumors of the skull base, inclusion body myositis, and spinobulbar muscular atrophy (SBMA; Kennedy's disease) may mimic ALS symptoms, these diseases are important differential diagnoses and are mentioned in this chapter.

3.1.8 Spinal Muscular Atrophies

Spinal muscular atrophies (*SMAs*) are diseases which cause degeneration of spinal and sometimes also of bulbar motoneurons. There are four types of autosomal recessive SMAs affecting the proximal musculature (the distal types are not dealt with here), called SMA types I (Werdnig–Hoffmann disease), II, III, and IV (types III and IV correspond to the juvenile and the adult form of Kugelberg–Welander disease, respectively). According to Messina et al. (2008), in 122 persons with SMA type II (age between 1 and 47 years), chewing problems occurred in 34 patients (28%), impaired jaw opening in 36 patients (30%), and dysphagia in 30 patients (25%). Recently, Cha et al. (2010) described noninvasive treatment interventions against dysphagia in a 25-year-old man with SMA type II.

SBMA (*Kennedy's disease*) is an X-linked genetic disease (hyperexpansion of CAG repeats) which, therefore, occurs almost only in men. As compared with ALS, with which it shares some similarities, such as bulbar symptoms and fasciculations of the facial and body musculature, sensory impairment of spinal and cranial nerves may occur and the course of the disease is slow. Nevertheless, aspiration pneumonia seems to increase the mortality risk in SBMA patients. Laryngeal stridor is much more frequently in SBMA (about 50%) than in ALS (initially 2%, in the course about 19%) (Kühnlein et al. 2008). Because the androgen receptor gene is affected, gynecomastia and testicular atrophy may also occur.

3.1.9 Ataxias

Spinocerebellar ataxias (SCAs) are rare autosomal dominant genetic diseases. According to the chronological order of detection of the gene loci, 26 SCAs can be differentiated (SCA1 to SCA26); in Germany SCA3—also called Machado–Joseph disease—is the most frequent type. Dysphagia occurs most frequently in SCA1, SCA2, SCA3, SCA6, and SCA7; in the last four types mentioned, widespread neurodegeneration of swallowing-relevant brainstem nuclei was found (Rüb et al. 2006). Friedreich's ataxia, the most frequent inherited ataxia, is an autosomal recessive genetic disease (hyperexpansion of GAA repeats), with a prevalence of about 3/100,000. The onset is usually before the age of 20 years. Characteristic features are gait ataxia, dysarthria, sensory symptoms, flaccid pareses of the distal muscles, scoliosis, foot deformity, and hypertrophic cardiomyopathy. In the study of Dürr et al. (1996) on 140 persons with Friedreich's ataxia, dysphagia occurred in 27%. Sporadic ataxias comprise, e.g., alcoholic or paraneoplastic cerebellar atrophy. In sporadic ataxia of unknown origin, the frequency of dysphagia is 38% (Abele et al. 2002).

3.1.10 Tumors of the Brain or the Skull Base

Whether a brain tumor causes neurogenic dysphagia depends on many variables, such as the exact site of the tumor, pressure exerted by the tumor on neighboring structures, and radiation injury of the brain. In the prospective study of Newton et al. (1994) on 117 patients with primary brain tumors, dysphagia occurred in 14.5% (30% of the dysphagias were present before the operation, 30% developed immediately after the intervention, and 40% developed in the course afterwards). In a retrospective study, Wesling et al. (2003) studied 38 patients with brain tumors as compared with a sample of stroke patients who were matched for age, site of lesion, and initial composite cognitive functional independent measure score. Primary (80% malignant) and secondary (metastatic) brain tumors accounted for 83% and 17%, respectively. With regard to outcome(length of stay, total hospital charges, and swallowing status), no statistically significant difference between the tumor and stroke patient groups was found. The authors' conclusion was that patients with brain tumors, including malignant ones, "should be afforded the same type and intensity of rehabilitation for their swallowing that is provided to patients following a stroke."

Tumors of the posterior fossa (fourth ventricle) such as ependymomas and cerebellar pilocytic astrocytomas may cause neurogenic dysphagia after neurosurgical intervention, since during detachment of these tumors from the posterior region of the medulla oblongata, medullary (venous?) bleeding may occur. Owing to consecutive bilateral affection of the dmCPGs, the resulting dysphagia is often very severe (Prosiegel et al. 2005a, b). On the basis of clinical findings after operations of posterior fossa tumors in 121 children, Kirk et al. (1995) described a postoperative syndrome in 19 children, labeled "posterior fossa syndrome" involving mutism or speech disturbances, dysphagia, decreased motor movement, cranial nerve palsies, and emotional lability; these signs and symptoms developed from an average range of 24–107 h after surgery and took weeks to months to resolve.

The outcome of 12 patients with dysphagia after excision of tumors of the skull base was described by Jennings et al. (1992) (five glomus jugulare tumors, one glomus vagale tumor, three acoustic neuromas, and three meningiomas). Aspiration occurred in 75% of patients, and after 2 weeks 58% of the patients were able to tolerate oral intake by use of compensatory swallow techniques and diet modifications.

3.1.11 Multiple Sclerosis

Multiple sclerosis (MS) is an inflammatory CNS disease with high incidence and prevalence rates of 6/100,000 persons per year and 100/100,000, respectively, in industrial countries of the northern hemisphere. Although the cause is still unknown, the autoimmune pathogenesis may be briefly described as follows. Activated lymphocytes penetrate the blood–brain barrier and initiate immunological events such as activation of certain proinflammatory cytokines. Besides demyelination of axons in the white (and gray) matter of the brain and spinal cord, even axonal loss occurs. In about 80% of patients, the disease shows a relapsing–remitting onset, whereas 20% of patients suffer from a primary-progressive course. After some years, about half of the patients with relapsing–remitting MS develop a secondary–progressive MS. Pharmacological approaches include intravenous corticosteroid treatment, intravenous immunoglobulin treatment, and plasmapheresis in the case of relapses; chronic treatment comprises immunotherapy with interferon-β preparations or glatiramer acetate, but also with natalizumab and mitoxantrone in more severe cases. Dysphagia is rarely an isolated, predominant symptom in MS. The prevalence of dysphagia accounts for about 30% of persons with MS and is associated with overall disability and with brainstem signs; about 15% of persons with mild disability may, however, also suffer from dysphagia. There are no swallowing disturbance patterns which are typical for MS; aspiration pneumonia due to dysphagia is among the leading causes of death in persons with MS (Prosiegel et al. 2004).

3.1.12 Central Pontine and Extrapontine Myelinolysis

In *central pontine myelinolysis* (*CPM*), a so-called osmotic demyelination of white matter in the central pons occurs owing to rapid correction of hyponatremia. Also brain areas outside the pons (basal ganglia, cerebellum, thalamus, etc.) may be affected, which is called *extrapontine myelinolysis* (*EPM*). The most frequent disease underlying CPM or EPM is alcoholism. But also liver transplant patients may develop CPM or EPM; in these cases the development of the disease is particularly attributed to the immunosuppressive agent cyclosporine (Lampl and Yazdi 2002). Besides spastic tetraparesis with dysarthria, neurogenic dysphagia occurs very frequently and usually has a good prognosis.

3.1.13 Infectious Diseases of the Central Nervous System

In herpes simplex encephalitis, dysphagia rarely occurs, since the virus affects predominantly the temporal lobes. Stickler et al. (2003) described a patient with dysphagia due to bilateral lesions of the insula and the adjacent operculum caused by viral encephalitis of unknown origin.

Acute encephalitis of the lower brainstem (rhombencephalitis) caused by *Listeria monocytogenes*—a food-borne Gram-positive bacterium—is commonly associated with severe dysphagia. Overall mortality is about 50%, 100% of untreated patients die, and more than 70% of patients treated early with ampicillin or penicillin survive; neurological sequelae develop in about 60% of survivors (Armstrong and Fung 1993; Smiatacz et al. 2006).

Poliomyelitis is a viral disease affecting the motor nuclei of the brainstem and/or the spinal cord. Global polio immunization resulted in eradication of the disease caused by wild-strain polio virus type 2, which has not been detected worldwide since 1999. In polio-free countries, cases and outbreaks are reported owing to imported wild-strain polio virus type 1 or wild-strain polio virus type 3 because of unbroken localized circulation of these types in four polio-endemic countries (Afghanistan, India, Nigeria, and Pakistan). Postpolio syndrome is a condition which develops about 30–40 years after an acute paralytic polio infection in about 50% of formerly affected people. It is characterized by exacerbation of preexisting symptoms or development of new symptoms, including muscle weakness, general fatigue, pain, cold intolerance, and swallowing problems. Sonies and Dalakas (1991) examined 32 patients with postpolio syndrome, among whom 14 persons had new swallowing difficulties; 12 persons had bulbar involvement during acute polio infection. Interestingly, 31 patients had "some abnormality on detailed testing of oropharyngeal function" and "only 2 patients had any signs of aspiration." The authors' conclusion was that "in patients with the post-polio syndrome, the bulbar muscles often have clinical or subclinical signs of dysfunction. These abnormalities suggest that in bulbar neurons there is a slowly progressive deterioration similar to that in the muscles of the limbs."

Human immunodeficiency virus (HIV)—with its two types HIV-1 and HIV-2—belongs to human T-cell lymphotropic virus type III retroviruses. Dysphagias may be due to many causes in infected persons: (1) directly by HIV-based diseases such as HIV-associated encephalopathy, AIDS dementia complex, HIV neuropathy, and HIV myopathy; (2) indirectly by meningitis/encephalitis/encephalopathy caused by fungi (e.g., *Cryptococcus neoformans* and *Candida albicans*), *Toxoplasma gondii*, cytomegalovirus, herpes simplex virus, varicella-zoster virus, mycobacterium, or *Treponema pallidum* or by the JC virus causing progressive multifocal leukoencephalopathy. One should also keep in mind primary CNS lymphomas caused by the Epstein–Barr virus and esophagitis due to candida, cytomegalovirus, and/or herpes simplex virus.

Neuroborreliosis is caused by *Borrelia burgdorferi* transmitted by ticks. In the second and third stages of the disease, dysphagia may occur (Velázquez et al. 1999). Neuroborreliosis can mimic symptoms of other diseases such as MS and is, therefore, an important

differential diagnosis. It can successfully be treated by use of antibiotics.

3.1.14 Chiari Malformations

Most important in the context of adult patients with dysphagia is type I Chiari malformation with herniation of the cerebellar tonsils below the foramen magnum and elongation of the medulla oblongata. Dysphagia may occur as the sole manifestation of adult type I Chiari malformation and may mimic a bulbar palsy in ALS; probably, in those cases dysphagia is caused by pressure exerted by the cerebellar mass on the hypoglossal nuclei and/or on the CPGs (Paulig and Prosiegel 2002). Neurosurgical posterior fossa decompression is necessary in symptomatic cases.

3.1.15 Syringomyelia and Syringobulbia

Syringomyelia is a congenital or acquired (e.g., after trauma) cavitation of the central part of the spinal cord, in most cases in its cervical region; syringobulbia may be an isolated idiopathic form or caused by the extension of a cervical syrinx (Greek word for "flute") into the medulla oblongata. In syringobulbia, the most frequent symptoms are headache, vertigo, dysphonia, dysarthria, trigeminal paraesthesia, diplopia, and dysphagia; dysphagia is caused by atrophy and weakness of the soft palate, the pharynx, or the tongue owing to pressure exerted by the syrinx on the ambiguous or hypoglossal nuclei. Neurosurgical intervention is necessary depending on the severity of the symptoms.

3.1.16 Paraneoplastic Syndromes of the Central Nervous System

With respect to dysphagia, paraneoplastic brainstem encephalitis is of special importance. Most frequently in patients with small cell lung carcinoma, an anti-Hu syndrome may occur with positive anti-Hu antibodies—also called antineuronal nuclear autoantibody type 1. Saiz et al. (2009) reported on 22 patients with anti-Hu-associated brainstem encephalitis, of whom seven suffered from dysphagia. Paraneoplastic brainstem encephalitis due to anti-Ri antibodies (antineuronal nuclear autoantibody type 2) is in most cases found in women with breast cancer or persons with small cell lung carcinoma and may also cause dysphagia (Pittock et al. 2003). Patients with anti-Ma2-associated (brainstem) encephalitis suffer frequently (more than 50%) from testicular germ-cell tumors. Stiff-person syndrome is characterized by rigidity of the trunk and proximal limb muscles, intermittent spasms, and increased sensitivity to external stimuli. Antibodies against glutamic acid decarboxylase are frequently found. Stiff-person syndrome of paraneoplastic origin accounts for about 5% of cases and is associated with antiamphiphysin, antigephyrin, and anti-Ri antibodies. Dysphagia may occur in stiff-person syndrome, but reports on its prevalence are lacking (Bhutani 1991, Chen 1992).

3.2 Diseases of the Cranial Nerves

3.2.1 Guillain–Barré Syndrome and Variants

Guillain–Barré syndrome (GBS) is an acute, acquired, monophasic autoimmune disorder of peripheral nerves including cranial nerves such as cranial nerve VII. GBS develops frequently about 2 weeks after respiratory (e.g., caused by cytomegalovirus) or gastrointestinal (e.g., caused by *Campylobacter jejuni*) infections, operations or less frequently after vaccination (influenza, hepatitis B, or rabies vaccine; Souayah et al. 2007). GBS is the most common cause of acute ascending flaccid sensorimotor paralysis. An elevated cerebrospinal fluid protein level without elevation of the level of lymphocytes is typically found (albuminocytological dissociation). The most frequently occurring type of GBS is acute inflammatory demyelinating polyradiculoneuropathy. After *Campylobacter jejuni* enteritis, the prognosis of GBS seems to be worse than after other infections, since there is acute motor axonal damage (acute motor axonal neuropathy). Chen et al. (1996) found in a videofluoroscopic study on 14 GBS patients neurogenic dysphagia in all cases; five patients with moderate–severe dysphagia were reexamined and showed a light–moderate dysphagia 4–8 weeks later. Variants of GBS (1–5%) are Miller–Fisher syndrome and polyneuritis cranialis. Miller–Fisher syndrome is characterized by an external ophthalmoplegia, cerebellar ataxia, areflexia, and frequently also by neurogenic dysphagia. In polyneuritis cranialis, a bilateral affection of the caudal cranial nerves with consecutive neurogenic dysphagia occurs. In Miller–Fisher syndrome and polyneuritis cranialis, serum antiganglioside antibodies (against GQ1b or GT1a) are often present. In a chronic variant of GBS, the so-called *chronic inflammatory demyelinating polyradiculoneuropathy*, cranial nerves are involved in up to 20% of patients, but neurogenic dysphagia occurs rarely (Mazzucco et al. 2006). Therapeutic options in GBS and its variants include intravenous administration of immunoglobulins (5-day course of 0.4 g/kg/day) and plasma exchange.

3.2.2 Tumors

Tumors of cranial nerves IX, X, or XII such as glossopharyngeal, vagal and hypoglossal neurinomas cause mild–moderate dysphagia including palatal, pharyngeal, and lingual hemiparesis, respectively (Prosiegel et al. 2005b). Dysphagia may be more severe in cases of affection of more than one caudal cranial nerve; examples are tumors of the skull base including the region of the jugular foramen (Oestreicher-Kedem et al. 2010) such as meningiomas, chondromas, and glomus jugulare tumors (see Sect. 3.1.10).

3.2.3 Eagle's Syndrome

An elongated styloid process (unilaterally or bilaterally) occurs in about 2–4% of healthy persons; only 4–10% of these persons are, however, symptomatic (Murtagh et al. 2001) and develop symptoms of the so-called Eagle's syndrome: masticatory pain, globus sensation, neuropathic pharyngeal or facial pain, odynophagia, and dysphagia. Eagle's syndrome may follow tonsillectomy or trauma. Diagnosis is confirmed by lateral cervical radiograph, (three-dimensional) computed tomography scan, palpation of the styloid process in the tonsillar fossa, and/or infiltration with anesthesia. Therapy depends on the predominant symptoms, i.e., analgesic therapy in the case of pain or—provided that pain relief by local anesthesia is proven—surgical removal of elongated styloid processes. The severity of symptoms does not seem to correlate with the degree of elongation of the styloid processes (for a review, see Piagkou et al. 2009; for a case report with computed tomography scan, see Akhaddar et al. 2010).

3.3 Diseases of the Neuromuscular Junction

The two most important types are myasthenia gravis and Lambert–Eaton myasthenic syndrome.

3.3.1 Myasthenia Gravis

Adult-onset myasthenia gravis is an acquired autoimmune disorder. Antibodies against the acetylcholine receptor (AChR) of the muscle endplate are present in 80–90% of patients with generalized myasthenia gravis. These anti-AChR antibodies do not only block the AChRs, they are also able to destroy them. The incidence and prevalence of myasthenia gravis are about 0.2–0.5/100,000 persons per year and 5–20/100,000, respectively. The characteristic features are muscle weakness worsening on exertion/during the course of the day and improving with rest; typically, proximal muscles and muscles of the eyes as well as chewing and swallowing muscles are predominantly affected. Therefore, besides proximal muscle weakness also ptosis, diplopia, and dysphagia are frequent findings. Dysphagia occurs in about 20% of patients as the initial symptom and in about 50% of patients in the course of myasthenia gravis. In most cases, myasthenia gravis can be treated successfully by use of cholinesterase inhibitors such as pyridostigmine (by increasing the concentration of acetylcholine) with the aim of improving neuromuscular junction transmission, corticosteroids, and immunosuppressants, as well as intravenously administered immunoglobulins or plasmapheresis. In patients younger than 60 years or in patients with thymomas, thymectomy might be indicated. In some patients with predominant oculobulbar symptoms, the efficacy of pharmacological interventions seems to be less; the role of muscle-specific tyrosine kinase antibodies in these cases may play a role, which is, however, not fully understood (Farrugia and Vincent 2010).

3.3.2 Lambert–Eaton Myasthenic Syndrome

Lambert–Eaton myasthenic syndrome is rare and occurs more frequently in men than in women. Its origin is paraneoplastic in over 60% of cases (small cell lung cancer in most cases) and then caused by antibodies against voltage-gated calcium channels at presynaptic nerve endings with consecutive impaired synaptic release of acetylcholine. Proximal lower limb girdle weakness is a typical finding. In the course of the disease, ptosis, double vision, and dysphagia may occur. The frequency of dysphagia ranges in the literature between 24 and 34% (Payne et al. 2005). Use of 3,4-diaminopyridine, intravenously administered immunoglobulins, and immunosuppressants, plasmapheresis, and the removal of an underlying tumor are therapeutic options.

3.4 Diseases of the Muscles

This section deals with the most frequent muscle diseases which are frequently associated with dysphagia (for myopathies caused by endocrine or metabolic disorders and for rare types of myopathies including those due to mitochondrial respiratory chain disorders, see specialist literature).

3.4.1 Muscular Dystrophies

The most frequent late-onset muscular dystrophies are myotonic dystrophies. *Myotonic dystrophy type 1 (DM1; Curschmann–Steinert disease)* is an autosomal dominant disorder and is caused by an expansion of a CTG trinucleotide repeat (chromosome 19, long arm, subband 13.3); the European prevalence is 3–15/100,000. The disease affects distal skeletal muscles, smooth muscles, the eyes, the heart, the endocrine system, and the CNS. Depending on the severity of DM1, symptoms comprise cataract, myotonia (sustained muscle contraction), muscle atrophy, cardiac conduction abnormalities, and dysphagia. Myotonic dystrophy type 2 (Ricker syndrome) is also an autosomal dominant genetic disorder and is caused by an expansion of the CCTG repeat (chromosome 3, long arm, band 21), but occurs more rarely than DM1. Myotonic dystrophy type 2 affects predominantly proximal muscles and is, therefore, also called proximal myotonic myopathy. Dysphagia is common in DM1, with reported frequencies of about 70% and with frequently occurring UES opening deficits (Ertekin et al. 2001); esophageal motility disorders may also occur in DM1 (Eckardt et al. 1986).

The rare autosomal dominant *oculopharyngeal muscular dystrophy* (OPMD) is caused by expansion of GCG repeats (long arm of chromosome 14) and begins in the fifth or sixth decade of life (Brais et al. 1999). Oculopharyngeal muscular dystrophy is characterized by slowly progressive ptosis and dysphagia. The severity of dysphagia correlates positively with the progression of ptosis. This is mainly caused by retroflexion of the neck which compensates the ptosis ("astrologist's view"), but aggravates dysphagia (de Swart et al. 2006).

The X-linked *Duchenne muscular dystrophy* affects male children and is associated with high frequencies of dysphagia in the advanced stage—30 of 31 patients with a mean age of 19.9 years in the study of Hanayama et al. (2008). The X-linked

Becker–Kiener muscular dystrophy is rarer than Duchenne muscular dystrophy and has a much more benign disease course. The autosomal dominant facioscapulohumeral muscular dystrophy is a rare muscular dystrophy with slow disease progression and predominant affection of the muscles of the face and shoulder; according to the study of Stübgen (2008), dysphagia occurred in eight of 20 patients— with oropharyngeal symptoms in five patients and esophageal symptoms in three patients.

3.4.2 Inflammatory Muscle Diseases

In adult patients, the most frequent inflammatory muscle diseases are polymyositis, dermatomyositis, and sporadic inclusion body myositis.

Polymyositis and *dermatomyositis* belong to the so-called connective-tissue diseases comprising systemic lupus erythematosus, rheumatoid arthritis, diffuse systemic sclerosis/scleroderma, and Sjögren's syndrome. In mixed connective-tissue disease (Sharp's syndrome, overlap syndrome) features of various connective-tissue diseases coexist and overlap. Polymyositis and dermatomyositis are more frequent in women than in men and their onset is acute or subacute with weakness of proximal muscles (e.g., shoulder region); various types of antinuclear antibodies can be found. A paraneoplastic pathogenesis is more frequent in dermatomyositis than in polymyositis.

Sporadic inclusion body myositis, the most frequent myositis in adulthood, is associated with weakness and atrophy of distal muscles, a feature which may initially mimic ALS. Amyloid β_{42} is more cytotoxic than amyloid β_{40} and its concentration has been shown to be preferentially increased in sporadic inclusion body myositis muscle fibers; monoclonal antibodies against "amyloid-β-derived diffusible ligands" seem to play a pathogenic role (Nogalska et al. 2010). Dysphagia is very frequent in inclusion body myositis, where it occurs in about 80% of patients (Houser et al., 1998). Among 62 patients with dysphagia due to myositis, 26 patients suffered from inclusion body myositis, 18 patients suffered from dermatomyositis, nine patients suffered from polymyositis, and nine patients suffered from an overlap syndrome; in 13 patients (21%) dysphagia was the initial symptom (11 of these 13 patients suffered from inclusion body myositis)

(Oh et al. 2007). The response of polymyositis and dermatomyositis to therapeutic approaches including use of corticosteroids, immunosuppressants, and intravenously administered immunoglobulins is good as compared with inclusion body myositis with poor response.

Other inflammatory muscle diseases are rare at least in industrial countries of the western hemisphere. Examples are trichinosis and cysticercosis as well as viral (e.g., HIV myositis) or bacterial causes.

3.4.3 Complications of Prolonged Mechanical Ventilation and/or Sepsis

Ajemian et al. (2001) examined 48 patients by use of videoendoscopy in whom prolonged mechanical ventilation was performed for at least 48 h; 56% suffered from dysphagia, with silent aspirations in 25%. These results are similar to those of the study of Tolep et al. (1996), who found dysphagia in 80% of 35 patients with prolonged mechanical ventilation. The cause of dysphagia in these patients is unclear.

Critical-illness polyneuropathy and *critical-illness myopathy*, which are—owing to a lack of diagnostic criteria for each syndrome—also called *critical-illness polyneuromyopathy* (*CIPNM*) and *critical-illness myopathy and neuropathy* (*CRIMYN*), are monophasic and self-limited diseases occurring in about 50–70% of patients treated in intensive care units because of sepsis or systemic inflammatory response syndrome. Characteristic features of CIPNM/CRIMYN are delayed weaning from the respirator owing to weakness of respiratory musculature, flaccid tetraparesis, and a prolonged mobilization phase. In the pathogenesis, inflammatory factors mediating systemic inflammatory response syndrome as well as drugs such as steroids and neuromuscular blocking agents seem to be involved (for a review, see Hund 2001). Dysphagia occurs in CIPNM/CRIMYN, but there are no reports on incidence or prevalence rates. Since in patients with CIPNM/CRIMYN septic encephalopathy also occurs frequently, it is sometimes difficult to differentiate whether neurogenic dysphagia is caused by CIPNM/CRIMYN and/or by the encephalopathy. From my experience, the restitution of swallowing problems in patients with CIPNM/CRIMYN is rather good.

3.5   Iatrogenic Causes

3.5.1   Drugs

A lot of pharmacological interventions may cause dysphagia or aggravate preexisting swallowing problems. Sedatives such as benzodiazepines may suppress cortical or brainstem control of swallowing. Drugs which impair neuromuscular junction transmission can cause weakness of swallowing muscles or aggravate myasthenic symptoms; examples are aminogylosides and D-penicillamine. A drug-induced myopathy may be caused, e.g., by corticosteroids, colchicine, the antiretroviral drug ziduvidine, cholesterol-lowering agents such as statins and fibrates, amiodarone, cyclosporin, etc. (Walsh and Amato 2005). Certain neuroleptics (e.g., haloperidol) or the antiemetic agent metoclopramide may cause dysphagia via extrapyramidal symptoms due to dopamine antagonistic action. Anticholinergic agents or drugs with anticholinergic side effects (e.g., the antidepressant amitriptyline) may influence swallowing by CNS effects (e.g., confusion) or via xerostomia. Drug-induced esophageal injury may be induced by tetracyclines, nonsteroidal anti-inflammatory agents, potassium chloride, quinidine sulfate, and bisphosphonates (Zografos et al. 2009). Botulinum toxin may cause dysphagia after injection into neck muscles, e.g., in patients with torticollis, into the thyroarytenoid muscle in the case of adductor spasmodic dyshonia or into the cricopharyngeal muscle because of primary UES dysfunction (the author of this chapter knows three patients who developed bilateral vocal fold paresis after botulinum toxin injection into the cricopharyngeal muscle), into the lateral pterygoid muscle in patients with oromandibular motor disorders, and into the tensor veli palatini muscle in the case of essential palatal tremor. The probability of these complications is injection-site-specific (e.g., more common with injection into pterygoid or palatal muscles as compared with neck muscles). In the case of torticollis, dysphagia induced by botulinum toxin occurs in about 6% of patients on average 9.7 days after injection, with a duration of about 3.5 weeks (Kessler et al. 1999).

3.5.2   Carotid Endarterectomy

According to the study of Cunningham et al. (2004) on 1739 patients undergoing carotid endartectomy, 88 motor cranial nerve injuries occurred; since the deficit

had resolved in 23 patients by hospital discharge, 3.7% of patients had a residual cranial nerve injury: 27 hypoglossal, 17 marginal mandibular, 17 recurrent laryngeal, one accessory nerve, and three Horner syndrome; in nine patients the deficit was present at 4-month follow-up examination; none of the persisting deficits resolved during the subsequent follow up (1 year); duration of operation longer than 2 h was associated with an increased risk of cranial nerve injury. In the case of a postoperative combination of ipsilateral vocal cord and pharyngeal hemiparesis (with consecutive dysphagia), the term "double trouble" is used (hoarseness and dysphagia). According to a study on 14 patients with "double trouble" (AbuRahma and Lim 1996), after Teflon injections to medialize the paralyzed vocal cord and a cricopharyngeal myotomy to restore swallowing and alleviate aspiration, "13 of 14 patients had satisfactory outcomes, including normal voice and swallowing."

3.5.3   Anterior Cervical Spine Surgery

Martin et al. (1997) studied retrospectively 13 patients with new-onset dysphagia after anterior cervical spine surgery. They found the following dysphagia patterns: prevertebral soft tissue swelling near the surgical site with deficient posterior pharyngeal wall movement and impaired UES opening in two patients, absent or weak pharyngeal phase in five patients (with consecutive aspiration in three cases), problems in the oral preparatory and oral stages of swallowing, including deficient bolus formation and reduced tongue propulsive action in four patients, and impaired oral preparatory and oral phases with a weak pharyngeal swallow combined with prevertebral swelling in two patients. Owing to postoperative swelling/edema or hematoma, transitory odynophaga is frequent. The study of Lee et al. (2007) is very interesting, since the authors examined 310 patients over a period of 2 years. The frequencies of dysphagia were 54.0, 33.6, 18.6, 15.2, and 13.6% after 1, 2, 6, 12, and 24 months, respectively. Three negative predictors with regard to the onset of dysphagia within 2 years were found: female gender, revision surgeries, and multilevel surgeries. During history taking, it is important to ask for cervical spine surgery, even if it was performed many years ago: Vanderveldt and Young (2004) described a patient in whom many months after anterior cervical spine surgery a symptomatic esophageal stricture at the level of the cervical hardware was found (scar? graft extrusion?); in addition, the authors mentioned cases in the literature with new onset of dysphagia due to various complications after anterior cervical spine surgery.

3.5.4 Radiochemotherapy for Head and Neck Cancers

Irradiation of oropharyngeal tumors often causes xerostomia, mucositis, altered taste, edema and indurations of the soft tissue, altered sensation, and trismus. These side effects may lead to dysphagia or aggravate preexisting swallowing problems. Especially, subcutaneous indurations impair hyolaryngeal excursion with consecutive UES opening deficits and other problems.

In the pathogenesis of neurogenic dysphagia, however, radiation-related cranial nerve palsy plays the most important role. It is assumed that irradiation-induced fibroses of the affected tissue cause nerve lesions directly via pressure and/or secondarily by reduced vascular supply. Lin et al. (2002) studied 19 patients in whom tumors of the nasopharynx were irradiated. Cranial nerve XII (hypoglossal) was affected most frequently ($n = 17$; bilaterally, $n = 7$), cranial nerve X (vagal) was lesioned in 11 patients (bilaterally, $n = 2$), and affection of the recurrent laryngeal nerve occurred in six patients (bilaterally, $n = 5$) and that of cranial nerve XI occurred in two patients (bilaterally). The latency between irradiation and affection of cranial nerves showed a range between 12 and 240 months! An additional chemotherapy enhances the severity of radiation-related sequelae (Caudell et al. 2009). Nguyen et al. (2004) studied 55 patients with combined chemoradiation due to cancers of the oropharynx (29 patients), larynx (11 patients), oral region (six patients), hypopharynx (five patients), and nasopharynx (four patients); the frequencies of dysphagia and aspirations were 45 and 36%, respectively. New methods of radiation therapy such as intensity-modulated radiation therapy reduce the frequency and severity of chronic dysphagia and via parotid gland sparing also of xerostomia (Anand et al. 2008; van Rij et al. 2008).

3.6 Special Diagnostic Approaches

In neurogenic dysphagia of known origin, laboratory findings and other diagnostic results may help to confirm the diagnosis and more importantly to monitor the treatment. For example, in polymyositis serum creatine kinase level is usually elevated and the dose of corticosteroids and other drugs can be lowered in the case of normalization of this muscle enzyme.

In some cases the origin of neurogenic dysphagia is unknown; this occurs frequently when swallowing problems are the sole symptoms at disease onset, e.g., in inclusion body myositis. In suspected inclusion body myositis, a muscle biopsy is the next diagnostic step. In such situations it is highly recommended to use a checklist in order not to forget any of the many causes and the corresponding diagnostic tools.

In clinical routine, the following blood/serum parameters should be assessed: complete blood counts, besides routine serum values also creatine kinase (e.g., elevated level in myositis, temporal arteritis), calcium, potassium, sodium, and copper levels, erythrocyte sedimentation rate, and C-reactive protein level (both, e.g., usually elevated in temporal arteritis), vitamin B_{12} and folic acid levels, thyroid screening, and serologic tests for syphilis and Lyme disease (elevated IgG or IgM levels in the serum do not prove neuroborreliosis, which can only be conformed by cerebrospinal fluid examination).

For details see the checklist in Table 1, which does not of course contain all possible causes, but contains at least the most frequent ones.

3.7 Therapy

3.7.1 Interventions Against Dysfunction of the Upper Esophageal Sphincter

Primary UES dysfunction is caused by impaired/lacking relaxation of the UES, which occurs most frequently in brainstem lesions and Parkinson's disease (Williams et al. 2002). In such cases, cricopharyngeal myotomy may be indicated, dependent on certain videomanometric findings (Kelly 2000; Williams et al. 2002). Botulinum toxin injection into the cricopharyngeal muscle is a reversible alternative approach. The available data pool is much better with regard to cricopharyngeal myotomy as compared with botulinum toxin injection. In botulinum toxin studies, the patient groups are small; the largest and most recent study (Alfonsi et al. 2010) consisted of 34 patients with quite different neurological diseases (stroke, ten patients; PSP, nine patients; IPS, seven patients; MSA, five patients; MS, two patients; ataxia telangiectasia, one patient), of whom 50% "showed a significant improvement" after a transcutaneous injection of 15 Botox units into the cricopharyngeal muscle; the dose of botulinum toxin ranges in different studies between 30 and 360 Dysport equivalent units (Chiu et al. 2004). The assumption that effective cricopharyngeal botulinum toxin injection might predict good results after cricopharyngeal myotomy seems logical, but is not confirmed by study results. Balloon dilatation of the UES works best in patients with fibrosis of the sphincter (Kelly 2000) and can, therefore, not be recommended in patients with neurogenic dysphagia.

3.7.2 Pharmacotherapy and New Therapeutic Approaches

When causal therapy of the underlying disease (e.g., myasthenia gravis) is possible, dysphagia responds in most cases to about the same extent as the other symptoms. An exception is, e.g., IPS, where dopaminergic drugs are not very effective with regard to dysphagia and deep brain stimulation of the subthalamic nucleus does not influence swallowing problems at all as compared with other symptoms of the disease, since besides dopaminergic neurons also nondopaminergic swallowing-relevant cells of the brainstem are affected in IPS (see Sect. 3.1.2).

Unfortunately, specific pharmacological interventions against neurogenic dysphagia are not available. But for some years, research has focused on *substance P (SP)* and on drugs which enhance its concentration, because SP facilitates swallowing and protective cough. Its concentration is decreased in many body compartments (e.g., sputum, serum) in silent aspirators; therefore, drugs such as *angiotensin-converting enzyme (ACE) inhibitors*, which inhibit degradation of SP and thus cause an increase of its concentration, may be effective (for a review, see Ramsey et al. 2005). Also, dopamine stimulates the synthesis of SP and amantadin acts by releasing dopamine from dopaminergic nerve terminals. In a randomized, but not placebo-controlled study (100 mg *amantadine* per day vs. no therapy) on 163 dysphagic stroke patients, Nakagawa et al. (1999) compared the frequency of pneumonia 3 years after disease onset: the frequencies were 6% versus 28% in the treated versus the untreated group. In a randomized placebo-controlled multicenter trial with 6,105 patients with a history of stroke, the ACE inhibitor perindopril was compared with placebo with regard to pneumonia rate after a median follow-up of 3.9 years: in the whole study population, the frequency of pneumonia was 3.8% in the perindopril group and 4.7% under placebo (relative risk reduction of 19%; $p = 0.09$), whereas in participants of Asian origin there was a significant relative risk reduction of 47% ($p = 0.009$); this difference seems to be caused by ACE allele polymorphism (Ohkubo et al. 2004). According to the principles of evidence-based medicine, drugs such as amantadine, L-dopa, and perindopril can, therefore, be applied only in individual patients after stroke and with a low grade of recommendation.

With regard to pharmacotherapy, the main problem is that randomized placebo-controlled multicenter trials in large patient populations are still lacking. This underscores the necessity of swallowing therapy (see Chapter by S. Hamdy in this volume) as well a new approaches such as electrical stimulation of the pharynx and repetitive transcranial magnetic stimulation (see Chapter by S. Hamdy in this volume).

References

Abele M, Bürk K, Schöls L, Schwartz S, Besenthal I, Dichgans J, Zühlke C, Riess O, Klockgether T (2002) The aetiology of sporadic adult-onset ataxia. Brain 125:961–968

AbuRahma AF, Lim RY (1996) Management of vagus nerve injury after carotid endarterectomy. Surgery 119:245–247

Ajemian MS, Nirmul GB, Anderson MT, Zirlen DM, Kwasnik EM (2001) Routine fiberoptic endoscopic evaluation of swallowing following prolonged intubation: implications for management. Arch Surg 136:434–437

Akhaddar A, Elasri A, Zalagh M, Boucetta M (2010) Eagle's syndrome (elongated styloid process). Intern Med 49:1259

Alfonsi E, Merlo IM, Ponzio M, Montomoli C, Tassorelli C, Biancardi C, Lozza A, Martignoni E (2010) An electrophysiological approach to the diagnosis of neurogenic dysphagia: implications for botulinum toxin treatment. J Neurol Neurosurg Psychiatry 81:54–60

Anand AK, Chaudhoory AR, Shukla A, Negi PS, Sinha SN, Babu AA, Munjal RK, Dewan AK, Kumar K, Doval DC, Vaid AK (2008) Favourable impact of intensity-modulated radiation therapy on chronic dysphagia in patients with head and neck cancer. Br J Radiol 81:865–871

Armstrong RW, Fung PC (1993) Brainstem encephalitis (rhombencephalitis) due to *Listeria monocytogenes*: case report and review. Clin Infect Dis 16:689–702

Aviv JE, Kaplan ST, Thomson JE, Spitzer J, Diamond B, Close LG (2000) The safety of flexible endoscopic evaluation of swallowing with sensory testing (FEESST): an analysis of 500 consecutive evaluations. Dysphagia 15:39–44

Bader B, Walker RH, Vogel M, Prosiegel M, McIntosh J, Danek A (2010) Tongue protrusion and feeding dystonia: a hallmark of chorea-acanthocytosis. Mov Disord 25:127–129

Barritt AW, Smithard DG (2009) Role of cerebral cortex plasticity in the recovery of swallowing function following dysphagic Stroke. Dysphagia 24:83–90

Bath PM, Bath FJ, Smithard DG (2000) Interventions for dysphagia in acute stroke. Cochrane Database Syst Rev (2):CD000323

Bhutani MS (1991) Dysphagia in stiff-man syndrome. Am J Gastroenterol 86:1857–1858

Brais B, Rouleau GA, Bouchard JP, Fardeau M, Tomé FM (1999) Oculopharyngeal muscular dystrophy. Semin Neurol 19:59–66

Carnaby G, Hankey GJ, Pizzi J (2006) Behavioural intervention for dysphagia in acute stroke: a randomised controlled trial. Lancet Neurol 5:31–37

Caudell JJ, Schaner PE, Meredith RF, Locher JL, Nabell LM, Carroll WR, Magnuson JS, Spencer SA, Bonner JA (2009) Factors associated with long-term dysphagia after definitive radiotherapy for locally advanced head-and-neck cancer. Int J Radiat Oncol Biol Phys 73:410–415

Cha TH, Oh DW, Shim JH (2010) Noninvasive treatment strategy for swallowing problems related to prolonged nonoral feeding in spinal muscular atrophy type II. Dysphagia 25:261–264

Chen BJ (1992) Clinical analysis of 30 cases of stiff-man syndrome. Zhonghua Shen Jing Jing Shen Ke Za Zhi 25:363–365

Chen MY, Donofrio PD, Frederick MG, Ott DJ, Pikna LA (1996) Videofluoroscopic evaluation of patients with Guillain-Barré syndrome. Dysphagia 11:11–13

Chiu MJ, MD Chang YC, Hsiao TY (2004) Prolonged effect of botulinum toxin injection in the treatment of cricopharyngeal dysphagia: case report and literature review. Dysphagia 19:52–57

Cunningham EJ, Bond R, Mayberg MR, Warlow CP, Rothwell PM (2004) Risk of persistent cranial nerve injury after carotid endarterectomy. J Neurosurg 101:445–448

Daniels SK (2000) Swallowing apraxia: a disorder of the praxis system? Dysphagia 15:159–166

Daniels SK, McAdam CP, Brailey K, Foundas AL (1997) Clinical assessment of swallowing and prediction of dysphagia severity. Am J Speech Lang Pathol 6:17–24

de Swart BJ, van der Sluijs BM, Vos AM, Kalf JG, Knuijt S, Cruysberg JR, van Engelen BG (2006) Ptosis aggravates dysphagia in oculopharyngeal muscular dystrophy. J Neurol Neurosurg Psychiatry 77:266–268

Dennis MS, Lewis SC, Warlow C, FOOD Trial Collaboration (2005) Effect of timing and method of enteral tube feeding for dysphagic stroke patients (FOOD): a multicentre randomised controlled trial. Lancet 365:764–772

Doggett DL, Turkelson CM, Coates VC (2002) Recent developments in diagnosis and intervention for aspiration and dysphagia in stroke and other neuromuscular disorders. Curr Atheroscler Rep 4:311–318

Doty RW, Bosma JR (1956) An electromyographic analysis of reflex deglutition. J Neurophysiol 19:44–60

Dürr A, Cossee M, Agid Y, Campuzano V, Mignard C, Penet C, Mandel JL, Brice A, Koenig M (1996) Clinical and genetic abnormalities in patients with Friedreich's ataxia. N Engl J Med 335:1169–1175

Eckardt VF, Nix W, Kraus W, Bohl J (1986) Esophageal motor function in patients with muscular dystrophy. Gastroenterology 90:628–635

Edmonds C (1966) Huntington's chorea, dysphagia and death. Med J Aust 2:273–274

Ekberg O, Olsson R (1995) The pharyngoesophageal segment: functional disorders. Dis Esophagus 8:252–256

Ertekin C, Yüceyar N, Aydogdu Karasoy H (2001) Electrophysiological evaluation of oropharyngeal swallowing in myotonic dystrophy. J Neurol Neurosurg Psychiatry 70:363–371

Ertekin C, Aydogdu I, Seçil Y, Kiylioglu N, Tarlaci S, Ozdemirkiran T (2002) Oropharyngeal swallowing in craniocervical dystonia. J Neurol Neurosurg Psychiatry 73:406–411

Farrugia ME, Vincent A (2010) Autoimmune mediated neuromuscular junction defects. Curr Opin Neurol 23:489–495

Finestone HM, Greene-Finestone LS, Wilson ES, Teasell RW (1996) Prolonged length of stay and reduced functional improvement rate in malnourished stroke rehabilitation patients. Arch Phys Med Rehabil 77:340–345

Gariballa SE, Parker SG, Taub N, Castleden CM (1998) Influence of nutritional status on clinical outcome after acute stroke. Am J Clin Nutr 68:275–281

Hamdy S, Aziz Q, Rothwell JC, Singh KD, Barlow J, Hughes DG, Tallis RC, Thompson DG (1996) The cortical topography of human swallowing musculature in health and disease. Nat Med 2:1217–1224

Hamdy S, Rothwell JC, Brooks DJ, Bailey D, Aziz Q, Thompson DG (1999) Identification of the cerebral loci processing human swallowing with H2(15)O PET activation. J Neurophysiol 81:1917–1926

Hanayama K, Liu M, Higuchi Y, Fujiwara T, Tsuji T, Hase K, Ishihara T (2008) Dysphagia in patients with Duchenne muscular dystrophy evaluated with a questionnaire and videofluorography. Disabil Rehabil 30:517–522

Hankey GJ, Warlow CP (1999) Treatment and secondary prevention of stroke: evidence, costs, and effects on individuals and populations. Lancet 354:1457–1463

Higo R, Nito T, Tayama N (2005) Swallowing function in patients with multiple-system atrophy with a clinical predominance of cerebellar symptoms (MSA-C). Eur Arch Otorhinolaryngol 262:646–650

Hinchey JA, Shephard T, Furie K, Smith D, Wang D, Tonn S, Stroke Practice Improvement Network Investigators (2005) Formal dysphagia screening protocols prevent pneumonia. Stroke 36:1972–1976

Houser SM, Calabrese LH, Strome M (1998) Dysphagia in patients with inclusion body myositis. Am J Med 108(Suppl 4a):43S–46S

Huckabee ML, Deecke L, Cannito MP, Gould HJ, Mayr W (2003) Cortical control mechanisms in volitional swallowing: the Bereitschaftspotential. Brain Topogr 16:3–17

Humbert IA, Robbins J (2007) Normal swallowing and functional magnetic resonance imaging: a systematic review. Dysphagia 22:266–275

Hund E (2001) Critical illness polyneuropathy. Curr Opin Neurol 14:649–653

Jean A (2001) Brain stem control of swallowing: neuronal network and cellular mechanisms. Physiol Rev 81:929–969

Jennings KS, Siroky D, Jackson CG (1992) Swallowing problems after excision of tumors of the skull base: diagnosis and management in 12 patients. Dysphagia 7:40–44

Jones HN, Rosenbek JC (2010) Dysphagia in rare conditions. Plural, San Diego

Kelly JH (2000) Management of upper esophageal sphincter disorders: indications and complications of myotomy. Am J Med 108(Suppl 4a):43S–46S

Kessler KR, Skutta M, Benecke R (1999) Long-term treatment of cervical dystonia with botulinum toxin A: efficacy, safety, and antibody frequency. German Dystonia Study Group. J Neurol 246:265–274

Kirk EA, Howard VC, Scott CA (1995) Description of posterior fossa syndrome in children after posterior fossa brain tumor surgery. J Pediatr Oncol Nurs 12:181–187

Kraemer M, Berlit P (2010) Primary central nervous system vasculitis and moyamoya disease: similarities and differences. J Neurol 257:816–819

Kühnlein P, Gdynia HJ, Sperfeld AD, Lindner-Pfleghar B, Ludolph AC, Prosiegel M, Riecker A, Medscape (2008) Diagnosis and treatment of bulbar symptoms in amyotrophic lateral sclerosis. Nat Clin Pract Neurol 4:366–374

Lampl C, Yazdi K (2002) Central pontine myelinolysis. Eur Neurol 47:3–10

Lang IM, Shaker R (1997) Anatomy and physiology of the upper esophageal sphincter. Am J Med 103:50S–55S

Lang IM, Dantas RO, Cook IJ, Dodds WJ (1991) Videoradiographic, manometric and electromyographic assessment of upper esophageal sphincter. Am J Physiol 260:G911–G919

Lee MJ, Bazaz R, Furey CG, Yoo J (2007) Risk factors for dysphagia after anterior cervical spine surgery: a two-year prospective cohort study. Spine J 7:141–147

Levine R, Robbins JA, Maser A (1992) Periventricular white matter changes and oropharyngeal swallowing in normal individuals. Dysphagia 7:142–147

Lin YS, Jen YM, Lin JC (2002) Radiation-related cranial nerve palsy in patients with nasopharyngeal carcinoma. Cancer 95:404–409

Litvan I, Mangone CA, McKee A, Verny M, Parsa A, Jellinger K, D'Olhaberriague L, Chaudhuri KR, Pearce RK (1996) Natural history of progressive supranuclear palsy (Steele-Richardson-Olszewski syndrome) and clinical predictors of survival: a clinicopathological study. Neurol Neurosurg Psychiatry 60:615–620

Machado A, Chien HF, Deguti MM, Cançado E, Azevedo RS, Scaff M, Barbosa ER (2006) Neurological manifestations in Wilson's disease: report of 119 cases. Mov Disord 21:2192–2196

Mann G, Hankey GJ, Cameron D (2000) Swallowing disorders following acute stroke: prevalence and diagnostic accuracy. Cerebrovasc Dis 10:380–386

Martin RE, Neary ME, Diamant NE (1997) Dysphagia following anterior cervical spine surgery. Dysphagia 12:2–8

Mazzucco S, Ferrari S, Mezzina C, Tomelleri G, Bertolasi L, Rizzuto N (2006) Hyperpyrexia-triggered relapses in an unusual case of ataxic chronic inflammatory demyelinating polyradiculoneuropathy. Neurol Sci 27:176–179

Messina S, Pane M, De Rose P, Vasta I, Sorleti D, Aloysius A, Sciarra F, Mangiola F, Kinali M, Bertini E, Mercuri E (2008) Feeding problems and malnutrition in spinal muscular atrophy type II. Neuromuscul Disord 18:389–393

Miller AJ (1993) The search for the central swallowing pathway: the quest for clarity. Dysphagia 8:185–194

Mosier K, Bereznaya I (2001) Parallel cortical networks for volitional control of swallowing in humans. Exp Brain Res 140:280–289

Mu L, Sanders I (2007) Neuromuscular specializations within human pharyngeal constrictor muscles. Ann Otol Rhinol Laryngol 116:604–617

Müller J, Wenning GK, Verny M, McKee A, Chaudhuri KR, Jellinger K, Poewe W, Litvan I (2001) Progression of dysarthria and dysphagia in postmortem-confirmed parkinsonian disorders. Arch Neurol 58:259–264

Murtagh RD, Caracciolo JT, Fernandez G (2001) CT findings associated with Eagle syndrome. AJNR Am J Neuroradiol 22:1401–1402

Nakagawa T, Wada H, Sekizawa K, Arai H, Sasaki H (1999) Amantadine and pneumonia. Lancet 353:1157

Newton HB, Newton C, Pearl D, Davidson T (1994) Swallowing assessment in primary brain tumor patients with dysphagia. Neurology 44:1927–1932

Nguyen NP, Moltz CC, Frank C, Vos P, Smith HJ, Karlsson U, Dutta S, Midyett FA, Barloon J, Sallah S (2004) Dysphagia following chemoradiation for locally advanced head and neck cancer. Ann Oncol 15:383–388

Nogalska A, D'Agostino C, Engel WK, Klein WL, Askanas V (2010) Novel demonstration of amyloid-β oligomers in sporadic inclusion-body myositis muscle fibers. Acta Neuropathol 120:661–666

Oestreicher-Kedem Y, Agrawal S, Jackler RK, Damrose EJ (2010) Surgical rehabilitation of voice and swallowing after jugular foramen surgery. Ann Otol Rhinol Laryngol 119:192–198

Oh TH, Brumfield KA, Hoskin TL, Stolp KA, Murray JA, Bassford JR (2007) Dysphagia in inflammatory myopathy: clinical characteristics, treatment strategies, and outcome in 62 patients. Mayo Clin Proc 82:441–447

Ohkubo T, Chapman N, Neal B, Woodward M, Omae T, Chalmers J, Perindopril Protection Against Recurrent Stroke Study Collaborative Group (2004) Effects of an angiotensin-converting enzyme inhibitor-based regimen on pneumonia risk. Am J Respir Crit Care Med 169:1041–1045

Oommen ER, Kim Y, McCullough G (2010) Stage transition and laryngeal closure in poststroke patients with dysphagia. Dysphagia. doi:10.1007/s00455-010-9314-0

O'Sullivan SS, Massey LA, Williams DR, Silveira-Moriyama L, Kempster PA, Holton JL, Revesz T, Lees AJ (2008) Clinical outcomes of progressive supranuclear palsy and multiple system atrophy. Brain 131:1362–1372

Paulig M, Prosiegel M (2002) Misdiagnosis of amyotrophic lateral sclerosis in a patient with dysphagia due to Chiari I malformation. J Neurol Neurosurg Psychiatry 72:270

Payne S, Wilkins D, Howard R (2005) An unusual cause of dysphagia. J Neurol Neurosurg Psychiatry 76:146

Penfield W, Boldrey E (1937) Somatic motor and sensory representation in the cerebral cortex of man as studied by electrical stimulation. Brain Res 60:389–443

Perry L (2001a) Screening swallowing function of patients with acute stroke. Part one: identification, implementation and initial evaluation of a screening tool for use by nurses. J Clin Nurs 10:463–473

Perry L (2001b) Screening swallowing function of patients with acute stroke. Part two: detailed evaluation of the tool used by nurses. J Clin Nurs 10:474–481

Pfeiffer RF (2003) Gastrointestinal dysfunction in Parkinson's disease. Lancet Neurol 2:107–116

Piagkou M, Anagnostopoulou S, Kouladouros K, Piagkos G (2009) Eagle's syndrome: a review of the literature. Clin Anat 22:545–558

Pittock SJ, Lucchinetti CF, Lennon VA (2003) Anti-neuronal nuclear autoantibody type 2: paraneoplastic accompaniments. Ann Neurol 53:580–587

Power ML, Hamdy S, Singh S, Tyrrell PJ, Turnbull I, Thompson DG (2007) Deglutitive laryngeal closure in stroke patients. J Neurol Neurosurg Psychiatry 78:141–146

Prosiegel M, Schelling A, Wagner-Sonntag E (2004) Dysphagia and multiple sclerosis. Int MS J 11:22–31

Prosiegel M, Höling R, Heintze M, Wagner-Sonntag E, Wiseman K (2005a) The localization of central pattern generators for swallowing in humans—a clinical-anatomical study on patients with unilateral paresis of the vagal nerve, Avellis' syndrome, Wallenberg's syndrome, posterior fossa tumours and cerebellar hemorrhage. Acta Neurochirurg 93:85–88

Prosiegel M, Höling R, Heintze M, Wagner-Sonntag E, Wiseman K (2005b) Swallowing therapy—a prospective study on patients with neurogenic dysphagia due to unilateral paresis of the vagal nerve, Avellis' syndrome, Wallenberg's syndrome, posterior fossa tumours and cerebellar hemorrhage. Acta Neurochirurg 93:35–37

Ramsey D, Smithard D, Kalra L (2005) Silent aspiration: what do we know? Dysphagia 20:218–225

Riecker A, Gastl R, Kühnlein P, Kassubek J, Prosiegel M (2009) Dysphagia due to unilateral infarction in the vascular territory of the anterior insula. Dysphagia 24:114–118

Robbins J, Levin RL (1988) Swallowing after unilateral stroke of the cerebral cortex: preliminary experience. Dysphagia 3:11–17

Rüb U, Brunt ER, Petrasch-Parwez E, Schöls L, Theegarten D, Auburger G, Seidel K, Schultz C, Gierga K, Paulson H, van Broeckhoven C, Deller T, de Vos RA (2006) Degeneration of ingestion-related brainstem nuclei in spinocerebellar ataxia type 2, 3, 6 and 7. Neuropathol Appl Neurobiol 32:635–649

Saiz A, Bruna J, Stourac P, Vigliani MC, Giometto B, Grisold W, Honnorat J, Psimaras D, Voltz R, Graus F (2009) Anti-Hu-associated brainstem encephalitis. J Neurol Neurosurg Psychiatry 80:404–407

Smiatacz T, Kowalik MM, Hlebowicz M (2006) Prolonged dysphagia due to *Listeria-rhombencephalitis* with brainstem abscess and acute polyradiculoneuritis. J Infect 52:165–167

Sonies , Dalakas (1991) Dysphagia in patients with the post-polio syndrome. N Engl J Med 324:1162–1167

Souayah N, Nasar A, Suri MF, Qureshi AI (2007) Guillain-Barre syndrome after vaccination in United States a report from the CDC/FDA vaccine adverse event reporting system. Vaccine 25:5253–5255

Stickler D, Gilmore R, Rosenbek JC, Donovan NJ (2003) Dysphagia with bilateral lesions of the insular cortex. Dysphagia 18:179–181

Stübgen JP (2008) Facioscapulohumeral muscular dystrophy: a radiologic and manometric study of the pharynx and esophagus. Dysphagia 23:341–347

Suiter DM, Leder SB (2008) Clinical utility of the 3-ounce water swallow test. Dysphagia 23:244–250

Teismann IK, Dziewas R, Steinstraeter O, Pantev C (2009) Time-dependent hemispheric shift of the cortical control of volitional swallowing. Hum Brain Mapp 30:92–100

Thexton AJ, Crompton AW, German RZ (2007) Electromyographic activity during the reflex pharyngeal swallow in the pig: Doty and Bosma (1956) revisited. J Appl Physiol 102:587–600

Tolep K, Getch CL, Criner GJ (1996) Swallowing dysfunction in patients receiving prolonged mechanical ventilation. Chest 109:167–172

van Rij CM, Oughlane-Heemsbergen WD, Ackerstaff AH, Lamers EA, Balm AJ, Rasch CR (2008) Parotid gland sparing IMRT for head and neck cancer improves xerostomia related quality of life. Radiat Oncol 3:41

Vanderveldt HS, Young MF (2004) The evaluation of dysphagia after anterior cervical spine surgery: a case report. Dysphagia 18:301–304

Velázquez JM, Montero RG, Garrido JA, Tejerina AA (1999) Lower cranial nerve involvement as the initial manifestation of Lyme borreliosis. Neurologia 14:36–37

Walsh RJ, Amato AA (2005) Toxic myopathies. Neurol Clin 23:397–428

Wesling M, Brady S, Jensen M, Nickell M, Statkus D, Escobar N (2003) Dysphagia outcomes in patients with brain tumors undergoing inpatient rehabilitation. Dysphagia 18:203–210

Williams RBH, Wallace KL, Ali GN, Cook IJ (2002) Biomechanics of failed deglutitive upper esophageal sphincter relaxation in neurogenic dysphagia. Am J Physiol Gastrointest Liver Physiol 283:G16–G26

Yamaguchi M, Arai K, Asahina M, Hattori T (2003) Laryngeal stridor in multiple system atrophy. Eur Neurol 49:154–159

Zografos GN, Georgiadou D, Thomas D, Kaltsas G, Digalakis M (2009) Drug-induced esophagitis. Dis Esophagus 22:633–637

Gastroesophageal Reflux Disease, Globus, and Dysphagia

Jacqui Allen and Peter C. Belafsky

Contents

J. Allen (✉)
Department of Otolaryngology,
North Shore Hospital, Takapuna,
Auckland, New Zealand
e-mail: jeallen@voiceandswallow.co.nz;
Jacqueline.Allen@waitematadhb.govt.nz

P. C. Belafsky
Center for Voice and Swallowing,
University of California, Davis, Sacramento,
CA 95817, USA

Abstract

Gastroesophageal reflux disease (GERD) is a highly prevalent disorder in Western society and closely linked with the production of two common symptoms—dysphagia and globus pharyngeus. The interrelationship of these symptoms with GERD and with each other is complex but critical to an understanding of patients' complaints, underlying pathological mechanisms and appropriate treatment planning. In this chapter we explore these relationships, related diagnostic methodology and options for treatment of reflux disorders, dysphagia and globus.

1 Introduction

As the population continues to age and medical science enables longevity of life that has previously been unheard of, we are now seeing the emergence of chronic disease processes. Prominent among these are diseases affecting deglutition. Largely (but not exclusively) experienced by our elderly community, dysphagia and its consequences have a marked effect on quality of life. Almost one in two adults over the

O. Ekberg (ed.), *Dysphagia*, Medical Radiology. Diagnostic Imaging, DOI: 10.1007/174_2011_340,
© Springer-Verlag Berlin Heidelberg 2012

age of 65 years will complain of swallowing problems (Meng et al. 2000; Robbins et al. 2002; Belafsky 2010). The incidence is much higher in those with neurologic disease and head and neck cancer (Altman et al. 2010; Ramsey et al. 2003; Nguyen et al. 2003, 2006). Dysphagia is the most common symptom following stroke and was estimated to be present in 16.5 million Americans in 2010 (Belafsky 2010). It is associated with mortality in rest home residents and people in long-term care (Belafsky 2010; Altman et al. 2010). Dysphagia however, is only a symptom and may range from the isolated sensation of a lump in the throat to profound oropharyngeal dysphagia and complete dependence on nonoral tube feeding. Dysphagia may be mild or severe, temporary or permanent, improve or progress over time, and may be due to solids, liquids, or pills alone or any combination of these. Swallowing is an extraordinarily complex function that integrates centers from the brainstem and spinal cord with vagally controlled musculature and the neurenteric plexi of the gut. Dysfunction at any point in the pathway or task will impact function proximally and distally, and may lead to symptoms. One of the most common causes of dysphagia is gastroesophageal reflux (GER).

GER disease (GERD) has increased in prevalence dramatically over the past 50 years, outstripping even the obesity epidemic, with which it is closely correlated (Lien et al. 2010; He et al. 2010; Tutuian 2011). Estimates of prevalence in Western populations exceed 20% (Orlando 2011). Population studies have reported that more than 6% of the population of the Western world suffer daily heartburn or regurgitation, with 14% having symptoms weekly (Ronkainen et al. 2006; Lacy et al. 2010). Prevalence estimates in China range from 3.1 to 5.2% using the symptom-based Montreal definition of GERD (He et al. 2010; Vakil et al. 2006). Although 20% of the population in Western societies are said to suffer from GERD, in most cases it is an intermittent phenomenon, which waxes and wanes in a seemingly random fashion (Lacy et al. 2010; Chassany et al. 2008). The relationship between GERD and dysphagia is well established. Over 35% of patients with esophagitis report dysphagia. The presence of swallowing impairment has been associated with the severity of esophageal erosion, and dysphagia resolves in over 80% of patients with erosive esophagitis who are treated with a proton pump inhibitor (PPI) for with

4 weeks (Vakil et al. 2004). It has become clear that GER affects not only the esophagus but also extra-esophageal sites. A wide range of symptoms are now attributed to reflux-mediated mechanisms from heartburn and regurgitation (so-called typical symptoms) to dysphonia, dyspnea, postnasal drip, cough, and pharyngeal irritation (atypical symptoms). Reflux has been implicated in disorders including sinusitis, otitis media, globus pharyngeus, pharyngitis, hyperactive airway disease, chronic cough, chronic laryngitis, and laryngeal cancer (Johnston et al. 2003; Pearson and Parikh 2011; Allen et al. 2011; Wilson 2005; Wight et al. 2003; Ozulgedik et al. 2006). The lifetime point prevalence of globus pharyngeus alone is nearly 50%. Despite improved understanding of reflux-mediated injury, controversy still remains over diagnosis, classification, and treatment of GER. The rapidly expanding prevalence of reflux and swallowing dysfunction demands that the clinician have an advanced understanding of these disorders. The purpose of this chapter is to review the current understanding of GERD, dysphagia, and globus and the interrelationship between these disorders.

2 Dysphagia

Difficulty swallowing (dysphagia) affects all ages. Dysphagia may be due to food, fluid, or pills or any combination of these. Dysphagia impacts food choices, meal durations, and quality of life (Meng et al. 2000; Altman et al. 2010). Many patients complaining of dysphagia believe their condition to be untreatable. Patients experience embarrassment and social isolation owing to inability to eat normally (Meng et al. 2000; Altman et al. 2010; Farri et al. 2007). Swallowing disorders are associated with serious health consequences including malnutrition, weight loss, aspiration, pneumonia, pulmonary abscess, and even death (Meng et al. 2000; Robbins et al. 2002; Altman et al. 2010). In the elderly, the prevalence of dysphagia approaches 50% (Schroeder and Richter 1994). High-risk groups include those with neurologic disease, including stroke and progressive neurodegenerative conditions such as Parkinson's disease, Alzheimer's disease, amyotrophic lateral sclerosis, inclusion body myositis, and multisystem atrophy. Poststroke dysphagia is reported in more than 80% of patients (Meng et al. 2000). Sufferers of head and neck cancer and

Table 1 Causes of dysphagia

Cause	Example	Type
Neurologic	Cerebrovascular accident	A, C
	Parkinson's disease	C, P
	Cranial nerve injury, e.g., postschwannoma resection	A, C
Autoimmune/neurologic	Guillain–Barré disease	A, C
Neuromuscular	Myasthenia gravis	A, C
Muscular	Muscular dystrophy	C, P
	Myopathies	A, C
Metabolic	Lysosomal storage disorders, e.g. Hunter's/Hurler's syndrome	C, P
Neoplastic	Oropharyngeal cancer	C, P
	Postradiation therapy	A, C, P
Infectious	Tonsillitis and pharyngitis	A
	Viral—cytomegalovirus, HSV	A
	Candidiasis	A, C
Inflammatory	Gastroesophageal reflux	C, P
	Caustic ingestion	A, C
Traumatic	Postsurgical defect, e.g., tumor resection	A, C
	Blunt force trauma, e.g., motor vehicle accident	A, C
Allergic	Eosinophilic esophagitis	C, P

A acute, *C* chronic, *P* progressive, *HSV* herpes simplex virus

treatment thereof also exhibit increased prevalence of dysphagia, with prolonged feeding tube dependence in 45% of patients and detectable aspiration in up to 59% of patients (Nguyen et al. 2004, 2006).

3   Etiology

The cause of dysphagia is expansive (see Table 1). Dysfunction may be central or peripheral. Central neurologic insults will affect afferent and efferent inputs, disrupt central patterning and processing, affect coordination, and result in end-organ neuromuscular deficits. Peripheral disruption will affect local tissue, peripheral neuromuscular connections and functions, and sensation. These are not mutually exclusive, and different disorders may have both central and peripheral consequences. The cause of acute-onset dysphagia differs with age. The most common pediatric disorders causing sudden-onset dysphagia are infectious pharyngitis and tonsillitis, foreign body ingestion, caustic ingestion, and Guillain–Barré syndrome (acute inflammatory demyelinating polyradiculoneuropathy). Chronic dysphagia

is uncommon in children but may be due to an inherited condition such as muscular dystrophy or metabolic disorders such as lipid and lysosomal storage diseases, e.g., Gaucher's disease, Neimann–Pick disease, Hunter's syndrome, and Hurler's syndrome. Eosinophilic esophagitis may cause prolonged and recurring dysphagia in both children and adults, and is one of the most prevalent swallowing disorders in children (Furuta et al. 2007; Hurtado et al. 2011; Ricker et al. 2011). The population-based prevalence is estimated between 0.003 and 0.06%, whereas the prevalence in symptomatic adults and children ranges between 6.5 and 22.5% (Furuta et al. 2007; Ricker et al. 2011; Sealock et al. 2010; Prasad et al. 2009; Kanakala et al. 2010). Misdiagnosis and underdiagnosis may occur because the diagnosis requires biopsy of esophageal mucosa and some debate remains regarding diagnostic criteria (Furuta et al. 2007; Kanakala et al. 2010).

Adults presenting with acute-onset dysphagia may have a variety of underlying conditions. Painful swallowing (odynophagia) is usually associated with infective causes, e.g., deep neck space abscess, tonsillitis, or quinsy. Infective esophagitis, for example, candidal or herpes esophagitis, may result in

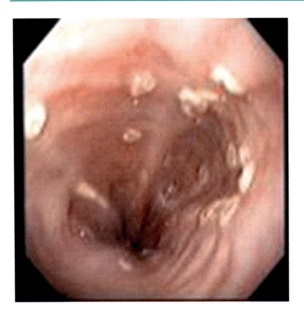

Fig. 1 Endoscopic view of herpetic viral esophagitis. Multiple macular lesions are seen across the esophageal mucosal surface

odynophagia with localization of pain to both the chest and the cervical region (Fig. 1). Both immune-competent and immunocompromised individuals may present with infective esophagitis. Painless acute dysphagia is often neurologic in origin—acute cerebrovascular event (stroke), neoplastic neural invasion or compression, postsurgical defects or injuries. Eosinophilic esophagitis in adults presents with solid food impactions in otherwise healthy adults. It is now the most common cause of solid food impaction in adults (Furuta et al. 2007; Sealock et al. 2010). Diabetes mellitus negatively impacts esophageal motility. This may result in delayed bolus transit and significant reflux and dysmotility (Kinekawa et al. 2008). The presence of diabetic neuropathy increases the prevalence of GERD symptoms and chronic cough (Wang et al. 2008). Here the interrelationship between reflux and dysphagia is well illustrated. GER may cause or exacerbate dysphagia through multiple pathways—by induced esophageal dysmotility secondary to prolonged exposure to refluxate, by pharyngoesophageal mucosal inflammation and esophageal stricture formation, or through cricopharyngeal dysfunction and pharyngeal outlet obstruction. Slow-onset dysphagia in adults may be due to progressive neurologic conditions, among them Parkinson's disease being most common, neoplastic

growth, posttreatment changes, e.g., after radiotherapy to the head and neck, or intrinsic muscular conditions, e.g., myasthenia gravis. At times, malignancy may also cause odynophagia, particularly when there is surface ulceration or erosion, or neural invasion. Other features may be present, such as change in voice, airway compromise, and difficulty managing secretions. Dysphagia may be a predictable consequence of treatment or disease progression. In these cases early intervention, rehabilitation, or frequent reassessment is suggested to limit the negative consequences of dysphagia.

4 Assessment of Dysphagia

4.1 History and Patient Reported Measures

Clinical history is crucial in understanding both the possible cause of dysphagia and its impact. Which types of food or fluid are difficult to manage, how long the symptom has been present, its onset, aggravating or alleviating factors, self-modification of diet, weight loss, and hospitalizations with pulmonary problems are all relevant in assessing the type of dysphagia and its impact. A patient self-assessment tool can be helpful for assessing self-perceived impairment and change over time. Several self-assessment tools are available, including the 40-item SWAL-QOL and the MD Anderson Dysphagia Inventory, which is specific for dysphagia related to head and neck cancer (McHorney et al. 2000a, 2000b, 2002, 2006; Chen et al. 2001). Because of its brevity and extensive validation studies, we use the ten-item Eating Assessment Tool (EAT-10). The EAT-10 is a validated, self-administered symptom questionnaire for dysphagia (Belafsky et al. 2008) (see Appendix). Items are rated on a five-point Likert scale (0 for no problems, 4 for severe problem), and the sum total is calculated for an estimation of severity. Validation studies in both dysphagic subjects and normal adults identified a score greater than 3 as lying more than two standard deviations outside the normal range. The survey takes just a couple of minutes to complete, is easy to interpret, and has been demonstrated to be responsive to treatment intervention and to be able to differentiate patient groups on the basis of disease (Belafsky et al. 2008).

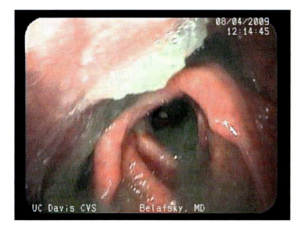

Fig. 2 Endoscopic view during functional endoscopic evaluation of swallowing in a patient with gross aspiration of puree into the subglottis and trachea

4.2 Examination and Instrumental Assessment

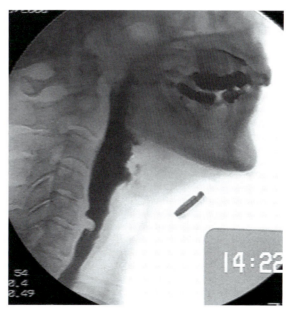

Fig. 3 Lateral videofluoroscopic image demonstrating a moderately obstructing cricopharyngeal bar

Examination must include cranial nerves, neck architecture, and visualization of the laryngeal apparatus. A simple bedside examination of swallowing involves feeding patients and observing them. A palpation of laryngeal structures during swallowing will allow the clinician to evaluate laryngohyoid elevation. Listening to vocal quality and auscultating for fluid in the trachea may help improve the sensitivity to detect swallowing dysfunction (Leslie et al. 2004; Borr et al. 2007). The bedside examination is inexpensive and requires no specialized instruments. Although it can be helpful in guiding dietary recommendations, it is limited by its inability to detect silent aspiration, which may be present in more than 30% of neurologically impaired patients (Ramsey et al. 2003; Bours et al. 2009). Instrumental examinations are more sensitive and specific for detecting violation of the airway, and offer increased information regarding anatomical, mechanical, and physiological aberrations. This may be achieved by videoendoscopy, which gives magnified images of pharyngeal and laryngeal structures, enables laryngeal function testing (motor and sensory), and may incorporate a functional endoscopic evaluation of swallowing (FEES) with sensory testing (FEESST) or without sensory testing. FEES involves administering small measured quantities of food and fluid (usually colored with food dye to improve visualization) to the patient while maintaining

endoscopic views of the pharynx during deglutition. Despite a short period of "whiteout" when the endoscopic view is obscured by pharyngeal contraction and epiglottic retroversion, this is a very sensitive method for identifying airway violation, and observing completeness of bolus transfer (Langmore et al. 1991; Langmore 2003) (Fig. 2). Additionally, the anatomy of the vocal folds may be seen and compensatory maneuvers may be tested with immediate feedback to the patient. Endoscopic examination may also demonstrate signs of laryngeal inflammation that in combination with the history may suggest reflux-mediated damage. FEESST allows quantitative testing of laryngopharyngeal sensation by delivering controlled puffs of air to the mucosa at selected sites in the laryngopharynx (Aviv et al. 2000). Sensory deficiencies are correlated with swallowing problems and with reflux injury, and FEESST may provide a way to document improvement over time.

The most commonly used instrumental assessment of deglutition is a videofluoroscopic swallowing study (VFSS). Various quantities and consistencies of barium contrast material are administered to the patient and real-time dynamic fluoroscopic images are obtained of the passage of the contrast material during the swallow, from the oral cavity to the stomach (Fig. 3). This technique is sensitive and specific for violation of the airway, and excellent for delineating

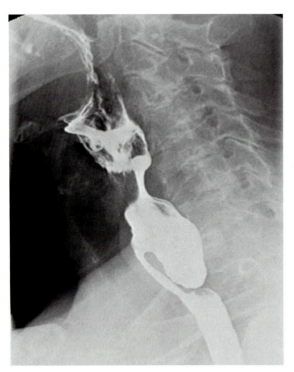

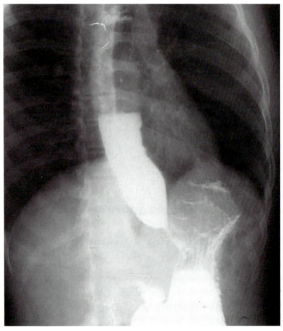

Fig. 5 Videofluoroscopic image demonstrating typical findings in achalasia with a barium air–fluid level in the distal esophagus and a "bird's beak" tapering at the lower esophageal sphincter

Fig. 4 Lateral videofluoroscopic view of a hypopharyngeal (Zenker) diverticulum. Note the pouch filled with barium posteriorly and the narrowed pharyngoesophageal segment anteriorly

anatomical features such as cricopharyngeal impressions or bars, webs, strictures, rings, hypopharyngeal diverticuli, hiatal herniae, esophageal dysmotility, and gastroesophageal, intraesophageal, and occasionally esophagopharyngeal reflux (Figs. 4, 5). Disadvantages of VFSS include radiation exposure, expensive machinery needed to perform the study, and lack of anatomical detail of the vocal folds.

4.3   Advanced Endoscopic Evaluation

Endoscopic techniques have advanced significantly in recent years. The development of thin-caliber endoscopes with working channels has ushered in an era of unsedated, in-office transnasal esophagoscopy (TNE). Endoscopes with 5.5-mm outer diameter and 2-mm working channels can be passed through the nasal cavity and into the pharynx, then through the esophageal inlet, esophagus, and ultimately to the stomach. In-office TNE has demonstrated equivalent diagnostic precision when compared with traditional sedated esophagogastroduodenoscopy, but has the advantages of avoiding sedation (and its attendant problems),

being performed in an upright patient (anatomical position), being cheaper, faster, and safer, and being preferred in most patients (Postma et al. 2002, 2005; Rees 2007; Belafsky and Rees 2009). Biopsies may be obtained and therapeutic procedures are also possible using TNE (e.g., balloon dilatation of strictures and rings, botulinum toxin injection) (Belafsky and Rees 2009). A guided observation of swallowing in the esophagus allows the clinician to observe transit of bolus through the pharyngoesophageal segment and into the stomach using TNE. Administering different food textures may identify areas of functional stenosis or holdup and affords the opportunity for targeted biopsies (Belafsky and Rees 2009). The authors employ early TNE in the assessment of patients presenting with dysphagia (and/or GERD as detailed later), as it is a safe, expeditious, and cost-effective method to rule out organic disease and guide further investigation and management.

4.4   Additional Studies

Additional studies that may be relevant to assessment of dysphagia include esophagram, computed tomography of the neck, chest, and brain, MRI of the neck and brain, ultrasonography of the neck and thyroid, and pH and manometry testing. These will each have a role depending on the presenting symptoms of the patient in addition to dysphagia, and relevant earlier examination findings.

5 Treatment

Treatment of dysphagia will depend on the cause and the specific characteristics of each patient, i.e., age, comorbidities, dietary goals, and cognition. The treatment plan should progress in a stepwise fashion, and is greatly enhanced by multidisciplinary cooperation and input. Vital members of the swallowing team include the speech–language pathologist, respiratory therapist, dieticians, geriatricians, otolaryngologists, nursing staff, rehabilitation service, and occupational therapist. Many other services may also be involved. Patients with significant swallowing dysfunction need frequent reassessment and review to ascertain the benefit of therapy and diet allocation.

Where possible, direct amelioration of causative factors is preferred, e.g., oral antifungal medication to treat *Candida* pharyngitis/esophagitis, and topical steroid treatment in allergic eosinophilic esophagitis. In most cases, however, it is a combination of symptomatic treatment and compensatory or rehabilitative strategies that offers the best outcomes. For example, in patients who have received radiotherapy and surgery for head and neck cancer, a combined approach is required. Dietary modifications plus swallowing rehabilitation during and after treatment can be combined with directed balloon dilatation of strictures. Consideration of dysphagia and planning prior to treatment are also important, e.g., use of intensity-modulated radiotherapy or conformal radiotherapy protocols that spare noninvolved and critical tissue such as the pharyngeal constrictor muscles. Peponi et al. (2011) reviewed 82 patients with advanced head and neck cancer treated with primary and postoperative radiotherapy with or without chemotherapy using an intensity-modulated radiotherapy protocol. At a mean of 32 months after treatment, only a single patient had persisting grade 3 (moderate) dysphagia, with no medial marginal failures seen due to sparing tissue (Peponi et al. 2011).

Intervention can be considered (1) prior to treatment or procedures, (2) during treatment, and (3) after treatment. It may be behavioral, medical, or surgical, often combining several therapies which are complementary.

5.1 Behavioral Therapy

Behavioral strategies include modification of diet, reformulation of medications, positioning strategies, compensatory maneuvers, and targeted rehabilitative exercises. Often patients will be treated by speech–language therapists and dieticians during this aspect of treatment. Biofeedback through endoscopic guidance or transcutaneous electrical stimulation has also been used with variable success (Ryu et al. 2009; Lim et al. 2009; Lin et al. 2011; Ludlow 2010). Positioning such as side lying to gravity-assist the food bolus, maneuvers such as chin tuck or head turn to exclude the bolus from the airway, and dietary manipulation such as thickening of fluids or soft, slippery diets may be helpful in maintaining oral intake. Ames et al. (2010) reported that continued oral intake of some sort during and after radiotherapy for head and neck cancer was associated with shortened gastrostomy tube duration and increased overall survival. A wide variety of targeted exercises and maneuvers can be utilized to increase safety of the swallow (particularly in preventing airway violation) and improve swallow efficiency (Table 2). Exercises may be tried out with the patient during FEES or videofluoroscopy to ensure safety and adequate response.

5.2 Medical Therapy

Directed medical therapy for an underlying condition may help symptoms of dysphagia. Anti-parkinsonian medications, antibiotics, antifungals, or antivirals may be employed in particular cases. Reducing polypharmacy is important, particularly in the elderly, where multiple medications may cause xerostomia and difficulty handling a bolus. Supportive nutrition by oral supplements or nasogastric tube is sometimes required. Tactile stimuli in the oral cavity and transcutaneous electrical stimulation have been used to enhance sensory detection and to increase efficacy of exercise regimes (Ryu et al. 2009; Lim et al. 2009; Lin et al. 2011). There is some debate regarding transcutaneous stimulation of suprahyoid muscles for assisted swallowing, with recent evidence suggesting

Table 2 Targeted maneuvers and exercises for dysphagia management

Maneuver	Method
Supraglottic swallow	Hold liquid in your mouth. Take a breath in and hold it and bear down. Swallow while holding your breath. Immediately after swallowing, exhale with a cough, then swallow again
Massako maneuver	Bite your tongue between your teeth (gently) and while holding it between your teeth, swallow
Mendlesohn maneuver	Palpate thyroid notch anteriorly. During swallow, when the larynx is at maximal elevation, hold this position for 10 s (or as long as instructed)
Shaker exercises	1. Lie supine without a pillow. Lift your chin off the bed, flexing your neck to look at your toes, keeping your shoulders on the bed. Hold your head in this position for 60 s (or as long as instructed). Relax your head back to the bed and rest for 60 s. Repeat as instructed 2. Lie supine without a pillow. Lift your chin off the bed, flexing your neck to look at your toes, keeping your shoulders on the bed. Immediately relax your head back to the bed. Repeat this 30 times in quick succession, then rest for 2 min
Effortful swallow	Moisten your oral cavity. Swallow as hard as possible, imagining you are swallowing a grape whole
Head turn and chin tuck	Turn your head to the side that is affected (as instructed by your clinician) and tilt your chin down as low as possible. Swallow in this position
Tongue resistance exercises	1. Tongue against fingers on cheek (both sides) for 10 s (or as long as instructed) 2. Tongue against roof of mouth for 10 s (or as long as instructed) 3. Hold a spoon in front of your mouth. Push your tongue against the bowl of the spoon for 10 s (or as long as instructed)
Tongue range of motion exercises	Holding your chin steady, protrude your tongue as far as possible and hold, then move your tongue from side to side to each commissure or as far as possible on each side

that instead of the desired laryngeal elevation, stimulation results in net downward motion of the larynx. Although this might provide "resistance training" to those with some residual swallow function, in patients unable to overcome this descent effect there is a risk of increased airway exposure and potential penetration or aspiration (Ludlow 2010).

5.3 Surgical Therapy

Surgical management of dysphagia is diverse, but broadly speaking is directed at improving bolus transit or preventing aspiration (or both) (Table 3). Intervention may be preoperative and preventative, incorporated into surgical plans, or instituted after onset of symptoms or progression of disease. A preventative approach is useful if one is embarking on a procedure known to cause dysphagia or that might have consequences for swallowing. The surgical plan may incorporate procedures to minimize postoperative dysphagia, protect the airway, or both. Early rehabilitation and swallowing therapy may help minimize posttreatment dysfunction. A slightly different surgical approach may be taken when a patient presents with dysfunctional swallowing due to disease

progression or previous intervention. The time after injury and previous efforts at rehabilitation then need to be taken into account in making the treatment plan.

Established surgical management options for improving bolus transit include cricopharyngeal muscle procedures such as dilation, botulinum toxin injection, myotomy with or without diverticulum management, pharyngoplasty, laryngeal suspension, and cervical osteophytectomy. Various laryngoplasty techniques and laryngeal framework surgery, tracheostomy and gastrostomy tube placement, laryngeal closure procedures, laryngotracheal separation, and total laryngectomy have been employed for prevention of aspiration. Innovative new techniques reported include hypopharyngeal pharyngoplasty, neuroprosthetic device implantation and cortical stimulation, and the swallowing expansion device (SED). We discuss selected procedures below.

5.3.1 Treatment of the Upper Esophageal Sphincter

The upper esophageal sphincter (UES), also called the pharyngoesophageal segment, acts as the valve mechanism between the hypopharynx and the cervical esophagus. Opening of this region is crucial to

Table 3 Surgical treatment of dysphagia

Reconstruction	Replace lost tissue with tissue of similar characteristics
	Preplan defect reconstruction
	Preserve superior laryngeal nerves if possible
	Sensate if possible
	Static vs dynamic reconstruction
	Prostheses
	Anastomotic closure considerations (tension-free)
Laryngeal suspension	Resuspension under neotongue helpful after resection
	Suspension in patients with abnormal hyolaryngeal elevation
Vocal fold medialization	Injection laryngoplasty
	Type I thyroplasty
	Arytenoid adduction
	Combination
Partial laryngeal surgery	Preserve competent valve mechanism
Cricopharyngeal procedures	Dilatation
	Botulinum toxin injection
	Myotomy—endoscopic (laser/stapler/harmonic scalpel) vs open
	Zenker diverticuli—excision, pexy, myotomy
Dental appliances	Dentures
	Dental implants
	Prostheses
Pharyngeal procedures	Tonsillectomy
	Pharyngoplasty (cleft lip)
	Hypopharyngeal pharyngoplasty (unilateral closure of piriform fossa)
	Cervical osteophytectomy or metalware removal
Laryngeal separation procedures	Total laryngectomy
	Biller laryngectomy/steamboat laryngectomy
	Laryngotracheal separation
Nonoral feeding	Percutaneous or open feeding tube placement
Esophageal procedures	Dilatation of strictures/rings/webs
	Botulinum toxin injection into UES/LES
	Heller myotomy
	Esophagectomy and gastric pull-up
	Esophageal stent
LES procedures	Fundoplication (Nissen, Toupet)
	Endoscopic suture plication
	Radio-frequency application
Novel procedures	Swallow expansion device
	Neuromuscular stimulation and pacing
	Deep brain stimulation

LES lower esophageal sphincter, *UES* upper esophageal sphincter

bolus transport. It is also plays a protective role preventing reflux or regurgitation of esophageal contents back into the pharynx. Reflux may result in cricopharyngeal hypertension. This may be expressed as globus or dysphagia. Reflux treatment may help ameliorate dysphagia, but if cricopharyngeal muscle hypertrophy becomes severe, surgery may be indicated. The cricopharyngeal muscle is often the target—by dilatation, chemical paralysis, or permanent surgical division. This region may also be the site of anastomotic strictures and posterior cricoid webs, which respond well to balloon dilation. Allen et al. (2010) demonstrated the effectiveness of balloon dilatation and botulinum toxin injection in relieving dysphagia due to cricopharyngeal bar. Although measured opening of the UES was less than that in patients treated surgically, patients treated with conservative therapies still noted improved swallowing

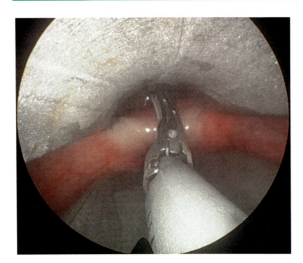

Fig. 6 Endoscopic image of harmonic scalpel across a crico-pharyngeal bar

(Allen et al. 2010). Lawson et al. (2003) reported success with CO_2 laser assisted cricopharyngeal myotomy in all of 29 patients with cricopharyngeal dysfunction. Kos et al. (2010) demonstrated resolution of dysphagia in 20 of 28 patients with chronic oropharyngeal dysphagia who underwent external cricopharyngeal myotomy. Ozgursoy and Salassa (2010) reported increased cricopharyngeal opening area and decreased intrabolus pressures after laser myotomy in 14 patients with radiographic cricopharyngeal bars. Despite concerns that division of the muscular sphincter may increase reflux in some patients, this does not appear to be borne out in practice. In patients with Zenker diverticulum the common denominator is a dysfunctional cricopharyngeal muscle, and cricopharyngeal myotomy is the most effective symptomatic treatment. Myotomy can be accomplished by endoscopic or open techniques. Risks of open procedures include recurrent laryngeal nerve injury, mediastinitis, and esophageal perforation. Endoscopic techniques are well tolerated. Patients demonstrate excellent symptomatic improvement, minimal complications, and shortened hospital stays. The greatest drawback of endoscopic approaches is difficult access. In a small number of patients, endoscopes cannot be placed to give adequate views. When visible, division of the party wall is accomplished by electrocautery, laser, stapler, or more recently, by the harmonic scalpel, particularly in shallow pouches or difficult anatomy (Allen et al. 2010; Lawson et al. 2003; Ozgursoy and Salassa

2010; Pitman and Weissbrod 2009; Wirth et al. 2006; Allen and Belafsky 2010) (Fig. 6).

Laryngeal elevation or suspension procedures help dysphagia in two ways. Suspension improves protection by moving the airway anterosuperiorly, and assists pharyngoesophageal segment opening by anterosuperior distraction. Combined with a myotomy, the UES will open, facilitating bolus transfer and reducing dysphagia. Suspension of the larynx involves mandibular anchoring, either in the midline or laterally. Suspension has been performed in patients with dysphagia after resection of cancer, trauma, and neurogenic dysphagia (Meurmann 1957; Herrmann 1992; Aviv et al. 1997; Fujimoto et al. 2007). Surgical suspension of the remaining laryngeal or hyolaryngeal apparatus under the neotongue assists in diverting material from the airway. Fujimoto et al. (2007) reported 62 patients with extensive oropharyngeal cancers who underwent resection with flap reconstruction, laryngeal suspension, and cricopharyngeal muscle myotomy. More than 85% achieved an oral diet. In all patients the superior laryngeal nerves were preserved bilaterally.

5.3.2 Laryngeal Procedures

A paralyzed or lateralized vocal fold inhibits closure of the airway, and can allow material into the airway. It also reduces effect cough responses. Repositioning of the vocal fold by augmentation or medialization helps to close the glottal gap and restore competence. Depending on the time since injury, a temporary or permanent implant may be chosen. Temporary implants allow spontaneous resolution of impaired vocal fold mobility, while helping achieve closure (and improve dysphagia) in the early postinjury phase. Hendricker et al. (2010) reported 20 patients treated with Gore-Tex thyroplasty for aspiration. Eleven of 20 were able to discontinue g-tube use postoperatively. Carrau et al. (1999) reported an 83% success rate in resolving aspiration and dysphagia in a series of 70 patients with unilateral vocal fold paralysis and dysphagia treated with silastic medialization. In some cases medializing the musculomembranous fold is inadequate to effectively close large gaps. These patients may benefit from repositioning of the arytenoid cartilage in combination with augmentation or medialization. Woodson (1997) described combined type I thyroplasty, arytenoid adduction, and cricopharyngeal myotomy in ten patients with severe

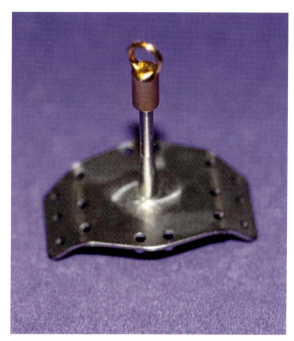

Fig. 7 Swallowing expansion device

unilateral vagal injury. All patients demonstrated improved swallow and resolution of aspiration.

When dysphagia leads to intractable aspiration, surgical options for treatment include laryngotracheal separation and narrow field laryngectomy. During laryngotracheal separation, the trachea is closed at the level of the second or third ring, creating a blind superior pouch, and requiring a tracheostoma for respiration. Phonation is severely affected. More recently, "steamboat laryngoplasty" has been described by Ku et al.(2009). This is a modification of a Biller laryngoplasty wherein the aryepiglottic folds are bisected along their length and approximated to each other in the midline, effectively closing off the airway below from the pharynx above except for a small hole for phonation. Leaving a small outlet passage allows continued glottal speech production, but prevents gross aspiration (Ku et al. 2009). Narrow-field laryngectomy is considered for end-stage intractable dysphagia and aspiration with no hope of recovery. In all cases of total laryngectomy the ultimate aspiration protection is installed—that of a separated airway and digestive tract. This is a permanent ablative surgery, also limiting phonation, and is only considered after failure of all conservative management protocols.

In planned total laryngectomy, cricopharyngeal myotomy may be helpful in minimizing postoperative dysphagia.

5.3.3 Novel Procedures

In 2010, Belafsky (2010) reported a novel device for treatment of oropharyngeal dysphagia. The SED allows manual control of the UES via an implanted shim that is attached to the anterior cricoid ring. The implant may be manipulated either by use of an external magnet or by traction on a projecting rod (Fig. 7). The average distraction possible in cadaver studies was 11.6 mm and in an ovine model was 14.2 mm. These are supraphysiologic values for adults on small boluses. Assisted opening of the UES eliminated aspiration of barium in the sheep model (Belafsky 2010).

The advantages of this device are that it is easy to implant, through a small skin incision, maintains reflux protections, and appears to result in minimal gross disturbance to the cricoid cartilage. However, as yet it is unclear whether this device would be accepted in irradiated tissue with the same success, the magnet is not compatible with MRI, there is a small infection risk, and some degree of manual dexterity and cognitive function is required to use it. The research group has now produced a modified device which lacks the iron core and instead has a projecting rod which passes transcutaneously and may be used to manipulate the implant. Human trials are pending (Fig. 7) (Belafsky 2010).

Several groups are looking at novel electrical stimulation devices that can elicit aspects of the swallow patterns. Lowell et al. (2008) and Broniatowski et al. (2010) have investigated myostimulation and triggered vocal fold closure through neurostimulation of the larynx, respectively. Triggering of action coordinated to the rest of swallow, particularly aimed at preventing aspiration, is still in progress. These novel avenues will offer new options for patients otherwise unresponsive to treatment.

In summary, the surgical management of dysphagia is extremely diverse. Treatment may be preventative and proactive or rehabilitative and restorative. Treatment is largely dependent on the cause, and identification of the cause will guide targeted therapy. Most importantly, successful management of dysphagia is best achieved in a multidisciplinary setting, where tailored treatment plans can be developed and implemented.

6   Gastroesophageal Reflux Disease

GER is the retrograde transit of material from the stomach into the esophagus. The Montreal Consensus meeting agreed that GERD was present when symptoms resulted from this transit or there was endoscopically discernable mucosal damage (Vakil et al. 2006). The prevalence of this disorder is estimated at greater than 20% of Western adults (Orlando 2011; Francis et al. 2011). The estimated costs of diagnostic efforts and medical treatment are in the billions of dollars, and yet we still lack a gold standard diagnostic test and gold standard treatment. GERD is one of the most common causes of dysphagia.

7   Pathophysiology

Reflux occurs in almost everyone to some degree. Physiological reflux is usually dealt with by intrinsic mechanisms. The esophagus has a three-tiered system of protection beginning with lower esophageal sphincter (and UES) closure resisting retrograde transit under neurohormonal control. This is supported by the extrinsic diaphragmatic pinch mechanism and differential pressures between intrathoracic and intra-abdominal portions of the esophagus. Material left in the esophagus or refluxed into its lumen is cleared by a combination of primary and secondary peristalsis. Primary peristalsis occurs with a swallow, begins in the pharynx, and will clear most of the bolus into the stomach. Secondary peristalsis is triggered by material left in the esophagus or refluxed into its lumen and may begin in the esophagus. Saliva buffers material by a dilution effect, and owing to its bicarbonate content helps neutralize acid reflux (Orlando 2011; Pearson and Parikh 2011). The esophagus is protected, in part, by an ill-defined coating of mucus and water rich in bicarbonate that resists penetration of acid and pepsin. The most robust barrier function is in the epithelium itself, which is specialized at the apical membrane. This membrane consists of a hydrophobic lipid bilayer and pH-sensitive cation channels that limit acid diffusion into the cell. The intercellular space is protected by apical junctional complexes consisting of tight junctions, adherens junctions, and desmosomes (Orlando 2011). Bridging proteins link cells at these junctions and

these intercellular bridges prevent diffusion of ions and fluid into the space. Additionally, the intercellular space contains buffering substances such as carbonic anhydrase enzyme that can respond to esophageal acidification by increasing neutralization (Orlando 2011; Rees and Belafsky 2008; Gill et al. 2005). Prolonged acid contact time or injury by other substances may disrupt these intercellular defenses, leading to ion diffusion accompanied by water and giving rise to dilated intercellular spaces—the pathognomonic sign of reflux damage on electron microscopy (Orlando 2011; Pearson and Parikh 2011). In laryngopharyngeal reflux (LPR), these protective mechanisms are lacking. The larynx lacks mucosal protection and peristalsis and demonstrates depletion of carbonic anhydrase and elevation of stress hormones when exposed to acid and pepsin (Johnston et al. 2004, 2007). This suggests that far fewer episodes of exposure to refluxate are required to cause tissue damage and symptoms (Little et al. 1985; Aviv et al. 2000; Postma 2000). Aviv et al. (2000) have demonstrated sensory deficits in patients with LPR and dysphagia. Furthermore, acid is not the only injurious substance present. Other factors contributing to tissue damage include pepsin, bile acids, and trypsin (Pearson and Parikh 2011; Wight et al. 2003; Galli et al. 2002; Johnston et al. 2004, 2006; Tack 2005; Strugala et al. 2009; Tang et al. 2005; Del Negro et al. 2008; Samuels and Johnston 2009). Prolonged or repeated exposures to activated pepsin, bile acids, and hydrochloric acid leads to inflammation, ulceration, metaplasia, dysplasia, and even frank carcinoma.

Recent work has examined the role of pepsin in esophageal and laryngeal injury (Allen et al. 2011; Gill et al. 2005; Johnston et al. 2006, 2007; Samuels and Johnston 2009; Samuels et al. 2008; Knight et al. 2005). Pepsin is the major enzyme in gastric juice and may reach concentrations of 1 mg/ml in the stomach. Pepsin is activated by acid and is most potent in a low-pH environment, but can retain proteolytic effect up to pH 6.5, and is not irreversibly inactivated until pH > 8 (Del Negro et al. 2008; Altman et al. 2010; Tack 2005; Nguyen et al. 2004). Some authors now support pepsin as the main etiological factor in esophageal and laryngeal reflux damage (Pearson and Parikh 2011; Johnston et al. 2006; Tack 2005; Strugala et al. 2009; Samuels and Johnston 2009; Samuels et al. 2008). Pepsin can adhere to the

Table 4 Differences between gastroesophageal reflux disease (*GERD*) and laryngopharyngeal reflux disease (*LPR*)

GERD	LPR
Supine reflux	Upright reflux
Postprandial	Throughout the day
Heartburn common	No heartburn in most
Obesity related	Usually normal BMI
Esophagitis more common	Esophagitis uncommon
LES dysfunction	UES dysfunction
Associated with esophageal dysmotility	Less common esophageal dysmotility
Multiple episodes required for symptoms (>50)	Few episodes required for symptoms (1–3)

laryngeal mucosa, or be absorbed into pharyngeal secretions. It may be inactive at that time, as the typical pH of the pharyngolarynx is 6.8; however, later exposure to low pH, as happens with a reflux episode, can reactivate sequestered pepsin, promoting inflammation and cell damage (Johnston et al. 2004, 2007; Tack 2005; Samuels and Johnston 2009). The laryngeal mucosa actively endocytoses pepsin, and the pepsin may remain viable within the cell cytosol, or may be transported to the Golgi apparatus and late endosomes. Pepsin can induce gene activation for inflammatory cytokines in human hypopharyngeal cells, and alter the production of protective mucus in these cells (Johnston et al. 2007; Samuels et al. 2008). Depletion of protective proteins such as carbonic anhydrase isoenzyme III and squamous epithelial stress protein Sep70 has been found in pepsin-exposed laryngeal tissue (Johnston et al. 2004, 2006). These findings strongly implicate pepsin as a key mediator in reflux-related tissue damage, and suggest a pathway through which pepsin/reflux injury may inhibit the cell's ability to cope with mutagenic insults.

8 Diagnosis

In adults, GERD is characterized by the symptoms of heartburn and regurgitation, but numerous other symptoms have been attributed to the effects of reflux, including chest pain, bloating, hoarseness, chronic cough, throat clearing, throat irritation, postnasal drip, globus sensation, and shortness of breath (Wilson 2005; Wight et al. 2003; Park et al. 2010; Frye and

Vaezi 2008). Disorders in which reflux is suspected to contribute to the cause include Barrett's esophagus, esophagitis, esophageal carcinoma and strictures, esophageal dysmotility, laryngeal edema, laryngeal cancer, cough, asthma and reactive airway disease, sinusitis, and otitis media (Allen et al. 2011; Wilson 2005; Francis et al. 2011; Little et al. 1985; Park et al. 2010; Frye and Vaezi 2008; Tauber et al. 2002; McCoul et al. 2011; Lewin et al. 2003; Maronian et al. 2001; El-Serag et al. 2001; Tasker et al. 2002; Vaezi et al. 2006). Children have a higher rate of GER and a different symptom profile compared with adults. Irritability, "spitting up," and food intolerance in infants are thought to be attributable to GER (Gold 2004). Numerous studies have linked reflux with pharyngeal and even otologic disease (McCoul et al. 2011; Tasker et al. 2002). McCoul et al. (2011) reported improved quality of life in children with otitis media with effusion treated for GERD (76% response rate) due to resolution of effusion and avoidance of tympanostomy tube insertion. The effects of refluxate are wide ranging and difficult to isolate. Diagnostic debate remains and controversy exists over what symptoms and signs may be attributed to GER or extraesophageal reflux. Debate even exists over whether LPR is a subset of GERD rather than a distinct disease entity (Rees and Belafsky 2008; Koufman 1991) (Table 4).

Physicians reach a diagnosis by pattern recognition. Rarely is a single symptom or finding diagnostic of any condition. Reflux is suggested by a symptom complex, like any other disease. The difficulty is that many of the features considered suggestive of reflux are also associated with other common diseases or risk behaviors. Diagnosis, therefore, is usually made on the basis of several different complementary sources of information.

8.1 Symptom Scores and Self-Reported Instruments

Use of patient-reported symptom scales and outcome scores can be helpful in quantifying disease severity and impact on the patient, as well as following disease progression over time or response to treatment. The sensitivity and specificity of scoring instruments for diagnosis of reflux disease is on par with other diagnostic tests e.g., trial of PPI, pH-metry, and endoscopy. Given that self-reported questionnaires are noninvasive, simple, and cheap, they may be instituted easily in practice. Broadly speaking, instruments may be symptom severity rating scales or quality of life scales. We will discuss only three scales as a representative sample.

8.1.1 Reflux Disease Questionnaire

Designed to act as a diagnostic tool for GERD, the 12-item Reflux Disease Questionnaire (RDQ) has now been used as both an outcome measure and a diagnostic tool (Shaw et al. 2001, 2008; Nocon et al. 2008; Dent et al. 2010) (see Appendix). Developed by Shaw et al. (2008), it is a 12-item scale grouped into three subscales—heartburn, regurgitation, and dyspepsia. It is validated and has been tested for responsiveness. The RDQ has subsequently been translated and validated in Swedish and Norwegian. It has been used as a symptom survey to monitor symptom severity over time in patients enrolled in the ProGERD study in Europe, showing useful stability and reproducibility (Nocon et al. 2008) and in the Diamond study comparing diagnostic tools in reflux disease (Dent et al. 2010). One interesting aspect of this survey instrument is the lack of use of the word "heartburn." Initial development suggested that this word was poorly understood by patients, and that a "word picture" was better in conveying the symptom, i.e., burning rising up from the stomach behind the breastbone (Dent et al. 2010). The primary advantages of this survey are its conciseness, short completion time, adapted patient wording describing symptoms clearly, and cross-cultural validation. The primary limitations are inclusion of more than one disease profile (i.e., GERD and dyspepsia), long recall period, uncontrolled treatment in the patient validation population, a diagnostic accuracy equal to that of physician assessment, and variable scoring system.

8.1.2 Gastro-oesophageal Reflux Disease Impact Scale

Jones et al. (2007) proposed the Gastro-oesophageal Reflux Disease Impact Scale (GIS) as a management tool for primary care physicians (see Appendix). The survey aims to assist patients in conveying GERD severity and impact, and to prompt clinicians to enquire about reflux-related symptoms. GIS is a nine-item scale with a 1-week recall period that can be completed in a matter of minutes. It has been validated, and tested for responsiveness. Primary care physicians using the scale found it helped direct treatment decisions and assess treatment effectiveness. It has been utilized and reported by Gisbert et al. (2009), as part of the multinational European RANGE (Retrospective Analysis of GERD) study. Louis et al. (2009) reported the GIS correlated well with physician-assessed GERD severity, and was sensitive to treatment changes over time. The primary advantages of this survey are the multidimensionality of the survey (symptoms and impact of GERD) and the brevity of the survey. The primary limitations of this survey are the tendency for results clusters and lack of diagnostic precision (GER vs dyspepsia vs functional heartburn).

8.1.3 Reflux Symptom Index

The Reflux Symptom Index (RSI) is a nine-item self administered survey that asks patients to rate on a scale of 0–5, with 0 being no problem and 5 being all the time, how much a particular symptom bothered them over the past month (Belafsky et al. 2002) (see Appendix). Total scores range from 0 to 45. In validation studies, the upper limit of 95% confidence intervals in normal controls was 13.6. Scores greater than 13 may suggest LPR playing a significant role in symptom production. Despite conflicting studies in support of and against the use of the RSI, it remains a simple, cheap, and reproducible tool, which most patients can answer in an expeditious fashion. It includes most of the accepted symptoms that are thought to be associated with LPR. Criticisms of the RSI have included the lack of frequency modifiers and missing symptom items such as throat pain and burning, and bundling of more than one symptom together. The review of Musser et al. (2010) of rating scales in extraesophageal reflux, although critical of the predictive value of the RSI, actually demonstrated significant correlation of the RSI with reflux area index at pH 4, a new proposed measure that normalizes frequency, duration, and acidity of reflux episodes for the total time of the study.

The greatest contribution of self-reported scales is their role in reflecting changes over time in the same patient, whether treatment is given or not. Subjectivity of symptom reporting differs hugely between patients, but will be more consistent in the same patient, and reflects the patient's level of disease burden. Reflux is a symptom-driven disease and what matters most is how the patient feels. Use of symptom indices and endoscopic grading systems in treatment outcome studies is necessary to allow comparison of relative disease severity (in selected test and control populations), and response to intervention.

8.2 pH Studies

Currently considered the gold standard for diagnosing both GERD and LPR, the pH study is expensive, relatively hard to perform or at least time-consuming, and not by any means 100% sensitive or specific for reflux disease (Vaezi et al. 2006; Arevalo et al. 2011). Inclusion of impedance studies is now advocated for detection of nonacid reflux and volume reflux that may cause symptoms aside from those due to drop in pH (Arevalo et al. 2011). pH and impedance studies may be more specific but are poorly sensitive in this remitting disease, and the appropriate diagnostic criteria remain unclear. Detection of these conditions in the pharynx is poor, and the study may be poorly tolerated in many patients. Patients may find the probe uncomfortable and unsightly and may alter daily behaviors, which reduces the reliability of the test. One in eight patients will remove the probe before a complete study can be recorded (Kotby et al. 2010). In the performance of the study, placement of the probe remains controversial, and probe-related artifacts from drying can be an issue. In diagnosis of GERD, established normative data suggest that prolonged acid times (more than 4% of 24 h spent at pH < 4) are associated with increasing mucosal injury (Vaezi et al. 2006; Arevalo et al. 2011). However, it is apparent that a group of patients with normal acid contact times still have symptoms related to reflux, and this group has been termed "sensitive esophagus" (Arevalo et al. 2011). Furthermore, abrupt esophageal distension that may occur in liquid or gaseous/liquid reflux may also give rise to symptoms via mechanoreceptors (Arevalo et al. 2011), and without impedance testing these episodes are unlikely to be detected. In a recent metanalysis, Kotby et al. (2010) quoted an overall sensitivity of pH studies in the range of 50–80%. Almost one third of patients with endoscopically visualized esophagitis will have completely normal findings in a pH study. Are the norms asserted for the esophagus applicable to the pharynx? The increasing body of literature in this

area suggests not. It is likely that much higher pHs (i.e., those closer to neutral) are still injurious to the laryngopharynx (Postma 2000; Merati et al. 2005).

8.3 Proton Pump Inhibitor Trial

Empirical trial of PPI medication may appear to be an appealing option. If acid production and its reflux were the cause of symptoms, then a potent inhibitor of gastric acid secretion should produce definitive symptom control. Good quality, randomized controlled trials of PPI in treatment of pH-documented GER still fail to show an unequivocal benefit in terms of symptoms or objective endoscopic findings. Only 60% of patients with erosive esophagitis treated with PPI show a complete symptomatic response (Arevalo et al. 2011). In patients with nonerosive esophagitis, the response rate is a dismal 40% (Arevalo et al. 2011; Mainie et al. 2006). In a multicenter study using combined multiluminal impedance and pH monitoring, 37% of 168 patients with persisting symptoms despite twice daily PPI treatment had a significant symptom association with nonacid reflux episodes (Mainie et al. 2006). Even more important, 11% of patients demonstrated symptoms with continued acid reflux on combined multiluminal impedance and pH monitoring, suggesting that PPI cannot control gastric acid secretion completely in some individuals (Mainie et al. 2006). Numans et al. (2004) undertook a meta-analysis of studies reporting the "PPI test." This demonstrated that the PPI test showed a low likelihood ratio and specificity of only 54% in diagnosing GERD (Numans et al. 2004). Qadeer et al. (2006) undertook a meta-analysis of randomized controlled trials of PPI in treatment of reflux. They found only a modest nonsignificant improvement in symptoms with PPI therapy (Qadeer et al. 2005, 2006).

Acid is not the only component of refluxate that may cause injury. Other gastric refluxate components, including bile acids and pepsin, and the mere volume itself may result in dysfunction (Johnston et al. 2004, 2007; Galli et al. 2002; Tack 2005; Strugala et al. 2009). PPI will not abrogate the effects of these components. Johnston et al. (2007) have demonstrated endocytosis of pepsin into laryngeal epithelium, and activity of pepsin up to pH 6.5. In fact, pepsin is not irreversibly deactivated until it is exposed to pH 8. This may explain some of the negative effects of nonacid or weakly acid reflux. There is ongoing debate about the dose and duration of treatment of PPI medication, and more concerning, new evidence suggesting that PPIs are not as benign as we once thought. Significant decrease in calcium absorption has been documented in women receiving long-term treatment, with increase in osteoporosis and hip fracture risk in those taking PPI for prolonged periods. These medications interact with some drugs, including the platelet inhibitor clopidogrel, and alone they have a side effect profile that includes gastric upset, bloating, rash, myalgia, and depressed mood. They also remain expensive medications, especially newer-generation formulations.

Finally, it has now become clear that use of a PPI can result in reflex acid hypersecretion when treatment is terminated, which then leads to false-positive reinforcement to the patient that he or she is indeed suffering from acid reflux (Reimer et al. 2009). This rebound effect may last as long as 4 weeks and may be induced by only 8 weeks of therapy. Trial of medications (primarily PPI) runs the risk of medication side effects, lack of therapeutic effect in nonacid reflux or with other gastric refluxate components, and inducing rebound hypersecretion.

8.4 Endoscopy and Biopsy

Looking at tissue from the area affected at a microscopic and cellular level would, on the face of it, appear to be a definitive diagnostic process. However, ulceration, inflammation, eosinophilia, fibrosis, metaplasia, and dysplasia may be suggestive of reflux damage but are not pathognomonic or diagnostic of reflux on light microscopy (Wada et al. 2009). Many biopsies from patients with typical reflux symptoms show completely normal findings. Endoscopy has weak correlation with symptoms. It is a good screen for reflux complications but has low diagnostic sensitivity. The site of biopsy—the pharynx, upper esophagus, distal esophagus—may affect findings. Acquiring tissue is mildly uncomfortable, may require sedation, is relatively time intensive and expensive, and requires highly specialized tools and practitioners. Esophageal electron microscopy studies suggest that dilated intercellular spaces are correlated with GER (Park et al. 2010; Fox 2011). Park et al. (2010)

have demonstrated characteristic dilated intercellular spaces in esophageal biopsies of patients with laryngeal symptoms only, and with both laryngeal and typical GER symptoms, compared with normal controls. Identification of pepsin in tissue or fluid aspirates (e.g., from middle ear, lung) has been suggested as a surrogate marker for reflux, and may well prove to be useful over time (Johnston et al. 2003, 2004, 2004; Knight et al. 2005; Tasker et al. 2002; Fox 2011). A new test kit, the Peptest lateral flow device (RD Biomed, Hull, UK) uses a latex bead monoclonal antibody to identify pepsin in saliva in the manner of a pregnancy test. Results take only 5 min to obtain and it may be more useful in primary practice as a diagnostic tool for reflux (Fox 2011). Further testing is awaited.

A history consistent with GERD or LPR and examination findings of laryngopharyngeal inflammation or complications of reflux disease support a clinical diagnosis of reflux. At this point clinicians differ in their view as to what is the most appropriate next step.

9 Investigation

The options for investigation include those mentioned earlier—pH-metry, manometry, endoscopy, and VFSS. Peng et al. (2010) reported 469 Chinese patients presenting with typical symptoms of GERD (heartburn or regurgitation). All patients underwent early endoscopic evaluation, with 38.4% demonstrating clinically significant endoscopic findings (esophagitis, Barrett's metaplasia, peptic ulcer, carcinoma). Peng et al. (2010) recommended early endoscopy for both diagnosis and identification of complications. In-office endoscopic screening is well tolerated, safer, and cheaper than a sedated esophagoscopy, and these findings support early TNE in the management of GER and LPR (Postma et al. 2005; Rees 2007; Belafsky and Rees 2009). Contrast imaging studies are widely used in the diagnosis of dysphagia. Videofluoroscopy for diagnosis of GERD, however, is poorly sensitive and its use is not routinely indicated without other symptoms being present. Provocative testing during VFSS may demonstrate active GER but will rarely demonstrate LPR.

Table 5 Lifestyle modifications recommended in gastro-esophageal and laryngopharyngeal reflux disease

Elevate head of bed (more than 10 cm)	Avoid refluxogenic foods
Smoking cessation	Alcohol
	Fatty foods
Avoid lying down within 2 h of meal	Chocolate
	Spicy food
Sleep on left side	Tomato products
	Peppermint
Weight loss and regular exercise	Citrus fruits
Chew gum (sugar free)	
Small frequent meals	

10 Management

Therapeutic options for reflux disease begin with lifestyle modifications (Table 5). Avoidance of refluxogenic foods, alcohol, caffeine, and smoking is recommended. Positioning with the head elevated during sleep, ensuring gastric emptying by not lying down for at least 2 h after meals, and regular exercise with weight loss may help symptomatic reflux. As yet there are no randomized controlled trials demonstrating efficacy of lifestyle changes alone.

10.1 Medications

The most potent and effective medications for GERD are PPIs. These reduce stomach intraluminal acid secretions by blocking end-organ function (H^+/K^+ ATPase pumps). No tolerance effect is seen; however, rebound hypersecretion can occur if use of these medications is discontinued abruptly, leading to a flare of symptoms. This may occur after only 8 weeks of therapy (Qadeer et al. 2005). The dose and duration of therapy are debated and different depending on whether the patient is deemed to have GERD or LPR. In GERD, response to therapy is seen at lower doses often with once daily regimens; however, in LPR patients twice daily administration is usually required, with higher doses at each time point (Park et al. 2005). The rate of response in nonerosive reflux disease may be lower than expected, with one study demonstrating only 40% response to PPI treatment in patients diagnosed with nonerosive reflux disease (Dean et al. 2004). Randomized controlled trials have failed to show unequivocal improvement in LPR patients

receiving PPIs however, and debate remains over the appropriate duration of treatment (ranging from 4 to 12 weeks) (Postma et al. 2002; Koufman 2002; Noordzij et al. 2001; Steward et al. 2004). Histamine type 2 receptor antagonists (H2RA) reduce gastrin secretion and therefore overall acid secretion in the stomach. H2RAs have a short onset of action (less than 1 h) but also reduced effective period (less than 12 h). They are effective in healing esophagitis in approximately 50% of cases, but are less effective than PPIs in the resolution rate of symptoms, ulcer healing, and relapse of both mucosal disease and symptoms (Meneghelli et al. 2002; Caro et al. 2001; Farley et al. 2000). Patients taking these medications develop tachyphylaxis or a drug tolerance effect with long-term usage. Instituting a "drug holiday" such as a week off therapy every 3 weeks may limit this effect.

Although acid suppression with PPI treatment is profound, these medications do not prevent reflux—rather they only make it nonacid. Physical reflux barriers such as magnesium sulfate or aluminium sulfate suspensions, alginates, and sucralfate may provide protection against volume reflux (Strugala et al. 2009; Tang et al. 2005; McGlashan et al. 2009; Dettmar et al. 2006). McGlashan et al. (2009) demonstrated equivalent success in treating symptoms of LPR with liquid alginate alone compared with PPIs. Dettmar et al. (2006) demonstrated faster onset of action with liquid alginate than with either H2RAs or PPI. Alginates are polysaccharide copolymers that form a meshlike gel structure which can act as a biological sieve (Strugala et al. 2009). The properties of the gel can be altered by changing the relative proportions of guluronic acid and mannuronic acid in the mix. This adjusts the cross-linking and changes the pore sizes within the gel mesh, critically changing the permeability of the substance (Strugala et al. 2009; Tang et al. 2005). Tang et al. (2005) demonstrated that adhered alginate gel significantly reduced both proton (acid) diffusion and pepsin diffusion in a dose-dependent fashion. Strugala et al. (2009) showed reduced pepsin diffusion in alginate, by up to 82% compared with controls. Furthermore, the alginate used in their study significantly retarded diffusion of bile acids as well. They simulated repeated reflux events by using multiple 5-ml-aliquot exposures of pepsin and bile acids. Even after ten exposures, alginate gel absorbed 50% of pepsin in the sample (Strugala et al. 2009). Alginate gel will coat mucosal

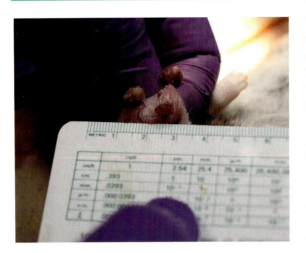

Fig. 8 Photomicrograph of hamster cheek pouch demonstrating three squamous cell carcinomas induced by pepsin and 7,12-dimethylbenz[*a*]anthracene, a known carcinogen

surfaces and can stay adherent for up to 60 min without being washed off by saliva flow (Tang et al. 2005). Thus, alginate gel may act like gastric mucus, forming a physical barrier to diffusion of acid and pepsin, and preventing contact with the cell surface and subsequent damage (Strugala et al. 2009; Tang et al. 2005). Allen et al. (2011), using a hamster model of carcinogenesis, demonstrated a significant reduction in tumor growth and proliferation in hamsters treated with alginate versus controls (Fig. 8).

Use of prokinetics agents or γ-aminobutyric acid B agonists is under investigation. Treatment with baclofen has demonstrated increased lower esophageal sphincter tone and reduced transient lower esophageal sphincter relaxations (Ciccaglione and Marzio 2003; Koek et al. 2003). Side effects include nausea, dizziness, and drowsiness which may improve over time.

10.2 Surgery

In refractory cases of GERD or LPR where medical therapy is unhelpful, or in cases complicated by large herniae, subglottic stenosis, brittle airway disease, or cancer, consideration of surgical intervention is warranted. Fundoplication is successful in reducing symptoms in the vast majority of patients with typical GER symptoms (Mainie et al. 2006). In those with extraesophageal symptoms, there is debate as to the role of fundoplication. Studies have demonstrated

both no effect and a significantly beneficial effect of fundoplication in selected patients presenting with extraesophageal manifestations (Westcott et al. 2004; Lindstrom et al. 2002; Swoger et al. 2006; Luostarinen 1993; Shaw et al. 2010; Catania et al. 2007). Fundoplication may play an increasing role in treatment of nonacid reflux (Arevalo et al. 2011). Novel procedures to reduce GER such as endoscopic suture plication, radio-frequency energy treatment, and injection of the lower esophageal sphincter are under investigation but there are no long-term data to support their implementation at this time.

11 Globus

Globus is a symptom rather than a diagnosis. Previously considered a hysterical manifestation, it is now recognized as being a symptom generated from largely organic dysfunction. This is reflected by a change in terminology to globus pharyngeus. Globus pharyngeus may be used to describe a "lump in the throat" sensation, throat irritation, fullness in the throat, or even effortful swallowing. The cause of this symptom is likewise varied. There may be an association with esophageal reflux and particularly proximal esophageal refluxate excursion. Both the presence of material in the proximal esophagus and slow distension of the proximal esophagus are known to result in reflex contraction of the UES (Szczesniak et al. 2010; Lang et al. 2001), whereas rapid distension may result in UES relaxation (Szczesniak et al. 2010). This protective contraction acts to prevent refluxate escaping into the pharynx and subsequently threatening the airway, whereas the relaxation of the UES enables eructation. It is suggested that intermittent recurrent reflux episodes result in a state of hypertension or hyperactivity in the UES, particularly the cricopharyngeal component. This mechanism is also proposed as the cause of cricopharyngeal bar. Szczesniak et al. (2010) have demonstrated an enhanced esophago-UES relaxation response in patients with symptoms of reflux laryngitis and suggested that this heightened belch response may contribute to symptoms. The sensation of a lump in the throat may be due to a lump in the throat. Vallecula cysts, lingual tonsillar hypertrophy, long uvula, and lingual thyroid tissue may all cause globus sensation.

12   Investigation

Patients presenting with globus as a symptom require full evaluation to ensure no obstructive lesion is responsible. This may entail endoscopy, contrast imaging studies, e.g., VFSS, or computed tomography, depending on other symptoms. If the findings are normal, consideration of pH/manometry studies to examine the UES region looking for a hypertensive or poorly compliant UES may be helpful. Esophageal disease commonly results in a feeling of discomfort in the cervical region. Smith et al. (1998) demonstrated that 58% of patients with a marshmallow impacted at the distal esophagus complained of cervical dysphagia. One third of patients with globus, cough, or cervical dysphagia have an esophageal cause (Smith et al. 1998).

13   Treatment

Treatment should be directed at the underlying cause of globus. If there is a mass lesion present, this should be addressed. Patients may benefit from reassurance, behavioral changes such as sipping water, or reflux lifestyle modifications. In many cases patients require aggressive antireflux therapy with medication. Muscle relaxant medications such as diazepam have been used successfully in some patients and there are anecdotal reports of empiric balloon dilation of the UES showing promise (C.J. Rees, unpublished data). If investigations suggest a cricopharyngeal bar or hypertensive UES, consideration of balloon dilation, botulinum toxin injection, and rarely cricopharyngeal myotomy may be required.

14   Conclusion

Swallowing disorders are common and will increase in prevalence in the coming decades. Dysphagia is intimately related to GERD and globus, and investigation and treatment of all conditions is best accomplished by thorough investigation and appropriate multidisciplinary-team-based therapy.

15   Appendix

Table A.1 Ten-item Eating Assessment Tool (EAT-10) (Belafsky et al. 2008)

My swallowing problem has caused me to lose weight	0 = no problem	1 = slight	2 = mild	3 = moderate	4 = severe
My swallowing problem interferes with my ability to go out	0 = no problem	1 = slight	2 = mild	3 = moderate	4 = severe
Swallowing liquids takes extra effort	0 = no problem	1 = slight	2 = mild	3 = moderate	4 = severe
Swallowing solids takes extra effort	0 = no problem	1 = slight	2 = mild	3 = moderate	4 = severe
Swallowing pills takes extra effort	0 = no problem	1 = slight	2 = mild	3 = moderate	4 = severe
Swallowing is painful	0 = no problem	1 = slight	2 = mild	3 = moderate	4 = severe
The pleasure of eating is affected by my swallowing	0 = no problem	1 = slight	2 = mild	3 = moderate	4 = severe
When I swallow food sticks in my throat	0 = no problem	1 = slight	2 = mild	3 = moderate	4 = severe
I cough when I eat	0 = no problem	1 = slight	2 = mild	3 = moderate	4 = severe
Swallowing is stressful	0 = no problem	1 = slight	2 = mild	3 = moderate	4 = severe

Table A.2 Reflux Symptom Index (RSI) (Belafsky et al. 2002)

In the last month how did the following problems affect you? (1 = no problem, 5 = all the time)	
Hoarseness or a problem with your voice?	0–5
Clearing your throat	0–5
Excess throat mucus or postnasal drip	0–5
Difficulty swallowing food, liquids, or pills	0–5
Coughing after you ate or after lying down	0–5
Breathing difficulties or choking episodes	0–5
Troublesome or annoying cough	0–5
Sensation of something sticking in your throat or a lump in your throat	0–5
Heartburn, chest pain, indigestion, or stomach acid coming up	0–5

Reflux Disease Questionnaire (RDQ) (Shaw et al. 2001)

Three domains (heartburn, regurgitation, dyspepsia)
Acid taste frequency
Acid taste severity
Movement of materials severity
Movement of materials frequency
Frequency of pain behind the breastbone
Frequency of burning behind the breastbone
Severity of burning behind the breastbone
Severity of pain behind the breastbone
Upper stomach burning severity
Upper stomach burning frequency
Upper stomach pain frequency
Upper stomach pain severity

Gastro-oesophageal Reflux Disease Impact Scale (GIS) (Jones et al. 2007)

Subjects make one of four responses—daily, often, sometimes, or never:
1. How often have you had the following symptoms:
   Pain in your chest or behind the breastbone?
   Regurgitation or acid taste in your mouth?
   Pain or burning in your upper stomach?
   Sore throat or hoarseness that is related to your heartburn or acid reflux?
2. How often have you had difficulty getting a good night's sleep because of your symptoms?

3. How often have your symptoms prevented you from eating or drinking any of the foods you like?
4. How frequently have your symptoms kept you from being fully productive in your job or daily activities?
5. How often do you take additional medication other than what the physician told you to take (such as Tums, Rolaids, Maalox)?

References

Allen J, Belafsky PC (2010) Endoscopic cricopharyngeal myotomy for Zenker diverticulum using the harmonic scalpel. Ear Nose Throat J 89:216–218

Allen J, White CJ, Leonard RJ, Belafsky PC (2010) Effect of cricopharyngeal muscle surgery on the pharynx. Laryngoscope 120:1498–1503

Allen J, Tinling SP, Johnston N, Belafsky P (2011) Effects of pepsin and alginate in an animal model of squamous cell carcinoma. Aliment Pharmacol Ther 33(Suppl 1):21–28

Altman KW, Yu GP, Schaefer SD (2010) Consequence of dysphagia in the hospitalized patient. Impact on prognosis and hospital resources. Arch Otolaryngol Head Neck Surg 136:784–789

Ames JA, Karnell LH, Gupta AK, Coleman TC, Karnell MP, Van Daele DJ, Funk GF (2011) Outcomes after the use of gastrostomy tubes in patients whose head and neck cancer was managed with radiation therapy. Head Neck 33(5):638–644. doi:10.1002/hed.21506

Arevalo LF, Sharma N, Castell DO (2011) Symptomatic non-acid reflux—the new frontier in gastro-oesophageal reflux disease. Aliment Pharmacol Ther 33(Suppl 1):29–35

Aviv JE, Mohr JP, Blizter A, Thomson JE, Close LG (1997) Restoration of laryngopharyngeal sensation by neural anastomosis. Arch Otolaryngol Head Neck Surg 123:154–160

Aviv JE, Kaplan ST, Thomson JE, Spitzer J, Diamond B, Close LG (2000a) The safety of flexible endoscopic evaluation of swallowing with sensory testing (FEESST): an analysis of 500 consecutive evaluations. Dysphagia 15:39–44

Aviv JE, Liu H, Parides M, Kaplan ST, Close LG (2000b) Laryngopharyngeal sensory deficits in patients with laryngopharyngeal reflux and dysphagia. Ann Otol Rhinol Laryngol 109:1000–1006

Belafsky PC (2010) Manual control of the upper esophageal sphincter. Laryngoscope 120:S1–S16

Belafsky PC, Rees CJ (2009) Functional oesophagoscopy: endoscopic evaluation of the oesophageal phase of deglutition. J Laryngol Otol 123:1031–1034

Belafsky PC, Postma GN, Koufman JA (2002) Validity and reliability of the Reflux Symptom Index (RSI). J Voice 16:274–277

Belafsky PC, Mouadeb DA, Rees CJ, Allen JE, Leonard RJ (2008) Validity and reliability of the Eating Assessment Tool (EAT-10). Ann Otol Rhinol Laryngol 117:919–924

Borr C, Hielscher-Fastabend M, Lücking A (2007) Reliability and validity of cervical auscultation. Dysphagia 22:225–234

Bours GJ, Speyer R, Lemmens J, Limburg M, de Wit R (2009) Bedside screening tests vs videofluoroscopy or fibreoptic endoscopic evaluation of swallowing to detect dysphagia in patients with neurological disorders: systematic review. J Adv Nurs 65:477–493

Broniatowski M, Moore NZ, Grundfest-Broniatowski S, Tucker HM, Lancaster E, Krival K, Hadley AJ, Tyler DJ (2010) Paced glottic closure for controlling aspiration pneumonia in patients with neurologic deficits of various causes. Ann Otol Rhinol Laryngol 119:141–149

Caro JJ, Salas M, Ward A (2001) Healing and relapse rates in gastroesophageal reflux disease treated with the newer proton-pump inhibitors lansoprazole, rabeprazole, and pantoprazole compared with omeprazole, ranitidine, and placebo: evidence from randomized clinical trials. Clin Ther 23:998–1017

Carrau RL, Pou A, Eibling DE, Murry T, Ferguson BJ (1999) Laryngeal framework surgery for the management of aspiration. Head Neck 21:139–145

Catania RA, Kavic SM, Roth JS, Lee TH, Meyer T, Fantry GT, Castellanos PF, Park A (2007) Laparoscopic Nissen fundoplication effectively relieves symptoms in patients with laryngopharyngeal reflux. J Gastrointest Surg 11:1579–1588

Chassany O, Holtmann G, Malagelada J, Gebauer U, Doerfler H, Devault K (2008) Systematic review: health-related quality of life (HRQOL) questionnaires in gastro-oesophageal reflux disease. Aliment Pharmacol Ther 27:1053–1070

Chen AY, Frankowski R, Bishop-Leone J, Hebert T, Leyk S, Lewin J, Geopfert H (2001) The development and validation of a dysphagia-specific quality-of-life questionnaire for patients with head and neck cancer. Arch Otolaryngol Head Neck Surg 127:870–876

Ciccaglione AF, Marzio L (2003) Effect of acute and chronic administration of the GABA B agonist baclofen on 24 hr pH metry and symptoms in controls subjects and in patients with gastroesophageal reflux disease. Gut 52:464–470

Dean BB, Gano AD Jr, Knight K, Ofman JJ, Fass R (2004) Effectiveness of proton pump inhibitors in nonerosive reflux disease. Clin Gastroenterol Hepatol 2:656–664

Del Negro A, Araújo MR, Tincani AJ, Meirelles L, Martins AS, Andreollo NA (2008) Experimental carcinogenesis on the oropharyngeal mucosa of rats with hydrochloric acid, sodium nitrate and pepsin. Acta Cir Bras 23(4):337–342

Dent J, Vakil N, Jones R, Bytzer P, Schoning U, Halling K, Junghard O, Lind T (2010) Accuracy of the diagnosis of GORD by questionnaire, physicians and a trial of proton pump inhibitor treatment: the Diamond Study. Gut 59: 7114–7721

Dettmar PW, Sykes J, Little SL, Bryan J (2006) Rapid onset of effect of sodium alginate on gastro-oesophageal reflux compared with ranitidine and omeprazole, and relationship between symptoms and reflux episodes. Int J Clin Pract 60:275–283

El-Serag HB, Hepworth EJ, Lee P, Sonnenberg A (2001) Gastroesophageal reflux disease is a risk factor for laryngeal and pharyngeal cancer. Am J Gastroenterol 96(7): 2013–2018

Farley A, Wruble LD, Humphries TJ (2000) Rabeprazole versus ranitidine for the treatment of erosive gastroesophageal reflux disease: a double-blind, randomized clinical trial. Rabeprazole Study Group. Am J Gastroenterol 95:1894–1899

Farri A, Accornero A, Burdese C (2007) Social importance of dysphagia: its impact on diagnosis and therapy. Acta Otorhinolaryngol Ital 27:83–86

Fox M (2011) Identifying the causes of reflux events and symptoms—new approaches. Aliment Pharmacol Ther 33(Suppl 1):36–42

Francis DO, Maynard C, Weymuller EA, Reiber G, Merati AL, Yueh B (2011) Reevaluation of gastroesophageal reflux disease as a risk factor for laryngeal cancer. Laryngoscope 121:102–105

Frye JW, Vaezi MF (2008) Extraesophageal GERD. Gastroenterol Clin North Am 37:845–858

Fujimoto Y, Hasegawa Y, Yamada H, Ando A, Nakashima T (2007) Swallowing function following extensive resection of oral or oropharyngeal cancer with laryngeal suspension and cricopharyngeal myotomy. Laryngoscope 117:1343–1348

Furuta GT, Liacouras CA, Collins MH, Gupta SK, Justinich C, Putnam PE, Bonis P, Hassall E, Straumann A, Rothenberg ME, (FIGERS) subcommittee (2007) Eosinophilic esophagitis in children and adults: a systematic review and consensus recommendations for diagnosis and treatment. Gastroenterology 133:1342–1363

Galli J, Cammarota G, Calò L, Agostino S, D'Ugo D, Cianci R, Almadori G (2002) The role of acid and alkaline reflux in laryngeal squamous cell carcinoma. Laryngoscope 112:1861–1865

Gill G, Johnston N, Buda A, Pignatelli M, Pearson J, Dettmar P, Koufman J (2005) Laryngeal epithelial defenses against laryngopharyngeal reflux: investigation of E-cadherin, carbonic anhydrase isoenzyme III, and pepsin. Ann Otol Rhinol Laryngol 114:913–921

Gisbert JP, Cooper A, Karagiannis D, Hatlebakk J, Agréus L, Jablonowski H, Zapardiel J (2009) Impact of gastroesophageal reflux disease on patients' daily lives: a European observational study in the primary care setting. Health Qual Life Outcomes 7:60

Gold BD (2004) Epidemiology and management of gastroesophageal reflux in children. Aliment Pharmacol Ther 19(Suppl 1):22–27

He J, Ma X, Zhao Y, Wang R, Yan X, Yan H, Yin P, Kang X, Fang J, Hao Y, Dent J, Sung JJY, Wallander MA, Johansson S, Liu W, Li Z (2010) A population-based survey of the epidemiology of symptom-defined gastroesophageal reflux disease: the Systematic Investigation of Gastrointestinal disease in China. BMC Gastroenterol 10:94

Hendricker RM, deSilva BW, Forrest LA (2010) Gore-Tex medialization laryngoplasty for treatment of dysphagia. Otolaryngol Head Neck Surg 142:536–539

Herrmann IF (1992) Surgical solutions for aspiration problems. J Jpn Bronchoesophageal Soc 43:72–79

Hurtado CW, Furuta GT, Kramer RE (2011) Etiology of esophageal food impaction in children. J Pediatr Gastroenterol Nutr 52:43–46

Johnston N, Bulmer D, Gill G, Panetti M, Ross P, Pearson J, Pignatelli M, Axford S, Dettmar P, Koufman J (2003) Cell biology of laryngeal epithelial defenses in healthy and disease: further studies. Ann Otol Rhinol Laryngol 112:481–491

Johnston N, Knight J, Dettmar P, Lively M, Koufman J (2004a) Pepsin and carbonic anhydrase isoenzyme III as diagnostic markers for laryngopharyngeal reflux disease. Laryngoscope 114:2129–2134

Johnston N, Knight J, Dettmar PW, Lively MO, Koufman J (2004b) Pepsin and carbonic anhydrase isoenzyme III as diagnostic markers for laryngopharyngeal reflux disease. Laryngoscope 114(12):2129–2134

Johnston N, Dettmar PW, Lively MO, Postma GN, Belafsky PC, Birchall M, Koufman JA (2006) Effect of pepsin on laryngeal stress protein (Sep70, Sep53, and Hsp70) response: role in laryngopharyngeal reflux disease. Ann Otol Rhinol Laryngol 115(1):47–58

Johnston N, Wells CW, Blumin JH, Toohill RJ, Merati AL (2007) Receptor-mediated uptake of pepsin by laryngeal epithelial cells. Ann Otol Rhinol Laryngol 116(12):934–938

Jones R, Coyne K, Wiklund I (2007) The Gastro-oesophageal Reflux Disease Impact Scale: a patient management tool for primary care. Aliment Pharmacol Ther 25:1451–1459

Kanakala V, Lamb CA, Haigh C, Stirling RW, Attwood SE (2010) The diagnosis of primary eosinophilic esophagitis in adults: missed or misinterpreted? Eur J Gastroenterol Hepatol 22:848–855

Kinekawa F, Kubo F, Matsuda K, Kobayashi M, Furuta Y, Fujita Y, Okada H, Muraoka T, Yamanouchi H, Inoue H, Uchida Y, Masaki T (2008) Esophageal function worsens with long duration of diabetes. J Gastroenterol 43:338–344

Knight J, Lively MO, Johnston N, Dettmar PW, Koufman JA (2005) Sensitive pepsin immunoassay for detection of laryngopharyngeal reflux. Laryngoscope 115(8):1473–1478

Koek GH, Sifrim D, Lerut T, Janssens J, Tack J (2003) Effect of the GABA(B) agonist baclofen in patients with symptoms and duodeno-gastro-oesophageal reflux refractory to proton pump inhibitors. Gut 52:1397–1402

Kos MP, David EF, Klinkenberg-Knol EC, Mahieu HF (2010) Long-term results of external upper esophageal sphincter myotomy for oropharyngeal dysphagia. Dysphagia 25:169–176

Kotby MN, Hassan O, El-Makhzangy AMN, Farahat M, Shadi M, Milad P (2010) Gastroesophageal reflux/laryngopharyngeal reflux disease: a critical analysis of the literature. Eur Arch Otorhinolaryngol 267:171–179

Koufman J (1991) The otolaryngologic manifestations of gastroesophageal reflux disease (GERD): A clinical investigation of 225 patients using ambulatory 24-hr pH monitoring and an experimental investigation of the role of acid and pepsin in the development of laryngeal injury. Laryngoscope 101(Suppl 53):1–78

Koufman JA (2002) Prevalence of esophagitis in patients with pH-documented laryngopharyngeal reflux. Laryngoscope 112:1606–1609

Ku PK, Abdullah VF, Vlantis AC, Lee KY, van Hasselt AC, Tong MC (2009) 'Steam-boat' supraglottic laryngoplasty for treatment of chronic refractory aspiration: a modification of Biller's technique. J Laryngol Otol 123:1360–1363

Lacy B, Weiser K, Chertoff J, Fass R, Pandolfino JE, Richter JE, Rothstein RI, Spangler C, Vaezi MF (2010) The diagnosis of gastroesophageal reflux disease. Am J Med 123:583–592

Lang IM, Medda BK, Shaker R (2001) Mechanisms of reflexes induced by esophageal distension. Am J Physiol Gastrointest Liver Physiol 281:G1246–G1263

Langmore SE (2003) Evaluation of oropharyngeal dysphagia: which diagnostic tool is superior? Curr Opin Otolaryngol Head Neck Surg 11:485–489

Langmore SE, Schatz K, Olson N (1991) Endoscopic and videofluoroscopic evaluations of swallowing and aspiration. Ann Otol Rhinol Laryngol 100:678–681

Lawson G, Remacle M, Jamart J, Keghian J (2003) Endoscopic CO$_2$ laser-assisted surgery for cricopharyngeal dysfunction. Eur Arch Otorhinolaryngol 260:475–480

Leslie P, Drinnan MJ, Finn P, Ford GA, Wilson JA (2004) Reliability and validity of cervical auscultation: a controlled comparison using videofluoroscopy. Dysphagia 19:231–240

Lewin J, Gillenwater A, Garrett J, Bishop-Leone J, Nguyen D, Callender D, Ayers G, Myers J (2003) Characterization of laryngopharyngeal reflux in patients with premalignant and early carcinomas of the larynx. Cancer 97:1010–1014

Lien HC, Wang CC, Hsu JY, Sung FC, Cheng KF, Liang WM, Kuo HW, Lin PH, Chang CS (2010) Classical reflux symptoms, hiatal hernia and overweight independently predict pharyngeal acid exposure in patients with suspected reflux laryngitis. Aliment Pharmacol Ther. doi: 10.1111/j.1365-2036.2010.04502.x

Lim KB, Lee HJ, Lim SS, Choi YI (2009) Neuromuscular electrical and thermal-tactile stimulation for dysphagia caused by stroke: a randomized controlled trial. J Rehabil Med 41:174–178

Lin PH, Hsiao TY, Chang YC, Ting LL, Chen WS, Chen SC, Wang TG (2011) Effects of functional electrical stimulation on dysphagia caused by radiation therapy in patients with nasopharyngeal cancer. Support Care Cancer 19:91–99

Lindstrom D, Wallace J, Loehrl T, Merati A, Toohill R (2002) Nissen fundoplication surgery for extraesophageal manifestation of gastroesophageal reflux (EER). Laryngoscope 112:1762–1765

Little F, Koufman J, Kohut R, Marshall R (1985) Effect of gastric acid on the pathogenesis of subglottic stenosis. Ann Otol Rhinol Laryngol 94:516–519

Louis E, Tack J, Vandenhoven G, Taeter C (2009) Evaluation of the GERD Impact Scale, an international, validated patient questionnaire, in daily practice. Results of the ALEGRIA study. Acta Gastroenterol Belg 72:3–8

Lowell SY, Poletto CJ, Knorr-Chung BR, Reynolds RC, Simonyan K, Ludlow CL (2008) Sensory stimulation activates both motor and sensory components of the swallowing system. Neuroimage 42:285–295

Ludlow CL (2010) Electrical neuromuscular stimulation in dysphagia: current status. Curr Opin Otolaryngol Head Neck Surg 18:159–164

Luostarinen M (1993) Nissen fundoplication for reflux esophagitis Long-term clinical and endoscopic results of 109 of 127 consecutive patients. Ann Surg 217:329–337

Mainie I, Tutuian R, Shay S, Vela M, Zhang X, Sifrim D, Castell DO (2006a) Acid and non-acid reflux in patients with persistent symptoms despite acid suppressive therapy: a multicentre study using combined ambulatory impedance-pH monitoring. Gut 55:1398

Mainie I, Tutuian R, Agrawal A, Adams D, Castell DO (2006b) Combined multichannel intraluminal impedence-pH monitoring to select patients with persistent gastro-oesophageal reflux for laparoscopic Nissen fundoplication. Br J Surg 93:1483

Maronian N, Azadeh H, Waugh P, Hillel A (2001) Association of laryngopharyngeal reflux disease and subglottic stenosis. Ann Otol Rhinol Laryngol 110:606–612

McCoul ED, Goldstein NA, Koliskor B, Weedon J, Jackson A, Goldsmith AJ (2011) A prospective study of the effect of gastroesophageal reflux disease treatment on children with otitis media. Arch Otolaryngol Head Neck Surg 137:35–41

McGlashan JA, Johnstone LM, Sykes J, Strugala V, Dettmar PW (2009) The value of liquid alginate suspension (Gaviscon Advance) in the management of laryngopharyngeal reflux. Arch Otorhinolaryngol 266:243–251

McHorney CA, Bricker DE, Kramer AE, Rosenbek JC, Robbins J, Chignell KA, Logemann JA, Clarke C (2000a) The SWAL-QOL outcomes tool for oropharyngeal dysphagia in adults: I. Conceptual foundation and item development. Dysphagia 15:115–121

McHorney CA, Bricker DE, Robbins J, Kramer AE, Rosenbek JC, Chignell KA (2000b) The SWAL-QOL outcomes tool for oropharyngeal dysphagia in adults: II. Item reduction and preliminary scaling. Dysphagia 15:122–133

McHorney CA, Robbins J, Lomax K, Rosenbek JC, Chignell KA, Kramer AE, Bricker DE (2002) The SWAL-QOL and SWAL-CARE outcomes tool for oropharyngeal dysphagia in adults: III. Documentation of reliability and validity. Dysphagia 17:97–114

McHorney CA, Martin-Harris B, Robbins J, Rosenbek JC (2006) Clinical validity of the SWAL-QOL and SWAL-CARE outcomes tool with respect to bolus flow measure. Dysphagia 21:141–148

Meneghelli UG, Boaventura S, Moraes-Filho JP, Leitão O, Ferrari AP, Almeida JR, Magalhães AF, Castro LP, Haddad MT, Tolentino M, Jorge JL, Silva E, Maguilnik I, Fischer R (2002) Efficacy and tolerability of pantoprazole versus ranitidine in the treatment of reflux esophagitis and the influence of Helicobacter pylori infection on healing rate. Dis Esophagus 15:50–56

Meng NH, Wang TG, Lien IN (2000) Dysphagia in patients with brainstem stroke: incidence and outcome. Am J Phys Med Rehabil 79:170–175

Merati A, Lim H, Ulualp S, Toohill R (2005) Meta-analysis of upper probe measurements in normal subjects and patients with laryngopharyngeal reflux. Ann Otol Rhinol Laryngol 114:177–182

Meurmann Y (1957) Suspension of the larynx with fascial strips on the hyoid bone for removal of deglutition disorders after trauma [in German]. Arch Ohren Nasen Kehlkopfbeilkd 172:96–104

Musser J, Kelchner L, Neils-Strunjas J, Montrose M (2011) A comparison of rating scales used in the diagnosis of extraesophageal reflux. J Voice 25(3):293–300

Nguyen NP, Moltz CC, Frank C, Vos P, Smith HJ, Karlsson U, Dutta S, Midyett FA, Barloon J, Sallah S (2004) Dysphagia following chemoradiation for locally advanced head and neck cancer. Ann Oncol 15:383–388

Nguyen NP, Frank C, Moltz CC, Vos P, Smith HJ, Bhamidipati PV, Karlsson U, Nguyen PD, Alfieri A, Nguyen LM,
Lemanski C, Chan W, Rose S, Sallah S (2006) Aspiration rate following chemoradiation for head and neck cancer: an underreported occurrence. Radiother Oncol 80:302–306

Nocon M, Labenz J, Jaspersen D, Leodolter A, Richter K, Vieth M, Lind T, Malfertheiner P, Willich SN (2008) Health-related quality of life in patients with gastro-oesophageal reflux disease under routine care: 5-year follow-up results of the ProGERD study. Aliment Pharmacol Ther 29:662–668

Noordzij J, Khidr A, Evans B, Desper E, Mittal R, Reibel J, Levine P (2001) Evaluation of omeprazole in the treatment of reflux laryngitis: a prospective, placebo-controlled, randomized, double-blind study. Laryngoscope 111: 2147–2151

Numans ME, Lau J, de Wit NJ, Bonis PA (2004) Short-term treatment with proton-pump inhibitors as a test for gastroesophageal reflux disease. Ann Intern Med 140:518–527

Orlando RC (2011) Oesophageal tissue damage and protection. Aliment Pharmacol Ther 33(Suppl 1):8–12

Ozgursoy OB, Salassa JR (2010) Manofluorographic and functional outcomes after endoscopic laser cricopharyngeal myotomy for cricopharyngeal bar. Otolaryngol Head Neck Surg 142:735–740

Ozulgedik S, Yorulmaz I, Gokcan K (2006) Is laryngopharyngeal reflux an important risk factor in the development of laryngeal carcinoma? Eur Arch Otorhinolaryngol 263: 339–343

Park W, Hicks DM, Khandwala F, Richter JE, Abelson TI, Milstein C, Vaezi MF (2005) Laryngopharyngeal reflux: prospective cohort study evaluating optimal dose of proton-pump inhibitor therapy and pretherapy predictors of response. Laryngoscope 115:1230–1238

Park S, Chun HJ, Keum B, Uhm CS, Baek SK, Jung KY, Lee SJ (2010) An electron microscopic study—correlation of gastroesophageal reflux disease and laryngopharyngeal reflux. Laryngoscope 120:1303–1308

Pearson JP, Parikh S (2011) Nature and properties of gastro-oesophageal and extra-oesophageal refluxate. Aliment Pharmacol Ther 33(Suppl 1):2–7

Peng S, Xiong LS, Xiao YL, Lin JK, Wang AJ, Zhang N, Hu PJ, Chen MH (2010) Prompt upper endoscopy is an appropriate initial management in uninvestigated Chinese patients with typical reflux symptoms. Am J Gastroenterol 105:1947–1952

Peponi E, Glanzmann C, Willi B, Huber G, Studer G (2011) Dysphagia in head and neck cancer patients following intensity modulated radiotherapy (IMRT). Rad Oncol 6:1

Pitman M, Weissbrod P (2009) Endoscopic CO_2 laser cricopharyngeal myotomy. Laryngoscope 119:45–53

Postma G (2000) Ambulatory pH monitoring methodology. Ann Otol Rhinol Laryngol 109:10–14

Postma G, Johnson L, Koufman J (2002) Treatment of laryngopharyngeal reflux. Ear Nose Throat J 81(Suppl 2):24–26

Postma G, Cohen J, Belafsky P, Halum S, Gupta S, Bach K, Koufman J (2005) Transnasal esophagoscopy: revisited (over 700 consecutive cases). Laryngoscope 115:321–323

Prasad GH, Alexander JA, Schleck CD, Zinsmeister AR, Smyrk TC, Elias RM, Locke GR 3rd, Talley NJ (2009) Epidemiology of eosinophilic esophagitis over three decades in Olmstead County, Minnesota. Clin Gastroenterol Hepatol 7:1055–1061

Qadeer MA, Swoger J, Milstein C, Hicks DM, Ponsky J, Richter JE, Abelson TI, Vaezi MF (2005) Correlation between symptoms and laryngeal signs in laryngopharyngeal reflux. Laryngoscope 115:1947–1952

Qadeer MA, Phillips CO, Lopez AR, Steward DL, Noordzij JP, Wo JM, Suurna M, Havas T, Howden CW, Vaezi MF (2006) Proton pump inhibitor therapy for suspected GERD-related chronic laryngitis: a meta-analysis of randomized controlled trials. Am J Gastroenterol 101:2646–2654

Ramsey DJC, Smithard DG, Kalra L (2003) Early assessments of dysphagia and aspiration risk in acute stroke patients. Stroke 34:1252–1257

Rees C (2007) In-office transnasal esophagoscope-guided botulinum toxin injection of the lower esophageal sphincter. Curr Opin Otolaryngol Head Neck Surg 15:409–411

Rees CJ, Belafsky PC (2008) Laryngopharyngeal reflux: current concepts in pathophysiology, diagnosis, and treatment. Int J Speech Lang Pathol 10:245–253

Reimer C, Søndergaard B, Hilsted L, Bytzer P (2009) Proton-pump inhibitor therapy induces acid-related symptoms in healthy volunteers after withdrawal of therapy. Gastroenterology 137:80–87

Ricker J, McNear S, Cassidy T, Plott E, Arnold H, Kendall B, Franklin K (2011) Routine screening for eosinophilic esophagitis in patients presenting with dysphagia. Ther Adv Gastroenterol 4:27–35

Robbins J, Langmore S, Hinds JA, Erlichman M (2002) Dysphagia research in the 21st century and beyond: proceedings from Dysphagia Experts Meeting, August 21, 2001. J Rehabil Res Dev 39:543–548

Ronkainen J, Aro P, Storskrubb T, Lind T, Bolling-Sternevald E, Junghard O, Talley NJ, Agreus L (2006) Gastro-oesophageal reflux symptoms and health-related quality of life in the adult general population—the Kalixanda study. Aliment Pharmacol Ther 23:1725–1733

Ryu JS, Kang JY, Park JY, Nam SY, Choi SH, Roh JL, Kim SY, Choi KH (2009) The effect of electrical stimulation therapy on dysphagia following treatment for head and neck cancer. Oral Oncol 45:665–668

Samuels TL, Johnston N (2009) Pepsin as a causal agent of inflammation during nonacidic reflux. Otolaryngol Head Neck Surg 141(5):559–563

Samuels TL, Handler E, Syring ML, Pajewski NM, Blumin JH, Kerschner JE, Johnston N (2008) Mucin gene expression in human laryngeal epithelia: effect of laryngopharyngeal reflux. Ann Otol Rhinol Laryngol 117(9):688–695

Schroeder PL, Richter JE (1994) Swallowing disorders in the elderly. Semin Gastrointest Dis 5:154–165

Sealock RJ, Rendon G, El-Serag HB (2010) Systematic review: the epidemiology of eosinophilic esophagitis in adults. Aliment Pharm Ther 32:712–719

Shaw MJ, Talley NJ, Beebe TJ, Rockwood T, Carlsson R, Adlis S, Fendrick M, Jones R, Dent J, Bytzer P (2001) Initial validation of a diagnostic questionnaire for gastroesophageal reflux disease. Am J Gastroenterol 96:52–57

Shaw M, Dent J, Beebe T, Junghard O, Wiklund I, Lind T, Johnsson F (2008) The Reflux Disease Questionnaire: a measure for assessment of treatment response in clinical trials. Health Qual Life Outcomes 6:31

Shaw JM, Barnman PC, Callanan MD, Beckingham IJ, Metz DC (2010) Long-term outcome of laparoscopic Nissen and laparoscopic Toupet fundoplication for gastroesophageal reflux disease: a prospective, randomized trial. Surg Endosc 24:924–932

Smith DF, Ott DJ, Gelfand DW, Chen MYM (1998) Lower esophageal mucosal ring: correlation of referred symptoms with radiologic findings using a marshmallow bolus. Am J Roentgenol 171:1361–1365

Steward D, Wilson K, Kelly D, Patil M, Schwartzbauer H, Long D, Welge J (2004) Proton pump inhibitor therapy for chronic laryngo-pharyngitis: a randomized placebo control trial. Otolaryngol Head Neck Surg 131:342–350

Strugala V, Avis J, Jolliffe IG, Johnstone LM, Dettmar PW (2009) The role of an alginate suspension on pepsin and bile acids—key aggressors in the gastric refluxate Does this have implications for the treatment of gastro-oesophageal reflux disease? J Pharm Pharmacol 61:1021–1028

Swoger J, Ponsky J, Hicks DM, Richter JE, Abelson TI, Milstein C, Qadeer MA, Vaezi MF (2006) Surgical fundoplication in laryngopharyngeal reflux unresponsive to aggressive acid suppression: a controlled study. Clin Gastroenterol Hepatol 4:433–441

Szczesniak MM, William RBH, Brake HM, Maclean JC, Cole IE, Cook IJ (2010) Upregulation of the esophago-UES relaxation response: a possible pathophysiological mechanism in suspected reflux laryngitis. Neurogastroenterol Motil 22:381–389

Tack J (2005) Role of pepsin and bile in gastro-oesophageal reflux disease. Ali Pharmacol Ther 22(Suppl 1):48–54

Tang M, Dettmar P, Batchelor H (2005) Bioadhesive oesophageal bandages: protection against acid and pepsin injury. Int J Pharmaceutics 292:169–177

Tasker A, Dettmar PW, Panetti M, Koufman JA, Birchall J, Pearson JP (2002) Is gastric reflux a cause of otitis media with effusion in children? Laryngoscope 112:1930–1934

Tauber S, Gross M, Issing WJ (2002) Association of laryngo-pharyngeal symptoms with gastroesophageal reflux disease. Laryngoscope 112:879–886

Tutuian R (2011) Obesity and GERD: pathophysiology and effect of bariatric surgery. Curr Gastroenterol Rep. doi: 10.1007/s11894-011-0191-y

Vaezi MF, Qadeer MA, Lopez R, Colabianchi N (2006) Laryngeal cancer and gastroesophageal reflux disease: a case-control study. Am J Med 119:768–776

Vakil NB, Traxler B, Levine D (2004) Dysphagia in patients with erosive esophagitis: prevalence, severity, and response to proton pump inhibitor treatment. Clin Gastroenterol Hepatol 2(8):665–668

Vakil N, van Zanten SV, Kahrilas P, Dent J, Jones R, Global consensus group (2006) The Montreal definition and classification of gastroesophageal reflux disease: a global evidence-based consensus. Am J Gastroenterol 101:1900–1920

Wada T, Sasaki M, Kataoka H, Ogasawara N, Kanematsu T, Tanida S, Nojiri S, Ando T, Okochi M, Joh T (2009) Gastroesophageal and laryngopharyngeal reflux symptoms correlate with histopathologic inflammation of the upper and lower esophagus. J Clin Gastroenterol 43:249–252

Wang X, Pitchumoni CS, Chandrarana K, Shah N (2008) Increased prevalence of symptoms of gastroesophageal reflux diseases in type 2 diabetics with neuropathy. World J Gastroenterol 14:709–712

Westcott C, Hopkins B, Bach K, Postma G, Belafsky P, Koufman J (2004) Fundoplication for laryngopharyngeal reflux disease. J Am Coll Surg 199:23–30

Wight R, Paleri V, Arullendram P (2003) Current theories for the development of nonsmoking and nondrinking laryngeal carcinoma. Curr Opin Otolaryngol Head Neck Surg 11:73–77

Wilson JA (2005) What is the evidence that gastro-oesophageal reflux is involved in the aetiology of laryngeal cancer? Curr Opin Otolaryngol Head Neck Surg 12:97–100

Wirth D, Kern B, Guenin MO, Montal I, Peterli R, Ackermann C, von Flue M (2006) Outcome and quality of life after open surgery versus endoscopic stapler-assisted esophago-diverticulostomy for Zenker's diverticulum. Dis Esophagus 19:294–298

Woodson G (1997) Cricopharyngeal myotomy and arytenoid adduction in the management of combined laryngeal and pharyngeal paralysis. Otolaryngol Head Neck Surg 116:339–343

Pediatric Aspect of Dysphagia

Pascale Fichaux Bourin, Michèle Puech, and Virginie Woisard

Contents

Abstract

Pediatric dysphagia is specific because of the different developmental stages from the neonatal period to the infancy. Diagnosis and treatment will be different if it concerns a newborn or a young child having already experienced oral feeding. Furthermore swallowing and feeding disorders, having a direct impact on the nourishment function of the parents, will have repercussions on the child-parents relationship. Swallowing disorders are frequently multifaceted and impairments can be morphological, functional or induced. The assessment of these disorders includes anamnesis (reviewing family, medical, developmental and feeding history), physical examination (searching for nutritional impact, cardiopulmonary state and looking for developmental anomalies or genetic dysmorphism), swallowing evaluation (analyzing oropharyngolaryngeal structure and function by observation, fiber-optic endoscopy, videofluoroscopy, ultrasonography) and feeding evaluation (implicating parents and caregivers). Management of these disorders is a complex task, thus an interdisciplinary team and recurrent assessments are required so as to match the child's development and capacities. Its main aims are to prevent repercussions on developmental milestones and to assure the safety of the child and the psychological balance of child-parents relationship.

P. Fichaux Bourin (✉) · M. Puech · V. Woisard
Unité de la Voix et de la Déglutition,
Department of Ear, Nose and Throat,
CHU de Toulouse, Hôpital Larrey,
31059 Toulouse Cedex 9, France
e-mail: fichaux-bourin.p@chu-toulouse.fr

O. Ekberg (ed.), *Dysphagia*, Medical Radiology. Diagnostic Imaging, DOI: 10.1007/174_2012_583,
© Springer-Verlag Berlin Heidelberg 2012

1   Introduction

The child's swallowing evolves; this is one of its principal characteristics. In adults, dysphagia is a loss of the abilities. In children, its evolution is modified, impacting on the morphological development of the organs like on the other functions of the aerodigestive tract such as breathing and speech.

The maturation of swallowing is organized over the first few years of life until 6 years as reported by most authors or 10 years as reported by some authors (Schindler et al. 2011), a date when mastication is fully controlled. This long evolution starts in utero. From 7 weeks' gestational age (GA), the brainstem receives the first sensory information from the pharyngolarynx. The sensory effectors are in place at the end of the embryonic phase. The principal anatomical structures develop as follows: the mandible at 4 weeks, the palate between the 6th and 12th weeks, and the esophagus at 7 weeks' GA. At this time the fetus starts to swallow the amniotic liquid. From 10 weeks' GA, pharyngeal deglutitions are observable on ultrasonography (Miller et al. 2003). Suction is mature from the 15th week. A sucking–swallowing pattern appears from 18 to 24 weeks' GA. It becomes functional from 34 to 37 weeks' GA. Fetal sucking and swallowing plays a significant role in the morphogenesis of the oropharyngeal cavities. It takes part in the development of the digestive tract, the fetal trophicity, and its fluid balance. It is also the period of the first food experiments, the olfactory particles crossing the placental barrier. The observation of this sucking and swallowing, on ultrasonographic examinations of the second and third quarters of pregnancy, can be used to predict the sucking and swallowing of the baby at birth (Couly et al. 2009; Miller et al. 2003).

All must be in place at birth to ensure good coordination between sucking, swallowing, and breathing. The primary reflexes allow the newborn to ensure its vital needs are met. By rooting, the newborn moves towards the nipple. By grasping it remains attached to its mother. At this stage, the baby is acquiring feeding behavior. The alternation of hunger and satiety gives a rhythm to the baby's days in relation to the alternation of wakefulness and sleep. These various steps are paramount in the psychoemotional structuring of the baby. The progressive contributions of the nutrients must be in agreement with the quantitative and qualitative needs for each age. Food diversification supports the progressive evolution as do textures and tastes, while respecting the organic and neurological evolution of the child and its sensorimotor abilities.

Any modification or obstacle in this long evolution may contribute to significant delays in the emergence of the other oromotor behaviors, including babbling, speech, and language production. The causes of swallowing disorders are multifaceted and their consequences will depend on the stage of the child's development.

This is why early and suitable evaluation and management are necessary to limit the functional effects of swallowing disorders on the aerodigestive crossroads.

2   The Different Developmental Stages

At birth, the newborn must pass from the liquid atmosphere into the air. The breath goes through the pharyngeal cavities, via the glottis, the trachea, and the bronchi. The alveoli become smooth, and the baby cries for the first time. Then the child starts to suck. The passageway for nutrients from the mouth to the digestive tract depends on the effectiveness and coordination of muscles and on a very precise synchronization (Amaizu et al. 2008).

2.1   The Neonatal Period

At this stage the baby will coordinate nutritive sucking, swallowing, and breathing.

2.1.1   Sucking

Sucking is an alternation of suction, intraoral negative pressure, and expression/compression, mouthing, or stripping of the nipple by the tongue against the hard palate. The two basic forms are nonnutritive sucking, on a finger or pacifier, and nutritive sucking, when a nutrient is ingested from a bottle or the maternal breast. The sucking pattern evolves. It is immature in preterm infants, consisting primarily of expression/compression. This is followed by the appearance of suction and the progressive establishment of the

Table 1 The five-point sucking scale (Lau et al 2000)

Stage	Description
1a	No suction; arrhythmic expression
1b	Arrhythmic alternation of suction and expression
2a	No suction; rhythmic expression
2b	Arrhythmic alternation of suction and expression; sucking bursts noted
3a	No suction and rhythmic expression
3b	Rhythmic suction and expression; suction amplitude increases, wide amplitude ranges, prolonged sucking bursts
4	Rhythmic suction and expression; well-defined suction, amplitude ranges decreased
5	Rhythmic, well-defined suction and expression; increasing suction amplitude; sucking pattern similar to that of a term infant

rhythmic alternation of suction and expression. The sucking pattern of term infants is characterized by the rhythmic alternation of suction and expression/compression. Lau et al. (2000) have demonstrated that the bottle-feeding performance is positively correlated with the development stage of sucking. They used a five-point scale to characterize the infant's oromotor skills. This scale evaluates the presence or absence of suction, and rates the rhythmicity of suction and expression/compression in preterm infants (Table 1).

The sucking efficiency can also be analyzed from the ingested milk flow in the preterm infant. It increases significantly between the 34th and 36th weeks' GA, exceeding 7 ml/min with the 35 weeks (Mizuno and Ueda 2003). The same holds for the pressure of suction and its duration. A functional maturation but also a good coordination of the muscle groups is essential. The coordination of the movement of the oromotor structures controls the changing intraoral pressures that occur during a suck cycle. Successful sucking is dependent on intact brainstem pathways and transmission of impulses through the cranial nerves to healthy musculature in the mouth, tongue, and pharynx.

The pace and alternation of suction and expression will vary during the first month of life in the term infant without a disorder. A 1:1 suck–swallow ratio is most frequent (78.8%), and then there will be bursts of two or three sucks for one swallow as if the child has adapted to be more effective (Qureshi et al. 2002). The normal feeding infant is reflexive without suprabulbar input (Stevenson and Allaire 1991). The maturation of

nutritive sucking progresses in a caudocephalad way in the brainstem (Bosma 1985). The baby then becomes able to modify these various paces and acquires new food strategies. The reflex behaviors become automatic functions strengthened by voluntary movements.

2.1.2 Breathing

During nonnutritive sucking the infant swallows only little saliva, and coordination of sucking and breathing is not important to avoid inhalation. The situation is different during nutritive sucking, the alternations between sucking, swallowing, and breathing being closely dependent. To be effective, the newborn must take milk without aspiration, desaturation, or bradycardia. The patterns most frequently encountered are 1:1:1 and 2:2:1 ratios of sucking, swallowing, and breathing (Lau et al. 2003). According to Lau et al., oral feeding difficulties in a preterm infant are more likely to result from a coordination defect between swallowing and breathing than from sucking–swallowing interaction. During nutritive sucking, the newborn swallows during apnea, preferentially at the beginning of the inspiratory phase or at the end of expiration, at low lung volume. However, during the first oral feeding experiments, it can also swallow at the end of inspiration/beginning of expiration or during the inspiratory phase. After 12 months, a swallowing pattern similar to that of an adult is most frequent: a swallow followed by expiration.

2.1.3 Airway-Protective Reflexes

Protection of the airway during swallow is a reflexive, multilevel function consisting of the apposition of the epiglottis and aryepiglottic folds and the adduction of the false and true vocal folds. The fetus is in an all-aqueous environment and can swallow and inhale amniotic fluid. For the newborn the challenge is to defend the airways from aspiration of liquid during feeding. Laryngeal chemoreflex includes reflexes such as startle, rapid swallowing, apnea, laryngeal constriction, hypertension, and bradycardia. Water or acidic liquids in contact with the laryngeal epithelium trigger these reflexes. The receptors involved are concentrated in the interarytenoid cleft, at the entrance of the larynx. Laryngeal chemoreflex can cause prolonged apnea in infants. But these responses are functional: swallowing removing fluid from the laryngopharyngeal airway and vocal chord constriction combined with apnea preventing aspiration (Thach 2008). As the infant matures, rapid swallowing and apnea become much less pronounced, whereas cough arousal and possibly laryngeal constriction become more prominent. These changes result from the maturation of the central processing of afferent stimuli rather than reduction of sensitivity.

2.1.4 Central Control

The neuromotor function of the child depends on the stages of motor control maturation. At birth, up to 6 weeks before and 6 weeks after the term of 40 weeks' GA, infant motricity is under brainstem control without suprabulbar input. At this stage feeding is reflexive. The functional development of the central nervous system progresses in an ascending way. The synaptogenesis begins around 6–8 weeks' GA. The development of dendrites and synaptic connections is a dynamic process whose maximum development occurs postnatally. The body structure of the neuronal circuitry is more dependent on the movements themselves than on the genetic program (Lagercrantz and Ringstedt 2001; Hanson and Landmesser 2004).

The wiring of the precise neural circuits seems to be dependent on neuronal activity, which could be stimulated either by sensory input or endogenously driven activity. The fetal swallowing movements will thus play a main role in the organization of specific neural pathways. Conversely sucking–swallowing disorders will have a negative effect on the good development of these circuits. As feeding development progresses, basic brainstem-mediated responses come under voluntary control through the process of encephalization, up to 2 years, going down from the cortex to the spinal cord. The sensory feedback of the gustatory and somatoesthesic stimulations gradually modulates the central patterning of lapping, sucking, swallowing, and chewing.

In summary, the neurophysiological control of feeding and swallowing is complex and involves sensory afferent nerve fibers, motor efferent fibers, paired brainstem swallowing centers, and suprabulbar neural input. Close integration of sensory and motor functions is essential to the development of normal feeding skills. Feeding development, however, depends on structural integrity and neurologicalmaturation. It is a learned progression of behaviors. This learning is heavily influenced by oral sensation, motor development, and experiential opportunities. Finally, the basic physiologic complexity of feeding is compounded by individual temperament, interpersonal relationships, environmental influences, and culture.

2.1.5 The Maturation of the Digestive Tract

The neuromuscular development of the gastrointestinal tract appears relatively early during the gestational period, but the ontogeny of the peristaltic coordination depends on digestive tract segments (Dumont and Rudolph 1994). The three esophageal portions do not have same maturation. In the median portion of the esophagus, the proximal part of the smooth musculature is acquired well before term. On the other hand, the peristalsis in the two other areas remains variable in half of swallows at full term if there are no disorders (Staiano et al. 2007). Two types of esophageal peristalsis have been described during the neonatal period (Gupta et al. 2009). The first one is initiated during swallowing, transferring the bolus from the pharynx through a relaxed upper esophageal sphincter into the esophageal segments. This primary peristalsis on the level of the striated muscles is under the control of central pattern generators, whereas for the smooth musculature it depends on interactions between central and peripheral neurological control mechanisms. The presence of this primary peristalsis has been observed as early as 32 weeks' GA in the fetus. The secondary peristalsis is described like an adaptation reflex to the esophageal distension. It is under the control of the vagus nerve. This peristalsis has also been described as early as 32 weeks' GA.

2.1.6 Postural Control

The full-term newborn without a disorder is in discreetly asymmetrical flexion. This passive tonicity associated with the primary reflexes (rooting, grasping) permits the newborn to remain fixed at the breast, thus allowing it to have an effective food catch (Radzyminski 2005). The ability to control the head position is also important in the first few days of life. In the study of Radzyminski (2005), letdown was significantly related to active tone. This is interpreted like an active tonicity allowing the baby to comprehend the exterior surroundings and thus to better manage its feeding with the maternal breast.

2.1.7 Neuroendocrine Control

The presence of an effective sucking–swallowing pattern after birth plays a main role in the feeding of the infant. Several hormones have been described as being fundamental in this control: leptin, already known as an orexigenic hormone, and more recently oxytocin. Schaller et al. (2010) showed the effectiveness of oxytocin in the treatment of feeding disorders in the Magel2-defective mouse (animal model of Prader–Willi syndrome). They hypothesized that oxytocin could be used to treat impaired feeding onset in the newborn.

The maintenance of energy homeostasis requires a balance between intake and expenditure. The alternation of hunger and satiety plays an important role in the regulation of food intake. Smith and Ferguson (2008) have well described the neurophysiology of hunger and satiety, which are regulated by complex central nervous system circuitries. Central feeding circuits are localized in hypothalamic nuclei which communicate with each other and project to an area in the brainstem. The regulation is under the control of hormonal and neural feedback. Gastrointestinal and gustatory feedback are the primary controls of ingestive behavior (Smith and Ferguson 2008).

2.2   From 2 Months to 2 Years

The child's swallowing abilities progress with its neuromotor development (Hedberg et al. 2005). This long period of sensorimotor acquisition, named encephalization time, follows the evolution of the corticobulbar tracts. The reflex becomes a voluntary gesture, then automatic motion. Suckling, tongue motions in an anteroposterior direction, corresponds to the abilities of the 6-month-old infant. The bending axial posture evolves gradually from the supine position to the sitting station. The jaw movement is then free, allowing the acquisition of sucking, upright movement of the tongue. Suckling and sucking are combined between 6 and 12 months. They form the bolus control in the oral cavity preceding chewing. The child evolves from a gross to an increasingly fine motricity, alternative pressure preceding malaxation then chewing. At 2 years, the phase of oral preparation starts to be in place (Table 2).

3   Etiologies in Children

Any obstacle in the evolution and the development of this set of complex processes can cause swallowing, feeding, and speech disorders. It is necessary to distinguish sucking–swallowing disorders in the neonatal period from feeding behavior disorders in a young child. Neonatal sucking–swallowing disorders, considering them according to the level of trouble, can be classified from the central nervous system to the peripheral nervous system (Fig. 1). The various impairments can be morphological, functional, or induced by enteral feeding, for example.

3.1   Suprabulbar Lesions

Between the basal nuclei and frontal cortex, the causes are classified as encephalopathy, congenital malformations, perinatal stroke, or asphyxia.

3.1.1   Encephalopathy

(a) Neonatal encephalopathy: Risk factors are maternal thyroid disorders, and placental anomalies more than neonatal asphyxia (Badawi et al. 2005; Nelson 2005). Neuroprotective treatments such hypothermia would appreciably decrease the risks in newborns suffering from moderate neonatal encephalopathy (Gluckman et al. 2005).

(b) Degenerative encephalopathy: Mucopolysaccharidosis, epileptic encephalopathy, and leukodystrophy.

3.1.2   Congenital Malformations

Gyration abnormalities and agenesis of corpus callosum and of vermis cerebellum are congenital malformations.

3.1.3   Perinatal Stroke or Asphyxia

In the case of cerebral palsy, the prognosis depends on the existence of associated neonatal encephalopathy (Badawi et al. 2005). Most perinatal strokes are not diagnosed during the neonatal period. It is necessary to think of stroke and perform neuroradiological investigations when neurological signs or dysphagia arise during the first few months after birth (Wu et al. 2004).

For Armstrong-Wells et al. (2009), neonatal encephalopathy and seizure are the clinical criteria of symptomatic perinatal stroke. In a study done between 1993 and 2003, of 323, 532 births, they found a prevalence of 6.2 per 100,000 infants.

3.2   Bulbar Lesions

Bulbar lesions cause neonatal sucking–swallowing disorders. They can be classified as follows.

Table 2 Neuromotor development in an infant

Age	Oral sensorimotor function for feeding	Oral structure	Neuromotor skills	Cognitive and communication skills
1st month	Suckling < latching, Incomplete lip closure Nasal respiration Unable to release nipple	Tongue fills oral cavity Relatively small mandible No distinct oropharynx Larynx high in neck	Rooting and grasping reflex Hands flexed across chest during feeding Asymmetrical flexion	Facial expression of fear or pain Differentiates vocal voice from other sounds Recognizes parents' voices
2nd month	Suckling with active lip movement > latching Range of movement for jaw Lip closure improved		Letdown Able to control head position VD: Asymmetrical position DD: Lifts head up at	Smile answer Fixes gaze on an object and follows moving ones too Start of labial consonant and [r]
3rd to 4th month	Introduction of spoon, but nipple feeds only Dissociation of movements of lips and tongue Effective and voluntary control of mouth	Chin tuck does not occur until this time	No more grasping reflex Midline orientation VD : Lifts chest and head up DD: Extended and flexed movements of legs	Incites smile Vocal plays and imitates vocalizations and clicks as "fish sound" and tongue clicks Blows bubbles with saliva
5th to 6th month (transition to feeding by spoon)	Sucking, but suckling pattern prominent Start of weaning Gag reflex on new textures Tongue reversal after spoon removal Teething	Growth of neck Larynx goes down in neck Rhinopharynx closed during swallowing	Can likely roll over Bears weight on its leg Able to sit with support Pulls itself up to a sitting position Holds on to a rattle	Perceives itself as different from its mother Smiles to its image in a mirror
7th to 9th month (cup drinking)	Coordinated lip, tongue, and jaw movements Movement of lateral tongue over solids Gag reflex becomes protective		Sits without support Bounces, pulls itself up, and crawls Mouth used to investigate the environment	Afraid of strangers Jabbers and imitates sounds Waves bye-bye Points
10th to 12th month	Self finger feeding Start of chewing, control of sustained bite Closes lips on spoon and uses them to remove food from the spoon	Tongue posteriorization Growth of vocal tract	Stand holding on to things First steps	Intonational jabber and first words Able to understand simple commands

(continued)

Table 2 (continued)

Age	Oral sensorimotor function for feeding	Oral structure	Neuromotor skills	Cognitive and communication skills
13th to 18th month	All texture taken Well-coordinated swallowing and breathing Lateral tongue motion Straw drinking		Walk acquired Climb up and down the stairs	Well-coordinated phonation Associates words, simple sentences Emotional instability: impatient, frustrated when it cannot communicate
19th to 24th month	Swallows with lip closure Up–down tongue movements precise Rotary chewing Independent feeding		Runs and jumps Shoots at balloon Climbs more surely Less likely to fall	Marked equilibrium, added maturity, and calm Symbolic plays Stock lexicon of 200 words, first sentences

Adapted from Arvedson and Brodsky (2001)
VD ventral decubitus, *DD* dorsal decubitus, < less than, > more than

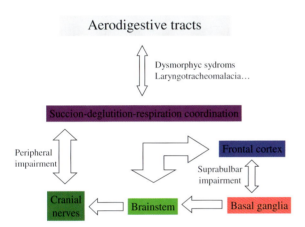

Fig. 1 Summary of various injuries

3.2.1 Neonatal Dysfunctions of the Brainstem

These cause sucking–swallowing–breathing disorders, glossopharyngolaryngoesophageal dysmotricity, and heart rate dysregulation. Neonatal dysfunctions of the brainstem were initially described in children with Pierre Robin syndrome. The metameric organization of the rhombencephalon explains facial malformations associated with failure of cranial nerves (Fig. 2). Moreover, lack of fetal sucking increases the facial dysmorphism observed, such as glossoptosis, microretrognathia, and ogival cleft palate. Other dysfunctions are involved in known genetic syndromes such Möbius syndrome (agenesis of nerves VI and VII) and Goldenhar syndrome (oculoauricular dysplasia usually affecting one side of the face with microtia and a missing eye).

Sometimes the clinical presentation is not complete "para Robin," with the dysfunction of the brainstem being without palatal anomalies but with typical facial characteristics according to genetic syndromes such DiGeorge syndrome, microdeletion of chromosome 22 (de Lonlay-Debeney et al. 1997), Kabuki syndrome, and Noonan syndrome, characterized by early eating disorders and a break in the growth curve. Finally, children with CHARGE syndrome (coloboma, heart malformation, atresia of choanae, retarded growth and development, genital hypoplasia, and ear abnormalities or deafness) have durable and complex feeding difficulties. Cranial nerve dysfunction impacts feeding development with weak sucking/chewing, swallowing difficulty, gastroesophageal reflux (GER), and aspiration (Dobbelsteyn et al. 2008).

3.2.2 Clastic

These lesions cause antenatal or perinatal anoxic ischemia of the brainstem.

3.2.3 Malformative

The lesions are visible on MRI and can cause olivopontocerebellar impairments or posterior fossa atrophy. They can cause Arnold–Chiari syndrome, occipitocervical malformations (Albert et al. 2010), or Dandy–Walker syndrome, cystic dilatation of the fourth ventricle.

3.3 Peripheral Causes

3.3.1 Neuromuscular Junction or Muscle Impairment

They are often hereditary as in the myotonia of Steinert, or motor and sensory neuropathy.

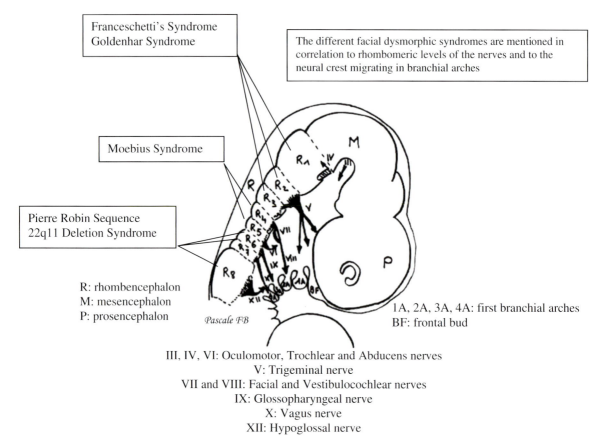

Franceschetti's Syndrome
Goldenhar Syndrome

The different facial dysmorphic syndromes are mentioned in correlation to rhombomeric levels of the nerves and to the neural crest migrating in branchial arches

Moebius Syndrome

Pierre Robin Sequence
22q11 Deletion Syndrome

R: rhombencephalon
M: mesencephalon
P: prosencephalon

Pascale FB

1A, 2A, 3A, 4A: first branchial arches
BF: frontal bud

III, IV, VI: Oculomotor, Trochlear and Abducens nerves
V: Trigeminal nerve
VII and VIII: Facial and Vestibulocochlear nerves
IX: Glossopharyngeal nerve
X: Vagus nerve
XII: Hypoglossal nerve

Fig. 2 Rhombomere diagram and cellular emergence of branchial nerves. (From Abadie et al. 1996)

3.3.2 Upper Respiratory Tract Disease

These diseases contribute to swallowing and breathing disorders. They include laryngotracheomalacia, diastema, and exceptionally laryngeal rhabdomyosarcoma of the larynx (Ferlito et al. 1999). In the case of laryngomalacia, laryngeal tone and sensorimotor integrative function of the larynx are altered (Thompson 2007). Thompson (2007) underlines the worsening role of GER, neurological disorders, and a low Apgar score.

3.3.3 Motility Disorders of the Digestive Tract

(a) GER is often incriminated. An increase of gastric liquid in the esophagus is frequent in healthy children. It is the consequence of anatomical characteristics (reduced length of the diaphragmatic portion and low capacity of the esophagus), diet (exclusively liquid feeding), position (mostly supine position). However, if pharyngitis is associated with inflammation of the esophagus or worse acid aspiration, this GER becomes pathological. The North American Society for Pediatric Gastroenterology, Hepatology, and Nutrition and the European Society for Pediatric Gastroenterology, Hepatology, and Nutrition have published guidelines for evaluation and management of GER (Vandenplas et al. 2009). The reflux is associated with upper airway symptoms in children. But from a review of the literature, the correlation and the risk of upper airway symptoms attributable to GER are difficult to determine (Rosbe et al. 2003). However, the presence of laryngopharyngeal reflux and respiratory symptoms may indicate the need for antireflux therapy (May et al. 2011).

(b) Esophageal transit disorders: A defect of contraction, an esophageal dyskinesia, a faulty upper esophageal sphincter relaxation, or a desynchronization of opening can be the origin of swallowing disorders with aspirations. An esophageal atresia is to be searched for in a systematic way. It is frequently associated with a tracheoesophageal fistula. Esophageal atresia and tracheoesophageal fistula are congenital malformations that occur in one in 3,500 births. The association is a multifactorial complex disease that involves genetic and environmental factors (de Jong et al. 2010).

(c) Finally a delay in gastric emptying can support backward flows and can impact on hunger–satiety balance.

3.3.4 All Morphologic Abnormalities from the Oral Cavity to the Stomach

Oropharyngeal lymphangiomas, cysts of the tongue, and facial clefts can be observed in the upper aerodigestive tract. At the level of the esophagus and stomach, one can encounter tracheoesophageal fistulas, esophageal atresia, and stricture (Castilloux et al. 2010; Till et al. 2008; Prasse and Kikano 2009). Microgastria, which will require exclusively enteral feeding, can also have long-term repercussions for the sensorimotor development of the aerodigestive tract.

3.3.5 Food Allergy and Sucking–Swallowing Disorders

These are encountered in an exceptional way as recalled by Abadie (2008). However, in the older child some can be the origin of eosinophilic esophagitis inducing vomiting and food blocking (Abu-Sultaneh 2010).

3.3.6 Induced Causes

These are multifactorial complex diseases involving environmental factors and consequences of the initial pathology. They follow from the lack of neonatal oral experimentation, with the traumatizing effect on the aerodigestive tract from suction probes, intubation, and an enteral feeding tube. Moreover, the mode of continuous enteral feeding or exclusive parenteral feeding will have noxious effects on the acquisition of pace by the child and in particular that of hunger–satiety. Finally, major disturbances in the link between the mother and child with an often traumatizing birth, an obligatory more or less long separation, and the impossibility for the mother to play her life-sustaining part are worsening factors. This is why most dysphagic infants had difficult perinatal antecedents, including prematurity (Salinas-Valdebenito et al. 2010).

3.4 The Young Dysphagic Child

All the causes previously mentioned can be encountered as can anorexia and feeding disorders as described in the following sections.

3.4.1 The Common Anorexia of Opposition in the Second Half of the Year

Anorexia arises in the first 3 years of life, most commonly between the ages of 9 and 18 months, as infants become more autonomous and make the transition to spoon feeding and self-feeding. The following are often found to have occurred: a traumatic event, aspiration during a mouthful, an infectious episode, especially as it required hospitalization, and a change in the child's life and its relationship with its mother (e.g., family death). The meal time is then marked by anxiety, the child is opposed to any attempt at spoon feeding, whereas often a feeding bottle is accepted just as drinking from a glass. The lack of interest in food contrasts with strong interest in exploration and interaction with caregivers. The child remains joyful, plays, and stays awake.

3.4.2 Severe Form of Infantile Anorexia

Children with infantile anorexia have an anxious neurosis, depression, or even maternal deprivation. The baby can only express its suffering through its body. Food refusal is accompanied by other signs, such as loss of contact, avoidance, irritability, sleep disorders, vomiting, and ruminations, which will worsen nutritional repercussions (Thouvenin et al. 2005). Failure to thrive is often associated with poorer cognitive development, learning disabilities, and long-term behavioral problems. Chatoor et al. (2004) described the importance of distinguishing between nonorganic forms of growth deficiency related to maternal neglect and growth deficiency that is related to dyadic conflict during feeding. They suggested that the concern for the nutritional needs has to be balanced with the management of feeding difficulties in young children.

3.4.3 Autism Spectrum Disorders

Although not revealing, anorexia or another feeding disorder is very frequently encountered in invading neurobehavioral alterations (Nicholls and Bryant-Waugh 2009).

3.4.4 Feeding Disorders

These involve problems in a range of eating activities that may or may not be accompanied by swallowing difficulties. These disorders may be characterized by disruptive mealtime behavior, rigid food preference, or food refusal:

(a) Pick eating: One can think of this as a child cherry picker who selects and eats only very modest amounts. There is no attachment disorder and the nutritional repercussion remains mild.

(b) Food phobias with behavior disorder: Selection of a color or an exclusive consistency, or the need to sniff at food before putting it in the mouth. They can also be the expression of an infantile neurosis beginner.

(c) Pica: Children who swallow in addition to food-stuffs nonnutritive substances such as stones and paper. This feature can be seen in a specific way between the ages of 9 and 12 months, and is then not pathological. On the other hand, it becomes abnormal if it continues, and is often associated with backwardness or behavior disorders in certain genetic syndromes such as Prader–Willi syndrome and also in autism spectrum disorders.

3.4.5 The Dyspraxia of Feeding

This is encountered in children with specific language impairments, oromotor dyspraxia, and during meals, difficulties in bolus formation. Tongue movement and chewing are limited. The child is described as a whole-food swallower when given mixed textures.

4 Assessment and Treatment of the Child with Swallowing Disorders

Diagnosis and treatment will be different if it concerns a newborn in a neonatology intensive care unit or a young child having already experienced oral feeding.

In the first case, it is necessary to be able to answer three main questions:

1. When should oral feeding be proposed?
2. What stimulations support a good maturation of oromotor abilities?
3. How can the functional consequences for food and verbal acquirements be avoided?

For the young dysphagic child, there will also be an etiologic diagnosis of the disorder, and an analysis of its consequences for feeding, hydration, and nutrition and the pulmonary repercussions. The evaluation must be able to inform about:

• The symptoms of the disorder and its evolution
• Whether or not there is an association with other dysfunctions and integration in a neurological or syndromic clinical presentation
• The somatic and psychogenic part of the feeding disorder (Abadie 2004).

4.1 The Premature Baby and the Infant in the Neonatology Service

The realization of the noxious effect of unfavorable surroundings on the morbidity of premature babies led to the installation of a mewborn individualized developmental care and assessment program (NID-CAP) in most neonatology intensive care units. This program aims at limiting stress by controlling the extraneous auditory, visual, vestibular, and tactile stimulations. It is achieved by putting the child in the fetal position with a soft application, with supporting presence of the two parents (mini isolated rooms). Its positive effects in the short and long term were objectified by many studies (McAnulty et al. 2009; Symington and Pinelli 2001; Ullenhag et al. 2009).

The premature baby is deprived of sensory stimulations normally tested by the fetus during the third quarter of pregnancy. They are replaced by noxious stimulations in the form of probe introductions such as intubation, suction, or enteral feeding tubes. To propose early positive stimulations of the oral sphere seems to be essential, as mentioned by Lapillonne (2010), but which ones can be proposed? Promoting breastfeeding as soon as it is possible seems to be most suitable for premature babies. It is necessary, however, that the preterm infant has the capacity to manage this. Acquiring a safe and efficient swallow and the capacity for oral feeding of infants in neonatology intensive care units are some of the prerequisites for the reduction of the consequences of the hospitalization. Safe swallowing is conditioned by sucking–swallowing–breathing coordination avoiding aspirations while allowing proper ventilation.

For the preterm infant, the principal difficulty is the integration of breathing in an already delicate sucking–swallowing pattern. Moreover, the respiratory condition is often precarious especially if it is associated with bronchodysplasia. Gewolb and Vice (2006) compared two cohorts of infants born between 26 and 33 weeks' GA. In the group with bronchodysplasia, they found a clear immaturity of acquisition and a greater incoordination of sucking, swallowing, and breathing.

The second difficulty is for the weary baby feed efficiently in a short time (about 20 min and no more than 30 min). Indeed the purpose is to feed so that the infant consumes sufficient volumes to gain weight appropriately. The transition from tube to oral feeding in the preterm infant depends on the teams. For some, any premature baby can manage the transition even for very tiny quantities. This is the technique of "kangoroo mother care" often associated with breastfeeding. The ability to make the transition from gavage to oral feeding depends on neurodevelopmental status, which is related to behavioral organization, cardiorespiratory regulation, and the ability to produce a rhythmic sucking–swallowing–breath pattern (Delaney and Arvedson 2008). The readiness of the infant for oral feeding may differ (Nyqvist et al. 2001; Delaney and Arvedson 2008; Lau et al. 2000).

4.1.1 The Different Means of Evaluation

(a) Morbidity assessment: This involves the awareness of the general state of the child according to the neonatal medical index, which has five stages, stage 1 being a baby without an intercurrent medical problem and stage 5 concerning serious complications. The birth weight and not the term are also part of the score. Delaney and Arvedson (2008) mentioned that it is important to differentiate "premature by date" from "premature by weight," for which the latter already has an important perinatal morbidity.

(b) Behavioral assessment: According to the NIDCAP, the reactions of premature babies can be staged in keeping with five behavioral subsystems: autonomic, motor, state regulation, attention, and self-regulation or regulatory system. Assessment of the infant's current functional competence and state of equilibrium determines if it is possible or not to propose oral feeding or oral stimulations. The infant must be either calm, awake, and in a stable cardiorespiratory state.

(c) Sucking behavior assessment: Some authors have linked oral feeding abilities with an effective nonnutritive sucking (Pinelli and Symington 2001). Others have shown that it is the oral feeding experimentation which improves the sucking capacities (Pickler et al. 2006). During nutritive sucking, two patterns exist, a continuous sucking and an intermittent sucking stopped by breathing. The continuous sucking, which is more common at the beginning of feeding, represents a long single sucking burst. Sucking does not automatically initiate swallowing. The preterm infant which has a respiratory rate from 40 to 60 inspirations per minute cannot have too frequent swallowing under penalty of interference with breathing. In a study of 88 preterm infants, Pickler et al. (2006) noted that experience in oral feeding may result in rapider maturation of sucking characteristics, increasing very quickly the numbers of sucks, sucking bursts, and the sucking rhythm. For them it is especially the infant's level of arousal and the neonatal medical index which will condition the possibilities of oral feeding, more than the capacities for sucking–swallowing–breathing coordination. Other authors prefer proposing oral feeding only when sucking–swallowing and breathing are well coordinated (Delaney and Arvedson 2008; Lau 2007).

For breastfed infants, Nyqvist et al. (1996) proposed an assessment using the preterm infant breastfeeding behavior scale. This scale evaluates the reflex activities (rooting, grasping), sucking, and swallowing. It also considers the number of sucks and sucking bursts. It considers, under the term "behavior," the awakening of the child, the influence of the surroundings, and the maternal behavior. Thoyre et al. (2005) described a method based on the assessment of early feeding ability of preterm infants. The ability is evaluated according to 36 items gathered in three domains: oral feeding readiness, oral feeding skills, and oral feeding recovery. The items require yes/no answers or rankings from 1 to 4 (Table 3).

(d) Surface electromyography. This is a noninvasive objective method for evaluating the muscle activity during oral feeding. Nyqvist (2008) recommends coupling it with observation of mouthing and sucking bursts and the trains of sucks to evaluate the infant's competencies during breastfeeding. The electrodes in this study were placed on orofacial

Table 3 Oral feeding readiness, skill, and recovery—example of items (Thoyre et al. 2005)

Oral feeding readiness				
Able to hold body in a flexed position with arms/hands toward midline	Yes	No		
Demonstrates energy for feeding, maintains muscle tone and body flexion through assessment period	Yes	No		
Oral feeding skill				
Ability to remain engaged in feeding				
Predominant muscle tone	Maintains flexed body position with arms toward midline	Inconsistent tone, variable muscle tone	Some tone consistently felt, but somewhat hypotonic	Little or no tone felt; flaccid, limp most of the time
Ability to organize oral–motor functioning				
Opens mouth promptly when lips are stroked at feeding onsets	All	Most	Some	None
Once feeding is under way, maintains a smooth rhythmic pattern of sucking				
Ability to coordinate swallowing and breathing				
Able to engage in long sucking bursts (7–10 sucks) without behavioral stress signs or an adverse or negative cardiorespiratory response				
Ability to maintain physiologic stability				
In the first 30 s after each feeding onset, oxygen saturation is stable, and behavioral stress cues absent				
Stops to breathe before behavioral stress cues appear				
Clear breath sounds; no grunting breath sounds (prolonging the exhale, partially closing glottis on exhale)				
Oral feeding recovery (during the first 5 min after feeding)				
Predominant state	Quiet alert	Drowsy	Sleep	Fuss/cry

muscles (orbicular, mylohioid, geniohyoid, stylohyoid, and digastric) and on pharyngeal muscles. Gomes et al. (2009) in a review of the literature underlined the significant role of the masseter muscle during breastfeeding. The feeding bottle was not tested in this study.

4.1.2 Management

(a) To support nonnutritive sucking: The observation that babies intubated orally maintained their sucking capacity and even sucked the intubation tube led many neonatology intensive care units to propose in a quasisystematic way the use of a pacifier (Delaney and Arvedson 2008). Nonnutritive sucking is a motor reflex activity which will make it possible to improve the capacity to control and coordinate nutritive sucking. A pacifier is proposed for any premature infant of more than 28 weeks' GA.

(b) To treat the infant by taking account of its level of vigilance of its physiological state of stability or instability according to the NIDCAP: The infant is allowed to regain the quiet state by keeping it in a flexed position during the transfer time, and bringing its hands back to the middle of the body near the mouth to help the self-regulation. The infant should be calm before nutritive sucking is attempted. Clinicians and caregivers have to structure and adapt the care and interaction to enhance the infant's own competencies and strengths, to prevent the infant being in pain, stress, or discomfort.

(c) To facilitate oral feeding: Many authors think that the systematic proposal of breastfeeding or bottle feeding is the most effective stimulation and that other sensitive stimulations are not necessary (Thoyre et al. 2005; Pieltain et al. 2007; Nyqvist 2008; Ullenhag et al. 2009). Facilitating means to mitigate the inefficiency of sucking having been proposed such as the feeding cup or using soft or perforated pacifiers. It is then necessary to be wary of too fast a flow, which may incur risks of inhaling and shock. This is why Lau and Schanler (2000) advise the use of a "vacuum-free bottle." For them, self-paced milk flow seems the technique most suitable for use with preterm infants. Delaney and Arvedson (2008) described the transition between enteral and oral feeding as difficult for the preterm infants of less than 32 weeks' GA because of neurological immaturity and cardiorespiratory instability.

(d) To complement feeding by parenteral feeding: Pieltain et al. (2007) described the importance of early efficient feeding, as in the first few days of life, in low-weight premature infants This is "aggressive feeding," i.e., rich in protein. The high proteinic contribution makes it possible to preserve the low weight of these infants and to limit their insulin resistance. Lapillonne (2010) prefers the term "optimal feeding." The aims of preterm management are multiple, and are to improve the growth and its quality, to preserve the cerebral, neurosensory, and pulmonary development, and to mitigate digestive diseases dominated by ulcero-necrotizing enterocolitis and GER disease.

Oral feeding, because of great neuromotor immaturity, often causes stress and increases the state of agitation and suffering of these fragile babies. In all cases, early clinical assessment and management of sucking–swallowing is one of the priorities. In this way, the long-term complications could be decreased as described by Buswell et al. (2009) in a cohort of preterm infants whose food functions were evaluated at 10 months of corrected age.

4.2 The Young Child

Assessment of infants and children with dysphagia and feeding disorders involves an interdisciplinary evaluation (Arvedson 2008). These disorders are multidetermined and need a multiaxial diagnosis. The interdisciplinary feeding/swallowing team approach allows optimal management decisions and understanding of health conditions and specific issues (Arvedson 2008). The parents are imperatively involved, and so are the child's caregivers. The anamnesis locates the disorder in the family context and the setting of the meal. Knowledge of the oral history of the child is essential to specify the origin of the disorder in its food and neurophysiological development.

When should a specific evaluation be requested? It will be systematic when personal autonomy during meals is impossible; this is the case for children with cerebral palsy or multiple disabilities. It is also the case for young patients with a disease with a high risk of feeding and swallowing disorders, e.g., in a genetic syndrome and in brainstem or cerebellum impairments.

A specific evaluation is necessary when the duration of feeding is abnormally prolonged, when mealtimes are stressful, and when there is increasing irritability of the child or on the contrary lethargy.

Food refusal might be diagnosed if there is any somatic cause.

Finally, vomiting, nasal food reflux, respiratory signs during or after meals, and frequent bronchopulmonary infections must also alert the physician to the need for a specific evaluation.

One is frequently confronted with a child who either does not chew or does not accept pieces of food during food diversification.

How should the child be approached? From 0 to 2 years it is necessary for the child to be closest to its usual situation. The friendly evaluation takes place during a meal or in a play context: grimaces resulting from mouth and vocal plays, linguistic situations adapted to its developmental age.

After 2 years, it is then possible to perform a morphological and dynamic evaluation of the child's oral functions and its swallowing, but before an examination of the mouth is undertaken, the child must have confidence in the physician.

4.2.1 Assessment Process

The assessment of infants or children with signs of feeding or swallowing disorders includes first the anamnesis reviewing family, medical, developmental, and feeding history, and then physical examination and swallowing evaluation. In some cases other diagnostic tests may be required:

1. The anamnesis: The findings of interviews of parents, medical and educational professionals, and caregivers specify the reason for the evaluation, the complaints, and the repercussions of the disorder. The taking of the anamnesis appreciates the medical and psychological context.

    (a) Grounds for evaluation: The most frequent difficulty for infants is a sucking–swallowing incoordination noticed by parents or caregivers. Bottle feeding or breastfeeding is slow and hard, often interrupted by the child crying. This also applies to weak suction, the baby sucking with difficulty and often stopping. A long period of apnea during feeding can be observed too. This is more alarming if all these signs are associated with hypoxia and bradycardia, implying oral feeding should be stopped. Oral or nasal regurgitations as well as episodes of cough at the time of the meals are often signs of a protective reflex from aspiration. Less specific signs are food refusal and prolonged feeding duration. Slow weight gain or worse weight loss is often one of the signs of the nutritional repercussion of a swallowing disorder. This evaluation may also be required to survey a disease with a risk of swallowing disorders such as a Pierre Robin sequence or cerebral palsy. Finally, the occurrence of repeated bronchopulmonary infections or severe asthma should lead one to suspect the existence of chronic aspiration.

    (b) The feeding history summarizes the main steps and in particular weaning, and specifies on which consistencies the disorder depends, its degree of severity, and its constancy with time. It also reflects the parents's difficulties to feed their child.

Assessment of the impact of feeding defines the consistencies given to the child, and specifies for liquids if they should be water, milk and fruit juice, and for pasty consistencies if they should be compotes or dairy produce. Does the child take semisolid foods such as blank or rice pudding? Does it accept soft solids (fruit cocktail) or tough solids (cookies and meats)? The symptoms, medical context, and evolution of the disorder are correlated with the oral-food trainings. The functional repercussion on the feeding makes it possible to envisage the upcoming risks. Limme (2011) stressed the importance of food diversification in the development of the masticatory function. This will allow the harmonious growth of the jawbones and the dentoalveolar structures.

It is also important to specify if it is or was necessary to resort to enteral, parenteral or ancillary feeding

2. Medical and developmental history can yield possible clues to the causes of dysphagia, in particularly prenatal birth, a genetic syndrome, and a neonatal accident.

(a) Physical examination: As Arvedson (2008) says, this is the prefeeding assessment.

    1. Assessment of nutritional impact notes the somatic growth patterns, in particular weight, height, and body mass index curves as well as the occipital frontal circumference and thoracic circumference (Lapillonne et al. 2011; Thibault et al. 2010). So recalled by Amiel-Tison (2005), "Increase in the volume of skull is particularly dramatic in the second part of gestation and the first 6 months of the life." A stagnation or a failure of growth is the unquestionable sign of a repercussion on good cerebral development. The thoracic circumference is a notable marker of the nutritional status of the child.

    2. Assessment of cardiopulmonary state: For the infant, bronchopulmonary infections and asthma are often markers of the repercussion of the dysphagia. But sometimes they can also be nasopharyngitis blocking the possibility of feeding. Moreover, one cardiopulmonary dyspnea interferes with the synchronization of breathing and swallowing and can be the cause of aspirations. This assessment is made to note deviations from normal expectations, in particularly respiratory patterns such as breathing rate at rest and during effort. Can the child breathe by nose and by mouth?

    3. Observation of developmental anomalies directed toward a genetic diagnosis. The developmental anomalies can be an epicanthus for the eyes,

a low implantation of the ears or abnormal lobules, or the characteristic form of the upper lip in Prader–Willi syndrome. In the same way, systematic observation is required for anomalies of the palmar folds, hands, feet, fingers, and toes. "Café au lait spots" will suggest a neurofibromatosis.

4. Neurodevelopmental examination: A semiological analysis according to the age and the neuromotor skills is essential. It can follow the scale of Amiel-Tison et al. (2005) or the Gesell stages in the revised test of Brunet-Lézine.

The observer notes the child's behavior and its spontaneous motility in resting posture and during interactions with its parents. The observations include the position, movement patterns, asymmetry or the stiffness of posture, response to sensory stimulation, temperament, and self-regulation abilities.

Then the examination of the child is performed in a dual situation, with the child lying on its back until 6 months of age or sitting on the examination bed or on the knees of a parent if it needs further reassurance. The physical examination appreciates axial and segmentary tonicity, proximal and distal muscle strength, and Babkin and jerk reflexes. Finally, the clinician should focus on cranial pairs V, VII, IX, X and XII.

(c) Oropharyngolaryngeal structure and function assessment

1. The oral examination must analyze the anatomical structures, the muscular functions, and symmetry at rest and in movement of the oral cavity and the face. The aspect of the lips, the jaw, the tongue position, and the shape and height of the palate are significant components that should be observed. In the infant oral reflexes (rooting, gagging) and nonnutritive sucking have to be noted. In general, laryngeal function is noted by voice quality.

2. Instrumental evaluation of swallowing: The visualization of oral, pharyngeal, and upper esophageal phases of swallowing is performed with fiber-optic endoscopic evaluation of swallowing and a videofluorosopic swallow study. Arvedson (2008) advocates the use of ultrasonography too. Although ultrasonography is not used routinely, it provides useful data on the temporal relationships between movement patterns of oral and pharyngeal

structures in the fetus, infant, and child during swallowing (Miller et al. 2003; Bosma et al. 1990; Fanucci et al. 1994).

Fiber-optic endoscopic evaluation of swallowing makes sure there is no morphologic or dynamic abnormality (Hartnick et al. 2000). The attempt to swallow is not always easy before 2 years of age, being dependent on the anatomical characteristics of the pharyngolarynx and the need to keep the rhinopharynx free. However, according to Sitton et al. (2011) it is practicable very early, as early as 3 days of life.

Sitton et al. (2011) propose collecting in a systematic way the outcomes of this analysis by specifying, according to textures, the level of release and the existence or not of penetration and aspiration. Temporal relationships of the different events and the efficiency of the mechanisms of expulsion are also noticed. It is a useful examination to visualize with the parents the pharyngolaryngeal structures, as well as to define some aspects of pharyngeal swallowing of secretions and food. The objective aspects of swallowing are noticed together, allowing the best following of oral feeding recommendations.

A *videofluoroscopic swallow study* allows visualization of the oropharyngeal and esophageal transit. It can be realized on very young children by respecting a suitable placement (Figs. 3, 4). The irradiation must obviously be controlled using reduced fields and short periods of radioscopy. The study provides information on the dynamics and the temporality of the various events of swallowing. It permits one to check the postures and adjustments of texture to avoid aspiration and to facilitate oropharyngeal transit. In all cases a functional suction must always be available in case aspiration occurs. In infants the observer notes the sucking efficiency. The movements of the jaws and the tongue are correlated to the neurodevelopmental level of the child. Pharyngeal time is analyzed as in the adult by considering the synchronization and the efficiency of the protection mechanisms and expulsion in the case of penetration. Arvedson (2008) proposes relating videofluorosopic swallow study findings to various swallowing disorders (Table 4). But it must be remembered that this examination captures only a brief window in time and does not simulate a real meal, and that is why it must be coupled with a observation of a meal.

3. Feeding observation: Observation of the child during meals allows one to collect useful information

Fig. 3 Installation during videofluoroscopy

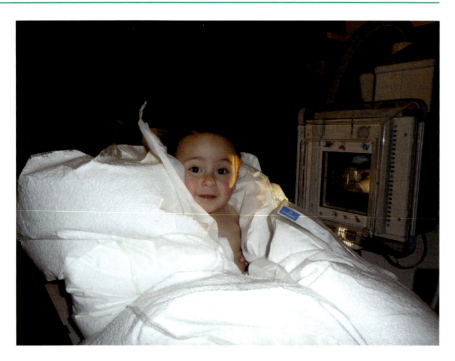

Fig. 4 Installation during videofluoroscopy

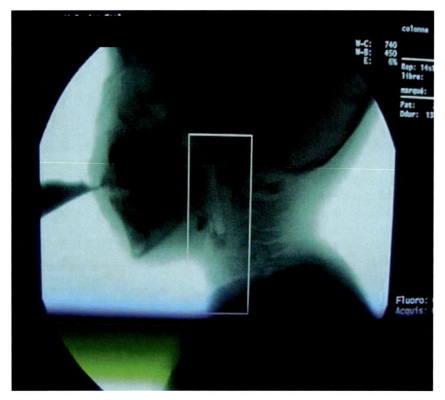

about eating and drinking (Table 5). Various observation grids can be used, such as the schedule for oral motor assessment (SOMA) (Reilly et al. 1999) and the nursing child assessment feeding scale (ratings of cognitive-growth fostering during meals) (Barnard 1978). The observation of feeding is made with a familiar feeder as typically as would be done with the child at home. The interactions between the parent and the child and positions adopted during feeding are observed. Food consistencies must be varied, starting with those which are usual and best controlled by the child. The child is observed for specific aspects of oral sensorimotor skills and the way of swallowing, in particular if multiple swallows are necessary to clear a single bolus. This feeding observation allows one to adjust the diagnosis and list the necessary adaptations.

(d) Other diagnostic tests are sometimes useful, for example, it is necessary to refer the child to a psychiatrist when the child has signs of a feeding disorder more prominent than swallowing disorders. Neurological, cardiopulmonary, and gastrointestinal functions often have to be explored by specialists.

An interdisciplinary approach with professionals across specialities communicating with parents and caregivers is important. This comprehensive assessment has to include the World Health Organization concepts (WHO 2001), involving information related to participation (society level), activities (person level), and impairment (body function level) . Management and decisions will be made taking into account:

• Oral sensorimotor and swallowing deficit
• Nutrition status
• Interactions between parents and the child
• Medical and neurodevelopmental status.

4.2.2 Decision Making and Management

At the end of the assessment process, the most important question is: Can this child drink and eat without risk? Then if it can do so, other questions are: What consistencies, what volumes, and what adaptations are possible?

The neurological examination evaluates the central and peripheral tools necessary for oral feeding.

The evaluation of the developmental stage of the child specifies its capacities for training, and its oral, feeding, and speech skills.

The oro-facial examination and instrumental swallow examination define the child's physiological swallowing status.

Finally, the examination delineates underlying causes and diagnoses because treatment will differ according to history, current status, and possible evolution.

The different treatment approaches include oral motor exercises, mealtime adaptations, and feeding adaptations:

(a) Oral motor exercises: Active exercises are used to increase strength and endurance and modify muscle tone by inhibiting or eliciting stretch reflex. Slow stretching reduces muscle tone and quick stretching increases it.

Passive exercises are applied to provide sensory input. They may include tapping, vibrations, and massage. They might reduce abnormal oral reflex such as biting reflex or gag reflex.

Sensory applications may be used to enhance a swallow response and to increase closure of the lips.

Arvedson et al. (2010) emphazize that a treatment exercise should closely parallel the desired task and that "age matter" and "time matter" have implications for the timing of intervention. The exercise protocol will depend on the developmental stage and skills of the child.

(b) Mealtime adaptations: The goal is to increase comfort, security, and pleasure. "Successful oral feeding must be measured in quality of meal time experience with best possible skills while not jeopardizing a child functional health status or the parent–child relationship" (Arvedson 2008). The adaptations concern posture and position, adapted equipment (spoons, glass, etc.), and broad adaptations (quiet conditions, no TV or too much noise, etc.).

(c) Feeding adaptations: These may concern the taste, consistency, texture, and temperature of food and liquid. It is also useful to schedule meals and to respect mealtimes to facilitate hunger. Otherwise, ancillary feeding is sometimes required.

Indications depend on clinical observations: Abadie (2008) proposed the following classification:

• Sucking disorder
• Swallowing disorder
• Velopharyngeal dysfunction
• Ventilation disorder
• Disorder of sucking–swallowing coordination
• Feeding disorder
• Oral dyspraxia.

For the organization of management plans with parents and caregivers, it seems more relevant to us to separate the various disorders encountered into:

• Child who does not know how to; this is like a maturation disorder.

Table 4 Videofluorosopic swallow study findings for various swallowing disorders

	Radiographic finding	Possible common swallowing disorder
Bolus formation	Loss of food or liquid from mouth	Loss of lip closure
	Material in anterior sulcus	Loss of lip tension or tone
	Material in lateral sulcus	Loss of buccal tension or tone
	Material pushed out with tongue	Tongue thrust, loss of tongue control
	Limited/immature chewing	Loss of jaw and tongue control
	More than 3 sucks per swallow	Loss of suck strength or coordination
Oral transit	Searching tongue movements	Apraxia of swallow, loss of oral sensation
	Forward tongue to move bolus	Tongue thrust
	Material remains in anterior sulcus	Loss of lip tone and tongue control
	Material remains in lateral sulcus	Loss of tongue movement or strength
	Material remains on tongue	Loss of tongue movement or strength
	Material remains on hard palate	Loss of tongue strength, or high and narrow palate
	Limited tongue movement	Loss of tongue coordination or disorganized AP movement
	Tongue–palate contact incomplete	Loss of tongue elevation
	Oral transit > 3 s	Delayed oral transit
Pharyngeal phase initiation	Material in valleculae, preinitiation	If brief, no delay in pharyngeal initiation
	Material in piriform sinuses, preinitiation	Delayed pharyngeal initiation
	Material in/on tonsil tissue	Tonsils blocking bolus transit, delayed pharyngeal initiation
	Material on posterior pharyngeal wall	Delayed pharyngeal phase initiation
Pharyngeal phase	Nasopharyngeal backflow/reflux	Loss of velopharyngeal closure or of UES opening
	Penetration to underside of superior part of epiglottis	Incoordination or loss of pharyngeal contraction
	Penetration into airway entrance	Loss of closure of airway entrance
	Residue after swallows in valleculae	Loss of tongue base retraction
	Residue in piriform sinuses	Loss of pharyngeal contractions or of UES opening
	Aspiration before swallow	Delayed pharyngeal swallow initiation
	Aspiration during swallow	Unilateral vocal fold paralysis, incoordination
	Aspiration after swallow	Reduced pharyngeal pressure
	Residue in pharyngeal recesses which may be cleared or not cleared with the next swallow	Loss of tongue base retraction or of pharyngeal contractions or loss of UES opening
Upper esophageal phase	Slow bolus passage through UES	UES prominence, loss of UES opening, reduced pharyngeal pressures may contribute
	Residual on or in UES	Structural abnormality or UES opening
	Retrograde bolus movement from esophagus to pharynx or from the lower to the upper esophagus	Esophageal dysmotility, structural abnormality

Adapted from (Arvedson and Lefton-Greif (1998)
AP anteroposterior, *UES* upper esophageal sphincter

Table 5 Examples of observations that may relate to cranial nerve function according to Arvedson and Brodsky (2001)

Cranial nerve	Input	Normal answer	Overdrawn answer
V	Food on the tongue	Chewing	Bolus not formed
VII	Sucking Food on the lower lip Smile	Labial gripping Labial closing Labial retraction	Labial incontinence Limiting or asymmetry of moving Incomplete
IX and X	Bolus into posterior part of the oral chamber	Swallowing reflex initiated in less than 2 seconds	RDTP or no initiation
XII	Food on the tongue	Refinement of the apex and protrusion	Miss lateral contraction, of rise atrophies

RDTP Delayed pharyngeal phase initiation

- Child who cannot; this is a secondary disorder.
- Child who does not want to; this is a behavioral disorder.

Specific therapies are as follows:

(a) Child who does not know how to: The child does not know because of a shift of acquisition or impossibility to train the infant in the case of prematurity, dysmaturity, or lack of training. For example, in the case of tracheotomy, the larynx is deprived of sensory stimulation and the coordination of swallowing and respiration can be lost. For enteral feeding it may be the oral sensorimotor skills that are not trained and the lost of hunger feeling. It is necessary to stimulate the oral sensorimotor skills and psychological maturation. The child has to find again pleasure in suction and the sensation of hunger to avoid refusing food.

(b) Child who cannot: The child cannot do because of a genetic syndrome or malformations. In the foreground are neuromotor disorders, which of are central, peripheral, or muscular origins. According to the lesional level, there might be weak suction or a lack of sucking reflex. Feeding duration is prolonged, often associated with drooling, delayed initiation of pharyngeal swallow, and penetration. (Table 5). There can also be craniofacial anomalies with midline defects such as cleft palate or oropharyngeal tumor such as lymphangioblastoma. In this case, the oral phase of swallowing is generally disturbed and may result in airway obstruction, requiring a tracheotomy. Finally gastrointestinal tract disorders including motility problems may contraindicate oral feeding and sometimes even enteral feeding. Without appropriate stimulations, the child will not be able to perform the necessary experiments for a harmonious oral construction. So it may secondarily have a faulty knowledge skill. The treatment consists in adaptational strategies to counteract the neuromotor dysfunction or anatomical anomalies.

(c) Child who does not want to: The child does not want to eat, or to test other textures or tastes. This is rather a feeding disorder. The child swallows correctly but not for a long time, as if it were very quickly satisfied. The child refuses to continue by clamping its mouth shut, and turning its head away when the spoon approaches its mouth. Sometimes it may vomit purposefully. The meal is then stopped. Oral intakes remain insufficient. This may induce fractionation meals which can worsen GER. After 6 months it is essential in a healthy child to maintain almost 3 h between each meal. In older children, solid food refusal can occur for a variety of reasons, including but not limited to airway or gastrointestinal tract factors, oral sensorimotor deficits, and disordered parent–child interactions. The distinction has to be made between an early feeding problem possibly amenable to education and an entrenched eating disorder requiring systematic diagnosis and treatment. A compartmental therapy is indicated for the child and its parents. Throughout meal sessions the therapist points out to the parents the behaviors that can reinforce food refusal. As described by Borrero et al. (2010) these can include attention (coaxing, threats, praise, reprimands, etc.), escape (spoon or drink removal, allowing the child to leave the table), and tangible delivery (switching to a previously consumed food, to a drink following

Fig. 5 Decision making

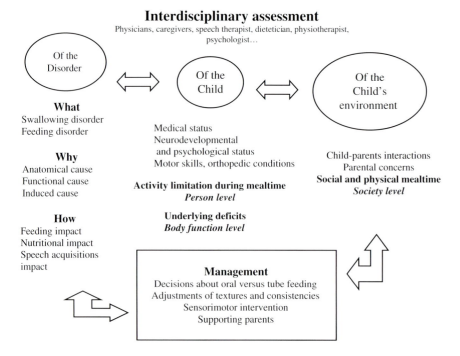

Interdisciplinary assessment

Physicians, caregivers, speech therapist, dietetician, physiotherapist, psychologist...

food presentation, etc.). The child trying new textures and tastes during playtime is indicated.

Swallowing and feeding disorders in a child, from sharing the direct impact on the nourishment function of the parents, will have repercussions on the parent–child relationship. A holistic assessment and management of these disorders cannot be done without the collaboration of the parents. This assessment involves considerations of the broad environment, parent–child interactions, and parental concerns. To be interested in dysphagia in children is to consider the child with its difficulties in its family circle and social environment. It is essential to enable the child to progress as well with the eating plan as in its socialization (Fig. 5).

The first support will be psychological support. The part of the interdisciplinary team is very important:

- To explain to the parents the swallowing disorder and the difficulties their child has
- To help them be more confident about their own capacities to manage these difficulties
- To reassure them and to trust in their child's competencies.

Then there will be educational support: they have to learn adaptational strategies, position, and broaderbased sensory and motor intervention to facilitate meal and feeding behavior.

5   Summary

To summarize, management of dysphagia in infants is a complex task based on several approaches. Indeed these disorders affect the safety of children, the psychological balance of parents, and the delay in developmental milestones. Therefore, an interdisciplinary team and recurrent assessments are necessary so as to match the child's development and capacities. The principal aims are to prevent feeding and speech disorders.

References

Abadie V (2004) Diagnostic approach in oral disorder in young children. Arch Pediatr 11(6):603–605

Abadie V (2008) Apparently isolated feeding behavior troubles in infant. Arch Pediatr 15(5):837–839

Abadie V, Cheron G, Lyonnet S et al (1996) Isolated neonatal dysfunction of brainstem. Arch Pediatr 3(2):130–136

Abu-Sultaneh SM, Durst P, Maynard V, Elitsur Y (2010) Fluticasone and food allergen elimination reverse subepithelial fibrosis in children with eosinophilic esophagitis. Dig Dis Sci 56(1):97–102

Albert GW, Menezes AH et al (2010) Chiari malformation Type I in children younger than age 6 years: presentation and surgical outcome. J Neurosurg Pediatr 5(6):554–561

Amaizu N, Shulman R et al (2008) Maturation of oral feeding skills in preterm infants. Acta Paediatr 97(1):61–67

Amiel-Tison C (2005) Neurologie périnatale, 3rd edn. Masson, Paris, pp 35–73

Amiel-Tison C et al (2005). Why is the neurological examination so badly neglected in early childhood? Pediatrics 116(4):1047; author reply 1047–1048

Armstrong-Wells J, Johnston SC et al (2009) Prevalence and predictors of perinatal hemorrhagic stroke: results from the Kaiser Pediatric Stroke Study. Pediatrics 123(3):823–828

Arvedson JC, Brodsky L (2001) Pediatric swallowing and feeding: assessment and management, 2nd edn. Singular Publishing Group, Albany, pp 283-388

Arvedson JC, Clark H et al (2010) Evidence-based systematic review: effects of oral motor interventions on feeding and swallowing in preterm infants. Am J Speech Lang Pathol 19(4):321–340

Arvedson JC, Lefton-Greif MA (1998) Pediatric video fluoroscopic swallow studies: a professional manual with caregiver guidelines. The Psychological Corporation, San Antonio

Arvedson JC (2008) Assessment of pediatric dysphagia and feeding disorders: clinical and instrumental approaches. Dev Disabil Res Rev 14:118–127

Badawi N, Felix JF et al (2005) Cerebral palsy following term newborn encephalopathy: a population-based study. Dev Med Child Neurol 47(5):293–298

Barnard K (1978) The family and you. MCN Am J Matern Child Nurs 3(2):82–83

Borrero C, Vollmer T et al (2010) Concurrent reinforcement schedules for problem behavior and appropriate behavior: experimental applications of the matching law. J Exp Anal Behav 3(93):455–469

Bosma JF (1985) Post natal ontogeny of performances of the pharynx, larynx and mouth. Am Rev Respir Dis 13(5):S10–5

Bosma JF, Hepburn LG et al (1990) Ultrasound demonstration of tongue motions during suckle feeding. Dev Med Child Neurol 32(3):223–229

Buswell CA, Leslie P et al (2009) Oral-motor dysfunction at 10 months corrected gestational age in infants born less than 37 weeks preterm. Dysphagia 24(1):20–25

Castilloux J, Noble AJ et al (2010) Risk factors for short- and long-term morbidity in children with esophageal atresia. J Pediatr 156(5):755–760

Chatoor I, Surles J et al (2004) Failure to thrive and cognitive development in toddlers with infantile anorexia. Pediatrics 113(5):e440–e447

Couly G, Aubry MC et al (2009) Fetal oral immobility syndrome. Arch Pediatr 17(1):1–2

de Jong EM, Felix JF et al (2010) Etiology of esophageal atresia and tracheoesophageal fistula: mind the gap. Curr Gastroenterol Rep 12(3):215–222

de Lonlay-Debeney P, Cormier-Daire V et al (1997) Features of DiGeorge syndrome and CHARGE association in five patients. J Med Genet 34(12):986–989

Delaney AL, Arvedson JC (2008) Development of swallowing and feeding: prenatal through first year of life. Dev Disabil Res Rev 14(2):105–117

Dobbelsteyn C, Peacocke SD et al (2008) Feeding difficulties in children with CHARGE syndrome: prevalence, risk factors, and prognosis. Dysphagia 23(2):127–135

Dumont RC, Rudolph CD (1994) Development of gastrointestinal motility in the infant and child. Gastroenterol Clin North Am 23(4):655–671

Fanucci A, Cerro P et al (1994) Physiology of oral swallowing studied by ultrasonography. Dentomaxillofac Radiol 23(4):221–225

Ferlito A, Rinaldo A et al (1999) Laryngeal malignant neoplasms in children and adolescents. Int J Pediatr Otorhinolaryngol 49(1):1–14

Gewolb IH, Vice FL (2006) Abnormalities in the coordination of respiration and swallow in preterm infants with bronchopulmonary dysplasia. Dev Med Child Neurol 48(7):595–599

Gluckman PD, Wyatt JS et al (2005) Selective head cooling with mild systemic hypothermia after neonatal encephalopathy: multicentre randomised trial. Lancet 365(9460):663–670

Gomes CF, Thomson Z et al (2009) Utilization of surface electromyography during the feeding of term and preterm infants: a literature review. Dev Med Child Neurol 51(12):936–942

Gupta A, Gulati P et al (2009) Effect of postnatal maturation on the mechanisms of esophageal propulsion in preterm human neonates: primary and secondary peristalsis. Am J Gastroenterol 104(2):411–419

Hanson MG, Landmesser LT (2004) Normal patterns of spontaneous activity are required for correct motor axon guidance and the expression of specific guidance molecules. Neuron 43(5):687–701

Hartnick CJ, Hartley BE et al (2000) Pediatric fiberoptic endoscopic evaluation of swallowing. Ann Otol Rhinol Laryngol 109(11):996–999

Hedberg A, Carlberg EB et al (2005) Development of postural adjustments in sitting position during the first half of life. Dev Med Child Neurol 47(5):312–320

Lagercrantz H, Ringstedt T (2001) Organization of the neuronal circuits in the central nervous system during development. Acta Paediatr 90(7):707–715

Lapillonne A (2010) Early nutrition and the development of the preterm infant. Arch Pediatr 17(6):711–712

Lapillonne A, Razafimahefa H et al (2011) Nutrition of the preterm infant. Arch Pediatr 18(1):313–323

Lau C (2007) Development of oral feeding skills in the preterm infant. Arch Pediatr 14(Suppl 1):S35–S41

Lau C, Alagugurusamy R et al (2000) Characterization of the developmental stages of sucking in preterm infants during bottle feeding. Acta Paediatr 89(7):846–852

Lau C, Schanler RJ (2000) Oral feeding in premature infants: advantage of a self-paced milk flow. Acta Paediatr 89(4):453–459

Lau C, Smith EO et al (2003) Coordination of suck-swallow and swallow respiration in preterm infants. Acta Paediatr 92(6):721–727

Limme M (2011) The need of efficient chewing function in young children as prevention of dental malposition and malocclusion. Arch Pediatr 17(Suppl 5):S213–S219

May JG, Shah P et al (2011) Systematic review of endoscopic airway findings in children with gastroesophageal reflux disease. Ann Otol Rhinol Laryngol 120(2):116–122

McAnulty GB, Duffy FH et al (2009) Effects of the newborn individualized developmental care and assessment program

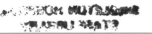
(NIDCAP) at age 8 years: preliminary data. Clin Pediatr (Phila) 49(3):258–270

Miller JL, Sonies BC et al (2003) Emergence of oropharyngeal, laryngeal and swallowing activity in the developing fetal upper aerodigestive tract: an ultrasound evaluation. Early Hum Dev 71(1):61–87

Mizuno K, Ueda A (2003) The maturation and coordination of sucking, swallowing, and respiration in preterm infants. J Pediatr 142(1):36–40

Nelson KB (2005) Neonatal encephalopathy: etiology and outcome. Dev Med Child Neurol 47(5):292

Nicholls D, Bryant-Waugh R (2009) Eating disorders of infancy and childhood: definition, symptomatology, epidemiology, and comorbidity. Child Adolesc Psychiatr Clin N Am 18(1):17–30

Nyqvist KH (2008) Early attainment of breastfeeding competence in very preterm infants. Acta Paediatr 97(6):776–781

Nyqvist KH, Farnstrand C et al (2001) Early oral behaviour in preterm infants during breastfeeding: an electromyographic study. Acta Paediatr 90(6):658–663

Nyqvist KH, Rubertsson C et al (1996) Development of the preterm infant breastfeeding behaviour scale (PIBBS): a study of nurse–mother agreement. J Hum Lact 12:207–219

Pickler RH, Best AM et al (2006) Predictors of nutritive sucking in preterm infants. J Perinatol 26(11):693–699

Pieltain C, Habibi F et al (2007) Early nutrition, postnatal growth retardation and outcome of VLBW infants. Arch Pediatr 14(Suppl 1):S11–S15

Pinelli J, Symington A (2001) Non-nutritive sucking for promoting physiologic stability and nutrition in preterm infants. Cochrane Database Syst Rev (3):CD001071

Prasse JE, Kikano GE (2009) An overview of pediatric dysphagia. Clin Pediatr (Phila) 48(3):247–251

Qureshi MA, Vice FL et al (2002) Changes in rhythmic suckle feeding patterns in term infants in the first month of life. Dev Med Child Neurol 44(1):34–39

Radzyminski S (2005) Neurobehavioral functioning and breastfeeding behavior in the newborn. J Obstet Gynecol Neonatal Nurs 34(3):335–341

Reilly SM et al (1999) Oral-motor dysfunction in children who fail to thrive: organic or non-organic? Dev Med Child Neurol 41:115–122

Rosbe KW, Kenna MA et al (2003) Extraesophageal reflux in pediatric patients with upper respiratory symptoms. Arch Otolaryngol Head Neck Surg 129(11):1213–1220

Salinas-Valdebenito L, Nunez-Farias AC et al (2010) Clinical characterisation and course following therapeutic intervention for swallowing disorders in hospitalised paediatric patients. Rev Neurol 50(3):139–144

Schaller F, Watrin F et al (2010) A single postnatal injection of oxytocin rescues the lethal feeding behaviour in mouse newborns deficient for the imprinted Magel2 gene. Hum Mol Genet 19(24):4895–4905

Schindler O, Ruoppolo G, Schindler A (2011) Deglutilogia, 2nd edn. Omega, Turin, pp 27–50

Sitton M, Arvedson JC et al (2011) Fiberoptic endoscopic evaluation of swallowing in children: feeding outcomes related to diagnostic groups and endoscopic findings. Int J Pediatr Otorhinolaryngol 75(8):1024–1031

Smith PM, Ferguson AV (2008) Neurophysiology of hunger and satiety. Dev Disabil Res Rev 14(2):96–104

Staiano A, Boccia G et al (2007) Development of esophageal peristalsis in preterm and term neonates. Gastroenterology 132(5):1718–1725

Stevenson RD, Allaire JH (1991) The development of normal feeding and swallowing. Pediatr Clin North Am 38(6):1439–1453

Symington A, Pinelli J (2001) Developmental care for promoting development and preventing morbidity in preterm infants. Cochrane Database Syst Rev (4):CD001814

Thach BT (2008) Some aspects of clinical relevance in the maturation of respiratory control in infants. J Appl Physiol 104(6):1828–1834

Thibault H, Castetbon K et al (2010) Why and how to use the new body mass index curves for children. Arch Pediatr 17(12):1709–1715

Thompson DM (2007) Abnormal sensorimotor integrative function of the larynx in congenital laryngomalacia: a new theory of etiology. Laryngoscope 117(6 Pt 2 Suppl 114): 1–33

Thouvenin B, d'Arc BF et al (2005) Infantile rumination. Arch Pediatr 12(9):1368–1371

Thoyre SM, Shaker CS et al (2005) The early feeding skills assessment for preterm infants. Neonatal Netw 24(3):7–16

Till H, Muensterer OJ et al (2008) Staged esophageal lengthening with internal and subsequent external traction sutures leads to primary repair of an ultralong gap esophageal atresia with upper pouch tracheoesophagel fistula. J Pediatr Surg 43(6):E33–E35

Ullenhag A, Persson K et al (2009) Motor performance in very preterm infants before and after implementation of the newborn individualized developmental care and assessment programme in a neonatal intensive care unit. Acta Paediatr 98(6):947–952

Vandenplas Y et al (2009) Pediatric gastroesophageal reflux clinical practice guidelines: joint recommendations of the North American Society for Pediatric Gastroenterology, Hepatology, and Nutrition (NASPGHAN) and the European Society for Pediatric Gastroenterology, Hepatology, and Nutrition (ESPGHAN). J Pediatr Gastroenterol Nutr 49(4): 498–547

WHO (2001) International classification of functioning, disability and health: world health assembly resolution WHA54.21, 54th session, 22 May 2001

Wu YW, March WM et al (2004) Perinatal stroke in children with motor impairment: a population-based study. Pediatrics 114(3):612–619

Dysphagia in Systemic Disease

Thomas Mandl and Olle Ekberg

Contents

O. Ekberg (✉)
Department of Diagnostic Radiology,
Skåne University Hospital,
205 02 Malmö, Sweden
e-mail: olle.ekberg@med.lu.se

T. Mandl
Department of Rheumatology,
Skåne University Hospital,
205 02 Malmö, Sweden

Abstract

Systemic disease may result in dysphagia through numerous mechanisms. For example, salivary gland impairment may result in xerostomia, which as well as resulting in painful mucosal blisters and ulcers may impair oral function. Acute or chronic inflammatory processes may result in strictures in the esophagus and/or pharynx. Furthermore, altered biomechanics of oral, pharyngeal, and esophageal musculature may be found in patients with rheumatoid arthritis with cervical spine abnormalities and in patients with scleroderma. Finally, systemic vasculitides involving the central nervous system may result in cortical and brainstem ischemia leading to neurological impairment hampering the swallowing process.

1 Primary Sjögren's Syndrome

Primary Sjögren's syndrome (PSS) is an autoimmune disease, primarily affecting the salivary and lacrimal glands. Impaired salivary and lacrimal secretion and mucosal dryness are the main symptoms. Nonexocrine organs, including the gastrointestinal tract and the nervous system, may also be involved.

PSS has an increased prevalence in patients with certain HLA-DR2 and DR3 genes. Several non-HLA genes may also be involved, including genes coding for cytokines and second messengers. An androgen/estrogen imbalance may also be of importance.

PSS is a rheumatic disease with lymphocytic infiltration and hypofunction in the salivary and lacrimal glands, resulting in dryness of the mouth and eyes, without coexisting connective tissue disease, whereas

O. Ekberg (ed.), *Dysphagia*, Medical Radiology. Diagnostic Imaging, DOI: 10.1007/174_2012_584,
© Springer-Verlag Berlin Heidelberg 2012

secondary Sjögren's syndrome is when the syndrome is associated with another connective tissue disease, such as scleroderma, systemic lupus erythematosus (SLE), or rheumatoid arthritis. Xerostomia is the most common gastrointestinal symptom in PSS patients (Türk et al. 2005; Kjellen et al. 1986; Anselmino et al. 1997a; Rosztóczy et al. 2001; Tsianos et al. 1986; Hradsky et al. 1967). Esophageal dysmotility and esophageal webs have also been reported (Anselmino et al. 1997a; Tsianos et al. 1986; Volter et al. 2004; Palma et al. 1994; Tsianos et al. 1985). Dryness of mucous membranes, due to lack of saliva, impairs swallowing by interfering with the sliding of the bolus on the mucous membranes. Sialometric measurements may be close to 0 ml/min. Esophageal dysmotility including weak contractions, aperistalsis, and tertiary contractions as well as abnormal peristaltic velocity and duration are seen in one third of PSS patients. A decrease in the lower esophageal sphincter pressure has also been reported (Anselmino et al. 1997b). A recent study showed that 65% of PSS patients have dysphagia (Mandl et al. 2007). They presented with solid and/or liquid food dysphagia. Also, a globus feeling was common. Other PSS patients had regurgitation and pyrosis. Some PSS patients had misdirected swallowing leading to coughing after swallowing, and haw king when eating. Others had experienced episodes of obstruction when swallowing. Many dysphagic patients had an increased liquid intake during eating.

In PSS patients a sialometric evaluation is of value (Liquidato and Bussoloti Filho 2005). Evaluation of pharyngeal and esophageal function is best done with barium swallow or fiber-endoscopic examination. Manometry of the esophagus can also be of value.

Treatment in PSS patients is in most cases symptomatic and local, aiming at reducing the symptoms and consequences of dryness. However, in some cases treatment may be systemic, including use of pilocarpine and cevimeline. These drugs stimulate the M3 receptors, causing an increased salivary flow. However, side effects of M3R stimulation may be abdominal distress, irritable bladder, and sweating (Thanou-Stavraki and James 2008). The use of biological agents is currently restricted to patients with severe nonexocrine disease, in whom especially B-cell-targeted biologicals, such as rituximab, have shown promising results (Ramos-Casals and Brito-Zerón 2007). The most important treatment is local, including an increased water intake in order to lubricate the dry mucosal surface. Lozenges and chewing gum stimulate the secretory function even in hypofunctioning salivary glands. Good dental hygiene is most important, since lack of saliva leads to tooth decay.

2 Rheumatoid Arthritis

Rheumatoid arthritis is an autoimmune disorder that is characterized by small joint synovitis resulting in swelling, pain, stiffness, and loss of function. Permanent damage to cartilage as well as bones and surrounding tissue may occur. The pathogenesis is multifactorial, and both genetic and environmental factors, especially smoking, are of importance for both the development and the severity of the disease. Lymphocytes activated by cytokines such as TNF invade the synovia and result in a swelling of the synovia and pannus formation. The disease may result in swallowing difficulties through various mechanisms. For example, temporomandibular joint involvement may cause mastication problems. Swelling of synovial membranes in the cricothyroid and cricoarytenoid joints may cause dysphagia (Chen et al. 2005). Medullary compression may result from subluxation of the atlantoaxial joint, causing brainstem compression by the odontoid process. The subluxation of the atlantoaxial joint may also cause altered biomechanics of the swallowing musculature. Pannus located in the anterior cervical spine may cause compression of the cervical esophagus. In addition, xerostomia may also occur in many patients with rheumatoid arthritis. In patients with juvenile rheumatoid arthritis, dysphagia may be due to micrognathia (Lindqvist et al. 1986; Ekberg et al. 1987). Dysphagia in rheumatoid arthritis may be due to dry mouth, delayed initiation of pharyngeal stage of swallow, and painful swallow (Geterud et al. 1991; Erb et al. 2001; Sun et al. 1974; Ekberg et al. 1987). The clinical evaluation includes imaging and should be done with a broad approach. Early initiation of treatment is important in rheumatoid arthritis patients. Of disease-modifying antirheumatic drugs (DMARDs), methotrexate is the most commonly used. Early initiation of treatment with DMARDs improves the prognosis and stops or delays the joint destruction process that otherwise is a consequence of the disease. In patients where there is an inadequate response to the first-line DMARDs, a combination of older DMARDs

Fig. 1 A patient with scleroderma. The esophagus is dilated owing to insufficiency of the lower esophageal sphincter that causes reflux. Acid reflux has caused a stricture in the distal esophagus seen in the single-contrast esophagram in (**a**) and in the double-contrast esophagram in (**b**). (Courtesy of Francis J. Scholz, Department of Diagnostic Radiology, Lahey Clinic, Burlington, MA, USA)

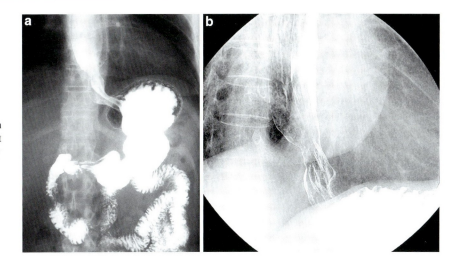

may be used or biological DMARDs may be used, of which TNF-α blockers are the most widely used. Corticosteroids and NSAIDs are today mainly used to alleviate symptoms while waiting for DMARDs to start exerting their effect, which may take a couple of weeks after treatment has started. Xerostomia usually causes increased water intake. Chewing gum and lozenges can have a beneficial effect. Other dysfunctions may be treated with direct or indirect therapies according to the underlying cause.

3   Scleroderma (Systemic Sclerosis)

Scleroderma, or systemic sclerosis (SSc), is a disorder resulting in functional and structural abnormalities of small blood vessels as well as leading to fibrosis of the skin and internal organs. The cause is unknown. Affected tissues show varying degrees of inflammation, fibrosis, and atrophy. The cutaneous lesions often appear symmetrically on the distal extremities and sometimes also on the truncal skin. Patients may show early involvement of internal organs. Raynaud's phenomenon is common. Findings of antinuclear antibodies with a centromere pattern as well as anti-ScL-70 antibodies support the diagnosis. Sclerosis of oral mucosa and masticatory muscles and salivary gland involvement may result in impaired mouth function and dysphagia (Ntoumazios et al. 2006; Rout et al. 1996). Microstomia, i.e., fibrosis of the perioral tissue, leads to a small mouth, which is a classic

finding of SSc (Pizzo et al. 2003; Menditti et al. 1990). Progressive destruction of smooth muscle in the esophagus leads to abnormal peristalsis or even aperistalsis. Usually, the tonicity in the lower esophageal sphincter is zero, leading to massive gastroesophageal reflux disease (GERD). Therefore, extensive fibrosis and strictures are common findings in these patients (Fig. 1).

Dysphagia is common in SSc patients. Intake of food is difficult owing to microstomia. Dysphagia is also caused by perioral muscle stiffness in the cheeks and tongue. Decreased elasticity is present in masticatory muscle. Decreased salivary production leads to xerostomia, i.e., secondary Sjögren's syndrome. Symptoms from esophageal dysfunction are also common. In patients with esophageal strictures, the characteristic symptom is obstruction of solid foods. The stomach and small bowel may also be involved, resulting in impaired transportation at various levels. Therefore, some of these patients have a very complex set of symptoms. In patients with discrete skin lesions, the diagnosis may be very difficult. In such cases, nail capillary microscopy can be of help in diagnosing the disease. If there are gastrointestinal symptoms, a biopsy can be of value and may show signs of degeneration of smooth muscles and fibrosis. It is important to bear GERD in mind and to do a barium examination of the esophagus and/or gastroscopy.

Current therapies for SSc are still disappointing and mainly consist of symptomatic treatment of the consequences of the disease. Various vasodilatory drugs such as gastrointestinal prokinetics and proton pump inhibitors are used. In addition, cyclophosphamide is used for the treatment of concomitant interstitial lung disease. No specific treatment is available for muscle fibrosis and muscle degeneration. It is very important to keep in mind that patients with GERD should be treated vigorously in order to avoid the development of strictures.

4 Systemic Lupus Erythematosus

Systemic lupus erythematosus (SLE) is an inflammatory, progressive systemic disease of connective tissue with an autoimmune cause and commonly affects the skin and various internal organs (Virella 1993; Goust and Tsokos 1993). Both antinuclear antibodies and the more specific anti-double-stranded-DNA antibodies may be found in patients with this systemic disease. Classically, patients present with a butterfly-shaped malar rash and photosensitivity, i.e., skin rash due to exposure to sunlight. Butterfly-shaped malar rashes usually appear on the cheeks and nose bilaterally in patients with SLE. The patients may present with oral and/or pharyngeal ulcers. Ulcers may also appear on the palate. Xerostomia appears when the salivary glands are involved. Dysphagia is present in 10% of patients with SLE (Pope 2005). Erythematous oral ulcers and xerostomia are usually the result of salivary gland involvement. Pharyngeal ulceration may extend into the nasopharynx and even into the larynx. Gastrointestinal dysmotility may include the esophagus but also the stomach and small bowel. This dysmotility may be caused by submucosal fibrosis. Cerebrovascular complications are not uncommon in patients with SLE and may cause motor and sensory impairment. The trigeminal and facial nerves may be involved. Assessment of the swallowing function is done with a thorough clinical examination and may also include barium swallow or fiber-endoscopic examinations. Endoscopy is used for assessment of mucosal lesions.

Treatment of SLE includes antimalarials and corticosteroids as well as various more potent immunomodulating drugs. In the era of biological treatments, B-cell-targeting therapies have shown beneficial effects in SLE patients. Other than the treatments used for specific dysfunctions, there is no specific treatment for swallowing impairment in SLE patients.

5 Pemphigus and Pemphigoid

Bullous pemphigoid is a subepidermal blistering skin disease of chronic character. The disease may also involve mucous membranes. Acantholysis is present in pemphigus but not in pemphigoid disease. Pemphigus and pemphigoid are both autoimmune diseases. Pemphigus has antibodies directed against desmosomes, whereas pemphigoid has antibodies directed against hemidesmosomes. These antibodies bind to their antigens and cause blistering by separation of the dermis and epidermis. The mucosa in the mouth and pharynx may also be affected (Yeh et al. 2003; International Pemphigus and Pemphigoid Foundation 2011). Mucosal abnormalities cause odynophagia, i.e., painful swallowing. Ruptured blisters may be secondarily infected, which aggravates the pain. Submucosal infection may cause fibrosis and strictures. Endoscopy and radiologic swallowing studies are often necessary in order to detect pharyngeal and esophageal involvement in the form of webs and/or strictures. Advanced diseases are treated with corticosteroids and immunosuppressive agents. Good oral hygiene is most important, since secondary infections must be prevented. When there is severe mucosal involvement, eating hard and crunchy foods, chips, raw fruits, or vegetables may be very painful. Local steroids can be of value.

6 Epidermolysis Bullosa Dystrophica

Epidermolysis bullosa dystrophica is an inherent autoimmune disease affecting the skin and the mucosa of the oropharynx. The cause is a genetic defect within the human COL-7A-1 that encodes the production of collagen. Collagen VII forms the structural link between the epidermal basement membrane and the collagen fibrils in the upper dermis. Sloughing of the mucosa causes ulcers that are easily infected and painful. Even though the oral mucosa is mostly affected, laryngeal, esophageal, and conjunctival mucosa can be involved. The blisters, erosions, and ulcers may lead to scars, webs, and strictures. It has even been reported that esophageal shortening can be caused by such scarring. This may cause hiatal hernia and GERD (Agah et al. 1983). The patient's symptom is by and large odynophagia.

Topical steroids are often used. Endoscopic dilatation may be necessary if esophageal strictures develop.

7 Lichen Planus

Lichen planus is a chronic mucocutaneous disease that causes papules or rashes involving the skin and mucous membranes but also the nails and genitals. It is likely to be an autoimmune disease that involves CD4+ and CD8+ T lymphocytes. Parakeratosis is present as well as atrophy of the esophageal epithelium. Strictures may have an appearance similar to those in GERD. The strictures are, however, localized in the proximal esophagus. This should raise the suspicion of the cause (Chandan et al. 2008; Madhusudhan and Sharma 2008; Sugerman and Porter 2010; Katzka et al. 2010). Endoscopically elevated lacy white papules, esophageal webs, and pseudomembranes are present. Erosions with and without stenosis may also be present. Strictures are present in advanced cases. Even though the disease is most frequent in the proximal and mid esophagus, the whole esophagus may be involved. The lichenoid lesions may be painful. Odynophagia may occur from lesions in both the oral cavity and the esophagus. Odynophagia is common for solids. Spicy food and liquids may cause pain.

Therapeutic options include systemic corticosteroids, cyclosporine, and azathioprine. Local steroids can be used. Endoscopic dilatation of strictures is usually needed.

8 Behçet Disease

Behçet disease is a vasculitis characterized by aphthous ulcers in the mouth and on the genitals. In addition, various skin lesions, e.g., erythema nodosum and folliculitis, eye lesions, arthritis, venous thrombosis in various locations, and CNS involvement may be encountered in these patients. The prevalence of the disease is highest in the eastern Mediterranean, the Middle East, and East Asia. In addition, the HLA-B51 gene has been reported to be a strong risk factor for the disease. The vasculitis causes recurrent oral and genital ulcers. Uveitis, erythema nodosum, folliculitis, thrombophlebitis, venous thrombosis,

meningitis or CNS vasculitis as well as arthritis may also be present (Brookes 1983; Levack and Hanson 1979; Demetriades et al. 2009; Messadi and Younai 2010). The ulcers are found on lips, tongue, and on the inside of the cheeks. Aphthous ulcers may occur as single lesions or in clusters. They may even be found in the esophagus. Ulcers in the oral cavity and mucosa and esophagus are often painful. These ulcers may be provoked by slight trauma. Treatment of the mucosal ulcers includes colchicine, whereas more systemic disease is treated with steroids and various immunomodulatory drugs. Good oral hygiene is important to prevent secondary infection of the ulcers. Strong-tasting food should be avoided as it may cause pain.

9 Sarcoidosis

Sarcoidosis is a granulomatous disease characterized by noncaseating epithelioid granulomas. The lungs and mediastinum are predominant locations, although virtually most other organs may be affected, including the gastrointestinal tract. An autoimmune cause has been suggested. A reduced delayed-type hypersensitivity response is found in many patients with sarcoidosis. The epitheloid granulomas may occur in the mucosa, where they cause superficial nodules and ulcerations that may be painful. Larger granulomas may cause irregular strictures which cause obstruction. They may be difficult to distinguish from malignant strictures on radiologic examination as well as on endoscopy (Bredenoord et al. 2010). Oral sarcoidosis may cause odynophagia. Also, esophageal involvement may be painful since esophageal strictures may cause obstruction of a solid bolus. Diagnosis is made by fiber endoscopy and/or barium/iodine contrast medium radiologic evaluation. A solid bolus test should usually be included (Levine et al. 1989; Hardy et al. 1967; Cook et al. 1970).

Oral corticosteroids are usually effective. Advanced disease can be treated with various immunomodulatory drugs and in severe refractory cases also with infliximab, a TNF-α blocker. Local steroids can be used in the treatment of oral mucosal involvement. Esophageal strictures can be treated with balloon dilatation or may at times have to be surgically resected.

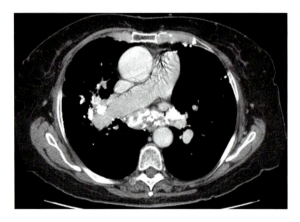

Fig. 2 An 82-year-old patient with berylliosis. CT of the upper thorax shows extensive fibrosis with calcifications in the upper lobes and in the mediastinum. In a patient like this, the esophagus is often encroached by the large lymph nodes. (Courtesy of Francis J. Scholz, Department of Diagnostic Radiology, Lahey Clinic, Burlington, MA, USA)

10 Berylliosis

Berylliosis, or chronic beryllium disease (CBD), is an immunologically mediated granulomatous lung disease due to beryllium sensitization (Flors et al. 2010). CBD is characterized by abnormal formation of inflammatory noncaseating granulomas that causes widespread scarring and most commonly interstitial pulmonary fibrosis. Mediastinal lymph nodes are also involved. A granuloma development may also occur in other organs, including extrapulmonary lymph nodes, skin, subcutaneous tissue, salivary glands, myocardium, liver, and skeletal muscle. Beryllium is a light-weight metal with variable physical and chemical properties that include stiffness, corrosion resistance, and electrical and thermal conductivity. Genetic predispositions seem to have a major role in the development of CBD. A variant of the major histocompatibility complex HLA-DPb1(Glu 69) has been found in many patients (Richeldi et al. 1993).

The symptoms of CBD are dry coughing, fatigue, weight loss, chest pain, increasing shortness of breath, and sometimes also dysphagia due to lymph node impingement on the esophagus. CBD has many similarities with other granulomatous diseases such as tuberculosis, syphilis, and fungal infection. The symptoms are mainly due to extrinsic compression of the esophagus leading to solid bolus dysphagia (Fig. 2).

Exposure to beryllium occurs particularly in miners. Other people are exposed in a variety of industries: aerospace, ceramics, dental supplies. The window in X-ray tubes often contains beryllium.

Beryllium exposure occurs primarily by inhalation of beryllium fumes or dust, but even contact through broken skin may occur. Most beryllium is excreted in urine, and the primary half-life ranges from several weeks to 6 months. Relatively insoluble chemical forms of beryllium may be retained for years.

After inhalation of beryllium, large numbers of CD4+ T lymphocytes accumulate in the lungs. These helper T lymphocytes demonstrate a marked proliferation response on exposure to beryllium. Beryllium seems to induce production of proinflammatory cytokines and growth factors that lead to granuloma formation.

Management of CBD includes cessation of beryllium exposure and the use of systemic corticosteroids. However, once pulmonary fibrosis has developed, corticosteroid therapy cannot reverse the scarring of lung tissue (Flors et al. 2010; Sood 2009).

11 Inflammatory Myopathies

Inflammatory myopathies include polymyositis, dermatomyositis, and inclusion body myositis (IBM) (Bella and Chad 1996). These inflammatory myopathies are characterized by mononuclear inflammatory cell infiltrates, myofibrillar necrosis, and regeneration. In polymyositis, T-lymphocyte cells, monocytes, and plasma cells are located in fascicles within the endomysial connective tissue. Dermatomyositis is characterized by the presence of atrophic fibres in the periphery of the fascicles. Unlike in polymyositis, the inflammatory cells are localized in the perivascular area and in the perimysial connective tissue and not in the endomysium. Microvascular changes are also common. Similarly to polymyositis, in IBM inflammatory cells are located in the endomysium. Patients with polymyositis, dermatomyositis, and IBM develop symmetric proximal muscle weakness. Muscle biopsy shows myositis. Patients also have elevated levels of serum creatine phosphokinase. Atypical EMG findings are also seen. In patients with dermatomyositis, there is also a characteristic skin involvement in the form of heliotrope exanthema or Gottron's papules on the knuckles.

Fig. 3 A 64-year-old woman with dermatomyositis and dysphagia. **a** Barium examination of the pharynx shows retention in the piriform sinuses. There is misdirected swallowing that reaches into the laryngeal vestibule. **b** Contrast medium also reaches up into the nasopharynx. There was very little contraction and movement of the pharyngeal wall

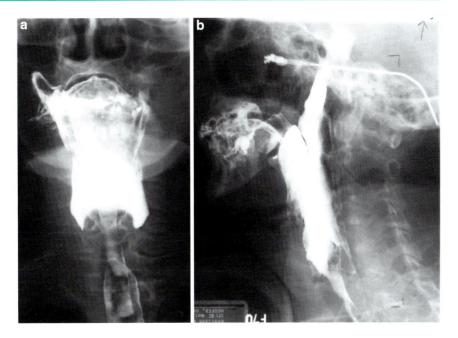

Patients with polymyositis, dermatomyositis, and IBM may have abnormal oropharyngeal and/or esophageal stages of swallowing (Darrow et al. 1992; Shapiro et al. 1996). Striated and smooth musculature is affected, leading to weakness of muscle strength but also fibrosis in the musculature. When the oral and pharyngeal stages are affected, this leads to retention with pooling in the vallecula and piriform sinuses. This may then lead to overflow aspiration (Selva-O'Callaghan et al. 2000). However, there is also usually laryngeal muscle involvement leading to defective closure of the airways as well (Fig. 3).

Abnormal upper esophageal sphincter opening is common in polymyositis, dermatomyositis, and IBM (Sonies 1997). Inflammation and edema in the cricopharyngeal muscle has been observed. Muscle fibrosis is often present. This has usually been treated by cricopharyngeal myotomy (Berg et al. 1985). Esophageal involvement leads to abnormal peristaltic transportation. This is similar to that seen in scleroderma. Injection of botulinum toxin into the cricopharyngeal muscle has also been recommended. Early treatment is important in order to avoid muscle atrophy. Treatment generally includes corticosteroids and immunosuppressive agents.

References

Agah FP, Francis IR, Ellis CN (1983) Esophageal involvement in epidermolysis bullosa dystrophica: clinical and roentgenographic manifestation. Gastrointest Radiol 8:111–117

Anselmino M, Zaninotto G, Constantini M, Ostuni P, Ianiello A, Boccu C et al (1997a) Esophageal motor function in primary Sjögren's syndrome. Dig Dis Sci 42:113–118

Anselmino M, Zaninotto G, Costantini M et al (1997b) Esophageal motor function in primary Sjögren's syndrome. Correlation with dysphagia and xerostomia. Dig Dis Sci 42:113–118

Bella JR, Chad DA (1996) Inflammatory myopathies. In: Samuel MA, Fekse SK (eds) Office practice of neurology, 2nd edn. Churchill-Livingstone, Philadelphia, pp 698–706

Berg HM, Persky MS, Jacobs JB, Cohen NL (1985) Cricopharyngeal myotomia: a review of surgical results in patients with cricopharyngeal achalasia of neurogenic origin. Laryngoscope 95:1337–1340

Bredenoord AJ, Jafari J, Kadri S et al (2010) Achalasia-like dysmotility secondary to oesophageal involvement of sarcoidosis. Gut. doi:10.1136/gut.2010.227868

Brookes GB (1983) Pharyngeal stenosis in Behcet's syndrome. The first reported case. Arch Otolaryngol 109:338–340

Chandan VS, Murray JA, Abraham SC (2008) Esophageal lichen planus. Arch Pathol Lab Med 132:1026–1029

Chen JJ, Branstetter BF IV, Myers EN (2005) Cricoarytenoid rheumatoid arthritis: an important consideration in aggressive lesions of the larynx. AJNR Am J Neuroradiol 26:970–972

Cook DM, Dines DE, Dycus DS (1970) Sarcoidosis: report of a case presenting as dysphagia. Chest 57:84–86

Darrow D, Hoffman H, Barnes G, Wiley C (1992) Management of dysphagia in inclusion body myositis. Arch Otolaryngol Head Neck Surg 118:313–317

Demetriades N, Hanford H, Laskarides C (2009) General manifestations of Behcet's syndrome and the success of CO_2-laser as treatment for oral lesions: a review of the literature and case presentation. J Mass Dent Soc 58:24–27

Ekberg O, Redlund-Johnell I, Sjöblom KG (1987) Pharyngeal function in patients with rheumatoid arthritis of the cervical spine and temporomandibular joint. Acta Radiol 28:35–39

Erb N, Pace V, Delamere JP, Kitas GD (2001) Dysphagia and stridor caused by laryngeal rheumatoid arthritis. Rheumatology 40:952–953

Flors L, Domingo ML, Leiva-Salinas C, Mazón M, Roselló-Sastre E, Vilar J (2010) Uncommon occupational lung disease: high-resolution CT findings. AJR Am J Roentgenol 194:W20–W26

Geterud A, Bake B, Bjelle A, Jonsson R, Sandberg N, Ejnell H (1991) Swallowing problems in the rheumatoid arthritis. Acta Otolaryngol 111:1153–1161

Goust J, Tsokos G (1993) Systemic lupus erythematosus. In: Virella G (ed) Introduction to medical immunology, 3rd edn. Dekker, New York, pp 437–450

Hardy WE, Tulgan H, Haidak G, Budnitz J (1967) Sarcoidosis: a case presenting with dysphagia and dysphonia. Ann Int Med 66:353–357

Hradsky M, Hybasek J, Cernoch V, Sazmova V, Juran J (1967) Oesophageal abnormalities in Sjögren's syndrome. Scand J Gastroenterol 2:200–203

International Pemphigus and Pemphigoid Foundation (2011) What is pemphigus? http://pemphigus.org/index.php?option=com_content&view=article&id=364&Itemid=100073/. Accessed 2 Aug 2011

Katzka DA, Smyrk TC, Bruce AJ, Romero Y, Alexander JA, Murray JA (2010) Variations in presentations of esophageal involvement in lichen planus. Clin Gastroenterol Hepatol 8:777–782

Kjellen G, Fransson SG, Lindström F, Sokjer H, Tibblin L (1986) Esophageal function, radiography and dysphagia in Sjögren's syndrome. Dig Dis Sci 31:225–229

Levack B, Hanson D (1979) Behcet's disease of the esophagus. J Laryngol Otol 93:99–101

Levine MS, Ekberg O, Rubesin SE, Gatenby RA (1989) Gastrointestinal sarcoidosis: radiographic findings. AJR Am J Roentgenol 153:293–295

Lindqvist C, Santavirta S, Sandelin J, Konttinen Y (1986) Dysphagia and micrognathia in a patient with juvenile rheumatoid arthritis. Clin Rheumatol 5:410–415

Liquidato BM, Bussoloti Filho I (2005) Evaluation of sialometry and minor salivary gland biopsy in classification of Sjögren's syndrome patients. Rev Bras Otorrinolaringol 71:346–354. doi:10.1590/S0034-72992005000300014

Madhusudhan KS, Sharma R (2008) Esophageal lichen planus: a case report and review of literature. Indian J Dermatol 53:26–27

Mandl T, Ekberg O, Wollmer P, Manthorpe R, Jacobsson LTH (2007) Dysphagia and dysmotility of the pharynx and oesophagus in patients with primary Sjögren's syndrome. Scand J Rheumatol 36:394–401

Menditti D, Palomba F, Rullo R, Minervini G (1990) Progressive systemic sclerosis (sclerodermal): oral manifestations. Arch Stomatol 31:537–548

Messadi DV, Younai F (2010) Aphthous ulcers. Dermatol Ther 23:281–290

Ntoumazios SK, Voulgari PV, Potsis K, Koutis E, Tsifetaki N, Assimakopoulos DA (2006) Esophageal involvement in scleroderma: gastroesophageal reflux, the common problem. Semin Arthritis Rheum 36:173–181

Palma R, Freire J, Freitas J, Morbey A, Costa T, Saraiva F et al (1994) Esophageal motility disorders in patients with Sjögren's syndrome. Dig Dis Sci 38:758–761

Pizzo G, Scardina GA, Messina P (2003) Effects of a nonsurgical exercise program on the decreased mouth opening in patients with systemic scleroderma. Clin Oral Invest 7:175–178

Pope J (2005) Other manifestations of mixed connective tissue disease. Rheum Dis Clin North Am 31:519–533

Ramos-Casals M, Brito-Zerón P (2007) Emerging biological therapies in primary Sjögren's syndrome. Rheumatology 46:1389–1396

Richeldi L, Sorrentino R, Saltini C (1993) HLA-DPB1 glutamate 69: a genetic marker of beryllium disease. Science 262:242–244

Rosztóczy A, Kovács L, Wittmann T, Lonovics J, Pokorny G (2001) Manometric assessment of impaired esophageal motor function in primary Sjögren's syndrome. Clin Exp Rheumatol 19:147–152

Rout PG, Hamburger J, Potts AJ (1996) Orofacial radiological manifestations of systemic sclerosis. Dentomaxillofac Radiol 25:193–196

Selva-O'Callaghan A, Sanchez-Sitjes L, Munoz-Gall X, Mijares-Boeckh-Behrens T, Solans-Laque R, Angel-Bosch-Gil J et al (2000) Respiratory failure due to muscle weakness in inflammatory myopathies: maintenance therapy with home mechanical ventilation. Rheumatology 39:914–916

Shapiro J, Marin S, DeGirolami U, Goyal R (1996) Inflammatory myopathy causing pharyngeal dysphagia: a new entity. Ann Otol Rhinol Laryngol 105:331–335

Sonies BC (1997) Evaluation and treatment of speech and swallowing disorders associated with myopathies. Curr Opin Rheumatol 9:486–495

Sood A (2009) Current treatment of chronic beryllium disease. J Occup Environ Hyg 6:762–765

Sugerman PB, Porter SR (2010) Oral lichen planus. http://emedicine.medscape.com/article/1078327-overview. Accessed 2 Aug 2011

Sun DCH, Roth SH, Mitchell CS, Englund DW (1974) Upper gastrointestinal disease in rheumatoid arthritis. Dig Dis 19:405–410

Thanou-Stavraki A, James JA (2008) Primary Sjögren's syndrome: current and prospective therapies. Semin Arthritis Rheum 37:273–292

Tsianos EB, Chiras CD, Drosos AA, Moutsopoulos HM (1985) Oesophageal dysfunction in patients with primary Sjögren's syndrome. Ann Rheum Dis 44:610–613

Tsianos EB, Vasakos S, Drosos AA, Malamou-Mitsi VD, Moutsopoulos HM (1986) The gastrointestinal involvement in primary Sjögren's syndrome. Scand J Rheumatol Suppl 61:151–155

Türk T, Pirildar T, Tunc E, Bor S, Doganavsargil E (2005) Manometric assessment of esophageal motility in patients with primary Sjögren's syndrome. Rheumatol Int 25: 246–249

Virella G (1993) Introduction. In: Virella G (ed) Introduction to medical immunology, 3rd edn. Dekker, New York, pp 1–8

Volter F, Fain O, Mathieu E, Thomas M (2004) Esophageal function and Sjögren's syndrome. Dig Dis Sci 49:248–253

Yeh SW, Ahmed B, Sami N, Ahmed AR (2003) Blistering disorders: diagnosis and treatment. Derm Ther 16:214–223

The Geriatric Pharynx and Esophagus

Olle Ekberg

Contents

Abstract

Dysphagia is common in the elderly. This is mainly due to neurodegenerative abnormalities in the central nervous system. The elderly may be able to compensate, to a certain degree, for deterioration of function but the reserve capacity is much less than in younger. Understanding of the normal aging process as well as disease processes common in the elderly is important for diagnosis and treatment of dysphagia in the elderly.

1   Introduction

There are several age-related alterations in oral, pharyngeal, and esophageal morphology and function. These variations in the healthy elderly (primary ageing) must be taken into account during clinical and radiological evaluation. In fact, these changes do not normally impair the swallowing process and are thereby not symptomatic. However, when disease processes (secondary ageing) add to primary ageing, they may result in significant impairment.

Deglutition disorders are common and costly in the elderly. The actual prevalence and natural history of such dysphagia is not very well known. Dysphagia is more commonly detected in the hospitalized and institutionalized elderly than in individuals who live in their own homes. In hospitals and nursing homes with predominantly an elderly population, the prevalence of dysphagia is up to 50% of the population (Groher and Bukatman 1986). Dysphagia is also much more common in the very old (over the age of 85)

O. Ekberg (✉)
Diagnostic Centre of Imaging and Functional Medicine,
Skåne University Hospital, 205 02 Malmö, Sweden
e-mail: olle.ekberg@med.lu.se

O. Ekberg (ed.), *Dysphagia*, Medical Radiology. Diagnostic Imaging, DOI: 10.1007/174_2011_389,
© Springer-Verlag Berlin Heidelberg 2012

than in any other group. Neurologic diseases such as stroke, dementia, and Parkinson's disease are common in these populations. The central nervous system regulates oropharyngeal function in an integrated complex sensory and motor activity pattern. Especially the coordination between the oral and pharyngeal stage, i.e., between a voluntary and an automatic function, is vulnerable. In the elderly this coordination is frequently impaired.

Many elderly people with dysphagia seem to be in reasonably good health, and are not frail or bedridden. They do not seem to suffer from clinically apparent neurologic disease. Oropharyngeal impairment is usually insidious and chronic in these individuals, although acute, transient cases do occur. A rational approach to understanding deglutition in the elderly requires that we differentiate expected, if not clearly predictable, senescent changes (primary ageing) from those caused by disease (secondary ageing). Unfortunately, subclinical disease, especially cerebral vascular disease, makes this distinction difficult.

From other organ systems we know that there is roughly a 1% yearly decline in function beginning at 30 years of age. Overall ageing is a progressive generalized impairment of function resulting in a loss of adaptive response to stress and in a growing risk of age-associated disease (Kirkwood 2000).

The morphodynamics of deglutition can be measured in terms of timing, movement of anatomical structures, pressure generation, and bolus movements (Tracy et al. 1989; Sonies et al. 1988; Shaw et al. 1990; Shaker et al. 1990). Senescent changes in oropharyngeal function can be characterized as "less efficient." However, the relationship between symptoms and morphodynamic abnormalities, especially in the context of compensation/decompensation, is very complex (Jones and Donner 1991).

One important feature of ageing is an inability to adapt to stress, and the videofluorographic examination is certainly a stressful situation. Abnormalities, or differences from younger, presumably normal individuals, may induce alterations that reflect senescent decline in function. Similarly, the examination itself may induce decompensation in those with existing dysfunction due to known disease and minor abnormalities may become major ones.

1.1 The Ageing Brain

In the central nervous system various alterations of the cytoarchitecture occur in ageing. For example, motor neuron counts in the spinal cord show that the number of cells declines by approximately 200 neurons per segment per decade (Schoenen 1991). A study that counted the pigmented neurons in the locus ceruleus in the brainstem found a decline averaging 2,000 cells per decade after the age of 60 years (Vijayashankar and Brody 1979). Cell counts in various glossopharyngeal and vagus nuclei within the brainstem are not available in humans, but a similar decline is likely.

1.2 Primary Ageing

The oral cavity undergoes important changes with age. Such changes include an increase in the amount of connective tissue in the tongue, loss of dentition, and reduced masticatory strength (Logemann 1990). In the pharynx it has been shown that the anterior elevation of the larynx is less pronounced in the elderly and that the pharyngeal swallowing phase is significantly slowed down (Sonies et al. 1988). The pharyngeal peristaltic motion has been shown to be slowed down above the age of 60 years (Tracy et al. 1989). However, another study showed that this is not the case but that there is instead a wider intrapersonal variability in the elderly (Borgström and Ekberg 1988a). However, there is no significant change in pharyngeal peak pressure, duration, or in the rate of propagation of contraction (Robbins et al. 1992). Healthy elderly subjects therefore do not have any residual accumulation in the pharynx after swallowing.

2 The Oral Stage

It has been shown that pressure that is generated during swallowing by the tongue does not change in the elderly compared with young individuals. However, when individuals are asked to apply maximal strength, the pressure recording increases considerably in the young, whereas in the elderly such reserve capacity does not seem to exist. Others have shown that lingual peristaltic pressure decreases with age (Shaker et al. 1988).

3 The Pharyngeal Stage

3.1 Misdirected Swallowing

Bolus misdirection into the airways is the most significant event observed during videofluoroscopy. The timing and level of bolus misdirection are important observations, but again may be extremely variable (Dodds et al. 1990; Logemann 1983; Groher 1983). In the elderly, it is not uncommon to see ingestion of too large a bolus volume or a rapid ingestion rate during uncontrolled administrations. This results in disruption of sequencing between bolus ingestion, delivery, propulsion, and laryngeal closure. Some patients aspirate only on the first liquid barium administration; others appear relatively normal until a small amount penetrates and then grossly deteriorate and aspirate before, during, and after some of the subsequent swallows. Particularly in the elderly bolus misdirection most often results from oral stage dysfunction even when it occurs during the pharyngeal stage.

Another common finding in the elderly is failure of containment during ingestion, oral processing of bolus holding. In these individuals the glossopalatal seal is inadequate. Lingual movements may be dyskinetic or disorganized and disrupt the glossopalatal seal. Alternatively, there may be no oromotor activity attempting to contain the bolus once it has been ingested. The third oral stage cause of misdirection is transitional dissociation. This means that the bolus is positioned at the wrong place at the wrong time.

In young individuals the hyoid bone starts to move anteriorly (from its posterior position) before the apex of the bolus passes the level of the faucial isthmus as it can be seen in a true lateral projection during swallowing. With increasing age, the start of this anterior hyoid bone movement is delayed. It is common in the elderly (over 75 years of age) to observe a delay of the anterior movement of the hyoid bone for more than 0.5 s after the apex of the bolus has passed the faucial isthmus (Feinberg and Ekberg 1991). In that study using the previously outlined pattern analysis, it was found that aspiration was due to oral stage dysfunction in 50% of patients, pharyngeal dysfunction in 30% of patients, and combined dysfunction in 20% of patients. The most common oral stage abnormality was failure of containment. Transitional dissociation was seen in many patients.

Almost as common was large bolus ingestion or rapid ingestion rate. The most common pharyngeal stage abnormality was incomplete transportation, i.e., retention. A mere defective laryngeal closure was seen less frequently (Feinberg and Ekberg 1991). There is, however, no significant relationship between a patient's specific disease and the pattern of abnormalities during barium swallow. This means that the observed dysfunctions are nonspecific in terms of their cause. The high frequency of oral dysfunction indicates that oral stage abnormalities must be routinely looked for during videofluoroscopy.

The presence of anterior osteophytes larger than 10 mm that impinge on the pharynx may explain aspiration in dysphagic patients (Strasser et al. 2000). Coexisting clinical conditions and diseases such as stroke and partial laryngeal resection increase the risk of aspiration in patients with smaller osteophytes of the cervical spine.

Pneumonia is common in the elderly and it may be due to defective closure of the airways during swallowing, i.e., penetration/aspiration. However, the cause and effect relationship is complex and few studies have addressed this accordingly (Doggett et al. 2001; Feinberg et al. 1996). The most plausible explanation is that infected saliva reaches the lower airways by means of the larynx and causes the infection (Langmore et al. 1998).

3.2 Pharyngeal Constrictors

There are conflicting opinions concerning the effect of ageing on deglutitive pharyngeal pressures. Whereas one study showed that there was no pressure difference (Robbins et al. 1992), other studies have shown differences (Tracy et al. 1989; Perlman et al. 1993; Shaker et al. 1993). However, there are a multitude of methodological differences that makes comparison difficult. In fact, one of the studies (Shaker et al. 1990) showed that the amplitude and duration of the peristaltic pressure wave were significantly greater in the elderly than in the young. Such alterations with age, alterations that actually could be seen as improvements, may actually be regarded as compensatory responses to, for instance, reduced cross-sectional area of the deglutitive pharyngoesophageal segment (PES) opening in the elderly (Shaw et al. 1990). A study supporting this theory was presented by Shaker (1993). In this study he found that intrabolus pressure in the pharynx was significantly higher in the elderly than in young patients, on swallowing in both upright and supine positions and with both liquid and mashed potatoes. This again may indicate that there is lack of distension of the PES in the elderly.

3.3 The Pharyngoesophageal Segment

The PES pressure has also been studied in the elderly and has been compared with that in younger subjects. Cook et al. (1989) did not find significant age-related changes in resting PES pressure measured with a sleeve device; however, they only studied individuals under 55 years of age. Wilson et al. (1989) made the same observation in healthy subjects under 62 years of age. On the other hand, Fulp et al. (1990) showed that normal elderly subjects over 62 years of age have lower resting PES pressure than younger controls. Shaker et al. (1993) studied the effect of ageing (70 years and over) on the resting PES pressure and its response to esophageal air and balloon distension. The results of this study indicate that ageing significantly reduces the resting PES pressure. However, this latter study (Shaker et al. 1990, 1993) also showed that there were normal PES pressure responses to swallowing and esophageal distension by air and balloon in the elderly. Therefore, the protective role of the PES against pharyngeal reflux of gastric acid is preserved in the elderly.

Kendall and Leonard (2001) showed that there is pharyngeal weakness in the elderly dysphagic patient. They also concluded that poor pharyngeal constrictions suggestive of pharyngeal weakness contributed to 75% of cases of aspiration in their study. Feeding and respiratory pattern was studied in normal elderly people (Hirst et al. 2002). Hirst et al. found a fairly stable pattern. It has been shown that particularly in the elderly incoordination commonly leads to aspiration (Nilsson et al. 1997). Solid aspirators also have a lower oxygen saturation level compared with normal individuals (Colodny 2001).

4 Examination Techniques

The examination technique in the elderly does not differ from that in young individuals. However, many elderly people are severely impaired and cannot cooperate. The examination should be custom-tailored to the patient's symptoms, and in a very impaired elderly patient there are very few relevant clinical questions that should be addressed. Therefore, such an examination is usually very easy to perform.

5 The Nondysphagic Elderly

An important aspect is, of course, the prevalence of videofluorographic abnormalities in nondysphagic elderly patients. Ekberg and Feinberg (1991) found that only 16% of the elderly population (mean age 83) were normal. Oral and pharyngeal dysfunction was very prevalent in their study (63 and 25%, respectively) (Fig. 1). Combined dysfunction was present in 60% of patients. Sixty-five percent of patients showed bolus misdirection into the airways (20% showed penetration into the vestibule, 45% showed minor aspiration to the trachea). No major aspiration was observed. Misdirection was due to oral dysfunction 4 times as often as pharyngeal dysfunction and twice as often as combined oral and pharyngeal dysfunction. In that study 36% of patients had dissociation between the oral and pharyngeal stage. This was the pathophysiological process of oral dysfunction leading to misdirected swallowing. However, in that study, half of the patients had a history of neurologic disease such as dementia, Parkinson's disease, and stroke, although none had a history of dysphagia or swallowing impairment. Pharyngeal constrictor paresis and lingual dysfunction was much more common in those patients with neurologic disease. The high frequency of abnormalities that was observed in that study may have a number of explanations. Many elderly individuals do not admit to being dysphagic even when it is obvious that they are. Caregivers are relatively poor at detecting dysphagia unless they have been specifically trained (Ekberg et al. 2002).

Altered oropharyngeal function has been documented in asymptomatic elderly volunteers (Pontoppidan and Beecher 1960; Baum and Bodner 1983; Sonies et al. 1984; Borgström and Ekberg 1988b; Tracy et al. 1989; Ekberg and Feinberg 1991; Robbins et al. 1992). Such changes may be due to normal age-related changes in tissues, muscles, and neuromorphodynamics. It is not clear what is "normal decline" in oropharyngeal function among the elderly and what is really the result of disease processes

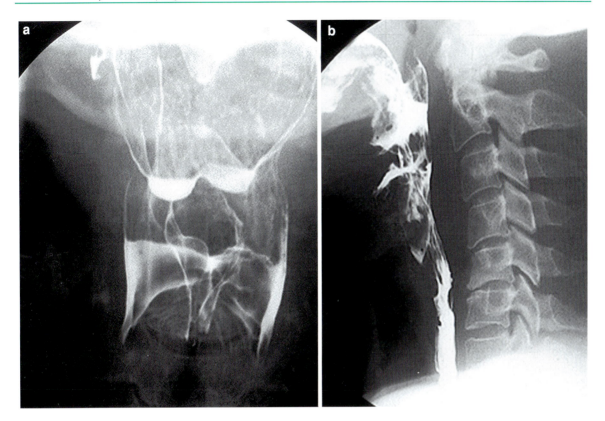

Fig. 1 Pharyngeal dysfunction is common in the elderly. Weak musculature leads to impaired clearance of the pharynx. This is mostly related to defective elevation of the pharynx. In this patient there is pooling of contrast medium in the vallecula and piriform sinus bilaterally. Contrast medium has reached into the laryngeal vestibule and is also seen between the arytenoids

which definitely are more common in the elderly, particularly in the central nervous system (Levine et al. 1992; Buchholz 1992). Again, it is very important to try to compare symptoms with morphodynamic findings (Sheth and Diner 1988; Donner and Jones 1991). There is a confusing overlap of clinical, videofluoroscopic, and magnetic resonance imaging findings in elderly individuals with and without oropharyngeal dysphagia/dysfunction (Figs. 2, 3, 4).

6   Dementia

Because dementia is the most common neurologic disease associated with misdirected swallowing, it is of interest to study such a population more closely (Feinberg et al. 1992). In the study of Feinberg et al., only 7% of patients were found to be normal during videofluoroscopy. Oral stage dysfunction was found in 73% of patients, pharyngeal dysfunction was found in 43% of patients, pharyngoesophageal abnormalities were found in 33% of patients, and combined dysfunction was found in 42% of patients. When only one stage was abnormal, again oral dysfunction (36%) was much more common than pharyngeal dysfunction (14%). Common neuropsychiatric features of dementia can explain the oral stage dysfunction that was observed in that study. Patients frequently seem to be displaying agnosia (inability to recognize familiar stimuli or situations), dyspraxia (inability to perform coordinated movements), and abulia (psychomotor retardation). Inappropriate ingestion behavior appears to be secondary to faulty judgment and lack of impulse control. Transitional phase dissociation was the most common oral abnormality, seen in 44% of patients. Volicer et al. (1989) have suggested that Alzheimer's disease patients "simply have forgotten how to initiate the swallowing reflex," and a high frequency of dissociation in the aforementioned study may reflect such a deficit.

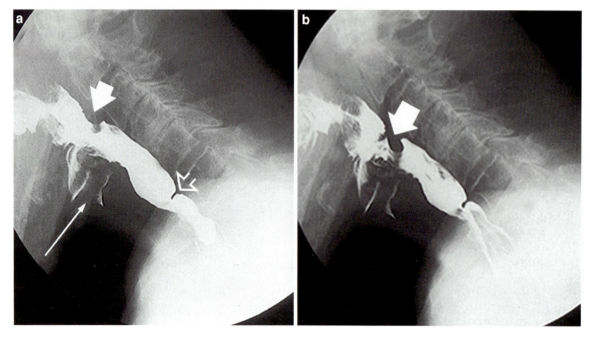

Fig. 2 Barium swallow in a 79-year-old woman with dysphagia. She coughs during eating. Compensation is often difficult to detect on barium swallow. This patient has increased activity in the middle pharyngeal constrictor (*broad arrow*). This is likely to be due to a weak tongue base pressure. In this patient there is also misdirected swallowing. Barium has passed through the vocal cords (*arrow*) into the subglottic area. There is also an incoordination of the opening of the pharyngoesophageal segment seen as an indentation of the cricopharyngeal muscle (*open arrow*). **a** Midpharyngeal stage of swallow. **b** One quarter of a second after **a**

A recent study found a correlation between the impairment of the oropharyngeal swallowing phase and the presence of unidentified objects observed incidentally on head magnetic resonance imaging performed on elderly subjects (Levine et al. 1992). Two other studies found alterations of pharyngeal clearance and swallowing pressure in patients with prominent cervical osteophytic formations (Ohmae et al. 1993; Strasser et al. 2000).

7 The Ageing Esophagus

The term "presbyesophagus" has been used to describe esophageal motility abnormalities in the elderly. However, studies have shown that dysmotility does not occur secondarily to ageing as such. However, esophageal diseases are common in all age groups, including the elderly. Some diseases have a relative frequency that increases with age, such as adenocarcinoma. One must also take into account that an elderly patient with suspected achalasia is much more likely than a younger one to have a distal esophageal malignancy. Moreover, long-standing achalasia that occurs in an elderly patient may develop a secondary malignancy.

Symptoms of well-known diseases usually have a more complex presentation in the elderly; therefore, chest pain due to esophageal dysmotility or gastroesophageal reflux disease may be much more difficult to distinguish from coronary artery disease. Moreover, chronic disorders present for a long time in the elderly are more likely to cause complications. This may be true for Barrett's esophagus and adenocarcinoma of the esophagus. Esophageal dysmotility is a major problem in the elderly. The symptoms are characteristically related to abnormal transportation of ingested material through the esophagus. Cardinal symptoms are chest pain and vomiting. The major differential diagnostic problem is to detect any underlying mechanical obstruction such as reflux (or other) stricture and malignancies. Characteristically strictures are symptomatic for solid foods but not for liquids. Dysmotility is usually equally symptomatic for liquids and solids. It is always important to consider endoscopy in this age group. If it is

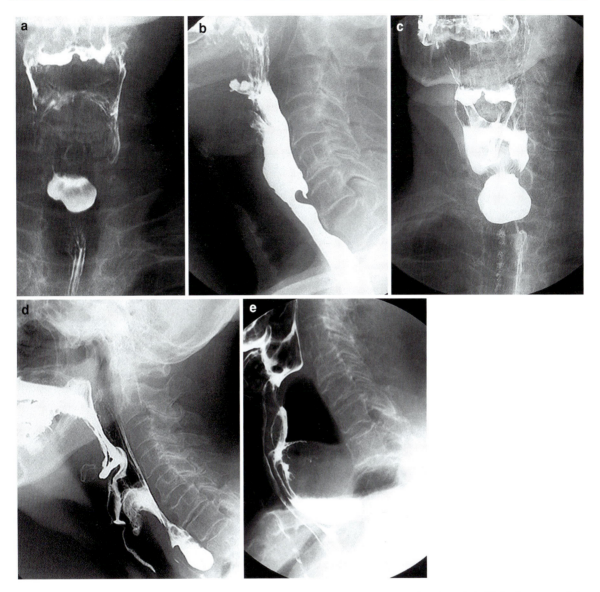

Fig. 3 Zenker's diverticula. These are usually asymptomatic in younger persons (as in **a**, **b**). In a young person, Zenker's diverticulum is usually the only abnormality found. This is in contrast to the situation in the elderly (as in **c**, **d**). In this patient there is concomitant dysfunction with pooling of contrast medium in the vallecula and in the piriform sinuses. There is also misdirected swallowing. Although the diverticulum is bigger in the young patient in **a**, it is likely that most of the symptoms are due to concomitant pharyngeal dysmotility. However, in elderly patients the diverticulum might be huge as in **d**. The diverticulum dislocates the cervical esophagus anteriorly, and it was obvious during the examination that there was an obstruction for bolus passage

contraindicated or not available, the radiologic study must include morphologic evaluation.

The effect of ageing on the esophageal motor function has been studied by several authors. Nonpropulsive, often repetitive contractions are numerous in the elderly (Soergel et al. 1964; Zboralske et al. 1964). Tertiary contractions and delay of the esophageal emptying, as well as dilatation of the esophagus, are also commonly seen. It has also been shown that the distal esophageal peristaltic amplitude is significantly higher in the elderly then in the young (Richter et al. 1987). Interestingly, however, the proximal esophageal contractile amplitude did not increase with age. Others have shown that the

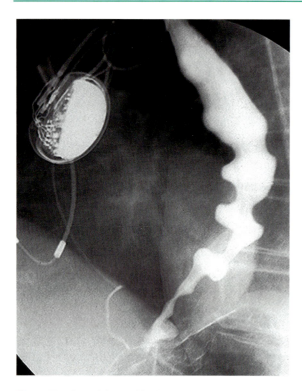

Fig. 4 Esophageal dysmotility is common in the elderly. This patient shows multiple nonpropulsive contractions of the distal esophagus. This may, as in this patient, be very symptomatic. This 81-year-old woman vomited halfway through every meal. The barium study shows retention due to the motor dysmotility. Other patients might show similar esophageal dysfunction but do not vomit and are not otherwise symptomatic either

lower esophageal sphincter resting pressure does not differ between the young and the elderly (Shaker 1993).

Esophageal dysmotility is one of the major reasons for drug-induced esophagitis. Commonly reported drugs are NSAIDs, tetracycline derivates, potassium chloride, and now also alendronate. Esophageal injury may be related to acidic pH with some of these drugs. However, potassium chloride causes injury by acting on smooth muscles, particularly on the small arteriole in the mucosa and submucosa, thereby causing an ischemic lesion which may lead to fibrosis and stricture. Such drug-induced esophagitis may be overcome if the patient takes precautions in terms of drinking before and after ingestion, and also to ingest in an upright position.

One common observation in the elderly is so-called corkscrew esophagus. It has a very impressive radiologic appearance. It may or may not be symptomatic. Control of motor activity in peristalsis in the esophagus is a complex interaction of excitatory and inhibitory stimuli. It should be remembered that denervation of smooth musculature leads to contraction. It may well be that these patients have lost contact between the dorsal motor nucleus of the vagus nerve and the smooth muscle of the esophagus and that we are observing the activity of the enteric nervous system. Such corkscrew esophagus is not the same as nutcracker esophagus seen in young patients. Nutcracker esophagus has normal transportation but an increased contraction pressure. Diffuse esophageal spasm (DES) and corkscrew contractions differ in such a way that it is considered that in the DES the peristaltic contraction obliterates the lumen, whereas in the corkscrew esophagus contraction does not obliterate the lumen. However, DES and curling or corkscrew dysfunction may be closely related. They both fall into the category of spastic esophageal dysfunction.

8   Gastroesophageal Reflux

It is important to realize that gastroesophageal reflux disease may cause strictures in the esophagus as frequently in the elderly as in younger patients. Key to the diagnosis here is, of course, endoscopy, and also double contrast examination. The history taking in these patients must focus on other classic symptoms or gastroesophageal reflux (Castell 1990; Fulp et al. 1990; Hey et al. 1982; Kikendall et al. 1983; McCord and Clouse 1990; Semble et al. 1989; Siebens et al. 1986; Tucker et al. 1978).

References

Baum BJ, Bodner L (1983) Aging and oral motor function: evidence for altered performance among older persons. J Dent Res 62:2–6

Borgström PS, Ekberg O (1988a) Pharyngeal dysfunction in the elderly. J Med Imaging 2:74–81

Borgström PS, Ekberg O (1988b) Speed of peristalsis in pharyngeal, constrictor musculature: correlation to age. Dysphagia 2:140–144

Buchholz D (1992) Editorial. Dysphagia 7:148–149

Castell DO (1990) Esophageal disorders in the elderly. Gastroenterol Clin North Am 19:235

Colodny N (2001) Effects of age, gender, disease, and multisystem involvement on oxygen saturation levels in dysphagic persons. Dysphagia 16:48–57

Cook IJ, Dent J, Collins SM (1989) Upper esophageal sphincter tone and reactivity to stress in patients with a history of globus sensation. Dig Dis Sci 34:672–676

Dodds WJ, Logemann JA, Stewart ET (1990) Radiologic assessment of abnormal oral and pharyngeal phases of swallowing. Am J Roentgenol 154:965–974

Doggett DL, Tappe KA, Mitchell MD, Chapell R, Coates V, Turkelson CM (2001) Prevention of pneumonia in elderly stroke patients by systematic diagnosis and treatment of dysphagia: an evidence-based comprehensive analysis of the literature. Dysphagia 16:279–295

Donner MW, Jones B (1991) Aging and neurological disease. In: Jones B, Donner MW (eds) Normal and abnormal swallowing: imaging in diagnosis and therapy. Springer, New York

Ekberg O, Feinberg MJ (1991) Altered swallowing function in elderly patients with dysphagia: radiographic findings in 56 patients. Am J Roentgenol 156:1181–1184

Ekberg O, Hamdy S, Woisard V, Wuttge-Hannig A, Ortega P (2002) Social and mental burden of dysphagia: Its impact on diagnosis and treatment. Dysphagia 17:139–146

Feinberg MJ, Ekberg O (1991) Videofluoroscopy in elderly patients with aspiration: importance of evaluating both oral and pharyngeal stages of deglutition. Am J Roentgenol 156: 293–296

Feinberg MJ, Ekberg O, Segall L, Tully J (1992) Deglutition in elderly patients with dementia: findings of videofluorographic evaluation and impact on staging and management. Radiology 183:811–814

Feinberg MJ, Knebl J, Tully J (1996) Prandial aspiration and pneumonia in an elderly population followed over 3 years. Dysphagia 11:104–109

Fulp SR, Dalton CB, Castell JA, Castell DO (1990) Aging-related alterations in human upper esophageal sphincter function. Am J Gastroenterol 85:1569–1572

Groher ME (1983) Mechanical disorders of swallowing. In: Groher ME (ed) Dysphagia: diagnosis and management. Butterworth, Worburn, pp 61–84

Groher ME, Bukatman R (1986) The prevalence of swallowing disorders in two teaching hospitals. Dysphagia 1:3–6

Hey H, Jorgensen F, Sorensen K et al (1982) Esophageal transit of six commonly used tablets and capsules. Br Med J 285:717

Hirst LJ, Ford GA, Gibson GJ, Wilson JA (2002) Swallow-induced alterations in breathing in normal older people. Dysphagia 17:152–161

Jones B, Donner MW (1991) Adaptation, compensation, and decompensation. In: Jones B, Donner MW (eds) Normal and abnormal swallowing: imaging in diagnosis and therapy. Springer, New York

Kendall KA, Leonard RJ (2001) Pharyngeal constriction in elderly dysphagic patients compared with young and elderly nondysphagic controls. Dysphagia 16:272–278

Kikendall JW, Friedman AC, Oyewole MA et al (1983) Pill-induced esophageal injury: case reports and review of the medical literature. Dig Dis Sci 28:174

Kirkwood TBL (2000) Biological origins of ageing. In: Grimley Evans J, Franklin Williams F et al (eds) Oxford textbook of geriatric medicine, 2nd edn. Oxford University Press, Oxford, pp 35–42

Langmore SE, Terpenning MS, Schork A, Chen YM, Murray JT, Lopatin D, Loeshe WJ (1998) Predictors of aspiration pneumonia: how important is dysphagia?. Dysphagia 13:69–81

Levine R, Robbins JA, Maser A (1992) Periventricular white matter changes and oropharyngeal swallowing in normal individuals. Dysphagia 7:142–147

Logemann JA (1983) Evaluation and treatment of swallowing disorders. College Hill Press, San Diego, pp 64–69

Logemann JA (1990) Effects of aging on the swallowing mechanism. Otolaryngol Clin North Am 23:1045–1056

McCord GS, Clouse RE (1990) Pill-induced esophageal strictures: clinical features and risk factors for development. Am J Med 88:512

Nilsson H, Ekberg O, Bülow M, Hindfelt B (1997) Assessment of respiration during video fluoroscopy of dysphagic patients. Acad Radiol 4:503–507

Ohmae Y, Inouye T, Kitahara S (1993) Relationship between cervical osteophytes and globus sensation: a study based on altered swallowing function. Nippon Jibiinkoka Gakkai Kaiho 96:379–386

Perlman AL, Guthmiller Schultz J, VanDaele DJ (1993) Effects of age, gender, bolus volume, and bolus viscosity on oropharyngeal pressure during swallowing. J Appl Physiol 75:33–37

Pontoppidan H, Beecher HK (1960) Progressive loss of protective reflexes in the airway with advance of age. JAMA 174:2209–2213

Richter JE, Wu WC, Johns DN, Blackwell JN, Nelson JL, Castell JA, Castell DO (1987) Esophageal manometry in 95 healthy adults volunteers. Dig Dis Sci 32:583–592

Robbins J, Hamilton JW, Lof GL, Kempster GB (1992) Oropharyngeal swallowing in normal adults of different ages:. Gastroenterology 103:823–829

Schoenen J (1991) Clinical anatomy of the spinal cord. Neurol Clin 9:503–532

Semble EL, Wu WC, Castell DO (1989) Nonsteroidal antiinflammatory drugs and esophageal injury. Semin Arth Rheum 19:99

Shaker R (1993) Effect of aging on the deglutitive oral, pharyngeal and esophageal motor function. DRS, 2nd annual scientific meeting, DRS, Lake Geneva, Wisconsin, Oct 22–24, 1993

Shaker R, Cook IJS, Dodds WJ, Hogan WJ (1988) Pressure-flow dynamics of the oral phase of swallowing. Dysphagia 3:79–84

Shaker R, Dodds WJ, Podursan MC et al (1990) Effect of aging on pharynx and upper esophageal sphincter (UES). Gastroenterology 98:A432 (abstract)

Shaker R, Ren J, Podvrsan B, Dodds WJ, Hogan WJ, Kern M, Hoffmann R, Hintz J (1993) Effect of aging and bolus variables on pharyngeal and upper esophageal sphincter motor function. Am J Physiol 264:G427–G432

Shaw DW, Cook IJ, Dent J, Simula ME, Panagopoulos V, Gabb M, Shearman DJ (1990) Age influences oropharyngeal and upper esophageal sphincter function during swallowing. Gastroenterology 98:A390

Sheth N, Diner WC (1988) Swallowing problems in the elderly. Dysphagia 2:209–215

Siebens H, Trupe E, Siebens A et al (1986) Correlates and consequences of eating dependency in institutionalised elderly. J Am Geriatr Soc 34:192

Soergel KH, Zboralske FF, Amberg JR (1964) Presbyesophagus: esophageal motility in nonagenarians. J Clin Invest 43:1472–1479

Sonies BC, Tone M, Shawker T (1984) Speech and swallowing in the elderly. Gerodontology 3:115–123

Sonies B, Parent L, Morrish K et al (1988) Durational aspects of the oropharyngeal phase in normal adults. Dysphagia 3:1–10

Strasser G, Schima W, Schober E, Pokieser P, Kaider A, Denk DM (2000) Cervical osteophytes impinging on the pharynx: importance of size and concurrent disorders for development of aspiration. Am J Roentgenol 174:449–453

Tracy JF, Logemann JA, Kahrilas PJ, Jacob P, Kobara M, Krugler C (1989) Preliminary observations on the effects of age on oropharyngeal deglutition. Dysphagia 4:90–94

Tucker HJ, Snape WJ, Cohen S (1978) Achalasia secondary to carcinoma: manometric and clinical features. Ann Intern Med 89:315

Vijayashankar N, Brody H (1979) A quantitativ estudy of the pigmented neurons in the neuclei locus coeruleus and subcoeruleus in man as related to aging. J Neuropathol Exp Neurol 38:490–497

Volicer L, Seltzer B, Rheaume Y et al (1989) Eating difficulties in patients with probable dementia of the Alzheimer type. J Geriatr Psychiatry Neurol 2:188–195

Wilson JA, Pryde A, Macintyre CCA (1989) Normal pharyngoesophageal motility: a study of 50 healthy volunteers. Dig Sis Sci 34:1590–1599

Zboralske FF, Amberg JR, Soergel KH (1964) Presbyesophagus: cineradiographic manifestations. Radiology 82:463–467

Voice and Dysphagia

Daniele Farneti

Contents

D. Farneti (✉)
Voice and Swallowing Center,
"Infermi" Hospital, Rimini, Italy
e-mail: lele_doc@libero.it

Abstract

The anatomical interaction between the upper respiratory and digestive tracts conditions the smooth running of their functions: breathing, swallowing and voice articulation. The phylogenetic evolution of our species has rendered possible the optimum integration of these functions, creating the conditions for an extremely refined timing. This functional optimization has facilitated the phonoarticulatory function with the possibility of highly skilled aesthetic results, as in artistic voice production. This anatomical integrity is essential for a proper and optimal functioning. Anatomical alteration may change a function, just as a functional alteration may facilitate, in the presence of comorbidity, anatomical changes. In singing, for example, the physiological adjustments required to produce a more resonant voice can alter, over time, the physiological characteristics of the structures involved in swallowing. The lowering of the laryngotracheal axis, which facilitates the mechanisms of articulation and vocal projection, may affect the timing of swallowing. The pressures usually required in singing can modify the functioning of the valves between the chest and abdominal cavities. The chapter reviews the main changes in the physiological and physiopathological characteristics of the upper respiratory and digestive tracts and the impact that artistic vocal performances have on swallowing. Similar considerations are made for other voice users. The chapter concludes with a review of the literature on the topic.

O. Ekberg (ed.), *Dysphagia*, Medical Radiology. Diagnostic Imaging, DOI: 10.1007/174_2011_341,
© Springer-Verlag Berlin Heidelberg 2012

1   Introduction

Under an anatomical and functional profile the assessment of interactions between upper respiratory and digestive tracts represents a field of great interest (Laitman and Reindenberg 1993). According to the natural indications derived from phylogenesis and ontogenesis, the interaction between the respiratory and digestive systems, in the head and neck, can actually be evaluated almost completely and at the various stages of life, including the intrauterine stage (Wolfson and Laitman 1990). Upper airways can be examined from the nostrils down to the cervicothoracic trachea and digestive pathways can be examined from the oral cavity down to the duodenum. The nasal–buccal–pharyngeal–laryngeal "apparatus" has thus become the site of functions that can be clearly identified: many actions and interactions can now be viewed, even though they are still not completely understood.

In the head and neck there are anatomically and functionally integrated activities responsible for performing vital functions, such as breathing and swallowing and other equally important non-vital functions, such as phonoarticulation. The phylogenetic evolution of the head and neck has favoured phonation, which is essential for the human species (differentiating it from other, equally developed but non-verbal species), but has penalized the other functions. So, if at birth the newborn baby can be fed and breathe at the same time, after the first months of life, the maturation of the larynx separates the two functions.

In the course of millennia the possibility of verbal communication has significantly fostered the evolution of our species, with an increasingly important role of verbal production (Purves and Litchman 1985). Only over the last few decades has the introduction of different communication modalities and systems (e.g. the Internet) reduced or at least modified the interest in such expression, typical of humans. The use of voice as an expression mode is, however, indispensable for various categories of operators, either as an essential part of their everyday working activity or because of its unique and powerful expressive connotations. This is the case in those professionals who use their voice while doing their usual job duties (e.g. teachers, call centre operators, telephonists, shop assistants, lawyers) or those who

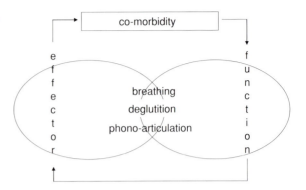

Fig. 1 Interaction among function, structure and comorbidity

use it according to "athletic" expressive modalities (e.g. professional classical singers, actors).

As regards the intimate anatomical–functional correlation between the head and neck, as mentioned above, it is quite evident that the unusual employment of the common effectors of breathing, swallowing and phonoarticulation may cause disjoint or joint alterations of the functions they perform. The alteration of such functions may, in the case of existing comorbidity conditions, result in openly pathological events, in the same way as pathological events modify functions (Fig. 1). A vicious cycle is started that may involve both the effectors and the functions according to subsequent and progressive levels of involvement. The alteration of the fine balances of vocal athletic exercises performed by vocal professionals may, for instance, on the one hand, enhance the amplification and capacity of sound, but, on the other, modify their swallowing patterns. The alterations of these events are such as to involve the artists' emotional sphere, making it more difficult for them to recover preexisting or modified balanced conditions.

2   Phylogenetic Development

A key element in the balance between respiration, deglutition and phonoarticulation is the position of the larynx inside the visceral space of the neck. In mammals, the cervical rachis consists of seven vertebrae: the larynx is usually placed between the first and the third cervical vertebra, with the epiglottis behind the velum of the palate allowing a sort of airway continuity (Soulié and Bardier 1907). In this way the animal can breathe and at the same time ingest food of various thicknesses. This high location of the larynx, which is also found in human newborns, as said above, strongly limits phonoarticulatory capabilities: the pharyngeal cavity is extremely reduced in size and consequently the tongue movements inside a relatively less wide cavity are limited. The oral cavity, widened by the lip movements, acts as a resonator for the laryngeal sound (Duchin 1990).

What happens in mammals occurs in the human species in the first months of life. After the sixth month, the larynx starts a descent that brings it to the level of the fourth to seventh cervical vertebrae (Kirchner 1993). This descent is accompanied by a progressive decrease in cranial base angle that in phylogenesis is found only in *Homo sapiens* (Negus 1949) and, in the development of our species, only after the second year of life. When the epiglottis leaves its narinal location, the child must be predisposed to swallowing in such a way as to protect the lower airways during the passage of the bolus into the pharynx. The laryngeal cavity opens up inside the pharyngeal cavity, thereby imposing the need for a sequential reconfiguration of the organ in relation to what passes through it (breathing configuration, swallowing configuration) (Cook and Kahrilas 1999). To facilitate the pharyngeal phase of swallowing and further protect the lower airways, the cervical region has increased its length so as to allow a sufficiently safe deglutition timing and has widened to enable the easy movement of structures (Arensburg et al. 1989). With respect to the phonoarticulatory capacity, these various changes have certainly represented a significant advantage. The sounds produced in the larynx are amplified in a series of wide and tortuous cavities (vocal tract) with several varieties of harmonic filtering, whereas the transit through the oral cavity allows a very fine articulation thereof (Houghton 1993).

In the aerodigestive crossroads, the hyoid bone plays an important role, since it acts as a kind of balance arm suspended from the skull base, providing insertion to the muscles of the tongue and subhyoid muscles, the suspensors of the laryngeal–tracheal axis. The hyoid bone anchors the oral floor to the cranial base, thereby optimizing the synchronization of the tongue movements with the movement of the jaw and palate. Such movements are important in breathing and phonoarticulation (Lieberman 1979).

2.1 Subglottic Pressure and Breathing

Verbal production is a complex anatomofunctional event that involves in parallel and in sequence several organs and systems (Sataloff 1992). The central impulse activates a series of cortical and subcortical areas that act as regulators of muscle effectors distributed in the organs involved to a different extent in the phonoarticulatory function (Jurgens 1974; Lotze et al. 2000).

The respiratory tract structures allow the movement of egressive airflow masses coming from the lungs, after gas exchanges (haematosis) (Jaeger and Matthys 1968). When the diaphragm, which is the main inspiratory muscle, contracts, it increases the size of the thoracic cavity. At the end of inspiration, the diaphragm relaxes, and the elastic structures of the chest return to a balanced state, thereby forcing out the previously inhaled air volume and supplying energy: under these circumstances the volumes (400–500 ml) and the times of the two acts are equivalent. However, the dynamics of the structures involved in breathing for the purpose of phonation change.

During phonation, inspiration is shorter and expiration is substantially longer, with some interruptions normally occurring during prosodic breaks within the utterance. The air volumes mobilized are greater. The inspiratory pressure and especially the expiratory pressure against the closed glottis are much higher and always require muscle activation. Fine adjustments are necessary to ensure the maintenance of adequate pressure levels according to the acoustic characteristics of the articulated vocal emission (Baken 1997).

2.2 Subglottic Pressure and Phonoarticulation

The subglottic pressure ranges from 2–5 cm H_2O in normal talking to 10–20 cm H_2O in projected voice up to 50–60 cm H_2O in singing. In thoracoabdominal breathing, the rib movements and the lowering of the diaphragm provide adequate air supply for any vocal need. In the diaphragm–abdominal muscles antagonism (the abdominal muscles push and the diaphragm remains in a state of tonic contraction) a precise amount of expiratory flow and pressure generated immediately below the vocal folds (subglottic

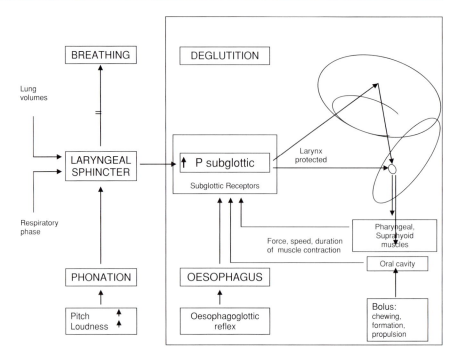

Fig. 2 Interaction of subglottic pressure between respiration, deglutition and phonation

pressure) is achieved, according to the specific vocal emission requirements (Fig. 2).

2.2.1 Laryngeal Sound

Sound is produced from the exhaled air at the level of the vocal folds. Current theories and models suggested to explain such activity derive from Ewald's myoelastic theory (1898). The contributions of Perello (1962), Hirano (1977), Dejonckère (1987) and Van den Berg (1954) have led to the formulation of the current myelastic aerodynamic theory of the vocal fold vibration. According to this theory, the vibration of vocal folds corresponds to the resolution of the elastic conflict between the air pressure and the closure force of the vocal folds.

When the pressure of the subglottic air exceeds the glottis resistance threshold, the vocal folds separate, the air flows out through the glottis and the subglottic pressure decreases. The vocal folds close back as a result of elastic recoil and mechanical suction ("Bernoulli effect"): a mucous wave is generated that propagates from the inferior aspect of the vocal fold down to the ventricle, reestablishing first glottis resistance and then subglottic pressure. Cyclic repetition of this mechanism takes place as long as energy is available, resulting in the formation of air

condensation and rarefaction areas in the glottis (vibratory mechanical wave). The recurrence of the event, in seconds, coincides with the fundamental frequency of the subject's voice.

The respiratory muscles may affect the fundamental frequency by regulating the subglottic pressure. The hyoid bone regulates the sagittal movements of the larynx: usually larynx lowering is observed during the production of low frequencies, whereas larynx raising occurs for higher frequencies. Larynx lowering is associated with a backward tilting of the thyroid cartilage with shortening, decrease in tension and increase in the thickness of the vocal folds, antagonizing the action of the cricothyroid muscle. Larynx lowering (controlled by subhyoid muscles) enhances low tones and lengthens the vocal tract.

The volume of the emitted sound is determined by the amplitude of the "airflow variation" during oscillation of the glottis. This variation is related both to the subglottic pressure and to the amplitude of the glottis movement. The "airflow" is the product of the duct section (glottic surface) and the velocity of the air outflow: the laryngeal muscles influence the quality of the fold closure, whereas the respiratory muscles regulate the subglottic pressure.

2.2.2 Articular Adaptation

The acoustic signal produced at the glottic level is a complex, quasi-periodic sound, characterized by a fundamental frequency, responsible for pitch perception, and by a series of harmonics at frequencies that are multiples of the fundamental frequency (Titze 1994). By passing through the supraglottic cavities (vocal tract), the laryngeal sound undergoes changes. The first change concerns the spectrum and refers to the energy reinforcement of groups of harmonics during their transit in a chamber, the resonance frequency of which is closer to their harmonic frequency. This energy reinforcement generates the formants that are at the basis of acoustic and perceptive recognition of the sound produced by the speaker. Such modification takes place in a passive way. The laryngeal sound can also undergo active changes by passing inside the vocal tract (Fant 1983). This occurs through the production of aperiodic signals (noise) that replace or are added to the glottic sound (periodic). Such activity as a whole is referred to as *articulation* and generates voiceless and voiced consonants, respectively: as a result thereof, consonants always have an oral (noise) and a laryngeal (sound) source. The sound of vowels, instead, has a laryngeal source, since vowels are articulated in the oral cavity from a mutual relationship of the tongue with the palate and posterior (pharynx wall) and anterior (lips) limiting structures.

2.3 Subglottic Pressure and Deglutition

Air under pressure, which is important in phono-articulation-related mechanisms, plays an equally important role in swallowing (Fig. 2). This occurs by stimulating mechanoreceptors localized in the subglottic region of the larynx (Ardzakus and Wyke 1979). This type of receptor has been identified, although the function of such receptors is not clearly known (Widdicombe 1986). Patients who have had a tracheotomy, for example, adequately ventilate; therefore, the role of such receptors in breathing can be considered as secondary. In addition to their function in breathing and voice production, these receptors are involved in swallowing. The stimulation of subglottic receptors may possibly act as a signal for the central nervous system that the larynx is "ready" (i.e. protected) for the bolus passage into the pharynx, and this signal may, at the same time, influence the low motor neurons of the brainstem innervating the pharynx.

The precise coordination of the respiratory and digestive systems is crucial in safe swallowing and this is reflected in the closed topographic organization of respiratory, deglutitory and branchial motor neurons (Larson et al. 1994). The localization, function and interaction of these neurons support the theory of an "online" processing of peripheral afferences both at a cortical and at a low brainstem level (Maddock and Gilbert 1993). As a result of the neuroanatomical connection between subglottic receptors and branchial motor neurons for the pharynx and larynx, the feedback from subglottic receptors may presumably affect the recruitment of motor neurons in the brainstem capable of activating the pharyngeal muscles during swallowing so that the force, speed and duration of the muscular contraction are regulated (normalized) by the closing of the larynx. The stimulation of this reflex arc increases the number of pharyngeal motor neurons, which, in turn, mediate a higher speed of the bolus transit, decreased time of pharyngeal contraction (resulting in a quicker pharyngeal clearing) and a stronger muscular contraction.

This feed-forward system may detect that a sensory input (subglottic pressure) has not been received and control a function (swallowing) by increasing the cortical processing, thereby ensuring safe passage of the bolus into the oesophagus. Cortical processing would thus account for a prolonged muscular contraction (Diez Gross et al. 2003).

Another possibility is that the segmental reflex is involved in bolus propulsion and therefore without said reflex the bolus is propelled more slowly. In this way, the pharyngeal muscles may increase the time of their contraction as a result of the increased latency of the bolus transit. This would partly explain why swallowing occurs in the later part of expiration. Swallowing during expiration helps the lungs fill with air before swallowing and it might be necessary to maximize the subglottic pressure and subsequent swallowing. In this way air is removed from the pharynx (thereby reducing air ingestion) and the exit of the bolus from the airways into the oesophagus is facilitated (Nishino et al. 1985).

3   Professional Voice Users

All those who use their voice within their professional activity may be deemed as voice professionals. This term makes us initially think of singers, actors or broadcasters, that is professionals who rely or have relied on their voice for their popularity or career. A wide variety of professional operators use their voice in their occupations: teachers, ecclesiastics, lawyers, telemarketers, receptionists and servicemen are just a few of the groups of people for whom oral communication is an essential part of their job. Then there are of course physicians, managers, call centre operators and many others. Although we live in the Internet and e-mail era, we can hardly imagine these professionals without an adequate voice for their professional tasks. In daily clinical phoniatric practice, however, voice disorders are also observed in housewives (Baitha et al. 2002).

Voice professionals can be divided into three main categories: top performers, such as opera singers, for whom any minimal voice alteration may sometimes have disastrous consequences; vocalists, including most other singers and actors; and finally all the other professionals mentioned above.

Workers who rely on their voice as an essential part of their occupation range from 25 to 35% of employees in the USA (Titze et al. 1997) and in other industrialized countries (Vilkman 2000) The professionals who are mostly affected by voice problems are teachers, with an incidence ranging from 38 (Smith et al. 1998) to 80% (Sapir et al. 1993), followed by telemarketers (68%) (Jones et al. 2002), aerobics instructors (44%) (Long et al. 1998) and salesmen (about 4%) (Coyle et al. 2001).

Among the 2,286 dysphonic patients reported by Brodnitz (1971), in 80%, dysphonia was due to vocal abuse or psychogenic factors causing dysfunction. Of these patients, 20% had organic lesions that in women were caused in 15% of cases by endocrine alterations. Other frequent causes were infectious laryngitis and reflux laryngitis.

Professional voice users complain of several problems, including hoarseness, vocal breaks, voice loss, hypophonia and vocal fatigue. Correlated symptoms may be phonatory dyspnoea, dry throat or sore throat, constricted sensation and pain. Chronic voice problems may be due to laryngitis and oedemas, benign cordal lesions, nodules, haemorrhage and cysts (Wingate et al. 2007).

4   Common Physiological Events

From the considerations illustrated in the previous sections, it appears evident that the respiratory, deglutitory, and phonoarticulatory functions are closely integrated and such integration resides in the integrity of the structures performing these functions.

4.1   Physical Adaptations in Artistic Voice Production

In singing, especially without amplification (classical or lyrical singing), the professional singer needs to exert greater pressures and maintain them for longer periods as compared with the pressures used in normal speech production. The need to obtain a product with a richer timbre (amplification) and carrying greater energy requires mutual adjustments of both the breathing dynamics and the vocal tract (Titze 1994). There is actually the need to realize a wider filtering resonating chamber while keeping the pressures at the lowest possible levels. This is achieved by lowering the larynx and the tongue and through a wider opening of the mouth. The forced and persistent lowering and anchoring of the larynx implies the downward movement of all related structures: hyoid bone and tongue root, with a strongly arched and raised soft palate. In romantic vocal productions all this goes to the benefit of the volume but to the detriment of articulatory capabilities and voice colouring that were so much appreciated in the previous musical period (Baroque).

As already said, in costal diaphragmatic breathing, during inspiration, the diaphragm contracts and the thoracic cavity becomes wider in its vertical and transverse diameters. During expiration, the breathing phase during which speech production and singing occur, the diaphragm is totally inactive and its rising is regulated only by other respiratory muscles (abdominal muscles, intercostal muscles, etc.). According to the need of producing low-intensity or high-intensity tones, high-pitched or low-pitched tones, or *filatura*, the behaviour of the respiratory muscles will affect the breathing dynamics. When full volume is reached, the elastic retraction forces of the lungs will spontaneously tend to empty them (as happens during quiet breathing). For most singing requirements, such retraction forces produce a sub-glottic air pressure that needs to be adjusted to the intensity of the sound to be emitted. A force capable of contrasting the elastic forces and reducing the sub-cordal pressure is therefore needed upon the attack of the sound, with an excessive impact on the vocal folds (brusque attack). This is what singers call "appoggio": the thorax is held in position by the action of external intercostal muscles, whereas the abdominal wall supports this activity. During a musical phrase, in order to keep the desired air pressure, the diaphragm starts rising, accompanied by a contraction of the abdominal muscles that provide the "support", which is constantly sought by the singer (Fussi 2003).

4.1.1 Valvular Activities

In these dynamics, diaphragm behaviour should be considered as an antireflux mechanism. Nowadays, it is clear that both the smooth muscle of the distal oesophagus (lower oesophageal sphincter) and the pillars of the diaphragm (crural diaphragm) represent the distal protection mechanisms of the oesophagus (Mittal and Balaban 1997). Changes in distal oesophageal pressures are correlated to contractions of the oesophagus and stomach (Dent et al. 1983), whereas crural contractions are related to the amount of inspiration or to the performing of activities increasing intra-abdominal pressure (e.g. Valsalva manoeuvre, cough, defecation, delivery) (Mittal et al. 1990): this mechanism is much more dynamic, pow-erful and effective in guaranteeing containment to the lower oesophageal sphincter. Furthermore, when the intra-abdominal pressure increases, a reflex is gener-ated that causes crural contraction and an increase in the lower oesophageal sphincter pressure (Shafik et al. 2004). The crura, however, consist of easily fatigable striated muscle fibres that are therefore inadequate for prolonged or too fast performances, which are quite often required in singing, for instance in supporting prolonged and sustained musical phrases or vocal exercises at extreme pitches. The air compression generated in the rib cage by the push action of the abdominal muscles and by the lowering of the ster-num increases the expiratory push but compresses the stomach, antagonizing the lower oesophageal sphincter. These dynamics may also account for the

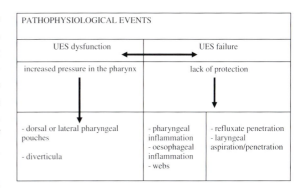

Fig. 3 Direct contact of refluxate with laryngeal structures. *UES* upper oesophageal sphincter

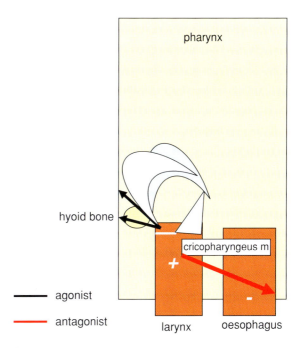

Fig. 4 Indirect involvement of laryngeal structure

increase in high-reflux episodes up into the pharynx during physical activity (Emerenziani et al. 2005) or with increased intra-abdominal pressure. Under these conditions there might be a direct contact of the refluxate with the laryngeal structures (direct mech-anism) (Fig. 3), which can also occur by means of a direct mechanism (Fig. 4).

Distal reflux through the lower oesophageal sphincter causes, through a neural or neurohumoral transmission route, a dysfunction in the upper oesophageal sphincter which may result in a reduced opening or early closure thereof (hypercompetence or hyperfunction). The insertion of the cricopharyngeal muscle into the cricoid cartilage determines, in the case of hypercontraction, an antagonism of the closing mechanisms of the laryngeal cavity, by reducing or preventing adequate facing of the arytenoids with respect to the epiglottis, thereby creating a predisposition to penetration episodes in the place of free inhalation. In 1,370 dysphonic patients, a high incidence of penetration (1,100 patients) was observed by Wuttge-Hannig and Hannig (2009) and was explained by the authors as a result of such an indirect mechanism. Posture can also differentiate patients with laryngopharyngeal reflux (LPR): in the standing position, and therefore while awake, the patients may experience reflux episodes during the day (Kouffman et al. 2000).

Some patients with LPR report reflux episodes only when they sing. In relation to what was stated above, we can add that patients with LPR also complain of motility disorders resulting in a delayed acid clearance or affecting the upper oesophageal sphincter with an increase in the basal pressure (Fouand et al. 1998). The experimental instillation of acid in the distal oesophagus of patients with LPR and in controls determines an increase in the tone of the upper oesophageal sphincter (Gerhardt et al. 1978).

4.1.2 Physiological Influences

In addition to the aforementioned influencing characteristics, singers often have dietary habits that promote reflux, with late dinners after evening performances and going to bed immediately after eating. Furthermore, the stress that is often part of the singer's career should also be taken into consideration. Oesophageal motility disorders or other reflux-related conditions (increased acid secretion, transient reduction in lower oesophageal sphincter pressure directly elicited by pharyngeal acid stimulation, decreased threshold of reflex gastric distension) have been described in psychophysical stress conditions (Castell 1999). The need to maintain their voices at optimal performance levels pushes these vocal professionals to take drugs or self-medication that may even worsen subjective or perceptive voice symptoms. Also the impact of an incorrect or inadequate diet on the genesis or maintenance of the reflux disease should not be neglected.

The most evident anatomical alterations of the laryngeal structures are caused by a direct contact with acid or alkaline juices and by the action of enzymes contained therein. In addition to erythema or oedema, a hacking cough can cause bleeding or mucosal tears responsible for obliteration of the lamina propria and the formation of adherences of mucosa to the vocal ligament. The inefficiency of the laryngeal vibrator associated with the decreased respiratory performance (potentially mediated by the aspiration of the refluxate into the lower airways) triggers vocal abuse and effort circuits that may lead to the onset of nodules or other lesions of the epithelial lining of vocal folds (Sataloff 1993; Spiegel et al. 1988).

5 Common Pathological Events

If the anatomical aspects are integrated into the various functions, such integration also characterizes pathological events that may affect effectors with a consequent impact on related functions (Fig. 1): in consideration of the high integration of these functions, dysfunctions may therefore be due to noxae localized at various levels and differently influenced by various pathological events.

Diseases related to voice and swallowing disorders may therefore be due to lesions of the nervous system in all of its components, autoimmune/dysreactive and iatrogenic (surgical operations, chemotherapy, radiotherapy, interaction of drugs) diseases as well as non-organic ones, if not overtly psychic or psychiatric components, which may sometimes explain certain clinical pictures. Table 1 briefly summarizes the events underlying voice production, whereas Table 2 illustrates the pathogenetic events that may affect it.

5.1 Vocal Alterations

Dysphonia is defined as a disorder characterized by altered vocal quality, pitch, loudness, or vocal effort that impairs communication or reduces voice-related quality of life (Schwartz et al. 2009). Voice disorders may be differently classified. In the literature there exist only a few works on the topic (Milutinovic 1966; Rosen and Murry 2000), but the most recent orientations identify two main categories: organic

Table 1 Events related to voice production

Site	Events
CNS	Planning, activation, control
PNS	Transfer of information
Thoracic bellows	Volume, pressures, flows
Larynx	Energy vibration: longitudinal and vertical direction
Vocal tract	Energy distribution in the speech spectrum

CNS central nervous system, *PNS* peripheral nervous system

Table 2 Pathophysiological events in voice disorders

Pathophysiological events	Site
Lack of planning, activation, control	CNS
Information transfer from centres to effectors	PNS, lack of motility, sensation
Breathing disorders (volumes, pressure, flows)	Thoracic bellows
Glottic insufficiency	Larynx, CNS, PNS
Vibratory alterations of the mucosa (qualitative and quantitative)	Larynx
Pathological posture of intrinsic and/or extrinsic laryngeal muscles	CNS, bellows, larynx, vocal tract
Breath–phonation incoordination	CNS, bellows, larynx
Phonation–resonance incoordination	Larynx, vocal tract
Incorrect posture	Posture, respiratory function

Table 3 Organic dysphonia

Thoracic bellows	Restrictive, obstructive, mixed lung disease
Laryngitis	Acute, chronic nonspecific and specific
Glottic plan alterations	Epithelium and lamina propria, arytenoid mucosa, anterior commissure
After surgery	Laryngeal structures (epithelium, muscles, framework)
Dysmobility	Ankylosis, peripheral nerves injury
Neurological disorders	Cortical, subcortical, cerebellar, peripheral nerve pathways
Muscle disease	Myasthenia, dystrophies, dermatomyositis, myofibromatosis, muscle tumours, intrachordal haematoma
Drugs	Testosterone, steroids, antihistamines, spasmolytics, atropine, drugs, high doses of vitamin C, diuretics
Hormonal disorders	Dysthyroidism, premenstrual hyperoestrogenism, dysmenorrhoea, pregnancy, menopause, andropause, hyperpituitarism, hypogonadism/hyperoestrogenism in prepubertal males and hyperandrogenism in prepubertal females, diabetes
Thesaurismosis	Amyloid, lipids, mucopolysaccharides
Pitch alterations	Primary (change of sex, androphonia), secondary
Vocal tract alterations	Nasality, volume resonators, feature walls

dysphonia (Table 3) (Blitzer et al. 1992; Bouchayer et al. 1985; Sataloff 1997; Schindler 1980; Segre 1976; Ursino 1995) and non-organic (dysfunctional or muscle tension) dysphonia (Table 4), characterized by structural or functional changes in the organs involved in voice production (Aronson 1980; Remacle and Lawson 1994; Sataloff 1997).

The interaction between form and structure (Fig. 1) explains the rich variety of related symptoms (dysphonia syndrome), including acoustic signs

Table 4 Non-organic (dysfunctional or muscle tension) dysphonia

Primary	Overuse, misuse, difficulties in pitch discrimination, imitation of incongruous vocal models
Secondary psychogenic	Conversion disorder, vocal cord dysfunction, disorders of the voice moult, pathological anxiety, depression
Secondary to organic disease	Audiogenic

Table 5 Conditions related to the onset of oropharyngeal dysphagia

Iatrogenic medication side effects (chemotherapy, neuroleptics, etc.)
Postsurgical muscular or neurogenic
Radiation
Corrosive (pill injury, intentional, cytolomegalovirus, candida, etc.)
Infectious: diphtheria, botulism, lyme disease, syphilis, mucositis (herpes)
Metabolic: amyloidosis, Cushing's syndrome, thyrotoxicosis, Wilson's disease, myopathic connective tissue disease (overlap syndrome)
Paraneoplastic syndromes
Neurological diseases
Myasthenia gravis, myotonic dystrophy, oculopharyngeal dystrophy dermatomyositis, polymyositis, sarcoidosis, cerebral palsy, Guillain–Barré syndrome
Metabolic encephalopathies
Neurological brainstem tumours
Head trauma
Stroke
Huntington's disease
Multiple sclerosis
Postpolio syndrome
Tardive dyskinesia
Amyotrophic lateral sclerosis
Parkinson's disease
Dementia
Elderly
Structural disease
Cricopharyngeal bar, Zenker's diverticulum, cervical webs
Oropharyngeal tumours
Osteophytes and skeletal abnormalities
Congenital (cleft palate, diverticula, pouches, etc.)

(alterations in volume, frequency, pitch, texture), clinical signs (endoscopic inspection with morphological and dynamic findings) and/or subjective physical signs (phonastenia, pharyngolaryngeal paraesthesia) and psychological signs (own voice perceived as unpleasant or inadequate), which are occasionally or constantly present in all or only in certain communication situations (Bergamini et al. 2002).

5.2 Deglutition Alterations

From a brief overview of the conditions that may be related to the onset of dysphagia, many common pathogenetic events can be identified, with a combination of swallowing and voice disorders (Table 5 (Cook and Kahrilas 1999)).

5.3   The Effects of Reflux

One of the main causes of comorbidity involved in voice and swallowing disorders is LPR, which is treated in a separate chapter in this volume. The topic will therefore be taken into account only as a concausal factor.

LPR involves different anatomical sites, including the lower oesophageal sphincter, oesophagus, upper oesophageal sphincter, laryngeal structures, oral cavity, trachea, and lungs. LPR represents the expression of the locoregional involvement of a gastro-oesophageal reflux (GOR) disease (GORD), whereas reflux laryngitis is a more circumscribed expression of the local problem. LPR was characterized as a nosological entity in the 1980s (Wiener et al. 1989; Koufman 1991) at the same time as laryngeal signs correlated with it gained greater attention (Belafsky et al. 2001, 2002). Hidden signs of GOR are an aetiological factor often reported in patients with ENT problems, especially in relation to voice. In 1989, Wiener et al. (1989) reported 78% of LPR cases documented with dual-probe pH monitoring in a series of 32 patients. This is a highly frequent problem in professional voice users and singers. In 1991, Sataloff et al. (1991) described reflux laryngitis in 265 of 583 voice professionals (45%), including singers, who had required medical treatment over the previous 12 months. However, reflux laryngitis is often an occasional finding during visits for other disorders and not the only cause of the voice problems of which the patient complains. The incidence of a posterior laryngitis is lower in patients without dysphonia, but posterior laryngitis is present in 78% of patients with hoarseness and in 50% of patients with general voice problems (Koufman et al. 1988). Other data on the prevalence of LPR were published in the following years (Koufman 1991; Koufman et al. 2002). LPR is often associated with aspiration. This may be clinically irrelevant or may be associated with chronic cough, reactive airway disease, difficulty in controlling asthma, distal phlogosis and bronchiectasias. Laryngeal involvement in GORD is often associated with hyperkinetic phonation in those patients who try

to compensate for an inflammatory condition of the larynx. Several issues are particularly interesting for voice professionals, above all, the age of the patients: many are young and need a long period of pharmacological treatment (pump inhibitors or H2 antagonists). The pharmacological agents used neutralize the refluxate and many related symptoms, but not the effect of neutral or alkaline substances (biliary salts) or enzymes that cause in any case damage to the larynx, pharynx and lungs. In professional voice users these substances may continue to cause local symptoms, such as clearing the throat, burning in the throat and cough (Sataloff et al. 2006).

6   Recent Contributions in the Literature

Although the correlations between the respiratory and digestive tracts are so closely interlinked and overlapping and in spite of the vast literature existing on voice and deglutition disorders when considered separately, only a few studies have been conducted on their association in specific populations and even less with respect to professional voice users.

A bibliography search using the major search engines confirmed the above. Results from a PubMed search for articles over the last 10 years including keywords such as "dysphagia" or "swallowing disorders" and "singing voice" or "professional voice" found only 25 articles in which sometimes the association between singing or professional voice and dysphagia is actually not strictly relevant. For instance, Sereg-Bahar et al. (2005) evaluated in a prospective study the acoustic characteristics of an /a produced by a sample of 43 patients with LPR before and after treatment with esomeprasol. The group was compared with another group of patients with vocal fold polyps. In addition to this acoustic parameter, further parameters were evaluated: medical history and laryngostroboscopic and oesophagogastroscopic findings. The conclusion was that the drug tested was effective for LPR management, whereas for LPR diagnosis, medical history and videolaryngoscopy proved to be superior to oesophagogastroscopy.

Acoustic voice analysis and laryngoscopic investigation can also be found in the work of Vashani et al. (2010), who evaluated the effectiveness of voice therapy in a group of 32 patients with GORD and dysphonia. The sample was subdivided into two groups: voice therapy combined with omeprazole and omeprazole alone, with follow-up evaluation after 6 weeks. Voice analysis included jitter, shimmer, harmonic-to-noise ratio and normalized noise energy. Oesophageal and laryngeal signs were assigned according to the reflux symptom index. The authors reported an improvement in all voice parameters and better results of the pharmacological treatment if it was combined with vocal therapy.

Similarly, Siupsinskiene et al. (2009) considered six parameters of the voice range profile and five parameters of the speech range profile in a group of 60 female dysphonic patients with LPR compared with a sample of 66 subjects with normal voice. In their conclusions the authors reported a reduced vocal capacity as documented by voice range profile measures in LPR patients and underlined the usefulness of these measures in the pre-post treatment quantitative assessment of voice performance. Similar conclusions were drawn by Oguz et al. (2007) and Pribuisienë et al. (2005). In an Italian study, the correlation between LPR and dysphonia was assessed in a sample of 62 patients without significant laryngoscopic findings and vocal abuse history by using a questionnaire validated for typical reflux signs versus a sample of subjects without voice problems. Electroacoustic, laryngostroboscopic and 24-h pH monitoring data of the two samples suggested a correlation between the amount and duration of the reflux (in patients with pH-metry suggestive of LPR) and a dysfunction of arytenoid muscles causing laryngeal compensatory stress, which was in turn responsible for chronic fatigue (Cesari et al. 2004). In contrast, no significant variation in electroacoustic parameters was found by Hamdan et al. (2001) in a sample of 22 patients with GOR-induced laryngeal signs treated for 4 weeks with pantoprazole (40 mg twice daily) and cisapride (20 mg twice daily). The treatment actually determined a quick disappearance of vocal symptoms (vocal fatigue and excess mucus production) and endoscopic signs.

The association between hoarseness and LPR was studied by Ozturk et al. (2006) in a sample of 43 subjects presenting with hoarseness for over 3 months and 20 control subjects. All subjects underwent videolaryngoscopic evaluation and 24-h double-probe pH monitoring. The results obtained by comparing data from the two methods in the two populations showed that in the study group 27 of 43 patients (62.8%) had laryngeal reflux episodes, whereas in the control group only six of 20 patients (30%) had laryngeal reflux episodes. The average of number of pharyngeal reflux episodes was 7 in 24 h (standard deviation, SD, 8.8) in the study patients versus 0.9 in 24 h (SD 1.9) in the control group, with $P = 0.003$. In the study group the average number of LPR episodes was 5.8 (SD 7.0) in an upright position versus 1.2 (SD 3.3) in a supine position, both values being significantly higher than those found in the control group ($P = 0.005$ and $P = 0.014$, respectively), thereby demonstrating that LPR is significantly greater in patients with hoarseness than in the control subjects, although they had LPR as well. The results of this study have further shown that the most common symptoms in the study group were heartburn and persistent throat clearing, whereas the endoscopic clinical finding was pachydermia. This may suggest that the severity of LPR rather than its presence may be the factor that triggers the onset of symptoms.

Some works found in the bibliography search are epidemiology studies. Among these, Roy et al. (2005) evaluated a random sample of 1,326 subjects interviewed with a questionnaire and reported that the lifetime prevalence of a voice disorder was 29.9%, with 6.6% of participants reporting a current voice disorder. The logistic regression correlated such data with some risk factors: sex (female), age (40–59 years), conditions and demands of vocal usage, oesophageal reflux, exposure to chemical agents and frequent colds and sinus infections. Paradoxically, the consumption of tobacco or alcohol was found not to increase the chances of developing a chronic voice disorder. Voice disorders proved to have a negative impact on work performance (4.3%) and work attendance: 7.2% of interviewees reported that they had been absent from work for 1 day or more in the course of the previous year and 2% of interviewees reported that they had been absent for more than 4 days because of voice problems.

Abnormal laryngeal findings that can be correlated to reflux were identified in a sample of 65 asymptomatic singing students who underwent videostroboscopic evaluation. Five students (8.3%) exhibited benign vocal fold lesions (two with nodules and three with cysts) and 44 students (73.4%) exhibited posterior erythema, suggesting possible reflux (Lundy et al. 1999). This correlation was considered useful to plan preventive measures in young singing professionals with high vocal demands.

Similar considerations were made by Elias et al. (1997) after observing 58% laryngeal abnormalities in six different clinical entities in a population of 65 professional singers who voluntarily underwent strobovideolaryngoscopic evaluation . The authors confirmed the usefulness of standardizing normal strobovideolaryngoscopic findings in professional singers, being aware of the variability of laryngeal behaviour in this population. Similarly, Heman-Ackah et al. (2002) studied 20 singing teachers who voluntarily underwent strobovideolaryngoscopic evaluation, of whom seven reported voice problems and 13 a normal voice. The presence of organic lesions (vocal fold masses) was a common finding in asymptomatic teachers, whereas reflux laryngitis was found in both symptomatic and asymptomatic teachers. Movement asymmetry was more common in singing teachers with voice disorders. Dysphonia and LPR findings were associated in a group of eight singers with bulimia, leading to the conclusion that LPR may be a factor that contributes to the development of vocal disorders in singers with bulimia (Rothstein 1998).

What is more interesting is the association between functional dysphonia and LPR. The correlation between the two entities has been investigated by several authors. Karkos et al. (2007) studied 23 subjects with dysphonia for over 3 months, by comparing them with eight healthy volunteers. Of the initial sample 22 dysphonic patients and six healthy subjects completed the protocol that included a 24-h dual-probe pH-metry. Of all the parameters studied, the longest duration (in seconds) of reflux episodes in the supine position and the time fraction in which the pH was below 4 in the supine position were significantly longer in dysphonic patients than in control subjects ($P < 0.05$). This led the authors to conclude that there is a correlation between LPR and the two parameters, although many more parameters may determine functional dysphonia, including "medical" and psychological causes.

A A 30-month retrospective review of 150 subjects (60% females and 40% males, mean age 42.3 years) with muscle tension dysphonia was conducted by Altman et al. (2005). Medical history showed the presence of GOR (49%), high stress levels (18%), vocal ablise (63%) and vocal misase (23%). Instrumental clinical evaluation performed in 82% of patients showed the presence of anatomical abnormalities in 52.3% of subjects (vocal fold oedema, or paralysis/paresis). Speech–language assessment identified a poor phonatory support to breathing, improperly low voice pitch and visible neck tension in most patients. Adequate voice volume was observed in 23.3% of patients. This range of factors indicates the presence of multiple factors in the genesis of muscle tension dysphonia.

The association between dysfunction factors, such as extrinsic laryngeal muscular tension and muscle misuse dysphonia, and GOR was investigated by Angsuwarangsee and Morrison (2002). A sample of 465 patients (65% females and 35% males) were sequentially evaluated and extrinsic laryngeal muscular tension results were analysed in relation to GOR diagnosis. A close relationship ($P \leq 0.01$) was found between the thyroid muscle in GOR patients and muscle misuse dysphonia, indicating that there might be a correlation between the extrinsic and intrinsic laryngeal muscular tension, which is useful in the diagnosis of muscle misuse dysphonia.

A professional susceptibility to GOR related to professional singing was suggested by several authors. The first work dates back to 2003 (Cammarota et al. 2003), reporting on the experience conducted with four professional singers who showed decreased respiratory muscle functioning during reflux episodes during performances. Reflux episodes were related to the quick and prolonged need to increase intra-abdominal pressure owing to the need to reduce subglottic pressure. According to the authors, this was the first case described in the literature of a worsening of GORD symptoms in professional singers during performances.

This study was followed by another work by the same lead author (Cammarota et al. 2007) with the purpose of studying the prevalence of GOR symptoms in a group of professional opera choristers versus a control group of non-singers. A total of 351 opera choristers belonging to professional lyrical choruses from various Italian regions were compared with 578 subjects resident in the same areas with a similar age and sex distribution. By means of a structured questionnaire, the occurrence of reflux symptoms in the course of the previous year, individual characteristics and life habits of the two groups were investigated. Prevalence rate ratios, adjusted for sex, age, body mass index, smoking status, alcohol consumption and other confounding factors, were computed.

In the sample of choristers, a statistically significant increase in heartburn, regurgitation, cough and hoarse voice was observed versus the control sample, with adjusted prevalent rate ratios of 1.60 [95% confidence interval (CI), 1.32–1.94], 1.81 (95% CI, 1.42–2.30), 1.40 (95% CI, 1.18–1.67) and 2.45 (95% CI, 1.97–3.04), respectively. Multivariate analysis correlated regurgitation in a consistent way with the cumulative duration of singing activity ($P = 0.04$) and weekly singing performances ($P = 0.005$). The authors concluded by reporting a greater prevalence of reflux symptoms in opera choristers versus control subjects. They also underlined the need for further investigation to clarify whether GOR in this population is stress-related and may be considered as a professional disease. As to the relation with stress, Marchese et al. (2008) described the case of a 49-year-old professional soprano with a 6-year history of regurgitation and pyrosis in association with an increased time to achieve adequate vocal warm-up, restricted vocal tone placement, and decreased pitch range. After the diagnosis of posterior laryngitis and negative oesophagogastroduodenoscopy findings, a functional study with oesophageal manometry and pharyngeal pH monitoring was conducted. Oesophageal manometry documented lower oesophageal sphincter incompetence and isolated episodes of upper oesophageal sphincter hypertonia. Pharyngeal pH monitoring (the patient was asked to perform her normal singing and vocal warm-up activity) reported, during singing, 69 episodes of pharyngeal reflux equivalent to 10% of the total reflux time, which is 10 times higher than that previously described as the upper limit (0.9%) in healthy volunteers. This finding suggested a correlation between pharyngeal acid exposure and singing, thereby indicating that such a condition may be considered related to this professional activity. The authors agreed that further data are required to support this conclusion.

The latest work on this topic was conducted by Pregun et al. (2009), who considered the prevalence of GOR symptoms in a population of professional opera choristers (202 subjects), wind players (71 subjects), glassblowers (43 subjects) and water polo players (54 subjects) in comparison with a sample of 115 subjects. By means of a questionnaire, the occurrence of reflux symptoms, individual characteristics and life habits of the two groups were investigated. Statistical processing of data showed a statistically higher prevalence of heartburn, regurgitation and hoarseness in professional choristers than in control subjects ($P < 0.001$). Among professional wind players, heartburn and regurgitation were significantly more frequent than in controls ($P < 0.05$ and $P < 0.01$, respectively). Glassblowers reported a significantly higher prevalence of acid regurgitation in comparison with controls ($P < 0.01$). The prevalence of reflux symptoms in water polo players was similar to that of controls. In opera choristers, wind players and glassblowers, reflux symptoms appeared to be significantly correlated with the cumulative lifetime duration of professional singing, playing and working activity, respectively ($P < 0.05$).

The results reported by the authors in agreement with the findings of Cammarota et al. (2007) demonstrated that professional opera choristers, professional wind players and glassblowers had a higher prevalence of reflux symptoms than control subjects. This work-related condition was found to have a negative impact on quality of life and professional performances.

References

Altman KW, Atkinson C, Lazarus C (2005) Current and emerging concepts in muscle tension dysphonia: a 30-month review. J Voice 19(2):261–267

Angsuwarangsee T, Morrison M (2002) Extrinsic laryngeal muscular tension in patients with voice disorders. J Voice 16(3):333–343

Ardzakus FK, Wyke B (1979) Innervation of the subglottic mucosa of the larynx and its significante. Folia Phoniatr (Basel) 31:271–283

Arensburg B, Tillier AM, Vandermeersch B, Duday H, Schepartz LA, Rak Y (1989) A middle palaeolithic human hyoid bone. Nature 338:758–760

Aronson AE (1980) Clinical voice disorders. An interdisciplinary approach. Thieme, New York

Baitha S, Raizada RM, Kennedy Singh AK, Puttewar MP, Chaturvedi VN (2002) Clinical profile of hoarseness of voice. Indian J Otolaryngol Head Neck Surg 54(I):14–18

Baken RJ (1997) Airflow and volume. In: Baken RJ (ed) Clinical measurement of speech and voice. Singual Publishing, San Diego

Belafsky PC, Postma GN, Koufman JA (2001) The validity and reliability of the reflux finding score (RFS). Laryngoscope 111(8):1313–1317

Belafsky PC, Postma GN, Koufman KA (2002) Validity and reliability of the reflux symptom index (RSI). J Voice 16:274–277

Bergamini G, Casolino D, Schindler O (2002) Inquadramento delle disfonie. In Casolino D (ed). Le disfonie: fisiopatologia, clinica ed aspetti medico-legali. Pacini Editore Medicina, Pisa

Blitzer A, Brin MF, Ramig LO (1992) Neurologic disorders of the larynx, 2nd edn. Thieme, New York

Bouchayer M, Cornut G, Witzing E, Loire R, Roch JB, Bastian R (1985) Epidermoid cysts, sulci and mucosal bridges of the true vocal cord. Laryngoscope 95:1087–1094

Brodnitz FS (1971) Hormones and the human voice. Bull N Y Acad Med 47(2):183–191

Cammarota G, Elia F, Cianci R, Galli J, Paolillo N, Montalto M, Gasbarrini G (2003) Worsening of gastroesophageal reflux symptoms in professional singers during performances. J Clin Gastroenterol 36(5):403–404

Cammarota G, Masala G, Cianci R, Palli D, Capaccio P, Schindler A, Cuoco L, Galli J, Ierardi E, Cannizzaro O, Caselli M, Dore MP, Bendinelli B, Gasbarrini G (2007) Reflux symptoms in professional opera choristers. Gastroenterology 132(3):890–898

Castell DO (1999) The esophagus, 3rd edn. Lippincott, Philadelphia

Cesari U, Galli J, Ricciardiello F, Cavaliere M, Galli V (2004) Dysphonia and laryngopharyngeal reflux. Acta Otorhinolaryngol Ital 24(1):13–19

Cook IJ, Kahrilas PJ (1999) AGA technical review on management of oropharyngeal dysphagia. Gastroenterology 116:455–478

Coyle SM, Weinrich BD, Stemple JC (2001) Shifts in relative prevalence of laryngeal pathology in a treatment-seeking population. J Voice 15:424–440

Dejonckère PH (1987) Physiologie phonatoire du larynx: le concept oscilloimpédantiel. Rev Laryng 108:365–368

Dent J, Wylie J, Dodds J et al (1983) Interdigestive phasic contractions of the human lower esophageal sphincter. Gastroenterology 84:453–460

Diez Gross R, Mahlmann J, Grayhack JP (2003) Physiologic effects of open and closed thacheostomy tubes on the pharyngeal swallow. Ann Otol Laryngol 112:143–152

Duchin LE (1990) The evolution of articulate speech: comparative anatomy of the oral cavity in Pan and Homo. J Hum Evol 19:687–697

Elias ME, Sataloff RT, Rosen DC, Heuer RJ, Spiegel JR (1997) Normal strobovideolaryngoscopy: variability in healthy singers. J Voice 11(1):104–107

Emerenziani S, Zhang X, Blondeau K et al (2005) Gastric fullness, physical activity, and proximal extent of gastroesophageal reflux. Am J Gastroenterol 100:1251–1256

Fant G (1983) The voice source: theory and acoustic modeling. In: Titze RI, Scherer R (eds) Vocal fold fisiology: biomechanics, acoustics and phonatory control. Center for Performing Arts, Denver

Fouand YM, Khoury RM, Hatlebakk JG et al (1998) Ineffective esophageal motility (IEM) is more prevalent in reflux patients with respiratory symptoms. Am J Gastroenterol 114(S1):A123 (abstract 0506)

Fussi F (2003) I parametri acustici nell'estetica e nella fisiologia del canto. In: Fusi F (ed) La voce del cantante, vol II. Omega, Turin

Gerhardt DC, Shuck TJ, Bordeaux RA, Winship DH (1978) Human upper esophageal sphincter: response to volume, osmotic and acid stimuli. Gastroenterology 75:268–274

Hamdan AL, Sharara AI, Younes A, Fuleihan N (2001) Effect of aggressive therapy on laryngeal symptoms and voice characteristics in patients with gastroesophageal reflux. Acta Otolaryngol 121(7):868–872

Heman-Ackah YD, Dean CM, Sataloff RT (2002) Strobovideolaryngoscopic findings in singing teachers. J Voice 16(1):81–86

Hirano M (1977) Structure and vibratory pattern of the vocald folds. In: Sawashima N, Cooper FS (eds) Dynamic aspects of speech production. University of Tokyo, Tokyo

Houghton P (1993) Neandertal supralaryngeal vocal tract. Am J Phys Anthropol 90(2):139–146

Jaeger MJ, Matthys H (1968) The pattern of flow in the upper human airways. Resp Physiol 6:113–127

Jones K, Sigmon J, Hock L, Nelson E, Sullivan M, Ogren F (2002) Prevalence and risk factors for voice problems among telemarketers. Arch Otolaryngol Head Neck Surg 128:571–577

Jurgens U (1974) On the elicitability of vocalisztion from the cortical lerynx area. Brain Res 81:564–566

Karkos PD, Yates PD, Carding PN, Wilson JA (2007) Is laryngopharyngeal reflux related to functional dysphonia? Ann Otol Rhinol Laryngol 116(1):24–29

Kirchner JA (1993) The vertrebate larynx: adaptation and aberrations. Laryngoscope 103:1197–1201

Kouffman JA, Amin MR, Panetti M (2000) Prevalence of reflux in 113 consecutive patients with laringea and voice disorders. Otolaryngol Head Neck Surg 123:385–388

Koufman JA (1991) The otolaryngologic manifestaton of gastroesophageal disease (GERD) a clinical investigation of 225 patients using ambulatory 24-pH monitoring and an experimental investigation of the role of acid and pepsin in the development of laryngeal injury. Laryngoscope 101(Suppl 53):1–78

Koufman JA, Wiener GJ, Wu WC, Castell DO (1988) Reflux laryngitis and its sequelae: the diagnostic role of ambulatory 24-h pH monitoring. J Voice 2(1):78–89

Koufman JA, Aviv JA, Casiano RR, Shaw GY (2002) Laryngopharyngeal reflux: position statement of the Committee on Speech, Voice, and Swallowing Disorders of the American Academy of Otolaryngology—Head and Neck Surgery. Otolaryngol Head Neck Surg 127:32–35

Laitman JT, Reindenberg JS (1993) Specializations of the human upper respiratory and upper digestive system as seen through comparative and developmental anatomy. Dysphagia 8:318–325

Larson CR, Yajima Y, Ko P (1994) Modification in activity of medullary respiratory-related neurons for vocalisation and swallowing. J Neurophysiol 71:2294–2304

Lieberman P (1979) Hominid evolution, supralaryngeal vocal tract physiology, and the fossil evidence for reconstructions. Brain Lang 7(1):101–126

Long J, Williford HN, Olson MS, Wolfe V (1998) Voice problems and risk factors among aerobics instructors. J Voice 12:197–207

Lotze M, Seggevies G, Erb M, Grodd W, Birbaumer N (2000) The representation of articulation in primary sensorimotor cortex. Neuroreport 11:2985–2989

Lundy DS, Casiano RR, Sullivan PA, Roy S, Xue JW, Evans J (1999) Incidence of abnormal laryngeal findings in asymptomatic singing students. Otolaryngol Head Neck Surg 121(1):69–77

Marchese M, Spada C, Costamagna G (2008) Stress-related esophagopharyngeal reflux during warm-up exercises in a singer. Gastroenterology 134(7):2192–2193; author reply 2193–2194 (Epub 16 May 2008)

Maddock DJ, Gilbert RJ (1993) Quantitative relationship between liquid bolus flow and laringea closure during deglutition. Am J Physiol 265:G704–G711

Milutinovic Z (1966) Classification of voice pathology. Folia Phoniatr Logop 48:301–308

Mittal RK, Balaban DH (1997) The esophagogastric junction. N Engl J Med 336:924–932

Mittal RK, Fisher M, McCallum RW et al (1990) Human lower esophageal sphincter response to increased abdominal pressure. Am J Physiol 258:G624–G630

Negus VE (1949) The comparative anatomy and physiology of the larynx. Heinemann, London

Nishino T, Yonezawa T, Honda Y (1985) Effects of swallowing on the pattern of continuous respiration in human adults. Am Rev Respir Dis 12:1219–1222

Oguz H, Tarhan E, Korkmaz M, Yilmaz U, Safak MA, Demirci M (2007) Acoustic analysis findings in objective laryngopharyngeal reflux patients. Ozluoglu LNJ Voice 21(2):203–210

Ozturk O, Oz F, Karakullukcu B, Oghan F, Guclu E, Ada M (2006) Hoarseness and laryngopharyngeal reflux: a cause and effect relationship or coincidence? Eur Arch Otorhinolaryngol 263(10):935–939

Perello J (1962) La théorie muco-ondulatoire de la phonation. Ann Oto Larynx 79:722–725

Pregun I, Bakucz T, Banai J, Molnár L, Pavlik G, Altorjay I, Orosz P, Csernay L, Tulassay Z, Herszényi L (2009) Gastroesophageal reflux disease: work-related disease? Dig Dis 27(1):38–44 (Epub 8 May 2009)

Pribuisienë R, Uloza V, Saferis V (2005) Multidimensional voice analysis of reflux laryngitis patients. Eur Arch Otorhinolaryngol 262(1):35–40

Purves D, Litchman JW (1985) Principles of neural development. Sinauer, Sunderland, p 340

Remacle M, Lawson G (1994) Troubles fonctionelle du larynx. Encycl Méd Chir Oto-rhino-laryngologie. Elsevier, Paris

Rosen AC, Murry T (2000) Nomenclature of voice disorders and vocal pathology. In: Rosen AC, Murry T (eds) The otolaryngologic clinics of North America (voice disorders and phonosurgery II). Saunders, Philadelphia

Rothstein SG (1998) Reflux and vocal disorders in singers with bulimia. J Voice 12(1):89–90

Roy N, Merrill RM, Gray SD, Smith EM (2005) Voice disorders in the general population: prevalence, risk factors, and occupational impact. Laryngoscope 115(11):1988–1995

Sapir S, Keidar A, Mathers-Schmidt B (1993) Vocal attrition in teachers: survey findings. Eur J Dis Commun 28:177–185

Sataloff RT (1992) The human voice. Sci Am 267:108–115

Sataloff RT (1993) The human voice. Sci Am 267:108–115

Sataloff RT (1997) Professional voice. The science and art of clinical care, 2nd edn. Singular Publishing, San Diego

Sataloff RT, Spiegel JR, Hawkshaw MJ (1991) Strobovideolaryngoscopy: results and clinical value. Ann Otol Rhynol Laryngol 100(9):725–727

Sataloff RT, Castell DO, Katz PO, Sataloff DM (2006) Reflux laryngitis and related disorders, 3rd edn. Plural Publishing, San Diego

Schindler O (1980) Afonie e disfonie. In: Schindler O (ed) Breviario della patologia della comunicazione. Omega, Turin

Schwartz SR, Cohen SM, Daily SH, Rosenfeld RM et al (2009) Clinical practice guideline: hoarseness (dysphonia). Otolaryngol Head Neck Surg 141:S1–S31

Segre R (1976) La comunicazione orale normale e patologica. Medico Scientifiche, Turin

Sereg-Bahar M, Jansa R, Hocevar-Boltezar I (2005) Voice disorders and gastroesophageal reflux. Logoped Phoniatr Vocol 30(3–4):120–124

Shafik A, El-Sibai O, Shafik AA et al (2004) Effect of straining on the lower esophageal sphincter: identification of the "strainingesophageal reflex" and its role in gastroesophageal competence mechanism. J Invest Surg 17:191–196

Siupsinskiene N, Adamonis K, Toohill RJ (2009) Usefulness of assessment of voice capabilities in female patients with reflux-related dysphonia. Medicina (Kaunas) 45(12):978–987

Smith E, Lemke J, Taylor M, Kirchner L, Hoffman H (1998) Frequency of voice problems among teachers and other occupations. J Voice 12:480–488

Soulié A, Bardier F (1907) Recherches sur le developpement du larynx chez l'homme. J Anat Physiol 43:137–240

Spiegel JR, Sataloff RT, Cohn JR, Hawkshaw M, Epstein J (1988) Respiratory function in singer: medical assessment, diagnosis and treatment. J Voice 2(1):40–50

Titze IR (1994) Control of vocal intensity and efficiency. In: Titze IR (ed.) Principles of voice production, Prentice hall, New Jersey

Titze I, Lemke J, Montequin D (1997) Populations in the U.S.Workforce who rely on voice as a primary tool of trade: a preliminary report. J Voice 11:254–259

Ursino F (1995) Le disfonie. In: Schindler O, Genovese E, Rossi M, Ursino F (eds) Foniatria. Masson, Milan

Van Den Berg J (1954) Sur lès théories myoélastique et neurochronaxique de la phonation. Rev Laryngol 75:492–512

Vashani K, Murugesh M, Hattiangadi G, Gore G, Keer V, Ramesh VS, Sandur V, Bhatia SJ (2010) Effectiveness of voice therapy in reflux-related voice disorders. Dis Esophagus 23(1):27–32 (Epub 22 Jun 2009)

Vilkman E (2000) Voice problems at work: a challenge for occupational safety and health arrangement. Folia Phoniatr Logop 52:20–125

Widdicombe J (1986) The neural reflexes in the airways. Eur J Resp Dis Suppl 144:1–33

Wiener GJ, Koufmann JA, Wu WC et al (1989) Chronic hoarseness secondary to gastroesophageal reflux disease: documentation with 24-pH monitoring. Am J Gasroenterol 84:1503–1508

Wingate JM, Brown WS, Shrivastav R, Davenport P, Sapienza CM (2007) Treatment outcomes for professional voice users. J Voice 21:433–449

Wolfson VP, Laitman JT (1990) Ultrasound investigation of fetal human upper respiratory anatomy. Anat Rec 227:363–372

Wuttge-Hannig A, Hannig C (2009) Diagnostica per immagini. In: Schindler O (ed) La voce. Fisiologia, patologia clinica e terapia. Piccin, Padua

Psychiatric Aspects of Dysphagia

Margareta Bülow

Contents

Abstract

Dysphagia with a psychiatric background is a rare condition, not so well understood, and presents with no structural or organic disease being detectable. Fear of swallowing and avoidance of swallowing specific foods, fluids, or pills seem to be the most frequent symptoms in psychogenic dysphagia, and may result in malnutrition and weight loss. When psychogenic dysphagia is suspected, a thorough swallowing evaluation is necessary, involving clinical as well as instrumental examinations. A multidisciplinary approach is required. Professionals from the fields of neurology, otolaryngology, speech–language pathology, radiology, and gastroenterology may be involved. The diagnosis of psychogenic dysphagia should, to avoid misdiagnosis, be reserved for patients with strong psychological symptoms and fear of swallowing. The most effective treatment of psychogenic dysphagia seems to be a combination of psychological treatment and dysphagia therapy. Antianxiety medications may be effective in some cases. Close collaboration between the dysphagia clinician and psychologists is necessary for the optimal management.

1 Introduction and Terminology

In the treatment of dysphagic patients with acute or chronic problems where no structural or organic disease could be diagnosed, the cause may be psychiatric. Dysphagia with a psychiatric cause is a rare condition, and not so well understood. In the literature,

M. Bülow (✉)
Neurological Department and Diagnostic Centre
of Imaging and Functional Medicine,
Skåne University Hospital, 205 02, Malmö, Sweden
e-mail: margareta.bulow@med.lu.se

O. Ekberg (ed.), *Dysphagia*, Medical Radiology. Diagnostic Imaging, DOI: 10.1007/174_2011_342,

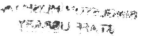

few reports could be found describing this condition. However, there are reports suggesting that persons with psychological conflicts in an attempt to reduce unacceptable emotional responses may convert them into more acceptable physical manifestations (Finkenbine and Miele 2004; Lehtinen and Puhakka 1976. It has also been suggested that patients with this condition may suffer from anxiety and depression (De Lucas-Taracena and Montanes-Rada 2006).

Several different terms are used to describe the condition of dysphagia with psychiatric origin, where "psychogenic dysphagia" is the most well known. Sometimes the term "sitophobia," from the Greek words *sito* ("food") and *phobia* ("fear," "aversion"), may be used to describe a condition with pathologic fear of swallowing. Other terms which may be used are "choking phobia or swallowing phobia" (Seems et al. 2009; De Lucas-Taracena and Montanes-Rada 2006; McNally 1994), "globus hystericus" (Finkenbine and Miele 2004; Ravich et al. 1989; Stacher 1983, 1986), "hysterical dysphagia" (Ciyiltepe and Türkbay 2006; Nicasso et al. 1981), "phagophobia" (Ciyiltepe and Türkbay 2006; Shapiro et al. 1997), and "pseudodysphagia" (Bradley and Narula 1987).

2 Symptoms in Psychogenic Dysphagia

Psychological factors which inhibit normal swallowing and result in inefficient and/or disorganized swallowing are thought to be related to signs of psychogenic dysphagia. Nicholson et al. (2010) think that psychogenic dysphagia is a problematic diagnosis. The psychological mechanism and how it differs from conscious simulation still remains unclear.

The most common complaint of patients with psychogenic swallowing problems is fear of swallowing manifested as difficulties initiating the swallowing and thereby sometimes avoidance of eating. Certain foods, fluids, and pills may cause huge problems for patients to swallow (Barofsky and Fontaine 1998; Ciyiltepe and Türkbay 2006; Leopold and Kagel 1997; Ravich et al. 1989; Shapiro et al. 1997). Also, abnormal oral behaviors, with repeated deviant tongue movements, a feeling of throat pressure, and complaint of globus were found in this patient group. Complaints reported by Bradley and Narula (1987) and Shapiro et al.

(1997) are a globus sensation, general difficulties in swallowing, breathing problems, and fear of choking. Also, malnutrition and weight loss may be associated with a swallowing condition with psychiatric origin (Barofsky and Fontaine 1998; Ciyiltepe and Türkbay 2006; Finkenbine and Miele 2004; Shapiro et al. 1997).

In some literature, psychogenic dysphagia has been described as a *conversion disorder*. Psychological conflicts and anxiety are transformed into somatic symptoms and are regarded as an unconscious process. Kanner (1935) described dysphagia as a primary conversion disorder. A case was presented of a 12-year-old boy who had developed dysphagia to solid foods owing to physical abuse by his father for eating improperly. In our swallowing clinic we have encountered similar cases. A young single mother, with a 5-year-old daughter, worked as a cashier in a grocer's shop. She was unable to take a normal lunch break because of customer demands, which was a high stress factor in her working conditions. After a period of time she was unable to eat and swallow in a normal way. Her complaints were primarily oral in nature, along with difficulties in initiating the swallow. Videofluoroscopic swallow evaluation (VFSE) showed signs of oral dysphagia with intact pharyngeal function. Another example is a middle-aged woman with an abnormal oral phase of swallowing and fear of initiating the swallowing. She told us during one of her therapeutic sessions that during her childhood she had been forced by a strict grandmother to always empty her plate. She experienced great fear when she visited her grandmother, especially when forced to eat with her. When exposed to stress later in life, she reacted with an inability to eat and swallow normally.

Another form of conversion disorder described as a manifestation of both a physiological disorder and psychiatric illness is the sensation of globus (Finkenbine and Miele 2004). Bradley and Narula (1987) described the sensation of a "lump" or "fullness" localized to the throat in association with globus hystericus, hysterical dysphagia, or pseudodysphagia. Their conclusion was that when no evident cause is found, the condition may be a "'primary globus pharyngeus', or a 'secondary globus pharyngeus' when the etiology was detectable" (p. 689). Okada et al. (2007) analyzed in a case study six children with phagophobia according to psycho-pathology and current treatment. Their results indicated that evaluation of premorbid personality is crucial to the prognosis.

Psychological factors have also been found to be associated with esophageal dysphagia. Esophageal contractions can result from psychological stress. Kronecker and Meltzer (1883) reported that esophageal contractions, not only due to emotional tension, but also in some cases due to cold or hot food could react with nonpropulsive contractions. Other interesting observations have shown that stimuli not related to ingestion such as intense short sounds may influence esophageal contraction and are likely to form part of the defense reaction of a healthy organism (Stacher 1983).

Abnormal oral swallowing behaviors in the presence of intact pharyngeal stage function may be revealed on radiological swallowing evaluations. In some cases, such oral abnormalities may be associated with psychogenic dysphagia. Diffuse esophageal symptoms may also be related to psychological factors. According to Jones (2003), patients with psychogenic dysphagia may demonstrate a variety of swallowing signs during VFSE, including the presentation of small boluses, multiple tongue movements, and "complex oral motions such as rocking, swirling, bunching and pumping" (p. 97). Also, the presence of a pharyngeal swallow delay without oral propulsion of bolus has been described by Jones (2003).

Even if reports regarding communicative symptoms associated with psychogenic dysphagia are not found in the literature, an interesting case study describes a 63-year-old male "deglutition stutterer." The man developed myoclonus of the tongue and contractions of the hypopharyngeal muscles in the moment of deglutition. The history was remarkable for pharyngeal spasms in his youth, which reemerged as described above in stressful situations (Escher 1983).

At our swallowing clinic, from 2002 to 2010 we completed 2,084 VFSE studies, and psychogenic dysphagia was diagnosed in 25 cases (0.01%). The most frequent complaints regarding swallowing signs and symptoms are listed in Table 1. The patients often presented with more than one symptom. Those patients with complaints of globus without pharyngeal dysfunction or with suspected esophageal dysfunction were referred to either an otolaryngologist or a gastroenterologist for further clinical or instrumental evaluation.

Table 1 The most frequent complaints in psychogenic dysphagia regarding swallowing signs and symptoms in our videofluoroscopic swallow evaluation (*VFSE*) studies

Complaint	No. of patients
Fear of swallowing	13 of 25
Experienced difficulties in swallowing specific consistencies	13 of 25
Problems in initiating the pharyngeal swallow. (The patient experienced a feeling of being unable to swallow. On VFSE we could document a normal pharyngeal swallow.)	10 of 25
Oral abnormalities (such as multiple tongue movements with difficulties in propelling the bolus posteriorly to pass the base of the tongue and initiating the pharyngeal swallow)	8 of 25
Globus complaints	6 of 25
Normal pharyngeal swallow	25 of 25

3 Epidemiology

From different swallowing clinics it has been reported that a minor group of the patients complaining of swallowing problems have psychogenic dysphagia. Among patients referred to the Johns Hopkins Swallowing Center, 13% had been diagnosed with psychogenic dysphagia or globus hystericus. However, when this group was later reevaluated, more than half of the group were found to have an organic cause of the dysphagia (Ravich et al. 1989). From a large sample of patients seen in a swallowing center and complaining of swallowing difficulties, a normal pharyngeal swallow revealed on VFSE (with additional abnormal oral behaviors in some cases) accounted for approximately only 3% of the group (Barofsky et al. 1993). Malcolmson (1966) diagnosed 231 patients with globus hystericus, and negative clinical and radiological evaluations were found in 20% of the patients. Patients with different psychosomatic disorders of gastrointestinal tract were studied (612 patients) by Korkina and Marilov (1995). In 70% of the 612 patients studied, relatives of the patient also had psychosomatic diseases, suggesting the possible influence of genetic and environmental factors in this condition. Choking phobia was found to be more frequent in females (two thirds of cases) and had a high comorbidity with anxiety disorders. Life events such as divorce, disease in the family, or unemployment, as well as traumatic eating antecedents, were also frequently present (De Lucas-Taracena and Montanes-Rada 2006). Prevalence studies have shown that 45% of young and middle-aged people are estimated to suffer from symptoms of globus, often in combination with strong emotion (Thompson and Heaton 1982).

4   Swallowing Evaluation

A diagnosis of psychogenic origin must be used with caution and only after a thorough evaluation. At the Johns Hopkins Swallowing Center, Ravich et al. (1989) performed a reevaluation of 23 patients with the diagnosis of psychogenic dysphagia or globus hystericus. They subsequently found that more than half of these patients had an underlying physical explanation for their difficulty swallowing. In 65% of the patients (15 of 23), pharyngeal dysfunction, structural obstruction, or esophageal dysmotility was found. Owing to those findings, they suggested that when any changes or progression of symptoms was reported, a careful reevaluation should be performed. Stacher (1986) also recommended caution when attributing symptoms of dysphagia to psychogenic origins and emphasized the importance of performing instrumental examinations:

> It is not justifiable to label dysphagic symptoms, for which no organic etiology can be detected, as psychogenic or psychosomatic. Patients with such symptoms should be studied by means of esophageal manometry and/or pH-metry to reveal the nature of their disorder and to enable adequate therapy (p. 502).

A careful and thorough evaluation must be completed, and may also include psychological assessment when a psychogenic dysphagia is suspected. Okada et al. (2007) studied psychopathology and treatment in children with phagophobia, and they found that an evaluation of premorbid personality was crucial to the prognosis. The diagnosis of psychogenic dysphagia should, to avoid misdiagnosis, be reserved for patients with strong psychological symptoms and/or fear of swallowing. (Jones 2003). A positive dysphagia history consisting of different complaints associated with the moment of swallowing is often found in patients with psychogenic dysphagia. The patients may report the feeling of a lump or pressure

in the throat, fear of choking, and/or the inability to swallow solids. A complete and careful medical history is crucial and should therefore be the first part of the swallowing evaluation (Castell and Donner 1987). Important considerations in the medical history include the patient's symptoms, when they occur, and under what circumstances; the duration of swallowing difficulty; and determination regarding a history of eating disorders, weight loss, and family history of dysphagia. Following the medical history, a physical examination should be performed to rule out any organic causes of the symptoms. A multidisciplinary approach may be required, involving professionals from the fields of neurology, otolaryngology, speech–language pathology, radiology, and gastroenterology. The next step, often indicated for a complete evaluation, is an instrumental assessment of swallowing (i.e., VFSE to evaluate oropharyngeal swallowing, barium swallow/esophogram to assess esophageal function). Esophagoscopy, manometry, pH monitoring, and endoscopy may also be of value. Laboratory tests to rule out disturbances as hypoglycemia or hyperglycemia, systemic infections, or toxins may also be of importance in establishing the diagnosis of psychogenic dysphagia. Another technique discussed by Vaiman et al. (2008) is to use surface electromyography (sEMG) of deglutition to investigate suspected psychogenic dysphagia (Table 2).

5   Treatment of Psychogenic Dysphagia

A multidisciplinary approach including professionals from the fields of psychiatry, psychology, otolaryngology, neurology, speech–language pathology, radiology, and gastroenterology may be required in the treatment of psychogenic dysphagia. A combination of psychological treatment and dysphagia therapy seems to be the most effective treatment of psychogenic dysphagia (Ball and Otto 1994; De Lucas-Taracena and Montanes-Rada 2006). In a case report by Ciyiltepe and Türkbay (2006), a 13-year-old boy suffering from psychogenic dysphagia treated with such an approach is described. A psychological behavior management program has to consist of behavior modification, insight-oriented therapy, and family therapy. The dysphagia therapy sessions should include therapeutic eating trials with

Table 2 Treatment of psychogenic dysphagia

Evaluation of psychogenic dysphagia	Professionals commonly involved
History	
A thorough history is often obtained in a multidisciplinary fashion emphasizing	Otolaryngologist
	Gastroenterologist
Patient complaints	Psychiatrist
Symptoms and when they occur and under what circumstances	Psychologist
Duration of swallowing difficulty	Speech–language pathologist
Determination regarding a history of eating disorders	Radiologist
Weight loss	Laboratory staff
Family history of dysphagia	
Clinical examinations	
Physical examinations may be performed by a multidisciplinary team of professionals including;	
Otolaryngologist	
Speech–language pathologist	
Gastroenterologist	
Psychiatrist	
Psychologist	
Instrumental examinations	
Radiology;	
VFSE	
Hypopharynx esophagus examination (a morpholgic swallowing examination)	
Videomanometry (examination for analysis of quantitative intraluminal pressure changes in the pharynx and the esophagus)	
Gastroenterology;	
pH-metry (24-h pH recording)	
Gastroscopy (assessment of the morphology in the esophagus and stomach	
Surface electromyography	
Different laboratory tests (to eliminate electrolyte disturbances, sideropenic anemia, or iron deficiency)	

various consistencies, as well as oral motor exercise programs. Also relaxation exercises, breathing support, and functional coughing could be of benefit for the patient. In a report by Shapiro et al. (1997), the benefit of behavioral techniques and the use of hypnosis in a single case were discussed. Also, other studies have emphasized the positive effect of behavioral therapy. For example, Nicasso et al. (1981) described behavioral therapy as a beneficial and even life-saving approach for hysterical behavior. The importance of explaining normal swallowing mechanisms, the role of emotions, and the use of a holistic approach was pointed out by Bretan et al. (1996). A relationship of trust between the patient

and the clinician is essential (Finkenbine and Miele 2004). In some cases, family therapy may be of benefit (Oberfield 1981).

To treat patients with psychogenic dysphagia may be a challenge. However, in our swallowing clinic we have also experienced that a combination of psychological treatment and dysphagia therapy may be a successful treatment for some patients with psychogenic dysphagia. We have found that it may be of benefit for patients if the dysphagia therapy sessions involve education regarding normal swallowing physiology combined with breathing exercises. Such training involving the coordination of breathing and swallowing necessary for safe swallowing could help the patient to understand the physiological process of the swallowing and thereby hopefully decrease the fear of swallowing. Therapeutic eating sessions starting with the consistency easiest to swallow may also be of benefit. Close collaboration between the dysphagia clinician and psychologists and psychiatrists is, in our experience, necessary for optimal management.

Pharmalogical treatment with antianxiety medications has been reported to be an effective treatment in some cases of psychogenic dysphagia (McNally 1994). De Lucas-Taracena and Montanes-Rada (2006) found that antipanic drugs (alprazolam, lorazepam, bromazepan, imipramine, clomipramine, fluoxefine, paroxetine) were of proven efficacy, with a remission rate of 58.5%.

Surgical treatment is not appropriate in the management of swallowing disorders of psychogenic origin, although psychogenic dysphagia has been reported to result from surgical intervention. Nicasso et al. (1981) described a 60-year-old man with postoperative hysterical dysphagia following esophagectomy and cervical esophagogastrostomy secondary to esophageal cancer. Postoperatively, the patient complained of globus, although instrumental evaluations revealed the patient was able to swallow safely and adequately.

6   Conclusion

Psychogenic dysphagia is an uncommon swallowing condition, most often characterized by fear of swallowing. On VFSE abnormal oral behaviors such as repeated deviant tongue movements may be present, but the pharyngeal stage swallowing is revealed to be normal. Also, esophageal dysfunction may at times be associated with psychogenic symptoms. To establish a diagnosis of psychogenic dysphagia, a thorough evaluation must be performed. The evaluation should involve careful taking of the medical history, clinical and instrumental examinations, and, if necessary, laboratory tests. The best therapeutic management approach appears to be a combination of a dysphagia therapy and psychological treatment. It has also been reported that patients, in some cases, have benefited from antianxiety medications. For best management of a patient with psychogenic dysphagia, evaluation and treatment should be performed with a multidisciplinary approach

References

Ball SG, Otto MW (1994) Cognitive-behavioral treatment of choking phobia: 3 case studies. Psychother Psychosom 62:207–211

Barofsky I, Fontaine KR (1998) Do psychogenic dysphagia patients have an eating disorder? Dysphagia 13:24–27

Barofsky I, Buchholz D, Edwin D, Jones B, Ravich W (1993) Characteristics of patients who have difficulties initiating swallowing [abstract]. In: Annual meeting of the Dysphagia Research Society, Lake Geneva, September 1993

Bradley PJ, Narula A (1987) Clinical aspects of pseudodysphagia. J Laryngol Otol 101:689–694

Bretan O, Henry MA, Kerr-Correa F (1996) Dysphagia and emotional distress. Arq Gastroenterol 3:60–65

Castell DO, Donner MW (1987) Evaluation of dysphagia: a careful history is crucial. Dysphagia 2:65–71

Ciyiltepe M, Türkbay T (2006) Phagophobia: a case report. Turk J Pediatr 48:80–84

De Lucas-Taracena MT, Montanes-Rada F (2006) Swallowing phobia: symptoms, diagnosis and treatment. Actas Esp Psiquiatr 34:309–316

Escher F (1983) A deglutition stutterer. Contribution on psychogenic inability to swallow. HNO 31:104–106

Finkenbine R, Miele VJ (2004) Globus hystericus: a brief review. Gen Hosp Psychiatry 26:78–82

Jones B (2003) Pharyngoesophageal interrelationship and reflexes involved in airway protection. In: Jones B (ed) Normal and abnormal swallowing: imaging in diagnosis and therapy, 2nd edn. Springer, New York, pp 91–96

Kanner L (1935) Child psychiatry. Thomas, Springfield

Korkina MV, Marilov VV (1995) Variants of psychosomatic personality development in disease of the gastrointestinal tract. Nevropatol Psikhiatr Im S S Korsakova 95:43–47

Kronecker H, Meltzer SJ (1883) Der Schluckmekanismus, seine Erregungen und seine Henimung. Arch Anat Physiol Physiol Abt 7:328–362

Lehtinen V, Puhakka A (1976) A psychosomatic approach to the globus hystericus syndrome. Acta Psychiatr Scand 53:21–28

Leopold NA, Kagel MC (1997) Dysphagia—ingestion or deglutition?: a proposed paradigm. Dysphagia 12:202–206

Malcolmson KG (1966) Radiological findings in globus hystericus. Br J Radiol 39:583–586

McNally RJ (1994) Choking phobia: a review of the literature. Compr Psychiatry 35:83–89

Nicasso PM, Arnold ES, Prager RL, Bryant PR (1981) Behavioral treatment of hysterical dysphagia in a hospital setting. Gen Hosp Psychiatry 3:213–217

Nicholson TR, Stone J, Kanaan RA (2010) Convension disorder: a problematic diagnosis. J Neurol Neurosurg Psychiatry. [Epub ahead of print: 29 Oct] doi:10.1136/jnnp.2008.171306

Oberfield RA (1981) Family therapy with adolescents: treatment of a teenage girl with globus hystericus and weight loss. J Am Acad Child Psychiatry 20:822–833

Okada A, Tsukamoto C, Hosogi M, Yamanaka E, Watanabe K, Ootyou K, Morishima T (2007) A study of psycho-pathology and treatment of children with phagophobia. Acta Med Okayama 61:261–269

Ravich WJ, Wilson RS, Jones B, Donner MW (1989) Psychogenic dysphagia and globus: reevaluation of 23 patients. Dysphagia 4:35–38

Seems S, Wielenska RC, Savoia MG, Bernik M (2009) Choking phobia: full remission following behavior therapy. Rev Bras Psiquiatr 31:257–260

Shapiro J, Franko DL, Gagne A (1997) Phagophobia: a form of psychogenic dysphagia. A new entity. Ann Otol Rhinol Laryngol 106:286–290

Stacher G (1983) Swallowing the psyche. Wien Klin Wochenschr 8:502–511

Stacher G (1986) Differential diagnosis of psychosomatic deglutition disorders. Wien Klin Wochenschr 98: 658–663

Thompson WG, Heaton KW (1982) Heartburn and globus in apparently healthy people. Can Med Assoc J 126:46–48

Vaiman M, Shoval G, Gavriel H (2008) The electrodiagnostic examination of psychogenic swallowing disorders. Eur Arch Otorhinolaryngol 265:663–668

The Clinical and Radiological Approach to Dysphagia

Peter Pokieser and Martina Scharitzer

Contents

Abstract

The intention of this chapter is to introduce a multi-disciplinary diagnostic work-up and, in particular, to present a practical and structured radiological approach. Swallowing disorders are common. U.S. statistics indicate that more than 5 % of the population has swallowing difficulties, and in hospitals up to 50% (Logemann 1995). The swallowing tract crosses many anatomic regions. Liquid and solid foods have to be transported properly from the oral cavity into the pharynx and through the esophagus into the stomach. Thus, a wide variety of diseases may affect deglutition, resulting in a multidisciplinary work-up of dysphagic patients. Videofluoroscopy (VF) of deglutition is the method of choice to investigate the whole swallowing tract in a "one-stop-shopping" fashion. VF can depict patho- logic findings of morphology and function as a basis to decide on a further specialized work-up.

1 Introduction

The intention of this chapter is to introduce a multidisciplinary diagnostic work-up and, in particular, to present a practical and structured radiological approach. Swallowing disorders are common. U.S. statistics indicate that more than 5 % of the population has swallowing difficulties, and in hospitals up to 50 % (Logemann 1995).

The swallowing tract crosses many anatomic regions. Liquid and solid foods have to be transported properly from the oral cavity into the pharynx and through the esophagus into the stomach. Thus, a wide variety of

P. Pokieser (✉) · M. Scharitzer
Department of Radiology, University of Vienna,
Währinger Gürtel 18-20, 1090 Vienna, Austria
e-mail: peter.pokieser@meduniwien.ac.at

O. Ekberg (ed.), *Dysphagia*, Medical Radiology. Diagnostic Imaging, DOI: 10.1007/174_2012_617,
© Springer-Verlag Berlin Heidelberg 2012

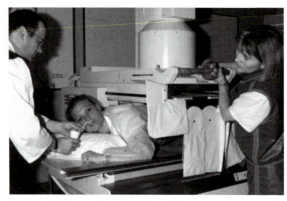

Fig. 1 Prone oblique position: Contrast material is given by a straw. Abnormal structural movements may be diagnosed. Further misdirection or retention of a bolus can be documented. The seven functional units may serve as a basis for the structured radiological report on deglutition

Table 1 Suggested protocol for the evaluation of symptoms

D	Difficulty swallowing?
Y	Yesterday compared with 2 years ago?
S	Solid, liquid or both?
P	Pattern of swallowing events?
H	Heartburn history?
A	Area of symptoms?
G	Gradual or sudden onset?
I	Interventions?
A	Auxiliary clues, such as weight loss?

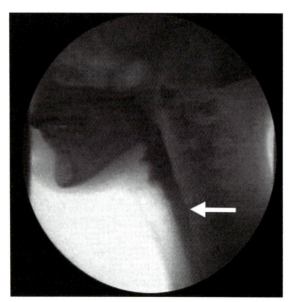

Fig. 2 First standard position. Overview of the lateral oral cavity and pharynx. In this position, the pharynx is shown in the largest possible section of the image in a way that the oral cavity and, in the caudal aspect, also the upper esophageal sphincter is included (*arrow*). The patient is examined in the upright position, either standing or sitting. Usually the patient is turned to the right side, slightly oblique. It is useful to repeat this scene after turning the patient to the left, if stenoses need to be ruled out

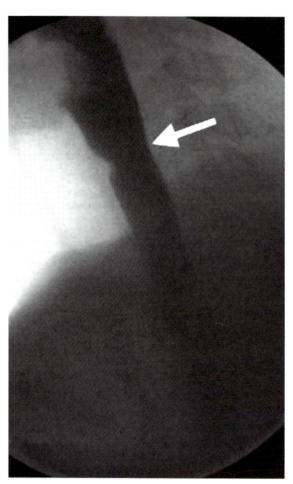

Fig. 3 Second standard position. This setting shows the upper esophageal sphincter in the lateral view, slightly oblique (*arrow*). The upper esophageal sphincter can be evaluated particularly well in this targeted image of the cervicothoracic junction

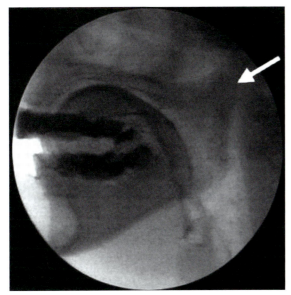

Fig. 4 Third standard position. Sometimes it is useful to view the oral cavity separately. In doing so, the movement of the soft palate during speech can be visualized. However, the pharyngeal phase is largely eliminated in this setting. While speaking, the soft palate rises up to the posterior wall of the nasopharynx, while the patient says "Kathy" (*arrow*)

diseases may affect deglutition, resulting in a multidisciplinary work-up of dysphagic patients. Videofluoroscopy (VF) of deglutition is the method of choice to investigate the whole swallowing tract in a "one-stop-shopping" fashion. VF can depict pathologic findings of morphology and function as a basis to decide on a further specialized work-up.

2   Symptoms of Swallowing Disorders

Establishing medical history is the first step in the investigation of patients with swallowing disorders, in order to individually tailor the examination and to correlate the specific radiological findings with the patient's symptoms. A questionnaire helps structure the patient's history and should include the onset and duration of swallowing disorders, the pattern of swallowing events, the location of symptoms, the consistencies of foods that lead to swallowing difficulties, as well as history of aspiration, regurgitation, coughing, pneumonia and

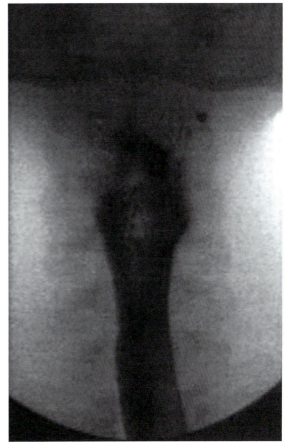

Fig. 5 Fourth standard position. Frontal view of the oral cavity, the pharynx and the cervical esophagus. The symmetry of the passage has to be documented

previous operations affecting the upper gastrointestinal tract and neurological diseases.

For an adequate work-flow of diagnostic tests and therapeutic concepts, the patient's history has to be differentiated into practical categories. With increasing experience with this patient group the investigator may step further into the "art and science of history-taking in the patient with swallowing difficulties" (Table 1) (Hendrix 1993).

For the imaging specialist, the patient's history guides the design of the VF examination and has to be integrated critically into the interpretation of the study. Do the VF findings or other test results explain the patient's symptoms? (Ekberg and Pokieser 1997). When

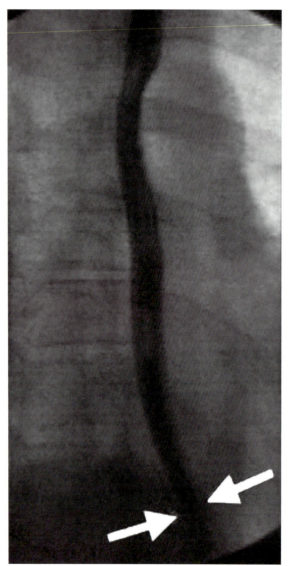

Fig. 6 Fifth standard position. This image shows the middle and lower esophagus in the erect left posterior oblique position. It is useful to repeat this scene in the right posterior oblique position to obtain two different projections of the esophageal phase. Gravity enforces the passage of contrast material in the erect position. With a single act of swallowing, the passage through the lower esophageal sphincter is shown (*arrows*). The patient is asked to swallow just once, to hinder repeated superimpositions of peristaltic waves. Practical advice: about 3 s after the pharyngeal phase in the first or second standard position, you develop the fifth standard position by following the bolus. This can be done when no abnormal findings were visible during the pharyngeal phase; then stop the movement of the central beam, when the esophagogastric junction is visible

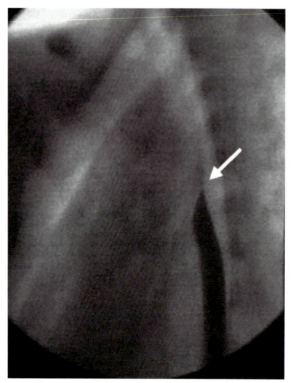

Fig. 7 Sixth standard position. The esophageal passage in prone position allows the peristaltic wave of the esophagus to be visualized. Repeated in the supine position, the esophageal transport is visualised in a different way. Hernias, rings and other findings are often seen in one position only—prone or supine. The cranially V-shaped peristaltic wave (*arrow*) is followed downwards from the top. As advised for the fifth standard position, you may follow the peristaltic wave with the central beam. The central beam should not be moved, during visualization of the dynamic movements of the esophagogastric junction

the patient has referred her problem, questions should focus on the presence of the symptoms or syndromes discussed in more detail in the following sections.

2.1   Dysphagia

Eating and drinking have to be executed without pulmonary compromise and should be for personal and social pleasure, nutrition and hydration. Any subjective feeling of disturbance is called dysphagia (Buchholz 1996).

In oropharyngeal dysphagia, the patient has difficulty swallowing. Isolated oral dysphagia is

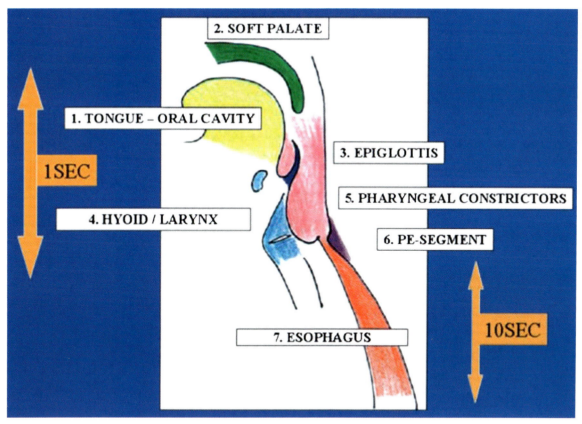

Fig. 8 This graph demonstrates the seven functional units of swallowing. Within 1 s, six of the units complete the pharyngeal stage of swallowing; then the esophagus bridges the long distance through the mediastinum to the stomach. A complete barium swallow of about 15 ml should reach the stomach within 10 s

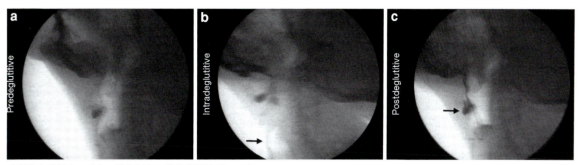

Fig. 9 **a** The oral phase is started by the intake of a beverage or the ingestion of food into the oral cavity. The lips close and seal the oral cavity anteriorly. To form the bolus, the substance is first loaded on the dorsum of the tongue. This process is under voluntary control. In this process, the tongue and soft palate together seal off the posterior part of the oral cavity (*arrows*). **b** When the involuntary act of deglutition is started, the tongue performs a wave-like movement and presses the manipulated bolus along the hard palate backwards into the pharynx. **c** Only the barium coating remains in the oral cavity

uncommon and based on neurogenic disorders or diminished salivary flow. Also, some drugs (anticholinergics, antihistaminics, antidepressants, antihypertensives, and diuretics) affect salivary flow, and neuroleptic drugs may slow or disrupt the oral phase of swallowing.

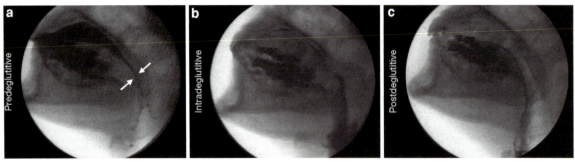

Fig. 10 a This 75-year-old woman with cerebral ischemia cannot control the bolus in the oral cavity. **b** The oral transit is achieved by tilting the head backwards. This causes some blurring and the spatial resolution is reduced. Only minimal amounts of material are transported. Aspiration occurs (*arrow*). **c** Contrast material has pooled in the lower oral cavity beneath the anterior parts of the tongue. Minor aspiration after the swallow (postdeglutitive) has occurred, and there is pooling in the valleculae (*arrow*)

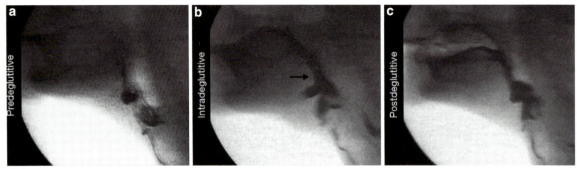

Fig. 11 a An 81-year-old woman suffers from Parkinson's disease. She has already aspirated material from previous swallows. Pooling in the valleculae is present. **b** The tongue fails to reach the hard palate and cannot propel the whole bolus into the oropharynx. Dorsal excursion of the tongue appears to be limited (*arrow*). **c** Barium mixed with mucus remains stuck to the hard palate and the tongue. Retentions in the valleculae have increased

Pharyngeal dysphagia is often described by the patient as a sensation of difficult passage of the bolus through the region of the suprasternal notch, most frequently caused by neuromuscular disorders causing weakness and/or incoordination of the striated muscles used for swallowing (Buchholz 1987). Less frequently, structural narrowings, such as neoplasms, postoperative defects, Zenker's diverticula, or mucosal webs, are found.

In esophageal dysphagia, the material seems to stick along the swallowing tract; the patient may localize the site anywhere from the suprasternal notch to the epigastrium. Usually the patient cannot differentiate between the proximal or distal site of an esophageal lesion (Edwards 1974). For example, a Schatzki ring at the level of the esophagogastric junction or achalasia often produce symptoms above the suprasternal notch. Intermittent esophageal dysphagia for solid food is typical for lower esophageal rings or strictures with a remaining lumen of less than 2 cm. Rapid progress of solid food dysphagia within 3 months is often found in esophageal carcinoma. If there is no sign or proof of aspiration, esophageal dysphagia for fluids only indicates esophageal motor disorders. Depending on the severity of the motility disturbance, the latter can produce solid food dysphagia as well. Regurgitation of previously ingested food can arise during a meal from any cause or location; late regurgitation of undigested food is typical of a Zenker's diverticulum or achalasia. Complaints of sour and/or bitter material with heartburn is pathognomonic for gastroesophageal reflux (GER). Furthermore, gastroesophageal reflux disease (GERD) is the most common cause of "non-cardiac chest pain." After exclusion of a cardiac cause, the esophagus has to be evaluated. A 3-week therapy with

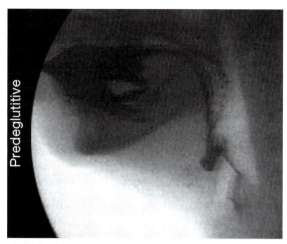

Fig. 12 In this 69-year old patient with cerebral ischemia, the dorsal closure of the oral cavity is disturbed and contrast medium prematurely passes into the pharynx—so-called "leaking"

proton pump inhibitors can be an effective diagnostic and therapeutic approach. Odynophagia means painful swallowing; the pain is described as "sharp," usually indicating ulcerative mucosal lesions of the pharynx or esophagus, whereas a dull or squeezing pain is associated with esophageal spasm.

2.1.1 Globus Sensation

Globus is a common problem, found in about 5 % of general otolaryngologic patients. A "lump in the throat," the sensation of a foreign body, sore throat, frequent throat clearing and fullness, are typical complaints of these patients. Symptoms tend to occur intermittently. Often the symptom improves during eating, while a combination with dysphagia is frequently found. In 75 % of 150 patients with globus as the only symptom, VF could depict pathological functional and/or morphologic findings; evidence of an esophageal motor disorder was present in 47 % of them (Schober et al. 1995). A high incidence of esophageal motility disorders in this setting was detected by manometry in 87 % (Moser et al. 1991). Globus sensation seems to be a symptom of laryngopharyngeal irritation, not specific to GERD, but in which GERD plays a role (Woo et al. 1996). There remains an open discussion about the pathogenesis of globus. However, the term "globus hystericus" should be avoided, and pharyngeal and/or esophageal pathologies should be ruled out according to the

specific history. If patients with chest pain do not show any evidence of cardiac disease, the term "non-cardiac chest pain" is often diagnosed.

2.2 Aspiration

Aspiration is defined as the entry of liquid or food into the airways below the level of the glottis. Choking and/or coughing immediately following a swallow, as well as recurrent pneumonia, is suspect of aspiration. Silent aspiration may occur if the cough reflex is absent or diminished. Persons who aspirate are at increased risk for serious respiratory sequelae, including airway obstruction and aspiration pneumonia. The quantity, the depth of aspiration (trachea or distal airways), and the physical properties of the aspirate influence the effects of aspiration (Palmer et al. 2000). Aspiration can occur anterograde, during or immediately after swallowing, or as retrograde aspiration of gastric or esophageal contents. The radiologist must be aware of patients at risk of aspiration. The tailored VF study avoids severe aspiration during the examination (Jones and Donner 1988).

3 Multidisciplinary Evaluation of Swallowing Disorders

The radiologist should be familiar with the specific techniques of different medical fields when investigating patients with swallowing problems. There is a considerable overlap in using different clinical tests by different clinical fields, with variations from country to country. We try to clarify the clinical interaction more than the borders between clinical specialties.

General patient status includes mental and social function and physical mobility, as well as his/her nutritional and hydration status.

Examination of the chest can reveal problems with the respiratory function related to aspiration or conditions in which aspiration might cause severe problems. The cardiovascular system has to be assessed for possible sources of emboli to the brain; impairment of the musculoskeletal system can affect normal mobility; and the swallowing mechanism can be affected by different systemic diseases, such as scleroderma or muscular diseases.

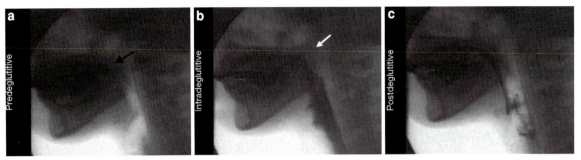

Fig. 13 **a** Before the act of swallowing, the soft palate, in conjunction with the tongue, seals off the oral cavity dorsally (*arrow*). **b** During the pharyngeal phase, the soft palate is raised to a right angle and tightens the oropharynx together with the posterior wall of the pharynx (*arrow*). The latter is called Passavant's cushion at this level, where the pharyngeal wall converges to the soft palate. Thus, food particles are prevented from entering the nasopharynx. One can test the elevation of the soft palate towards the posterior wall of the pharynx by having the patient utter words beginning with a "k", such as "Kathy". **c** After the act of swallowing, the soft palate returns to its original position

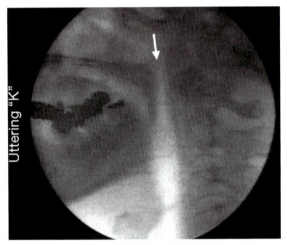

Fig. 14 In this 55-year-old patient with myasthenia, elevation of the soft palate is disturbed. A gap of air remains between the posterior wall of the pharynx and the soft palate (*arrow*) when the patient utters the "k" sound

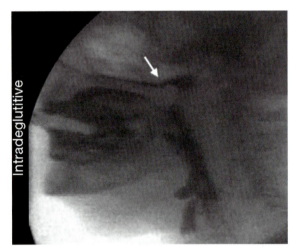

Fig. 15 This 53-year-old woman who had undergone surgery for a carcinoma of the right tonsil has a defect in the dorsal soft palate, that causes regurgitation. During swallowing, spillage of contrast material into the nasopharynx can be observed (*arrow*). Contrast material has penetrated into the larynx. The soft palate is shortened and deformed postoperatively. Aspiration has occurred

The status of otolaryngologists and speech/language pathologists includes a full head and neck examination. The neck should be evaluated for masses, especially for adenopathies, enlarged thyroid, and scars that indicate surgery on structures involved in swallowing. An inspection should be performed of the oral cavity, cranial nerve function, palate, pharynx and larynx, with indirect laryngoscopy or by fiberoptics to assess for tumors, mucosal integrity, vocal cord motion, pooling of secretions into the vallecula or the piriform sinus, as well as sensation and voice (Sonies et al. 1987). Stridor is a sign of upper airway obstruction and may be audible only on auscultation over the trachea; the sounds of swallowing motility and the palpation of the elevation of the hyoid and larynx are part of the dynamic clinical investigation. Fiberoptic endoscopic evaluation of swallowing (FEES) is a well-established diagnostic test and

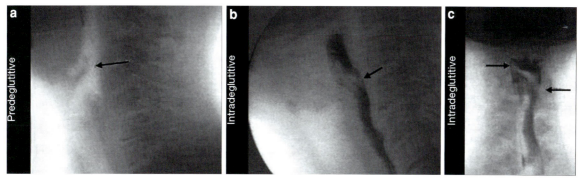

Fig. 16 a The epiglottis is usually seen even without contrast medium, in the lateral view of the pharynx (*arrow*). **b** The epiglottis should tilt below the horizontal plane. The complete tilt can be seen as a small longitudinal structure at the end of the bolus passage (*arrow*). **c** Even healthy individuals with a good swallowing function occasionally reveal asymmetrical tilting of the epiglottis. In frontal views, one side tilts more deeply than the other (*arrows*). Unilateral muscular weakness can cause the same finding but is often combined with abnormal radiological findings or other clinical signs of swallowing impairment

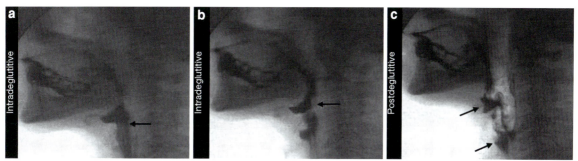

Fig. 17 a, and, **b** Incomplete epiglottic tilt (*arrow*). **c** This is combined with retention in the valleculae and piriform sinuses (*arrows*)

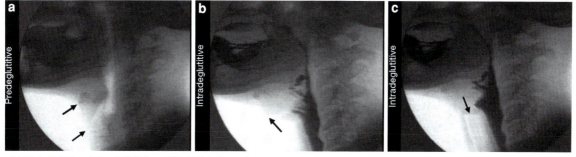

Fig. 18 a The hyoid bone and the air column in the lateral projection. The hyoid is visible as a bony structure, while the larynx is represented by an air column (*arrows*). **b** To protect the respiratory tract, the hyoid and larynx move cranially and ventrally at the beginning of the involuntary act of swallowing (*arrow*). The elevation of the larynx is visible fluoroscopically. It has to be emphasized that the pharyngeal muscles are elevating simultaneously, almost invisible for VF. **c** The opening of the larynx is tightly closed during the movement of the larynx, and the air column of the trachea is visible up to the horizontal end at the level of the vocal cord (*arrow*). During elevation, the hyoid and larynx come closer to each other. The upward movement of the larynx can be measured as an approximation. It varies widely and individually and with the volume of the bolus. If the elevation is less than 1 cm it can be described as abnormal. The height of a cervical vertebral body represents another approximation to estimate the minimum of laryngeal elevation

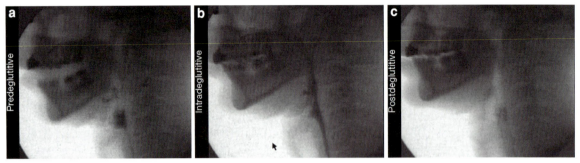

Fig. 19 **a** In this 45-year-old man who underwent resection of a tumor of the pharynx, retentions of contrast material in the hypopharynx from previous swallows are present. **b** The larynx rises very slightly, less than 1 cm and not even 50 % of the height of a cervical vertebral body (*arrow*). **c** After the swallow, some drops of contrast material have entered the larynx

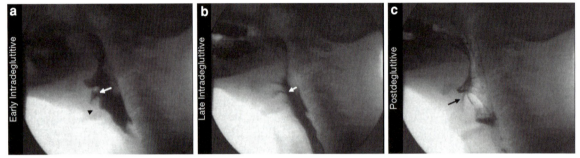

Fig. 20 **a** A 65-year-old man after a mild stroke. The opening of the larynx closes too late or in an incomplete manner. In this case, contrast medium enters the subepiglottic space (*arrow*). It may penetrate deeper into the supra-glottic space (*arrowhead*). **b** When this relatively mild disorder of closure is present, most of the material that enters is pressed back into the pharynx from the larynx (*arrow*). **c** Postdeglutitively, only the subepiglottic space is marked (*arrow*)

enables assessment of nasal, velopharyngeal, and laryngeal pathology of morphologic and functional changes as well. The flexible, light-weight instruments are inserted through the nose. Video documentation can be integrated. FEES is complementary to VF and the application and interpretation of results is the interdisciplinary task of otolaryngologists, speech/language pathologists and radiologists. FEES does not show the entire motion of essential foodway structures and the bolus during swallowing, but can identify aspiration and pharyngeal retentions. Firstly, results of FEES and VF are "diagnostic studies." Secondly, they allow the clinician to design an appropriate diet and compensatory maneuvers designed to improve pharyngeal clearance and reduce aspiration. This use of VF and FEES is called "therapeutic studies" it includes investigations that test the effectiveness of therapy.

FEES is also used by neurologists. However, the neurologic examination is a crucial part of the multidisciplinary approach to dysphagic patients. Cerebrovascular disease, Parkinson's disease, multiple sclerosis, amyotrophic lateral sclerosis, poliomyelitis, myasthenia gravis and dementia are examples of the wide spectrum of neurological disorders that may involve deglutition.

Invasive treatment of the upper esophageal sphincter (UES) is performed by otolaryngologists as well as general surgeons, and is frequently used as therapy for Zenker's diverticulum. Different surgical strategies are under continuous discussion. Myotomy of the UES with or without resection of the diverticulum itself, and myotomy with laser or with an endoscopic approach are applied to restore an adequate opening of the pharyngoesophageal segment.

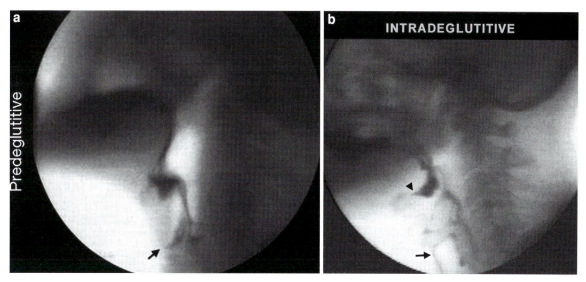

Fig. 21 **a** This 62-year-old man who had a stroke clearly aspirates before the involuntary act of swallowing, as the swallowing act begins too late and contrast medium has entered the larynx long before the initiation of swallowing (*arrow*).

b Mild aspiration of some drops of water-soluble contrast medium is visible (*arrow*). There is an incomplete epiglottic tilt and retentions in the valleculae (*arrowhead*)

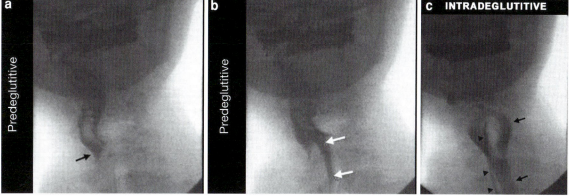

Fig. 22 **a** Frontal view of a 64-year-old man with fracture of the skull base and cerebral hemorrhage shows premature leakage and pooling of contrast material in the right piriform sinus (*arrow*). **b** Barium enters the larynx and the trachea before the involuntary swallow (*arrows*). **c** Intradeglutitive pharyngeal propulsion in the frontal projection when the patient tries to clear the retentions with repeated swallows (*arrows*). Less than 10 % of the bolus was aspirated before the involuntary swallow (*arrowhead*)

Gastroenterologists and surgeons are specialists in the diagnosis and treatment of esophageal disease. Endoscopy reveals even subtle mucosal details and can take biopsies for pathologic diagnosis. But endoscopy may overlook subtle rings or stenoses, that can be passed by the endoscope, but will hinder larger boluses of solid food. Furthermore, endoscopy cannot display the topographic relation of stenoses to the important anatomic landmarks in all cases and often cannot be forwarded distal to a narrow stenosis. VF is helpful in such instances, providing excellent topographic overviews, testing for subtle stenoses with solid bolus, and examining the esophagus distal to stenoses. Benign and malignant macromorphological changes of the esophageal tube are detected by endoscopy and VF (Scharitzer et al. 2002). In esophageal motility disorders, VF can detect a delayed

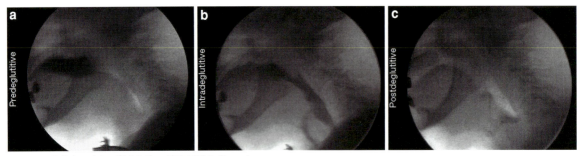

Fig. 23 a This 77-year-old woman after laser resection of a laryngeal carcinoma, presents with a competent seal of the oral cavity dorsally before swallowing. **b** The postoperative defect causes insufficient closure of the larynx and more than 10 % of the swallowed contrast medium is aspirated during the pharyngeal phase. **c** The aspirated contrast medium has reached the bronchial tree. Thus, after the swallow, only small amounts are visible in the trachea

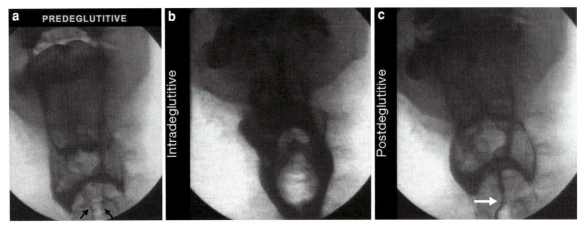

Fig. 24 a A 55-year-old man after a stroke, in frontal projection. Pharyngeal retentions in the valleculae and piriform sinuses are present. There is an intense coating of the pharyngeal walls. Aspiration from previous swallows is present (*arrows*). **b** Reduced movements of the lateral pharyngeal walls cannot propel the whole volume of 15 ml through the pharyngeal tube. **c** After swallowing, aspiration occurs (*arrow*), caused by retentions in the piriform sinuses. The retentions have caused an overflow at the laryngeal entrance, which has opened and moved caudally in the resting phase

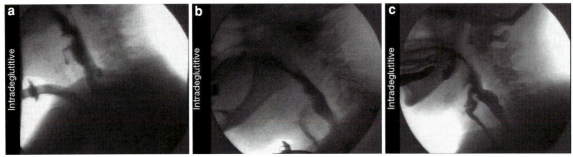

Fig. 25 a First, a slight grade I aspiration. This means that a few drops of contrast medium are aspirated. **b** Second, a moderate intradeglutitive aspiration, grade II. As far as can be seen, no more than 10 % of the bolus has been aspirated. **c** Third, a massive grade III aspiration with an aspirated volume of far more than 10 % of the ingested bolus

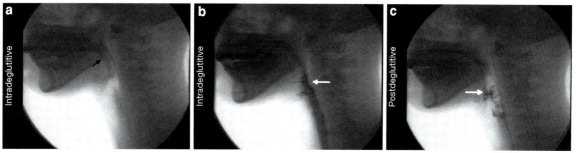

Fig. 26 a The right time point at which the pharyngeal contraction begins is very important for a physiological swallowing act. If the contrast medium has passed the angle of the jaw or has reached the valleculae, the involuntary act of swallowing should begin (*arrow*). **b** In the lateral view, the onset of pharyngeal wave of contraction can be seen as an indentation (*arrow*), that descends rapidly during the propulsion of the bolus. **c** After the passage, there should only be a coat of contrast medium in the valleculae and the sinus (*arrow*), but no residues with fluid levels

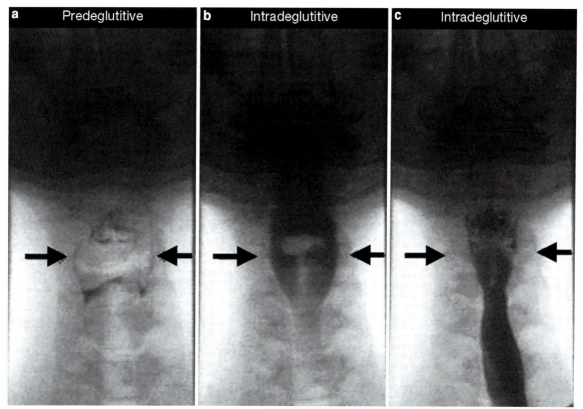

Fig. 27 a In the frontal view, the pharyngeal walls are delineated lateral convex without retentions in the piriform sinuses (*arrows*). **b** The lateral pharyngeal walls should move rapidly towards medial, with a symmetrical movement (*arrows*). **c** In the late intradeglutitive phase, the bolus is squeezed out of the pharynx (*arrows*)

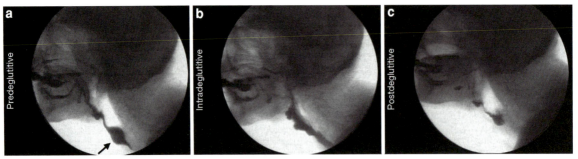

Fig. 28 **a** This 86-year-old man after a stroke has markedly delayed triggering. After the contrast medium enters the pharynx, the piriform sinuses (*arrow*) are filled before the involuntary act of swallowing begins. **b** Intradeglutitive phase of the same patient. **c** Retentions in the valleculae and in the hypopharynx after the swallow indicate pharyngeal weakness; no aspiration occurred

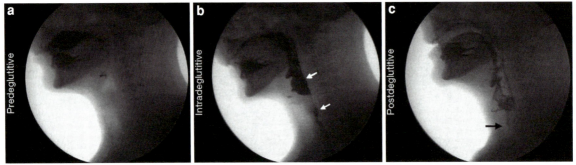

Fig. 29 **a** This 66-year-old woman with dermatomyositis has a high-grade pharyngeal weakness. Before the swallow, the bolus is controlled on the back of the tongue. **b** In the late intradeglutitive phase, a bolus of 15 ml is separated in two parts (*arrows*). The weak stripping wave is not able to propel the whole bolus into the esophagus, often also combined with a weak tongue movement. Meanwhile, a part of the bolus has entered the cervical esophagus. Drops of contrast medium have penetrated into the laryngeal vestibule. **c** Also note the aspiration from retentions after the involuntary swallow—postdeglutitive aspiration (*arrow*)

transport for liquids and solid food as well, complementary to manometry—the gold standard for diagnosing esophageal motility disorders. Manometry can be combined with VF as videomanometry. This method synchronizes the videofluoroscopic record of the bolus transport and the measurement of pressure. Evaluation of esophageal transport and gastric emptying is obtained by scintigraphy. Delayed gastric emptying, well known in diabetes, may interfere with esophageal transport and contribute to symptoms such as dyspepsia, epigastric fullness, or heartburn. pH probe studies can detect pathologic gastroesophageal reflux, while VF can describe the dynamic appearance of the esophagogastric junction during and after passage of a bolus. Intraluminal impedance monitoring is a relatively new technique offering the possibility of measuring bolus movement in the esophagus without radiation. Combined with manometry or pH, pressure changes and bolus transit as well as detection of all types of reflux episodes independent of the pH, can be evaluated. Therefore, these investigations offer additional new methods for patients with persisting GERD symptoms after acid suppressive therapy or with non-acid reflux. Comparisons of impedance and VF have shown almost identical volume clearance of the swallowed contrast media (Simren et al. 2003). Impedance measurements are also used for a new technique called "impedance planimetry," which measures cross-sectional areas in the esophagus in order to gradate esophageal stenosis. Hiatus hernia, cardiac insufficiency, the esophagogastric junction after surgery, such as fundoplication, myotomy, dilatation, gastric banding, and other operations, are studied

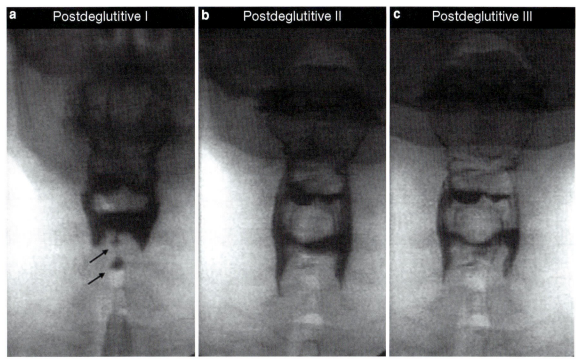

Fig. 30 **a** Same patient as in (Fig. 29) in the frontal projection. Symmetric retentions in the piriform sinuses are present, a fluid level at the laryngeal entrance indicates the potential of postdeglutitive aspiration, and contrast material has already entered the larynx (*arrows*). **b** Smaller retentions after a second swallow, which was performed by the patient to clear the hypopharynx from retention. **c** A third swallow succeeded, only slight retention remained, and no more material had penetrated into the larynx

videofluoroscopically to rule out early and late postoperative complications such as stenosis, leakage, or perforation. VF is the diagnostic test of choice to obtain a general overview of the whole swallowing tract, to detect macropathologic changes and disordered function as well. Pertinent to the clinical problem, a tailored VF examination can be designed to be the basis for other diagnostic tests or to complete their results in a complementary way.

4   Imaging of Swallowing Disorders

4.1   Technical Considerations

Videofluoroscopy is performed with a fluoroscopy unit connected to a video recorder. This dynamic examination studies motility of the oral, pharyngeal and esophageal phases, whereas the spot film examinations demonstrate morphology. Any fluoroscopic unit that offers remote control equipment is appropriate. By using the jog-wheel function, the videofluoroscopic study can be analyzed frame by frame, several times. Computer-based dynamic recording on hard disk, DVD, or CD is still under development and offers have to be evaluated carefully in case of interest. Continuously recording for 20 s seems to be the minimum, while inexpensive and easy storage of the examinations is mandatory.

The introduction of digital fluoroscopy and computer-based workstations offers a higher spatial resolution and new possibilities for the interpretation by lower radiation exposure at the same time. Digital images obtained during a dynamic study can be postprocessed and transmitted more easily.

4.2   Examination Technique

The approach as described by Ekberg and Pokieser (1997) is based on the patient's history, planning the investigation in detail. The radiographic examination

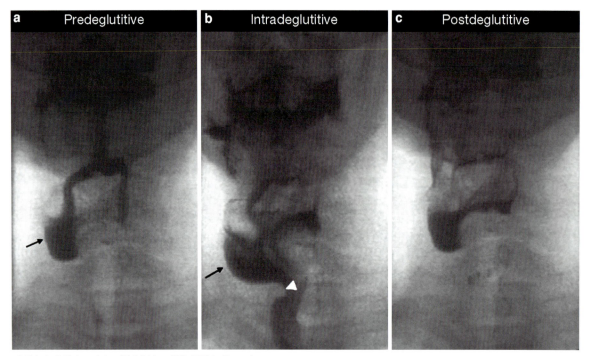

Fig. 31 **a** Ten years before the examination, this 62-year-old woman was operated on and underwent radiation on the right side for a floor-of-the-mouth carcinoma. Delayed triggering of the swallowing reflex is present. Contrast material runs over the valleculae into the discrete dilated right piriform sinus (*arrow*). **b** During swallowing, the bolus passes over the right side, causing the weak lateral pharyngeal wall to bulge (*arrow*) Ipsilateral, the pharyngoesophageal sphincter is visible as a lateral cricopharyngeal bar (*arrowhead*). **c** After swallowing, one sees the asymmetric or unilateral retention on the right—on the operated side

has to include all structures involved in swallowing, from the lips to the stomach. Nevertheless, it is important to focus the examination on specific areas. In any patient with a high suspicion of laryngeal or pharyngeal disease, the laryngeal vestibule should be included in the image from the beginning. It is very common that the first swallow is the worst swallow and that only the first swallow will reveal dysfunction.

It is certainly very important to realize that there are two fundamentally different examinations of swallow. One is customized for the diagnosis, i.e., the search for why the patient has a specific symptom (diagnostic study). It is basically concerned with finding that particular patient's worst swallow and therefore might include maneuvers for decompensation of a compensated swallow (Buchholz et al. 1985). This is in contrast to the diagnostic examination that is done when the dysfunction in a specific patient has been revealed; this test basically tries to reveal the patient's best swallow and therefore always includes maneuvers for compensation of a decompensated swallow (therapeutic study).

It is always important to observe as many swallows as possible, as dysfunction may be intermittent. Moreover, the benefits of therapeutic maneuvers are notoriously difficult to assess. The performance of dynamic studies turns the investigator from a photographer into both a film director and camera operator. Since FEES has gained raising availability and importance in the assessment of aspiration and the value of swallowing maneuvers, indications for a therapeutic videofluoroscopic swallow have decreased. In patients with suspicion of aspiration, FEES is increasingly the primary investigation method, and a radiological diagnosis of aspiration is mainly needed in the absence of videoendoscopic assessment.

No special preparation is needed for the radiological examination of the upper gastrointestinal tract. The patient is examined with his dentures or other oral appliances in place so that the patient's swallow is as normal as possible. Nasogastric feeding tubes should be removed prior to the investigation, but due to the discomfort during reinsertion of tubes, this has to be

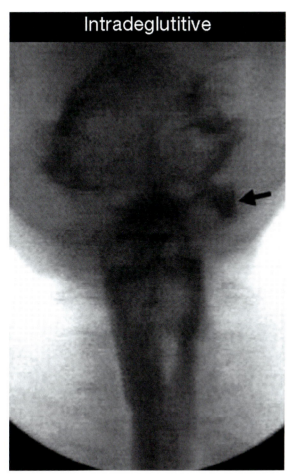

Fig. 32 A small pharyngocele on the left side, in an asymptomatic patient. On the left side, the pharyngocele has evaginated (*arrow*)

decided with regard to the clinical problem. The patient should stand or sit on the footboard of the fluoroscopic table. Esophageal motility can be depicted best in the horizontal position, when the contrast material is pushed mainly by esophageal motility (Fig. 1).

Debilitated patients can be examined on a specially designed chair. Patients should not experience stress during swallowing, and the investigator has to take care to provide a quiet, comfortable environment during the study.

4.2.1 The Seven Functional Units

The systematic analysis procedure known from X-ray reporting proved to be useful for reporting film sequences as well.

The radiological substrate of this analysis is the movements of anatomical structures that cause the formation and continuous propulsion of the bolus of contrast medium. Physiologically, the act of swallowing is divided into three phases: the oral, the pharyngeal and the esophageal phase. The duration of the oral phase may be determined arbitrarily. The pharyngeal phase takes less than 1 s. The esophageal phase takes approximately 10 s.

The esophageal phase is about 10 times as long as the pharyngeal phase.

For radiographic analysis of the act of swallowing, it is useful to summarize the involved anatomical structures into seven functional units (Pokieser et al. 1995).

The description of normal and pathological functional findings of the seven functional units of the act of deglutition is a simplification of the subject, but does include the most important clinical findings needed by those embarking on routine diagnosis of the act of swallowing (Fig. 1).

4.2.2 Design of Videofluoroscopic Scripts

A standard examination of these seven functional units is performed by lining up various film sequences of the video recording of the act of swallowing and fluoroscopy. During the pharyngeal phase of swallowing, the functional units should be filmed in a stationary position, as the recording will be blurred and rendered unusable for study if the central beam is moved. During the esophageal phase, the central beam may follow the bolus, because the esophageal propulsion is relatively slow (~ 4 cm/s).

4.2.2.1 Swallowing Disorders without Suspicion of Aspiration

Patients suffering from dysphagia, globus, chest pain, or other clinical conditions related to swallowing may have no clinical symptoms of aspiration. These patients should swallow boluses of normal size and should be investigated in all standard positions as mentioned below. The examination begins with films of the erect standard positions, followed by tests of esophageal motility in the horizontal, supine and prone positions. Plain films in double-contrast technique should be added, according to the clinical problem. Effervescent powder disturbs the standardized examination of the esophageal tube and should be given after studying the esophageal motility in the horizontal position. The passage of contrast material should be followed to the duodenojejunal junction.

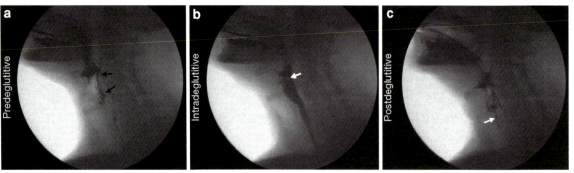

Fig. 33 **a** This 63-year-old man has pronounced ventral spond-ylophytes that narrow the pharynx at the level of the laryngeal entrance (*arrows*). **b** During the swallow, the epiglottic tilt is hindered (*arrow*). **c** After swallowing, some drops were aspirated from moderate retentions (*arrow*)

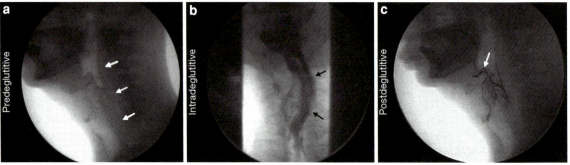

Fig. 34 **a** A further example of a pharyngeal space-occupying mass—here we see a recurring tumor of the hypopharynx in a 48-year-old man. The first photo shows broadening of the dorsal pharyngeal soft tissues in a lateral view (*arrows*). **b** In the frontal view, we see the tumor as a structure with irregular margins, in the right portion of the hypopharynx. The passage of the bolus is directed over the left side (*arrows*). **c** Retentions in the pharynx and a moderate postdeglutitive aspiration are present in lateral projection. The epiglottis is thickened (*arrow*) by tumor infiltration. The same appearance of a swollen epiglottis is found in epiglottitis, for example, postradiation in adults or of infectious origin in children

4.2.2.2 Swallowing Disorders with Suspicion of Aspiration

The investigation is restricted to erect standard projections, if aspiration occurs. With increasing amounts of contrast material, severe aspiration can be avoided by stopping any increase when the patient aspirates. Different consistencies are applied in diagnostic studies pertinent to the symptom, and in therapeutic studies to find out the best consistency without aspirating. This is best done in collaboration with a speech and language pathologist, who has complementary clinical information and interest in the therapeutic approach.

From a systematic point of view, every film scene may be defined by three characteristics: First, the selected section for imaging and the patient's *standard position*; second, the selected *type of contrast medium*; and third, the *amount* of contrast medium.

4.2.3 Standard Positions for Videofluoroscopy

Refer Figs. 2, 3, 4, 5, 6, 7.

4.2.4 Type of Contrast Medium

We use high-density barium suspension to visualize the morphology and function from the oral cavity to the esophagus.

Non-ionic iodinated low-osmolar or iso-osmolar water-soluble contrast material is necessary for patients with clinical suspicion of aspiration or perforation. Hyperosmolar iodinated contrast medium is contraindicated in patients with suspicion of

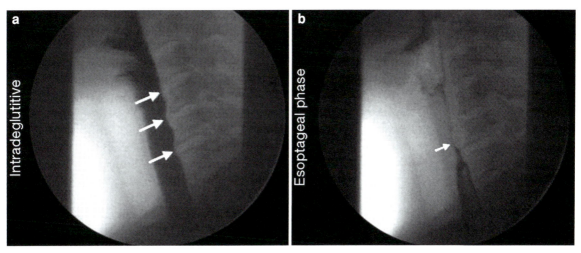

Fig. 35 a When the contrast bolus reaches the level of the PE segment, the dorsal pharyngeal wall should have smooth margins because the sphincter relaxes. A slight wave-like margin is normal–it is caused by the intervertebral disks (*arrows*). **b** After the passage of a normal-sized bolus, no residuals should be left in the pharynx, only coating of the pharyngeal and pharyngoesophageal wall is seen. Radiographically, a posterior indentation at the pharyngoesophageal junction during bolus passage indicates the level of the cricopharyngeal muscle, but may be seen also when the PE segment is closed (*arrow*)

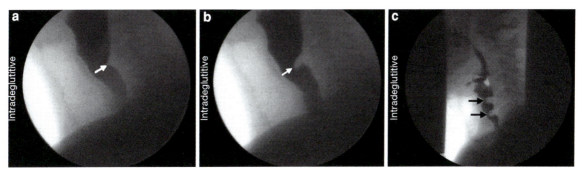

Fig. 36 a A 45-year-old woman with globus sensation and mild reflux disease for 3 years. The functional appearance of the sphincter is abnormal. There is a dorsal, rounded impression of the column of contrast medium at the level of the PE segment, representing a moderate cricopharyngeal bar with a narrowing of 30 % (*arrow*). **b** A 63-year-old man with dysphagia. Marked dysfunction of the PE segment, a cricopharyngeal bar shows 60 % narrowing. **c** Extreme incomplete opening. We find two indentations (*arrow*) in terms of a double sphincter, which can be found in various neuromuscular disorders. This 78-year-old woman suffers from muscular dystrophy

aspiration. In addition, solids are indicated to show a stricture, a solid-induced spasm or dysphagia, as well as for postoperative control studies. Therefore, a piece of bread with barium or placebo tablets with a 14 mm diameter can help in the evaluation of solid-induced abnormalities. The use of different consistencies is extremely helpful in patients with aspiration of only liquid boluses in order to assess the further therapeutic and dietetic management.

4.2.5 Amount of Contrast Medium

The normal amount of a single swallow of an adult patient is about 15 ml. However, a healthy adult can manage liquid boluses up to 50 ml and more. The amount of contrast material should be varied according to the individual capabilities. The examination includes up to 10 swallows of 15–30 ml of liquid barium sulfate. In the beginning, the amount of contrast media is 15 ml. In cases of suspected

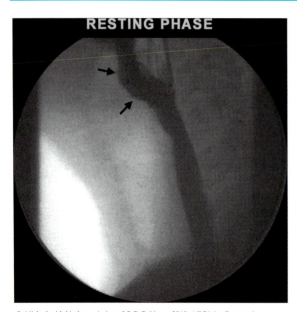

RESTING PHASE

Fig. 37 In this 55-year-old woman with mixed connective tissue disease, the PE segment remains open during all three phases of swallowing. In addition, one always finds a weakness of the pharynx and retentions (*arrows*) in such patients

aspiration, it is reduced to 3 ml for the first swallow. If this bolus volume is tolerated, the bolus size should be increased to 5 ml, and then up to 15 ml.

The contrast medium can be applied in many different ways, according to the abilities of the patient. Cups, drinking bottles, spoons or straws may suite. The best way to administer contrast material orally can be designed according to the feeding history and clinical presentation of the patient.

4.3 Reporting on the Seven Functional Units of Swallowing

The basic principles of the functional physiology and pathology of swallowing constitute the actual radiological basis for reporting VF.

The seven functional units are a radiological approach based on the dynamic radiological information (Fig. 8).

Often, there are several functional disorders of the same functional unit in a single patient. Countless combinations of findings occur, but typical "patterns of findings" are to be observed. Step by step, the

seven units may be analyzed for malfunction. The movements of the visible anatomical structures are the basis of the analysis, the passage of the bolus displays, and whether the function of the swallowing tract is adequate for the given amount and material. Each unit represents an area where the investigator can focus the analysis easily. Videofluoroscopy shows just a part of the complex structures below the barium coating. The strength of the method is the ability to see the entire swallowing action with its effect on bolus transport simultaneously.

4.3.1 Tongue—Oral Cavity

4.3.1.1 Normal Function of the Tongue
Incompetent Bolus Manipulation. An incompetence in manipulating the bolus summarizes many different dynamic findings (Fig. 9). The inability of the tongue to hold the bolus on its upper surface, fragmentation of the bolus, and uncoordinated movements such as tremor or undulations may be visible. When lip closure is insufficient and material runs out over the lips, this is called "drooling." (Fig. 10).

Weakness of the Tongue. Weakness of the tongue is often combined with pharyngeal weakness; retention in the valleculae can be caused by both, and overlaps cannot be differentiated (Fig. 11).

When weakness of the tongue is present, a high consistency of the contrast material proves to be more sensitive, such as barium paste or bread with barium. Water-soluble contrast material can be propelled more easily, thus masking a weakness of the tongue.

Incompetent Tongue-Palate Seal. Incompetence of the apposition of the soft palate, and the tongue leads to leakage of the bolus into the oropharynx (Fig. 12). Weakness or postoperative defects of the tongue, the soft palate or both, can cause this functional deficit. The differentiation between leakage and late triggering of the involuntary swallow can be difficult, when the oral transit time is short. This might be the case when the patient reclines the head to compensate for difficulties in oral transport.

4.3.2 Soft Palate

4.3.2.1 Normal Function of the Soft Palate

(a) Incomplete Elevation (Figs. 13, 14).
(b) Insufficient Velopharyngeal Closure (Fig. 15).

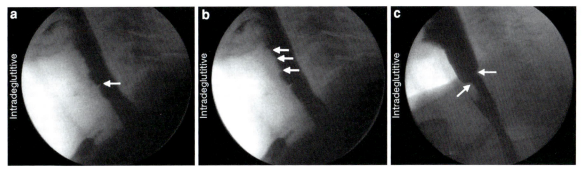

Fig. 38 **a** This 38-year-old man suffers from a globus sensation. A small web located ventrally in the lower PE segment (*arrow*) is only visible for parts of a second. The small membrane flap will hardly hinder the passage, yet is an indirect indication of other accompanying functional disorders. **b** Typical venous plexus at the postcricoid level. This normal dynamic appearance of an inconstant irregularity must not be misdiagnosed as a web (*arrows*). Webs are always thin and sharply delineated. This differentiates them from the retrocricoid venous plexus, which shows normal, movable, round mucosal folds. **c** This 81-year-old man with dysphagia for solids has a circular web with a marked jet phenomenon. The obstruction by a web may accelerate the flow after the narrowing. This functional finding is known as the "jet phenomenon"

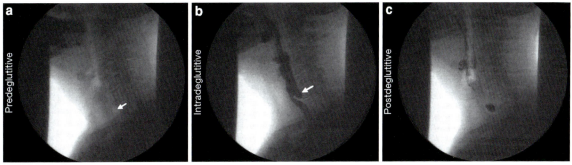

Fig. 39 **a** A 77-year-old woman with high-grade dysphagia for solid and liquid foods. Here we see a constant Zenker's diverticulum, a little more than 2 cm in size. Even without contrast medium, it can be detected by a small air bubble in the dorsal soft tissues of the pharynx (*arrow*). **b** Despite its small size of 12 mm, this diverticulum (*arrow*) causes a compression of the gastrointestinal pathway and hinders the bolus passage. **c** After swallowing, a constant 12 mm diverticulum is left

4.3.3 Epiglottis

4.3.3.1 Normal Function of the Epiglottis

Incomplete Epiglottic Tilt. An incomplete epiglottic tilt is almost always combined with retentions in the valleculae, and often with hypopharyngeal retentions and numerous other disturbances of the pharyngeal phase (Fig. 16). Tumors, swelling after radiation, or inflammatory diseases such as epiglottitis, and postoperative structural deficits up to total resection should be considered (Fig. 17).

4.3.4 Hyoid and Larynx

4.3.4.1 Normal Function of the Hyoid and the Larynx

Poor Elevation. Tracheostomy, pharyngeal or laryngeal resections, radiation therapy or muscular weakness are common causes of poor movements of the epiglottis and the larynx (Fig. 18). Over time, this condition contributes to pharyngeal retention and aspiration (Fig. 19).

The next four functional disorders are related to insufficient protection of the respiratory tract, namely,

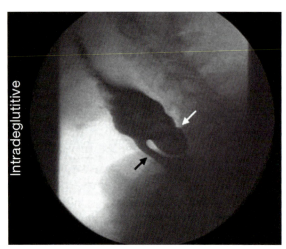

Intradeglutitive

Fig. 40 This 73-year-old woman with massive dysphagia has a Zenker's diverticulum approximately 4 cm in size, seen on lateral view. Very large Zenker's diverticula are usually visualized as obstructions of passage even on ordinary static images. On dynamic images, we see here an incorrect esophageal pathway—displayed by the characteristic ridge between the diverticulum and the esophagus. The point of entry into the diverticulum (*white arrow*) is markedly wider than the esophageal pathway (*black arrow*). Besides, the latter is compressed by filling of the diverticulum

penetration of contrast medium into the larynx and the three basic forms of aspiration into the trachea: pre-deglutitive, intra-deglutitive and post-deglutitive aspiration.

Penetration. After penetration, we will look at the basic forms of aspiration. The terms pre-, intra- and post-deglutitive refer to the involuntary act of swallowing, and the rapid, automatic motion of the larynx, hyoid and pharynx. Thus, aspiration may occur before, during or after the rapid swallowing movement (Fig. 20).

Pre-deglutitive Aspiration. The first type of aspiration occurs during preparation of the swallow and leads to an entry of bolus into the airway before triggering the pharyngeal phase of swallowing (Figs. 21, 22).

Intra-deglutitive Aspiration. The second important timing of aspiration is intra-deglutitive aspiration, which occurs during the rapid involuntary act of swallowing (Fig. 23).

Post-deglutitive Aspiration. The third basic form of aspiration is post-deglutitive aspiration after the involuntary act of swallowing. This form of aspiration occurs during incomplete swallowing, which causes retention in the pharynx (Fig. 24). Frequently, it is due to weak pharyngeal muscles.

Severity of Aspiration. An important aspect of the evaluation of aspiration is its severity. Video cinematography can be quite valuable here. However, it should be mentioned that any decision with regard to prognosis and therapy can only be made by taking all clinical data into account.

The simple gradation described in Fig. 25 is helpful for reporting the severity of aspiration. Several examples of intra-deglutitive aspiration of various grades of severity are also given in Fig. 25.

When the coughing attack has subsided or is entirely absent, it always signifies a high grade of aspiration and a great likelihood of broncho-pulmonary complications.

At the end of the examination, the bronchial tree should be documented with chest films or fluoroscopy. This facilitates an estimate of the depth of aspiration and the amount of aspirated material.

4.3.5 Pharyngeal Constrictors

Normal Function. The fifth functional unit includes the activity of the pharyngeal constrictors.

The pharyngeal wave of contraction starts at the level of C1 in lateral projection (Fig. 26). Here it has advanced up to C2–C3. The rapid upward movements of the hyoid and larynx also take place at the beginning of the involuntary act of swallowing. As the voluntary act smoothly passes into the involuntary one, the physiological beginning may be difficult to determine. In the normal act of swallowing, there should always be a rapid and continuous passage through the pharynx as soon as the angle of the jaw has been passed or the valleculae have been reached (Fig. 27).

Delayed Swallowing Reflex. Delayed triggering of the involuntary act of swallowing is an important and common finding (Fig. 28). Delay occurs when the contrast medium has reached the level of the valleculae before the involuntary act of swallowing is triggered. Pre-deglutitive aspiration may be present, when the closure of the laryngeal vestibule is also delayed. Several swallows can show a different length of the delay. Often, the delay is worst in the first swallow and may improve during the examination. An approximated simple measurement can be obtained with the time code of the video recorder or software, by counting the frames from the moment the contrast material passes the angle of the jaw until involuntary swallowing has begun. It is clinically useful to count in steps of 0.5 s. Delays from 0.5 s up to 3 s are frequent in neuromuscular disorders. The swallowing reflex is absent if the reflex does not trigger for 30 s.

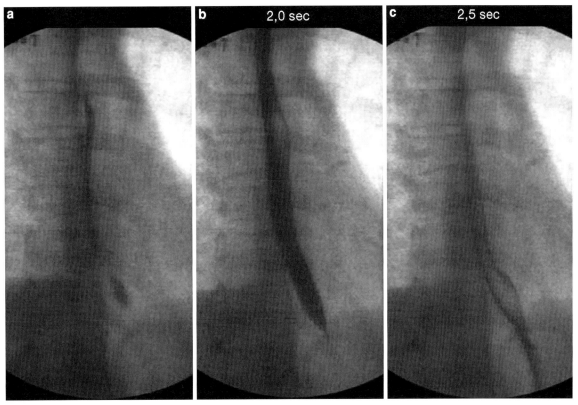

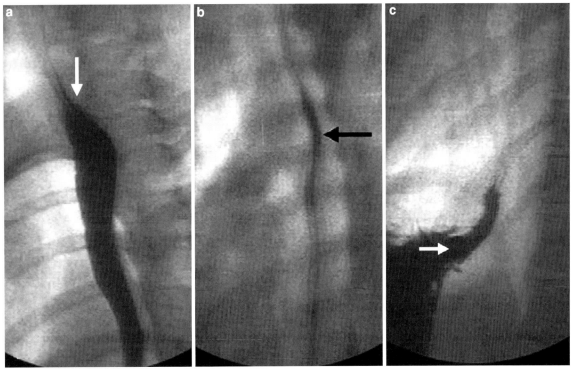

◀ **Fig. 41** **a** Left oblique projection of the lower esophagus before the esophageal phase. **b** At 2 s after initiation of the pharyngeal swallow. Here it is important to observe the timely, rapid emptying that occurs; 10 ml of barium should be able to pass immediately. The esophageal passage in the standing position takes place much faster than that in the horizontal position, because of gravity. **c** At 2.5 s later, the bolus has passed. This is normal when the bolus passes slowly through the esophagogastric junction. However, "10 ml barium—10 s" is a basic approximation of normal esophageal transport, in the erect and horizontal position (Schima et al. 1992). If the bolus takes between 5 and 10 s, a fluid level occurs for this short time span as a normal finding

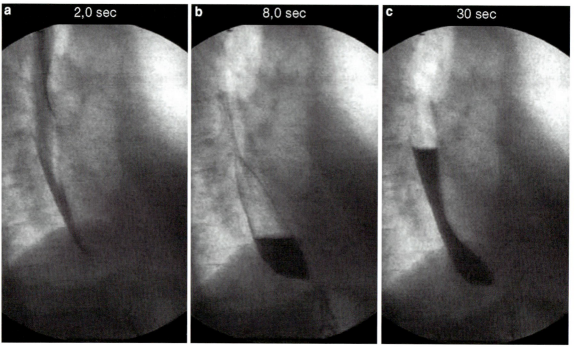

Fig. 43 **a** This 65-year-old woman suffers from achalasia of the lower esophageal sphincter. At 2 s after the pharyngeal phase, parts of the bolus reach the esophagogastric junction. **b** At 8 s after onset of swallowing, a little fluid level remains above the esophagogastric junction (EGJ). **c** The passage of 10 ml of barium takes more than 40 s in this case. The persistent fluid level in the distal esophagus, which is characteristically seen with the patient in standing position, moves up and down without completing the passage. This radiographic sign is also known as a "support level." Establishing a delayed esophageal transport in the erect position is a "must" when the esophagus is examined. Many patients with symptomatic achalasia without a marked dilatation of the tube, such as in this case, are reported as normal, many radiologists do not know about this valuable sign. A manometry should be performed in such cases

Symmetric Weakness of the Pharynx. The second important functional disorder of this functional unit, the pharynx, is weakness. It is present when residues of contrast medium remain in the piriform sinuses and the valleculae after swallowing.

The coating of the pharyngeal walls differs with the viscosity of contrast medium. Thus, the high viscosity of barium paste facilitates the detection of pharyngeal weakness (Figs. 29, 30).

◀ **Fig. 42** **a** A normal esophageal passage in right prone anterior oblique position with the left shoulder raised. At the beginning of the esophageal phase, a cranially V-shaped upper end of the bolus (*arrow*) defines the peristaltic contraction, which pushes the bolus caudally at a speed of 4 cm/s. Additionally, this view provides excellent delineation of the PE segment during the pharyngeal phase. **b** The bolus is followed through the middle third of the esophageal tube. Small residues of contrast medium that remain at the level of the aortic arch after the passage are normal (*arrow*). Radiologically detectable motility disorders are mainly depicted in terms of delayed passage, abnormal wall movements, and structural lesions. Delayed passage is by far the most common radiological functional finding in the upper gastrointestinal tract. **c** 10 ml of barium suspension are transported into the stomach at the end of the esophageal phase

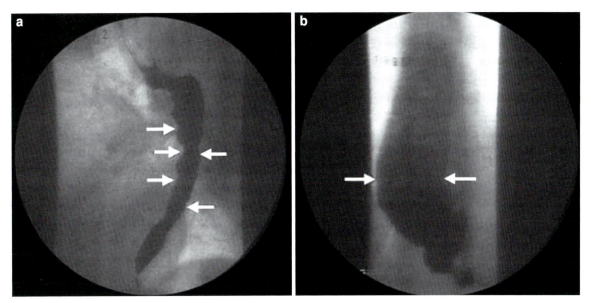

Fig. 44 **a** This 78-year-old man suffers from achalasia. In severe achalasia, a support level persists during the entire examination. Only small quantities of contrast medium are able to pass through a beak-like esophagogastric junction. In this case we also see strong non-propulsive contractions—a further important functional finding (*arrows*). **b** If the dilatation of the esophagus is severe (*arrows*), the diagnosis of achalasia is almost always reported on simple esophagrams. Note the inhomogeneous appearance of the material within the massively dilated esophagus. This is due to undigested food, that did not pass into the stomach

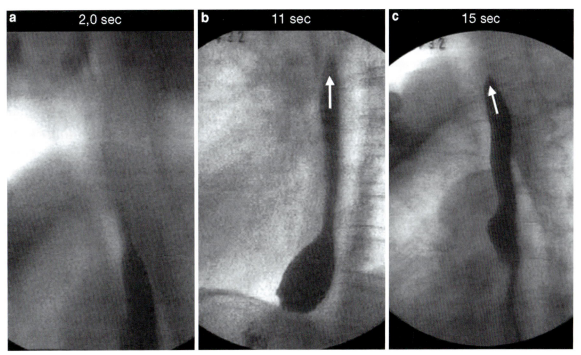

Fig. 45 **a** In this 65-year-old woman with achalasia, we have already seen the support level (see Fig. 44) while standing. In prone position, the contrast medium is initially transported. **b** Having reached the EGJ, the contrast medium now flows back in a proximal direction, because the esophageal contraction is too weak to propagate 10 ml of barium. This indirect sign of reduced contraction strength is known as "proximal escape." **c** The contrast material has reached the upper esophageal sphincter and flowed back to the upper esophageal sphincter. In gastroesophageal reflux, or even as a side effect of various medications, one frequently finds a motility disorder of the esophagus

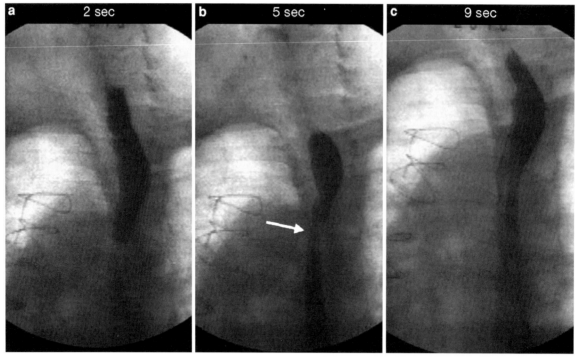

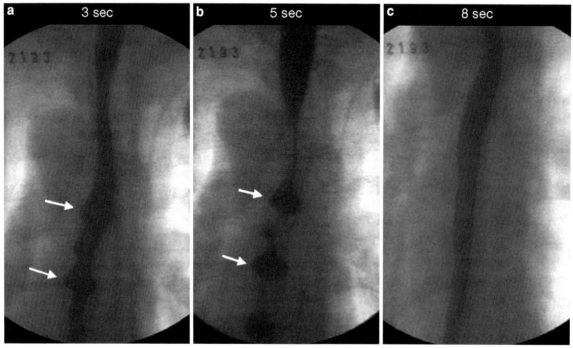

◀Fig. 46 **a** This 66-year-old post-bypass surgery patient takes several different medications for his heart and has suffered from reflux with mild dysphagia for a long time. The esophageal passage in prone position has already begun. **b** The bolus is segmented (*arrow*); the upper part of the bolus is left by weak esophageal contraction. **c** After the incomplete clearing of the bolus, the esophageal tube is filled with the contrast material, which had escaped proximally to the weak descending wave of primary peristaltic contraction

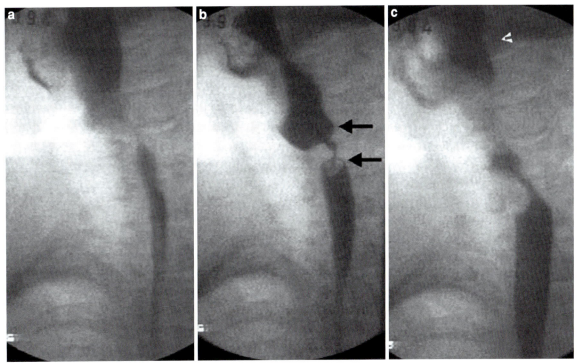

Fig. 48 **a** A 55-year-old woman with dysphagia and a carcinoma of the proximal esophagus. An endoscope could not be advanced; therefore VF was the first diagnostic test. Note that the carcinoma is invisible at the early esophageal phase. **b** For only 0.5 s, the narrow malignant stenosis is clearly depicted (*arrows*). **c** A few frames later, the lesion is obscured. The dynamic investigation is especially advantageous in this setting, and the lower spatial resolution of VF is compensated by the extraordinarily useful time resolution, when esophageal stenosis has to be diagnosed. At a frame rate of 3–4 spot films per second, digital recording proves to be an alternative technique for structural lesions, but not for dynamic evaluation of motility

Asymmetric Pharyngeal Weakness. In the case of pharyngeal weakness, it is important to distinguish between unilateral or mainly unilateral pharyngeal weakness and a bilateral symmetric pharyngeal weakness, as the therapeutic alternatives differ.

The frontal view is most suitable for radiographic diagnosis of a unilateral pharyngeal weakness, while in oblique views, asymmetric retentions can be seen with some experience (Fig. 31).

Pharyngoceles. Pharyngoceles are usually small, harmless, out-bulgings of the pharyngeal wall that may become symptomatic when they trap ingested food, which can cause mucosal irritation. Small pharyngoceles without retentions are common and harmless (Fig. 32). In rare cases, they can become enormous (trumpeter).

Space-Occupying Masses. Even large cervical osteophytes can be compensated without severe symptoms. A cerebrovascular accident may lead to a

◀ **Fig. 47** **a** This 53-year-old man who has suffered from severe dysphagia for solids for several years, has entirely constricting, non-propulsive contractions. Three seconds after the onset of the pharyngeal swallow, between the non-propulsive contractions, round segments of the tube do not contract (*arrows*). **b** Two seconds later the non-propulsive contractions have separated the non-contracting segments—"cork screw" or "rosary bead" esophagus are well known, but are non-specific descriptions of this severe esophageal motor disorder. Manometry is the gold standard to classify motor disorders of the esophagus. **c** Three seconds later, the esophagus shows smooth margins again. In patients with long-lasting motor disorders, the non-propulsive contractions may be shown constantly during all phases of swallowing

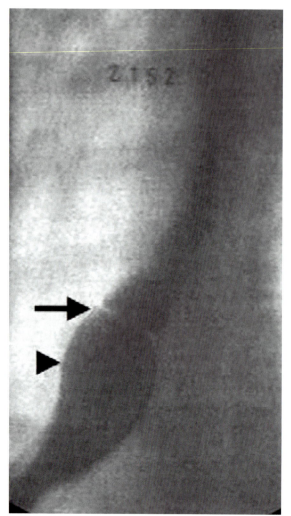

Fig. 49 The most common stenosis of the esophagus is the Schatzki ring; this shows a typical Schatzki ring in a 30-year-old man with dysphagia for solids (*arrow*). The ring is located exactly at the gastroesophageal junction and is nearly always combined with a hernia (*arrowhead*). It is crucial to investigate the patient both prone and supine, since rings and hernias of the EGJ may be seen in prone or supine position only. The Schatzki ring acts as a diaphragm and can cause impaction of solid food. During bolus passage, the ring is only visible for a second or two, depending on the bolus volume

decompensation in such cases. It is often very difficult to decide whether a resection of the osteophytic mass can improve a patient's swallowing function or not (Strasser et al. 2000) (Fig. 33).

Space-occupying masses may markedly hinder the pharyngeal passage (Fig. 34). It is rare that pharyngeal or laryngeal tumors are detected by VF or spot films; in symptomatic patients, endoscopy is usually performed first.

4.3.6 Pharyngoesophageal segment

Normal Function. We will now discuss the sixth functional unit of the swallowing act, namely the pharyngoesophageal sphincter or segment (PE segment). It is closed by its resting pressure between swallowing acts. Thus, it can be identified videofluoroscopically between the air column of the pharynx at rest and the air in the cervical esophagus. The PE segment consists of oblique parts of the inferior pharyngeal constrictor muscle, the cricopharyngeal muscle and parts of the cervical esophagus (Fig. 35).

Cricopharyngeal Bar. There are conflicting opinions about the percentage of narrowing allowing the diagnosis of a sphincter disorder, but more than 20–30 % seem to be pathological. Three different patients with varying degrees of incomplete opening of the upper esophageal sphincter are shown in Fig. 36.

In the case of mild dyskinesia, the dorsal indentation of the barium is discrete. The indentation of a cricopharyngeal bar may occur at various times during the passage of contrast medium. Furthermore, the indentation may be present for varying periods of time.

Gaping of the PE Segment. In cases of severe neuromuscular disease, the upper esophageal sphincter may reveal a gap, resulting from weakness. The resting pressure is no longer sufficient to close the sphincter (Fig. 37).

Web. The next is a morphological finding that is best seen on dynamic recordings. So-called membrane flaps or webs are solitary or multiple thin mucous membranes, most frequently located in the anterior wall of the upper esophageal sphincter. They are usually seen briefly on a few images (Fig. 38).

Zenker's Diverticulum. In the region of the pharyngoesophageal junction we find the clinically significant Zenker's diverticulum, which may substantially hinder bolus passage, depending on its size (Fig. 39).

Small Zenker's diverticula, or pseudodiverticula in combination with a sphincter dyskinesia, may also cause complaints (Fig. 40).

4.3.7 Esophagus

Normal Function. The esophagus, the seventh functional unit, is very different from the others. The esophageal passage takes about 10 s—about ten times the duration of the pharyngeal passage. The examination technique is

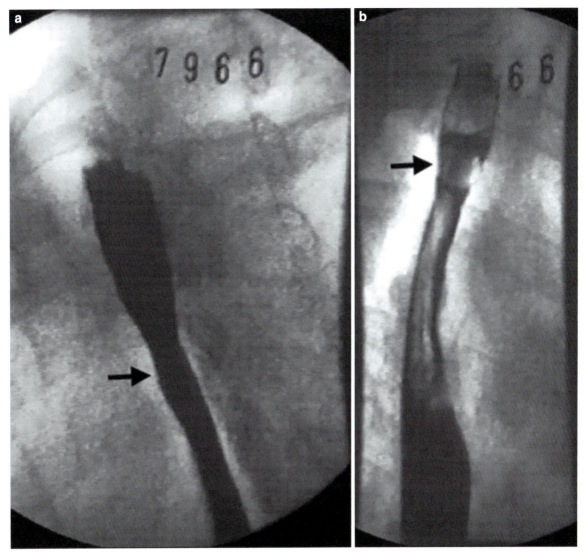

Fig. 50 a This 42-year old patient presented with recurrence of severe dysphagia and heartburn after repeated dilation of a laparoscopic Nissen fundoplication 6 years ago. Videofluoroscopy revealed a marked accentuation of the physiological narrowing at the level of the aortic arch (*arrow*). **b** After ingestion of a placebo tablet with a standardized diameter of 14 mm, the tablet gets stuck at this level, revealing a significant esophageal stenosis with an estimated lumen width of less than 1 cm (*arrow*)

also different, as one moves the device along with the slow peristaltic wave of the tubular esophagus from cranial to caudal. The device is kept stationary only at the beginning and the end of the esophageal passage. The analysis is focused on the dynamic movements of the esophageal walls (Figs. 41, 42).

hasis Type="Italic">Delay of Transport in the Erect Position. One should keep in mind that pseudoachalasia [tumor stenosis of the esophagogastric junction (EGJ)] cannot be differentiated videofluoroscopically from achalasia with certainty—endoscopy has to be performed (Figs. 43, 44).

Delay of transport in the Horizontal Position. The most frequent passage disorder is delayed esophageal transport in the prone or supine position. In oblique, prone RAO position, a single swallow of 10 ml is partially transported (Figs. 45, 46).

Non-propulsive Contractions. Non-propulsive or tertiary contractions are more or less strong constrictions of the esophagus that occur in addition to the wave

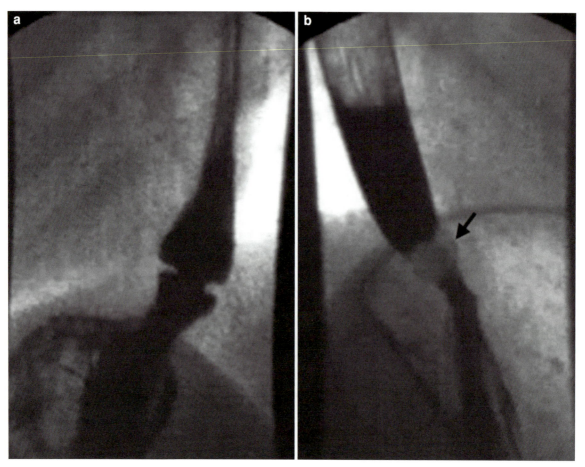

Fig. 51 **a** In this 15-year-old patient with solid food dysphagia and a history of three food impactions, drinking of several bolus of contrast media in the prone position revealed a thin ringlike narrowing in the distal esophagus. **b** The placebo tablet (*arrow*) could not pass this stenosis, suggesting a lumen width of less than 14 mm. Endoscopy confirmed the radiographic suspicion of eosinophilic esophagitis

of the contraction (Fig. 47). They are usually combined with a proximal escape or a support level.

Esophageal Stenoses. Stenoses of the esophagus, which are usually easier to diagnose on dynamic than static X-ray images, can be tested for their diameters (Fig. 48). Placebo tablets of 13–15 mm in diameter allow an exact measurement of the esophageal width. Furthermore, the tablet may produce symptoms that reproduce the patient's complaints.

If standard boluses of 10 ml do not obtain a clear delineation of the EGJ, about 150 ml of very thin barium can be applied by a straw—in the horizontal position. The patient may be advised to swallow repeatedly. This causes intradeglutitive inhibition of the peristaltic waves and the esophagus begins to fill up in monocontrast. This can help diagnose subtle stenoses and rings as an adjunct or alternative to a placebo tablet (Fig. 49). Videofluoroscopy enables the possibility of detecting subtle esophageal stenoses not diagnosed by endoscopy (Fig. 50, a–b). Especially in young patients with dysphagia and a history of recurrent impactions, VF can reveal a low-caliber esophagus and ringlike-stenotic margins, suggestive of eosinophilic esophagitis (Fig. 51, a–c).

Esophageal Diverticula. Diverticula of the upper digestive tract are an important diagnosis (Fig. 52). Whereas the Zenker's diverticulum may be easy to diagnose, the mid-esophageal and epiphrenic

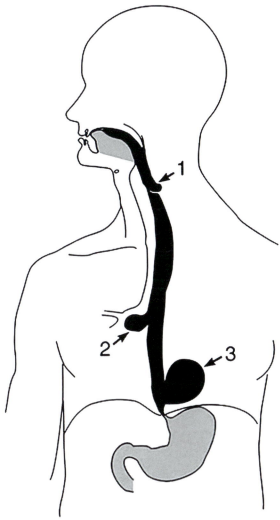

Fig. 52 1) Zenker's diverticulum; 2) mid-esophageal diverticulum; 3) epiphrenic diverticulum

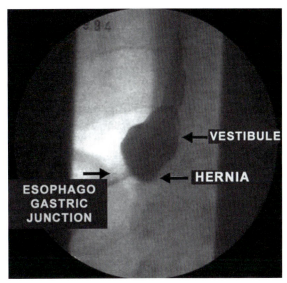

Fig. 53 The esophageal vestibule, a slight broadening of the gut distal to the muscular A-ring should end at the level of the diaphragm (see Fig. 56a). A hiatal hernia can be diagnosed when the vestibule ends at least 2 cm above the EGJ. The recess between the vestibule and the EGJ may be diagnosed as part of the stomach, protruding upward into the thorax—a hiatal hernia

Esophagogastric Junction. In 80 % of patients with reflux disease, a hiatal hernia is present, but only 50 % of patients with hiatal hernia suffer from reflux disease. The radiographic diagnosis of a small hiatal hernia is not of particular clinical importance; nevertheless, the radiographic examination of the esophagogastric junction is the method of choice for obtaining pertinent topographic information (Figs. 53–56).

The radiologic contributions to suggest reflux disease by means of functional observations, such as reflux or the dynamic appearance of the EGJ are controversial. This chapter does not intend to discuss provocative tests for reflux, such as the water-siphon test. Selected observations of authors, who had been interested in the dynamic appearance of the EGJ associated with gastroesophageal reflux, will be mentioned briefly. Reporting on the dynamic EGJ can enrich the view of VF and suggest a further work-up with pH monitoring or endoscopy. Topographic information can also help in planning surgical therapy.

diverticula can be obscured by severe non-propulsive contractions. The esophageal tube above and below a mid-esophageal diverticulum invariably shows a delayed esophageal transport and non-propulsive contractions. Incidentally, mid-esophageal diverticula may be found in non-dysphagic elderly people. It is crucial for further treatment, regardless of whether food impaction at the level of the diverticulum is present or not. Furthermore, it is important to note that epiphrenic diverticula are almost always combined with achalasia of the lower esophageal sphincter.

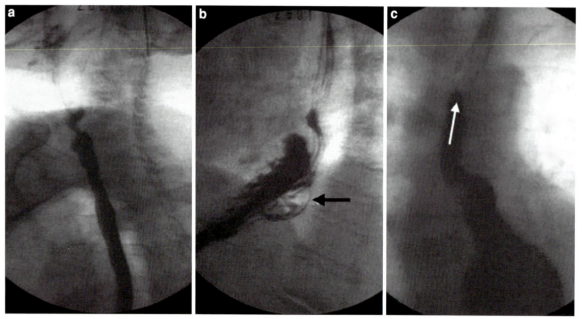

Fig. 54 a A 73-year-old woman with heartburn and mild dysphagia. In the prone right anterior oblique position, a cricopharyngeal bar is visible. **b** The end of the esophageal phase reveals an approximately 7 cm large hiatal hernia. **c** Turning the patient supine, gastroesophageal reflux to the upper third of the esophagus was present. pH monitoring is the gold standard for directly measuring reflux. However, if reflux to the upper esophagus can be demonstrated, a further clinical work-up is recommended

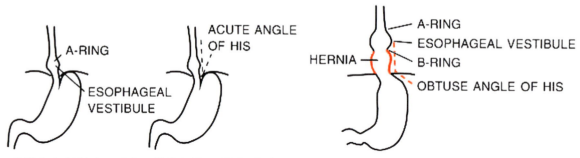

Fig. 55 The two graphs on the left represent the normal appearance of the esophagogastric junction, the graph on the right demonstrates an axial hernia and an obtuse angle of His (Fujiwara et al. 1998; Munzer 1997)

Most patients with heartburn can be managed symptomatically. With persistent, atypical symptoms, investigation may be required. The dynamic evaluation can diagnose the presence of a hernia, its topographic relations, abnormal esophageal peristalsis, cricopharyngeal dysfunction, and suggestive observations, such as the cardiac rosette, the angle of His and the width of the EGJ (Figs. 57–59).

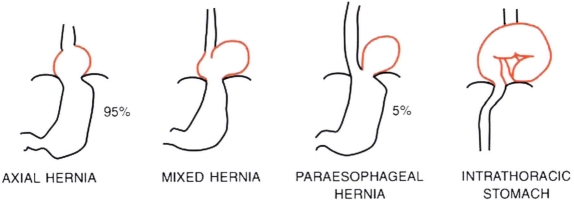

AXIAL HERNIA   MIXED HERNIA   PARAESOPHAGEAL   INTRATHORACIC
                                        HERNIA   STOMACH

Fig. 56 Axial hiatal hernia is common. When a part of the hernia reaches more cranially than the EGJ, it is called a "mixed hernia." Paraesophageal hernia is characterized by an EGJ at the level of the hiatus, and a hernia, which enters the thorax separately left and ventrally to the EGJ. An intrathoracic or upside-down stomach means a complete displacement of the stomach into the mediastinum

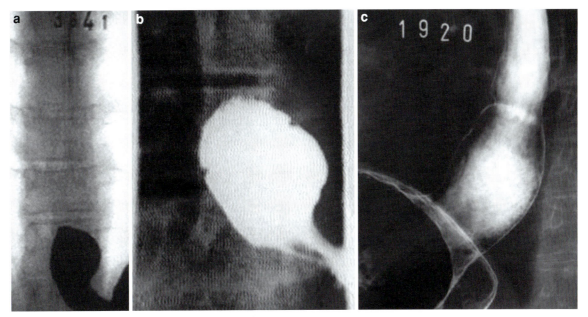

Fig. 57 **a** In the supine position, the esophageal vestibule should be cleared completely when a 10 ml bolus of barium has been swallowed with the single-swallow technique. **b** A subtle mucosal ring delineates the proximally sited esophageal vestibule and a 3 cm hernia between the vestibule and the EGJ. **c** Double-contrast radiography of a hernia can show a long-lasting gaping of the EGJ for several seconds

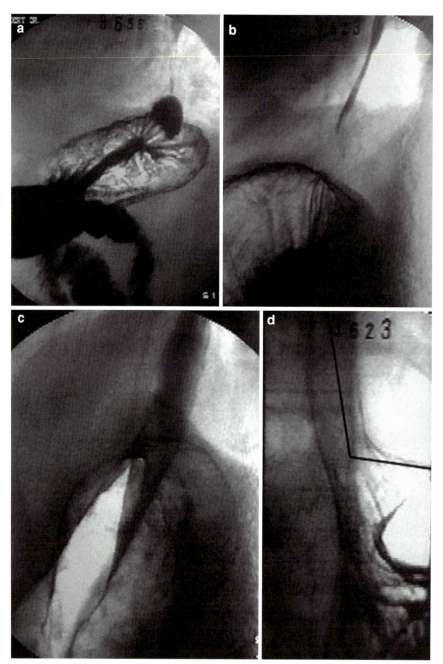

Fig. 58 **a** The cardia is anchored by surrounding phreno-esophageal membrane. The cardia is represented by stellate folds, radiating centrally as the cardiac "rosette"—the normal appearance. **b** Weakening of the ligaments can cause a funnel-shaped cardia due to laxity of ligamentous attachments (Herlinger et al. 1980). **c** In severe ligamentous laxity, a continuous gaping of the EGJ for a few seconds can be seen between the swallows. **d** The angle of His, first described in 1903, is the angle at which the esophagus enters the stomach. The angle is determined between the esophagus and the top of the fornix. The angle should be acute and not obtuse. After the application of effervescent powder, the His angle can be observed in the upright position

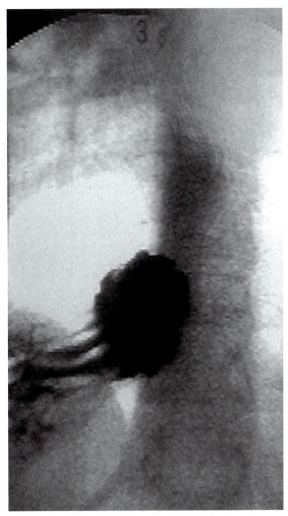

Fig. 59 A wide internal diameter of the esophagogastric junction of over 2.5 cm might be abnormal (Graziani et al. 1983)

References

Buchholz DW, Bosma JF, Donner MW (1985) Adaptation, compensation, and decompensation of the pharyngeal swallow. Gastrointest Radiol 10:235–239

Buchholz DW (1987) Neurologic evaluation of dysphagia. Dysphagia 1:187

Buchholz DW (1996) What is dysphagia? Editorial. Dysphagia 11:23–24

Edwards DAW (1974) History and symptoms of esophageal disease of the esophagus. In: Vantrappen G, Hellemans J (eds) Diseases of the esophagus. Springer-Verlag, New York

Ekberg O, Pokieser P (1997) Radiologic evaluation of the dysphagic patient. Eur Radiol 7:1285–1295

Fujiwara Y, Nakagawa K, Kusunoki M, Tanaka T, Yamamura T, Utsunomia J (1998) Gastroesophageal reflux after gastrectomy: possible significance of the angle of His. Am J Gastroenterol 93:11–15

Graziani L, De Nigris E, Pesaresi A, Baldellli S, Dini L, Montesi A (1983) Reflux esophagitis: radiographic-endoscopic correlation in 39 symptomatic cases. Gastrointest Radiol 8:1–6

Hendrix TR (1993) Art and science of history taking in the patient with difficulty swallowing. Dysphagia 8:69–73

Herlinger H, Grossmann R, Laufer I (1980) The gastric cardia in double contrast study: its dynamic image. AJR 135:21

Jones B, Donner M (1988) Examination of the patient with dysphagia. Radiology 167:319–326

Logemann JA (1995) Dysphagia: evaluation and treatment. Folia Phoniatr Logop 47:140–164

Moser G, Vacariu-Granser GV, Scneider C, Abatzi TA, Pokieser P, Stacher-Janotta G, Gaupmann G, Weber U, Wenzel T, Roden M, Stacher G (1991) High incidence of esophageal motor disorders in consecutive patients with globus sensation. Gastroenterology 101:1512–1521

Munzer D (1997) Angle of His in the cardioesophageal junction: is it a primordial factor in reflux esophagitis? Scand J Gastroenterol 32:847

Palmer JB, Drennan JC, Baba M (2000) Evaluation and treatment of swallowing impairments. Am Fam Physician 61:2453–2462

Pokieser P, Schober E, Schima W (1995) Videocinematographie des Schluckaktes: indikation, methodik und befundung. Radiologe 35:703–711

Scharitzer M, Pokieser P, Schober E, Schima W, Eisenhuber E, Stadler A, Memarsadeghi M, Partik B, Lechner G, Ekberg E (2002) Morphological findings in dynamic swallowing studies of symptomatic patients. Eur Radiol 12:1139–1144

Schima W, Stacher G, Pokieser P, Uranitsch K, Nekham D, Schober E, Moser G, Tscholakoff D (1992) Videofluoroscopic and manometric evaluation of esophageal motor disorders: Prospective study in 88 symptomatic patients. Radiology 185:487–491

Schober E, Schima W, Pokieser P (1995) Die radiologische Abklärung des Globus pharyngis. Radiologe 35:724–732

Simren M, Silny J, Holloway R, Tack J, Janssens J, Sifrim D (2003) Relevance of ineffective oesophageal motility during oesophageal acid clearance. Gut 52:784–790

Sonies BC et al (1987) Clinical examination of motor and sensory function of the adult oral cavity. Dysphagia 1:178

Strasser G, Schima W, Schober E, Pokieser P, Kaider A, Denk DM (2000) Cervical osteophytis impinging on the pharynx: importance of size on current disorders for the development of inspiration. AJR 174(2):449–453

Woo P, Noordzij P, Ross JA (1996) Association of esophageal reflux and globus symptom: comparison of laryngoscopy and 24 h pH monitoring. Otolaryngol Head Neck Surg 115:502–507

Imaging Techniques and Some Principles of Interpretation (Including Radiation Physics)

Olle Ekberg

Contents

O. Ekberg (✉)
Department of Diagnostic Radiology,
Malmö University Hospital,
205 02 Malmö, Sweden
e-mail: olle.ekberg@med.lu.se

Abstract

Radiologic examination of the oral cavity, pharynx, and esophagus should focus on bolus transportation as well as on registration of morphodynamic events. The examination should be custom-tailored to the patient's symptoms but should also be performed in a rather standardized way. The radiologic findings should always be compared to the patient's specific symptoms.

1   Introduction

In the dysphagic patient the radiologic examination of the oral cavity, pharynx, and esophagus should be regarded as an extension of the physical and neurologic examinations. The mouth and the pharynx and larynx can be reached only partially during more conventional clinical evaluation. The result of the radiologic examination should thus be put in a broader context together with the clinical history and the result of the clinical and neurologic examina-tions.

2   The Symptom Dysphagia

Dysphagia, i.e., any abnormal sensation during swallowing experienced by the patient, may be caused by either morphologic abnormalities or dysfunction. The clinical history is often spurious and careful workup must be considered. The swallowing apparatus consists of the oral cavity, pharynx, and esophagus and symptoms from any of these three compartments may be present. Morphologic evaluation of these three

O. Ekberg (ed.), *Dysphagia*, Medical Radiology. Diagnostic Imaging, DOI: 10.1007/174_2011_390,
© Springer-Verlag Berlin Heidelberg 2012

compartments can be done by direct inspection (the oral cavity), by indirect inspection (the pharynx and larynx) or by endoscopy (the esophagus). However, for a proper functional evaluation, radiology is necessary. For the evaluation of transportation through the oral cavity, pharynx, and esophagus, the barium swallow is without doubt the most reliable test. It is used extensively and its accuracy has been well shown.

Any clinician interested in patients with dysphagia needs to make sure that his consultant radiologist has the means and interest to perform a proper examination. A carelessly performed examination interpreted as showing normal findings may give the clinician a false impression that the examination has been completed and misinterpretation of the barium swallow may lead to unnecessary further workup and delay correct diagnosis.

2.1 Does the Patient Really Have Dysphagia?

When properly performed, the radiologic examination should start with a careful penetration of the clinical history. The examination should then be custom-tailored to each patient's specific complaints. The patient who complains of difficulties with certain foods should be examined with such food. The patient who complains particularly of choking during eating must be carefully examined for misdirected swallowing. The patient who complains of heartburn should be examined with respect to gastroesophageal reflux disease. Patients who complain of pain or obstruction during solid bolus swallow need to be examined with some kind of standardized solid bolus. Therefore, a clinical history is of crucial importance for the radiologist and he or she needs to state in his or her report for what symptoms/purposes the study was designed. However, it is also important to always examine all three compartments of the swallowing apparatus, namely, the oral cavity, the pharynx, and the esophagus. What the clinical history does is to help the radiologist focus on one particular segment and sometimes on a specific food consistency. If the patient has undergone a careful endoscopic examination, before being sent for the radiologic examination, this should focus not on morphology but merely on function. However, most patients with dysphagia do not undergo endoscopy of the esophagus. Therefore, in most patients with dysphagia, it is important that the radiologist perform both

a functional evaluation and a detailed double-contrast morphologic examination of the esophagus.

Most patients with swallowing symptoms have an abnormality that can be revealed during the radiologic examination whether it is morphologic or functional. However, many patients are sent for radiologic examinations of the swallowing apparatus without any real swallowing problems. These patients suffer from globus and their spontaneous clinical history always includes complaints or an inability to swallow. They feel a sensation of obstruction when swallowing and a constant feeling of a "lump" in the throat. This is the dominant and overwhelming symptom which bothers the patient considerably and this impresses many physicians. However, when a structured clinical history is taken, the patient admits that "he can eat and drink normally." This is the hallmark of globus. These patients localize their symptoms to the neck, but the symptoms should alert the radiologist to focus his or her examination on the lower esophagus in an attempt to reveal signs of gastroesophageal reflux disease. In fact, these patients, in addition to the inability to swallow "normally," also have heartburn and regurgitation. However, these symptoms are not the leading symptoms and are less alarming than the globus symptom. Therefore, globus should be taken seriously and these patients should be examined properly.

2.2 Findings Compared with Symptoms

The careful clinical history also serves another purpose, namely, to make an assessment of the clinical relevance of any radiologic finding. A comparison of the patient's symptoms and the radiologic finding should always be included in the radiologist's report. The radiologic examination may reveal a host of abnormalities, most of which are irrelevant in that particular clinical setting. In our experience, the radiologist experienced in dysphagia evaluation is best suited to make this comparison between symptoms and findings. The radiologist knows how the examination was performed and may also add to the clinical history after the examination has been done. It may be true that many patients with dysphagia do not undergo a proper functional evaluation of the swallowing apparatus. However, the result of many barium studies is at the same time misinterpreted and not put into a proper clinical context.

Fig. 1 A 46-year-old woman with solid bolus dysphagia. The findings of the initial barium examination were assessed as normal. A 13-mm-diameter antacid tablet used for stressing the esophagus became stuck in the proximal esophagus. A short asymmetric narrowing (assessed to be congenital in origin) was revealed by the tablet. Balloon dilatation made the patient become asymptomatic

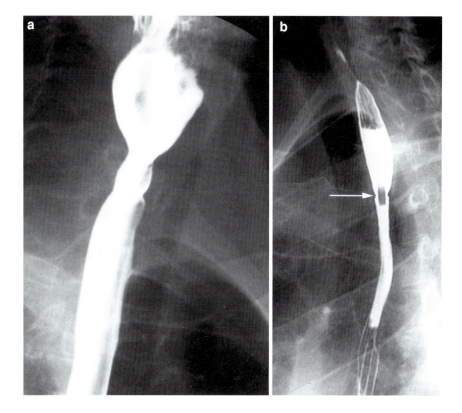

2.3 Dysphagia During the Radiologic Examination

As well as the importance of the clinical history concerning symptoms and signs, it is as important to register symptoms during the radiologic examination. If misdirected swallowing occurs, the radiologist needs to observe if cough or other signs of the patient's subjective experience of that misdirected swallowing event occur. By and large, patients who do not cough during even minor events of misdirected swallowing have a more advanced disease than those who cough and have an increased risk of airway disease (Figs. 1, 2). If a tablet is given to evaluate solid bolus dysphagia and if the patient does experience symptoms similar to the ones he or she experienced during normal eating and drinking, the tablet test can be considered diagnostic (van Westen and Ekberg 1993). However, even if the tablet gets stuck in the esophagus (excluding patients with strictures) for many minutes and the patient does not experience this, the tablet test has not revealed the cause of that particular patient's dysphagia. However, one needs to remember that patients usually do not spontaneously

comment on symptoms during the test. This is often because symptoms provoked during the radiologic examination are much milder than those that occur during normal eating and drinking. This circumstance should alert the radiologist to carefully but casually ask the patient about swallowing symptoms during this test.

2.4 The Radiologic Examination (Barium or Iodine Swallow)

In the team of professionals taking care of neurologically impaired patients with swallowing difficulties the radiologist plays an important role. He or she must choose the correct imaging technique which will most expediently and accurately answer the clinical questions. This is not always barium swallow. For instance, in patients with the combination/constellation of neck pain and dysphagia, MRI can reveal soft tissue disease, such as retropharyngitis (Ekberg and Sjöberg 1995). The radiologist in the swallowing team must be aware of the limitations of radiology for

Fig. 2 An elderly patient with solid bolus dysphagia. **a**, **b** Single-contrast examinations of the pharynx and the pharyngoesophageal segment (PES). There is an incoordination in the opening of the PES and also small weblike narrowings. There is no misdirected swallowing. **c** As the patient indicated solid bolus dysphagia, she was given an antacid tablet together with thin liquid barium. The tablet passed the pharynx and the PES and became stuck in the upper esophagus. The patient immediately indicated that this created the same dysphagia symptom as she had had before. She indicated the level of the symptoms with her left hand. There is a ring on her index finger. The location of the tablet is indicated with *arrows*. Further evaluation revealed decreased peristaltic contrast pressure in this area but there was no morphologic abnormality

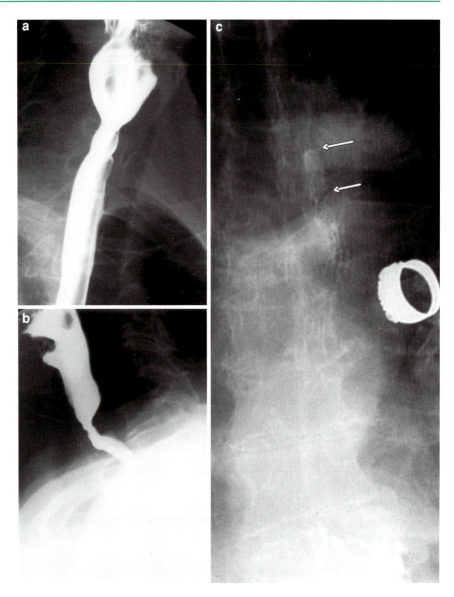

assessment of the course and treatment of the disease process.

Radiology therefore offers a unique possibility to screen patients with swallowing symptoms. The barium swallow allows evaluation of both morphology and function, which is unique to this technique.

2.4.1 How To Perform the Barium Swallow Examination

The radiologic examination should be performed as a biphasic examination, i.e., both function (single contrast) and morphology (double contrast) should be evaluated (Fig. 3). All patients with dysphagia can be accurately examined radiologically! Even in the severely ill stroke patient the relevant clinical questions can be answered. In the very impaired patient it is often enough to demonstrate whether or not the patient can elicit the pharyngeal stage of swallowing and maybe also the degree of aspiration if this occurs. Such an examination is usually easy to perform. Cumbersome and time-consuming are examinations in ambulatory, alert, otherwise healthy young patients who complain of vague or uncharacteristic symptoms during swallowing.

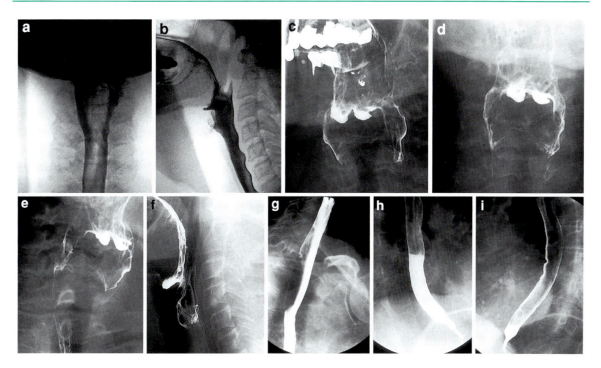

Fig. 3 Biphasic examination of the pharynx and esophagus. **a, b** Frontal and lateral projections of the pharynx. These images are digitally stored from the fluoroscopic images. **c** Double-contrast examination of the pharynx in slight left anterior oblique projection. **d** Frontal projection of the pharynx, double contrast. **e** Right anterior oblique projection of the pharynx examined with the double-contrast technique. **f** Lateral double-contrast examination of the pharynx. **g–i** Double-contrast examinations of the esophagus in different projections

The image should be centered at the important area whether this is the oral cavity, pharynx, or esophagus. Moreover, one should always use proper cone down, and most importantly, collimation. If wedge frames are available, they should always be used. A high voltage (110 kV) should always be used as this will shorten the exposure time, thereby minimizing movement artifacts.

The fluoroscopic intensifier should not be moved during exposure. Also, it should be kept steady during fluoroscopy. Moving the image intensifier around may save contrast medium but deteriorates image sharpness, thereby losing important morphologic information (Fig. 4).

Modern digital radiologic equipment offers the possibility to store the fluoroscopic image in digital form (Figs. 5, 6, 7). This reduces the radiation dose administered to the patient (and the radiologist!). A digital fluoroscopy system is configured in the same way as a conventional fluoroscopy system (tube, table, image intensifier, video system). The analogue video signal is converted to, and stored as, digital data.

A frame rate of 25–50 frames per second may be achieved, but most studies use 12 frames per second.

It is important to perform fluoroscopy and obtain images in standardized projections. Fluoroscopy is used for assessment of function, and also for positioning. Especially in the pharynx the importance of meticulous positioning and projection is important (Figs. 8, 9, 10).

All patients should be examined with them in an erect sitting or standing position if possible. We prefer to use high-density barium contrast medium (240 w/v) for the double-contrast evaluation of the oral cavity, pharynx, and esophagus. The high density of the barium contrast medium also makes it relatively easy to register penetration of barium into the laryngeal vestibule (Fig. 11). However, such high-density barium contrast medium, probably owing to its high viscosity, is less likely to reach into the vestibule in patients with a defective closure. Therefore, sometimes penetration is revealed only when low-density barium contrast medium (40% w/v) is

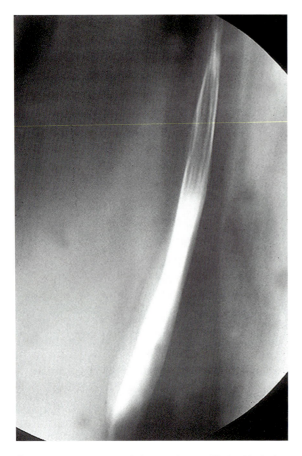

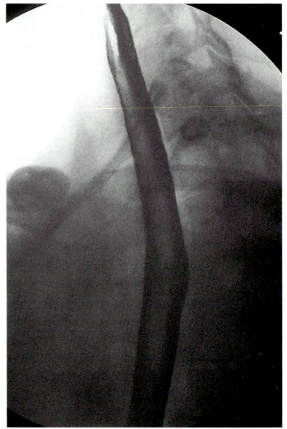

Fig. 4 The distal part of the esophagus filled with barium contrast medium and air. The image intensifier was moved during the exposure and this created lack of sharpness

Fig. 5 Digitally stored image of the esophagus. This gives an image with inferior spatial resolution compared with an exposed image, but the radiation dose is much lower

used. However, with the proper exposure technique, it should be possible to reveal even minute amounts of such contrast medium.

2.4.2 How To Perform the Iodine Swallow Examination

Only in patients in whom feeding must be strictly nonoral is it indicated to replace barium contrast medium with iodine contrast medium. The basic advantage with barium contrast medium is that it is radiopaque. It is also not harmful to the mucosa in the airways. It is readily transported cranially in the airways by the cilia. However, in patients with emphysema and other chronic obstructive lung diseases, the transportation might be delayed and even absent from the most distal parts, i.e., the alveoli and emphysematous bullae. In such patients it might also be indicated to use iodine contrast medium. Iodine

contrast medium generally used to be a hyperosmotic fluid with a very strong taste and smell. Nowadays, iodine contrast medium is usually nonionic, iso-osmolar, or has slightly higher osmolarity compared with plasma. Usually it has a sweet taste and no smell. The radiodensity of such a contrast medium (e.g., 350 mg I/ml) is appropriate for evaluation of morphology and function. Where iodine contrast medium has been chosen as the contrast medium, the clinical situation is usually that of a severely disabled patient with a very limited number of relevant clinical questions. One such question can be whether or not the patient can elicit a pharyngeal swallow. Therefore, the projections and number of swallows are much more individualized. It is usually sufficient to observe one or only a few swallows, and usually in lateral projection. Although double-contrast films may also be obtained with iodine contrast media, this is usually

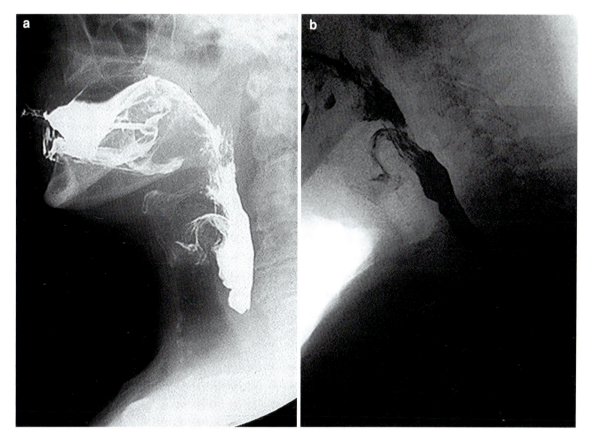

Fig. 6 The difference in image quality between the conventional (digital) exposure technique and the digital storage of a frozen fluoroscopic image is illustrated in this patient. **a** Exposure technique; **b** digitally stored fluoroscopic image. The spatial resolution is higher with an exposure technique. This is particularly important when assessing morphologic abnormalities. However, the detection of minor amounts of misdirected swallowing into the laryngeal vestibule can also be difficult using a fluoroscopic technique with digital storage only. However, the reduction in radiation dose is substantial

not indicated. However, even in a very limited examination it is important to ascertain that there is no obstruction for the bolus. Therefore, it is important to at least fluoroscopically examine the pharynx, PES, and esophagus in search for tumors or strictures. With the patient in the supine position, which is usually the only position that the patient can take, ample evaluation of esophageal motor function is also possible.

Other situations where iodine contrast medium is regularly used are in patients where there is a question of a leak and also in a postoperative situation where patency of anastomosis is evaluated (see Sect. 4.4).

2.5 The Oral Cavity and the Pharynx

As in most clinical circumstances the question of misdirected swallowing is the most crucial one and this should be carefully looked into. The patient should be in a lateral projection, preferably in an erect position, although the patient may also be recumbent. The field of imaging should include the oral cavity, soft palate, pharynx, and pharyngoesophageal segment (PES). In that position, the patient should be instructed to take a mouthful of liquid barium. The size of the ingestion should be according to the patient's own discretion. The radiologist should take time to explain this part of the examination. The volume ingested should then be evaluated and compared with the patient's swallowing capability. The ingested material should be observed in the oral cavity for at least 5–10 s. Any anterior or posterior leak should be observed during that period. It should also be possible to assess the volume of ingestion as many patients with oral apraxia or defective sensitivity ingest too big a bolus to be handled safely

Fig. 7 Comparison between different techniques. **a** The exposure and **b** the storage of the frozen fluoroscopic image

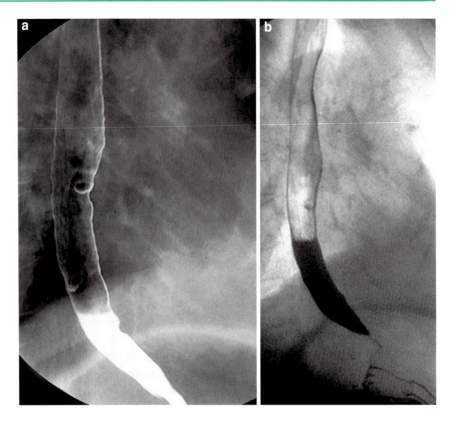

during swallowing. The fluoroscopy should be continued during the ingestion and until the bolus tail has passed into the cervical esophagus. Collimation and exposure techniques should be meticulously controlled and if possible wedged collimation should be used. This decreases flaring due to the air between the chin and the neck. A minimum of three swallows should be registered in this latter projection. However, if misdirected swallowing is a major concern and has not been revealed during these three swallows, it is important to observe additional swallows. We may observe at least 15 swallows in such patients (and even more if necessary). During such swallows provocation may be added. Patients may be able to compensate for defective closure of the laryngeal vestibule and/or misdirected swallowing. Alteration of the position of the head and neck may enable such a compensation to be decompensated, and thereby the cause of the patient's complaints is explained (Ekberg 1986). The easiest way to decompensate is to ask the patient to swallow with his or her neck extended. Patients with normal function should be able to close their laryngeal vestibule and misdirected swallowing

should not occur during swallowing even if the neck is extended. Patients who have partial malfunction may decompensate during this maneuvers.

We have found that it is much easier to assess the video recording if a soundtrack is also recorded during the examination. Therefore, we have installed a microphone conveniently mounted on the X-ray shield. During the video recording all pertinent information, such as bolus viscosity, bolus volume, patient positioning, and perhaps most importantly any symptoms reported by the patient during the examination, is recorded and can be easily assessed during the review if a loudspeaker is included in the reading room equipment.

2.6   The Esophagus

For a detailed description of how to examine esophageal function, see Sect. 5.1. A short introduction is given here. It is of the utmost importance to always include the oral cavity, the pharynx, and the esophagus in the radiologic examination. However, in each patient the focus is usually on only one or two compartments.

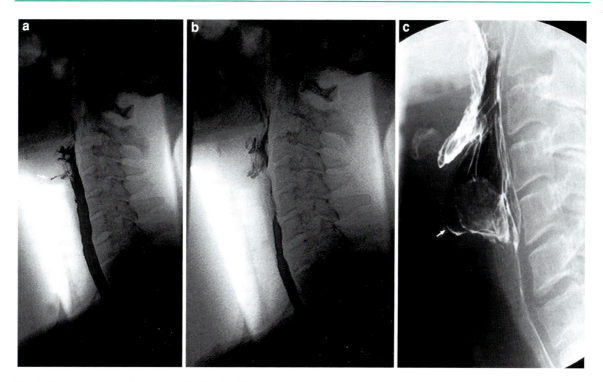

Fig. 8 The importance of correct projections/positioning.This patient was assessed to have contrast medium reaching into the laryngeal vestibule (*arrow*) (**a**). Contrast medium in one of the piriform sinuses in this slightly oblique projection mimics contrast medium in the laryngeal vestibule. However, this image was obtained in a slightly oblique projection. This was revealed during a more precise positioning of the patient (**b**).The same mistake can easily be made during double-contrast examination when contrast medium in one of the piriform sinuses may mimic contrast medium in the laryngeal vestibule (*arrow*) (**c**)

We prefer to perform the double-contrast examination of the esophagus after the functional evaluation of the pharynx. The esophageal examination starts with effervescent tablets and the patient is asked to rapidly drink the high-density barium contrast medium (240% w/v). Double-contrast radiograms are taken in left and right oblique projections. Patients with painful swallow should be evaluated for esophagitis such as *Candida* esophagitis. The radiologist should always be careful in evaluating the patient for neoplastic lesions such as superficial carcinomas.

Evaluation of esophageal function often needs to be done with the patient in a recumbent position. However, if esophageal dysfunction has already been revealed with the patient in an erect position, it is usually not warranted to place the patient in a recumbent position as dysfunction in the erect position is not known to become normal in the recumbent position.

3   Solid Bolus Examination

All patients with a history of obstruction during swallowing should be examined with a solid bolus, especially if solid bolus dysphagia is present (see Figs. 1, 2). The solid bolus used for the radiologic examination must be standardized. We prefer to use a radiolucent antacid tablet with a known diameter of 13 mm (van Westen and Ekberg 1993). This is swallowed together with thin liquid barium (40% w/v). Others have advocated the use of a barium tablet, a bread sphere, or a marshmallow (Curtis et al. 1987; Kelly 1961; Somers et al. 1986). Contraindications for tablet swallowing are known or suspected pharyngeal dysfunction with misdirected swallow. If this is suspected, the patient should first undergo evaluation of the pharyngeal stage and if misdirected swallowing is present with barium reaching below the

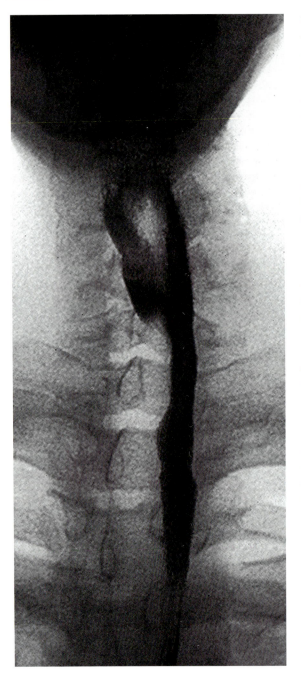

Fig. 9 Frontal projection of the cervical esophagus during barium swallow. There is a fusiform indentation from the right into the esophagus. This is the characteristic appearance of the effect of the kyphosis of a cervical spine. The esophagus is stretched over the kyphosis and deviates to the left. This gives a false impression of a "pseudotumor"

vocal folds, a solid tablet should not be given. This is because of the risk of choking. However, the best way to triage patients for the tablet test is to show them the

tablet and the thin liquid barium and ask them if they can swallow the tablet. In our experience this easily excludes patients who should not undergo the tablet swallow. In fact, that particular group of patients who do not think they can swallow the tablet are the ones who should be examined because of suspected stricture or other obstructions.

Tablet arrest may or may not be symptomatic. When the tablet becomes stuck above a stricture, symptoms are usually absent. This is in contrast to when the tablet arrest is due to dysmotility. In the latter cases, the patient is often symptomatic. However, the symptom is often much milder than the symptoms that arise during a meal.

Solid bolus arrest in the esophagus is due to either dysmotility or a narrowing. Dysmotility is due to either spasm or hyperperistalsis, two entities that are hard to separate fluoroscopically. As assessed by manometry, most of these patients have hypomotility and only rarely spasm.

4 Aspects of Radiation Physics/Safety

Radiologic examination relies on the ability of photons of a certain energy (X-rays) to penetrate opaque materials such as the human body. Since their discovery by Wilhelm Conrad Röntgen in 1895, they have made a major contribution to medicine as well as other industrial applications. However, such radiation means that energy is transported through the body. Only 1–20% of the given energy from the X-ray tube reaches the detector, i.e., the image-intensifying screen or the film–screen combination. The rest of the energy is absorbed in the patient. It is this absorbed energy, which is sometimes called radiation dose, that is the main hazardous aspect of radiation. Such ionized radiation, when absorbed in the body, might interfere with water molecules and cause free radicals to be produced. The ionizing radiation may also interfere with proteins and other important substances within the cell. This reaction may cause cell death or induce serious late side effects. It is therefore necessary that all radiations, including that used for swallowing studies, are used with care.

One important aspect to remember is that it is only when the X-ray tube is irradiating, namely, when the current is applied, that there is radiation from the tube

Fig. 10 a A single-contrast examination of the pharynx. The folded appearance of the epiglottis creates a hole in the contrast medium. This image also shows the medialization of the lateral pharyngeal wall as an indicator of normal function of the constrictors. **b** This is much more difficult to assess in lateral projection. **c** The characteristic, irregular in-bulging of the arytenoid region and the down-folded epiglottis is seen creating an irregular impression in the anterior wall of the midpharynx (*arrow*). **d** For proper evaluation of the PES, it is often necessary to obtain images in oblique projection

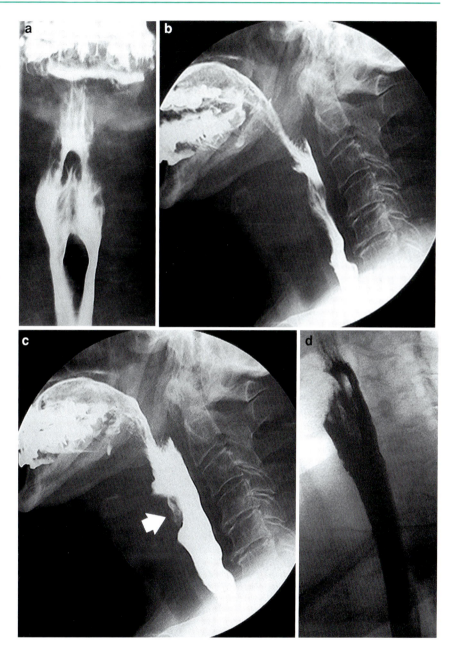

and in the room. At the same moment as the current stops, the radiation primarily from the X-ray tube (secondarily from the patient) stops and there is no hazard within the room or to the patient, nor to the personnel in the room. Radiation always and only traverses linearly, i.e., it does not bend around corners.

The X-ray equipment must undergo regular scheduled quality controls according to each country's regulations. It is also important that personnel responsible for the equipment ascertain that all functions are checked for proper function on at least a weekly basis.

The most important consideration is that an X-ray examination should never be performed unless it is necessary. It should be contemplated beforehand what the referring clinician is expecting to find and what therapeutic or prognostic consequences that may have. Once this is clear, the risk of radiation damage is always far smaller than the benefit that can be

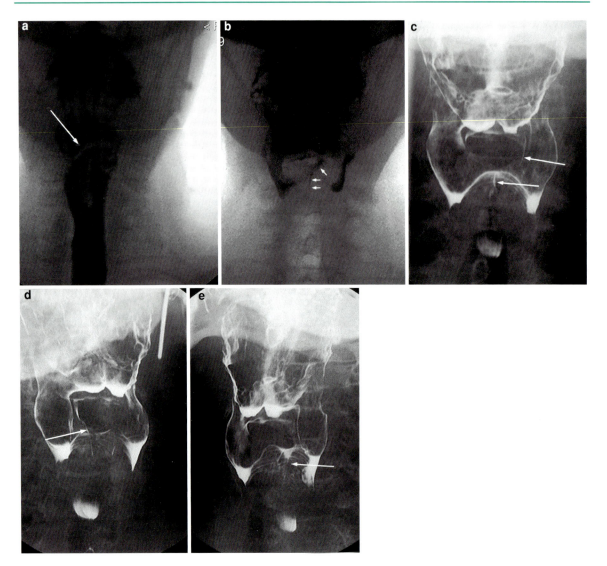

Fig. 11 It is important to be able to identify misdirected swallowing also in a frontal projection. During the full column examination, also called the single-contrast technique, the laryngeal vestibule is obscured in the frontal projection. **a** The oblique epiglottis (*arrow*) can be seen. This is per se not a functional abnormality. **b** Retention of barium in the pharynx showing that there is also contrast medium outlining the characteristic shape of the half-opened laryngeal vestibule (*arrows*). The shape resembles a tapered glass. **c** Contrast medium on the inside of the laryngeal vestibule up to the aryepiglottic folds (*arrows*). There is also contrast medium between the opposed arytenoids (*lower arrow*). The same is seen in left anterior oblique (**d**) and right anterior oblique (**e**) projections. Barium seen in the laryngeal vestibule, as in this patient, indicates misdirected swallowing. This finding is always abnormal but may or may not be symptomatic

achieved from the X-ray examination. This means that the X-ray examination needs to be necessary in the clinical setting and then that the performance of the study must be optimized. The risk of damage is far greater in children and young adults. In individuals older than 40 years, the risk is basically negligible. There is a positive correlation between patient dose and personnel dose. It is important to cone down on the pharynx and/or esophagus and thereby avoid irradiation of extensive volumes. The distance between the patient and the image intensifier/screen should be as small as possible.

You should try to stay as far away as possible from the patient; however, you must be close enough for assistance or manipulations. Lead aprons must be worn. Sometimes an apron over the thyroid or lead eyeglasses have been advocated. Most importantly, if you do not need to stand close to the patient, step away. If you double the distance from you to the patient, the radiation dose reduces to one quarter. Remember that it is not radiation from the X-ray tube that radiates the personnel in the room, it is the patient who radiates secondary radiation. It is also important to carefully perform the study, meaning that it is better to do one proper radiologic examination than to have to redo studies or even exposures because of bad technique. It is also important to realize that the fluoroscopy time contributes to most of the radiation dose. Fluoroscopy for 1 min is roughly equivalent to one exposure. This is, however, relative and depends on the situation. In a study by Chan et al. (2002), they found that if a videoradiographic swallowing study had a duration of 18 ± 8 min (and this is very long from my own perspective), the scattered radiation dose (measured 30, 60, and 100 cm from the patient's neck) received by the examiner varied tenfold, i.e., 34–3 μSv. This should then theoretically permit an examiner to perform 2,583 examinations per year given the annual effective dose limit of 20 mSv. It should be noted that since lead aprons are always worn, the additional protection they provide further reduces the scattered radiation dose to negligible levels.

If you have access to digital radiology, you may also have access to pulsed fluoroscopy. If possible, you should use as few pulses (usually two) per second as possible. However, this might sometimes be unsuitable for evaluation of function. It is better to use continuous fluoroscopy than to have to redo the swallowing studies. You should use a fluoroscopy time as short as possible. You should ensure that the patient does not move around, and if necessary you should have the patient hold his or her breath during exposures. You should avoid flaring by using wedge frames. Modern equipment also has the possibility to save the fluoroscopy image digitally. This may in fact lower the dose considerably in comparison with conventional exposures. These images may be enough for documentation of, for instance, misdirected swallowing. However, as stated above, it is better to make one proper exposure and to conduct one properly performed examination than to have to redo the study because of poor image quality. If studies are performed by speech-and-language pathologists, it is very important that they are familiar with radiation physics.

The effective dose of a radiologic dysphagia evaluation as described above is about 1 mSv. This can be compared with the effective doses for a chest X-ray (anteroposterior and lateral) of 0.1 mSv, an abdominal survey film (three images) of 5 mSv, and a barium colon examination of 5 mSv; the effective dose for coronary angiography with interventions as well as interventions in other parts of the body may easily exceed 100 mSv.

5   Other Techniques

Ultrasonography can be used for evaluation of the oral stage and hyoid bone movement (Hamlet et al. 1988; Brown and Sonies 1997). This technique is attractive because it does not rely on ionizing radiation. It can therefore be used unrestricted also in younger patients. It also enables visualization of the tongue surface. It could be the method of choice for monitoring oral function. However, the fact that the bolus is not visualized is a major drawback. Ultrasonography also requires considerable operator skills.

In recent years there has been growing interest in fiber-endoscopic evaluation of swallowing. During fiber-endoscopic evaluation of swallowing, the endoscope is inserted through one of the nostrils and the pharynx and larynx are observed before and after swallow (Langmore et al. 1988). Any posterior leak before swallowing over the tongue base can be observed, as well as movement of the pharyngeal wall. Also, laryngeal structures during breathing are observed. Sensitivity may be tested by touching the walls of the pharynx with the tip of the fiber endoscope. When the pharynx is elevated during swallowing and the bolus is brought into the pharynx, the endoscopist's view is obstructed. However, retention in the pharynx after swallowing can be observed and also whether or not the bolus has reached into the larynx. As a bolus one usually uses intensely colored water in order to better visualize the bolus.

The repetitive oral suction and swallowing test was introduced in the mid-1990s. With use of a multimodality and simultaneous technique (ultrasound, pressure, scale, temperature) it was possible to measure suction pressure, bolus volume, respiration and feeding–respiratory coordination and pharyngeal transit time (Nilsson et al. 1995).

A "swallowing safety index" can also be calculated (Nilsson et al. 1997); however, his technique has not gained widespread use.

The most promising "new technique" is MRI. With fast gradients and short acquisition times an "almost real-time" fluoroscopic technique is possible. This allows analysis of bolus transport but also, and more importantly, movements in anatomical structures, i.e., the tongue and pharyngeal constrictors (Buettner et al. 2001).

Dynamic cineradiography and videoradiography (videomanometry) of pharyngeal barium swallow provides morphological as well as qualitative functional information on the swallowing sequence. However, dynamic barium swallow relies mainly on functional qualitative judgment, failing to quantify the results. This is, for example, the case when trying to assess pharyngeal paresis in terms of the degree of barium retention in the pharynx.

In this context, intraluminal pharyngeal manometry is capable of providing a more quantitative analysis of pharyngeal muscle function in terms of intraluminal pressure registration (McConnel 1988; McConnel et al. 1988a, b; Olsson and Ekberg 1995; Olsson et al. 1994, 1995, 1996). Concurrent barium swallow and pharyngeal manometry combine qualitative assessment of bolus transport with quantitative registration of the contractions of the pharyngeal wall. Our experiences with this simultaneous technique have revealed that there is a substantial longitudinal asymmetry in pharyngeal pressure response in normal individuals. There is also a wide variety in the timing of PES opening/relaxation, where the pressure registration is extremely dependent on sensor positioning. Furthermore, the radiologic finding of a CP bar is often only an indicator of a more widespread dysfunction around the PES easily evaluated with the simultaneous technique. In many patients with a posterior CP bar the major abnormality is weak constrictors with outpouching of the lumen above and below.

The simultaneous technique provides new diagnostic information in dysphagic patients and we suggest the addition of pharyngeal solid-state manom-etry, preferably with simultaneous videoradiography, in cases where routine radiologic workup does not reveal any abnormality.

References

Brown BP, Sonies BC (1997) Diagnostic methods to evaluate swallowing other than barium contrast. In: Perlman AL, Schulze-Delrieu KS (eds) Deglutition and its disorders anatomy physiology, clinical diagnosis, and management. Singular Publishing Group, San Diego, pp 227–253

Buettner A, Beer A, Hannig C, Settles M (2001) Observation of the swallowing process by application of videofluoroscopy and real-time magnetic resonance imaging–consequences for retronasal aroma stimulation. Chem Senses 26: 1211–1219

Chan CB, Chan LK, Lam HS (2002) Scattered radiation level during videofluoroscopy for swallowing study. Clin Radiol 57:614–616

Curtis DJ, Cruess DF, Willgress ER (1987) Abnormal solid bolus swallowing in the erect position. Dysphagia 2:46–49

Ekberg O (1986) Posture of the head and pharyngeal swallow. Acta Radiol Diagn 27:691–696

Ekberg O, Sjöberg S (1995) Neck pain and dysphagia. MRI of retropharyngitis. J Comput Assist Tomogr 19:555–558

Hamlet SL, Stone M, Shawker TH (1988) Posterior tongue grooving in deglutition and speech: preliminary observations. Dysphagia 3:65–68

Kelly JE Jr (1961) The marshmallow as an aid to radiologic examination of the esophagus. N Engl J Med 265: 1306–1307

Langmore SE, Schatz K, Olsen N (1988) Fiberendoscopic examination of swallowing safety: a new procedure. Dysphagia 2:216–219

McConnel FMS (1988) Analysis of pressure generation and bolus transit during pharyngeal swallowing. Laryngoscope 98:71–78

McConnel FMS, Cerenko D, Hersh T, Weil LJ (1988a) Evaluation of pharyngeal dysphagia with manofluorography. Dysphagia 2:187–195

McConnel FMS, Cerenko D, Jackson RT, Hersh T (1988b) Clinical application of the manofluorogram. Laryngoscope 98:705–711

Nilsson H, Ekberg O, Olsson R, Hindfelt B (1995) Oral function test for monitoring suction and swallowing in the neurologic patient. Dysphagia 10:93–100

Nilsson H, Ekberg O, Bülow M, Hindfelt B (1997) Assessment of respiration during video fluoroscopy of dysphagic patients. Acad Radiol 4:503–507

Olsson R, Ekberg O (1995) Videomanometry of the pharynx in dysphagic patients with a posterior cricopharyngeal indentation. Acad Radiol 2:597–601

Olsson R, Nilsson H, Ekberg O (1994) Pharyngeal solid-state manometry catheter movement during swallowing in dysphagic and nondysphagic participants. Acad Radiol 1: 339–344

Olsson R, Castell JA, Castell DO, Ekberg O (1995) Solid-state computerized manometry improves diagnostic yield in pharyngeal dysphagia: simultaneous videoradiography and manometry in dysphagia patients with normal barium swallows. Abdom Imag 20:230–235

Olsson R, Kjellin O, Ekberg O (1996) Videomanometric aspects of pharyngeal constrictor activity. Dysphagia 11: 83–86

Somers S, Stevenson GW, Thompson G (1986) Comparison of endoscopy and barium swallow with marshmallow in dysphagia. J Can Assoc Radiol 37:72–75

van Westen D, Ekberg O (1993) Solid bolus swallowing in the radiologic evaluation of dysphagia. Acta Radiol 34: 332–375

Pharyngeal Morphology

Stephen E. Rubesin

Contents

Abstract

This chapter discusses the radiographic findings of structural abnormalities of the pharynx.

1 Introduction

There is no dividing line between morphologic and functional disorders of the pharynx. Structural abnormalities frequently cause abnormal pharyngeal motility. Motility disorders often are manifested by abnormal pharyngeal structure. Therefore, examination of the pharynx requires a dynamic examination of motility in combination with static images of morphology. The radiologist tailors the dynamic (videofluoroscopy) and morphologic (spot image) examination to the patient's clinical history, symptoms, and the initial fluoroscopic findings (Rubesin and Glick 1988; Rubesin and Stiles 1997). This chapter will discuss morphologic disorders of the pharynx.

2 Surface Anatomy Pertinent to Roentgen Interpretation

The principles of interpreting roentgen images of the pharynx are the same as in the evaluation of the remainder of the gastrointestinal tract (Rubesin and Laufer 1991). The shape of the pharynx is determined by the tongue, laryngeal cartilages (epiglottic, thyroid, cricoid, and arytenoid cartilages), the pharyngeal musculature, and the supporting skeleton. The normal surface of distended pharyngeal mucosa is smooth (Fig. 1), except in the regions of the palatine and

S. E. Rubesin (✉)
Department of Radiology,
University of Pennsylvania School of Medicine,
MRI Building 1-08, University of Pennsylvania
Medical Center, 3400 Spruce St.,
Philadelphia, PA 19104-4283, USA
e-mail: Stephen.Rubesin@uphs.upenn.edu

O. Ekberg (ed.), *Dysphagia*, Medical Radiology. Diagnostic Imaging, DOI: 10.1007/174_2011_344,
© Springer-Verlag Berlin Heidelberg 2012

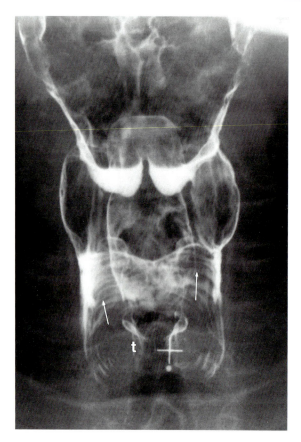

Fig. 1 Arcuate lines in hypopharynx. After the patient aspirated a small amount of barium, this spot radiograph of the pharynx shows the relationship of the barium-coated larynx (right true vocal cord identified with *t*) to the hypopharynx. The larynx acts as an extrinsic mass impression upon the lower hypopharynx. Arcuate lines (*arrows*) reflect redundant mucosa in the hypopharynx. As long as the arcuate lines are smooth and thin, no tumor or inflammatory process should be considered. (Reproduced with permission from Rubesin and Glick 1988, Fig. 11a)

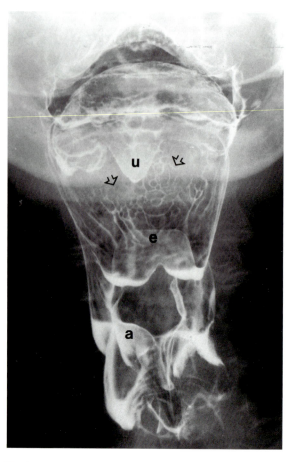

Fig. 2 Mucosal surface base of tongue. Spot radiograph of the pharynx demonstrating a reticular pattern (representative area identified by *open arrows*) reflecting barium filling the interstices of the fine nodular surface of the base of the tongue. The reticular surface reflects the underlying lingual tonsil. Disruption of the normal, relatively flat reticular surface of the tongue is abnormal. Also identified are the uvula (*u*) and epiglottic tip (*e*). The mucosa overlying the muscular processes of the arytenoid cartilages (right arytenoid cartilage identified by *a*) is elevated owing to radiation-induced edema. The left hypopharynx, the site of the radiated cancer, is contracted

lingual tonsils. The normal surface of the palatine and lingual tonsils is slightly nodular because of the underlying lymphoid tissue (Figs. 2, 3) (Gromet et al. 1982). When the pharynx is slightly collapsed, barium-coated striations may be seen (Fig. 4a) (Rubesin et al. 1987a). These lines reflect the underlying vertically oriented inner longitudinal muscle layer of the pharynx: the fibers and aponeurosis of the salpingopharyngeal, stylopharyngeal, and palatopharyngeal muscles (Fig. 4b). Transversely oriented lines are seen in the lower hypopharynx and reflect redundant epithelium overlying the muscular processes of the arytenoid cartilages and cricoid cartilage. Thus, any

nodularity or focal barium collection that disrupts the smooth mucosal surface of the lateral or posterior pharyngeal wall is suspicious for an inflammatory or neoplastic process.

During pharyngography, the mucosa behind the cricoid cartilage appears undulating (Fig. 5a). Although this prominent postcricoid mucosa was thought to reflect a venous plexus (Pitman and Fraser 1965), redundant squamous epithelium and submucosa explain the radiographic findings (Fig. 5b) (Rubesin et al. 1987a). As long as the postcricoid

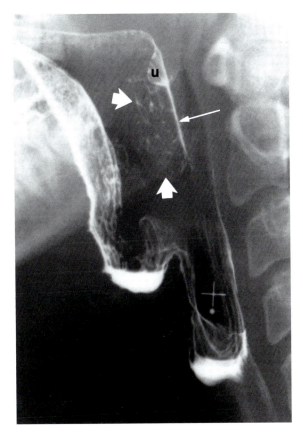

Fig. 3 Normal mucosal surface of the palatine tonsils. Spot radiograph of the pharynx showing barium filling the interstices of the normal lymphoid tissue of the palatine tonsil (*thick arrows*). Also note the uvular tip (*u*) of the soft palate and the palatopharyngeal fold (*long arrow*). (Reproduced with permission from Rubesin et al. 1987b, Fig. 2b)

mucosa changes size and shape during swallowing, a postcricoid tumor need not be considered.

3   Pouches and Diverticula

Pouches are transient protrusions at sites of anatomic weakness of the pharyngeal wall, whereas diverticula are persistent protrusions of pharyngeal mucosa and submucosa at these same sites (Perrot 1962).

3.1   Lateral Pharyngeal Pouches and Diverticula

The lateral pharyngeal wall most frequently protrudes in the region of the thyrohyoid membrane (Fig. 6), an area bounded superiorly by the greater cornu of the hyoid bone, inferiorly by the ala of the thyroid cartilage, anteriorly by the posterior border of the thyrohyoid muscle, and posteriorly by the superior cornu of the thyroid cartilage and the insertion of the stylopharyngeal muscle (Fig. 7) (DuBrul 1980). The unsupported portion of thyrohyoid membrane is perforated by the superior laryngeal artery and vein and the internal laryngeal branch of the superior laryngeal nerve (Pernkopf 1989). It is not known what happens to this space during swallowing, when the hyoid bone and thyroid cartilage are brought together by contraction of the thyrohyoid muscle.

Lateral pharyngeal pouches are extremely common, the incidence increasing with patient age. Only a small percentage (about 5%) of patients with lateral pharyngeal pouches are symptomatic, complaining of dysphagia, choking, or regurgitation of undigested food (Curtis et al. 1988; Lindbichler et al. 1998).

During swallowing, in the frontal view, lateral pharyngeal pouches are manifested as transient sac-like protrusions (Fig. 8) of the lateral wall above the notch in the lateral pharyngeal wall that denotes the junction of the ala of the thyroid cartilage and the thyrohyoid membrane. The neck of the sac changes size during swallowing when the thyroid cartilage is raised to appose the hyoid bone. On the lateral view, pouches are manifested as barium-filled sacs on the anterior hypopharyngeal wall just below the hyoid bone at the level of the valleculae. Barium retained in the pouches is spilled into the lateral swallowing channels just after the bolus passes.

Lateral pharyngeal diverticula are persistent protrusions at the level of the thyrohyoid membrane. These diverticula are barium-filled sacs which usually fill via a narrow neck. In contrast to lateral pharyngeal pouches, lateral pharyngeal diverticula are often unilateral (Fig. 9).

3.2   Branchial Cleft Cysts and Fistulas

Branchial clefts are grooves of ectodermal origin that develop on both sides of the neck in a 4-week-old embryo (Hyams et al. 1988; Maran and Buchanan 1978). The branchial pouches are four pharyngeal outpouchings of endodermal origin that meet the branchial clefts. The first branchial cleft forms the

Fig. 4 Lines of the pharynx. **a** Spot radiograph showing vertically oriented striations (*arrows*) in the lateral and posterior surface of the hypopharynx. These lines reflect the underlying longitudinal muscle layer. **b** Low-power photomicrograph of the lateral pharyngeal wall showing close apposition of the squamous epithelium (*short arrow*) to the longitudinal muscle layer (*long arrowhead*). Only a thin tunica propria (*long straight arrow*) separates the squamous epithelium from the longitudinal muscle layer. The constrictor muscle layer is identified by a curved arrow. (Reproduced with permission from Rubesin and Glick 1988, Figs. 5a, 6)

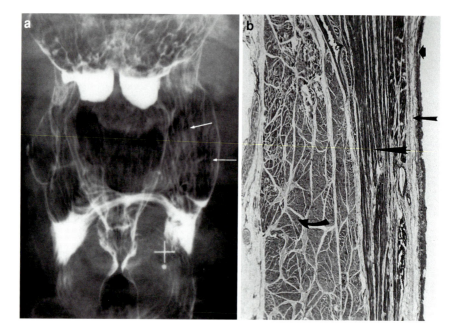

Fig. 5 Postcricoid mucosa. **a** Spot radiograph of the pharynx obtained while the bolus was passing through the pharyngoesophageal segment showing undulating mucosa (*arrows*) just behind the cricoid cartilage. **b** Low-power photomicrograph obtained at the level of the cricoid cartilage (*thick arrow*) showing a sinuous squamous epithelium (*curved arrows*) corresponding to the undulating mucosa seen in **a**. The submucosa (*long arrow*) is very thick at this level, reflecting the need for this area to move easily. Compare the thickness of the submucosa here with the thickness of the tunica propria in Fig. 4b. The cricoarytenoid muscle (*arrowhead*) lies posterior to the cricoid cartilage. (**a** Reproduced with permission from Rubesin 2000a, Fig. 47a; **b** reproduced with permission from Rubesin and Glick 1988, Fig. 8)

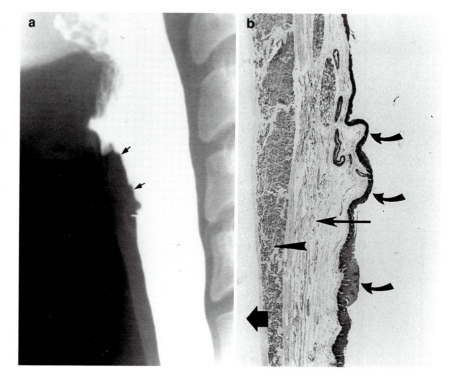

Fig. 6 The thyrohyoid membrane. **a** Spot radiograph of the pharynx showing focal indentation of the contour of the lateral hypopharyngeal wall (*arrow*). This marks the transition between the hypopharynx that lies above the ala of the thyroid cartilage and the portion of hypopharynx confined by the thyroid cartilage. **b** Corresponding line drawing demonstrating the point where the anterolateral hypopharyngeal wall becomes confined by the thyroid cartilage (*arrow*). The thyrohyoid membrane (*t*) bridges the space between the hyoid bone (*b*) and the thyroid cartilage (*c*). Also note the epiglottic cartilage (*e*) and cricoid cartilage (*Cr*). (Reproduced with permission from Rubesin et al. 1987a, Fig. 10a and b)

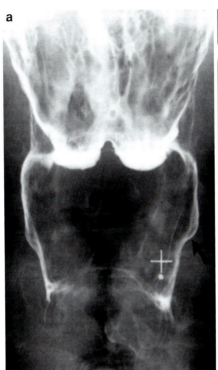
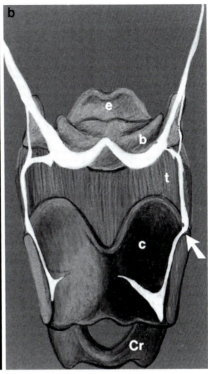

external auditory meatus. The second branchial cleft forms the middle ear, eustachian tube, and floor of the tonsillar fossa. The third and fourth branchial pouches form the piriform sinuses. Persistence of either a branchial cleft or a branchial pouch may result in a sinus tract or cyst.

The most common branchial vestige is a cyst arising from the second branchial cleft. Small second branchial cleft cysts lie anterior to the sternocleidomastoid muscle. Larger cysts may extend below the sternocleidomastoid muscle between the internal and external carotid arteries. These cysts only rarely communicate with the pharynx (Bachman et al. 1968).

Branchial pouch sinuses end blindly in the soft tissue of the neck. Branchial pouch fistulas extend to the skin. Branchial pouch sinuses and fistulas arise from the tonsillar fossa (second pouch), the upper anterolateral wall of the piriform sinus (third pouches), and the lower anterolateral wall of the piriform sinus (fourth pouches). Although most of these sinuses and pouches are present at birth, sinus tracts are occasionally detected for the first time in adults (Fig. 10).

3.3 Zenker's Diverticulum

Zenker's diverticulum (posterior pharyngeal diverticulum) is an acquired mucosal herniation through Killian's dehiscence, a gap in the region of the cricopharyngeal muscle, found in about one third of individuals on autopsy (Zaino et al. 1970). There is considerable variation in the anatomy of the thyropharyngeal muscle and the cricopharyngeal muscle. Thus, Killian's dehiscence has been described as arising either between the thyropharyngeal muscle and the cricopharyngeal muscle or between the oblique and transverse fibers of the cricopharyngeal muscle (Perrot 1962; Zaino et al. 1967, 1970).

The relationship between Zenker's diverticulum and the function of the cricopharyngeal muscle is not known. In some studies, upper esophageal sphincter (UES) pressure is normal (there is no spasm), the muscle relaxes completely during swallowing (there is no achalasia), and there is normal coordination between pharyngeal contraction and UES relaxation (Knuff et al. 1982; Frieling et al. 1988). Other studies have suggested that there is either abnormal

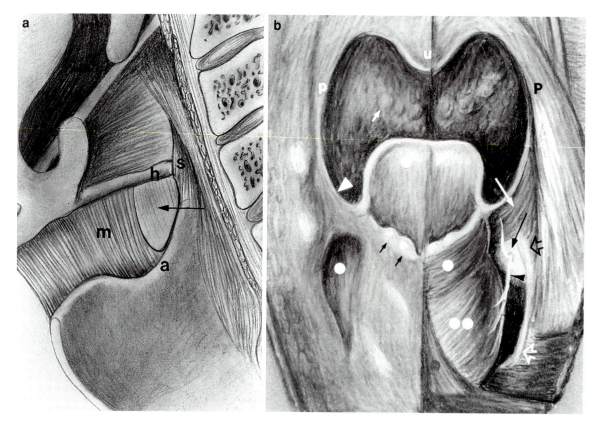

Fig. 7 Location of lateral pharyngeal pouches. **a** Line drawing performed in the lateral view showing the location of the unsupported portion of the thyrohyoid membrane (*arrow*): posterior to the thyrohyoid muscle (*m*) and membrane, anterior to the superior cornu of the thyroid cartilage and inserting fibers of the stylopharyngeal muscle (*s*), inferior to the hyoid bone (*h*), and superior to the ala of the thyroid cartilage (*a*). **b** Dissection of the pharynx viewed from behind showing the unsupported portion of the thyrohyoid membrane (*black arrow*) and the internal branch of the superior laryngeal nerve (*black*

arrowheads). The thyroid cartilage is identified by *open arrows*. Also identified are the palatopharyngeal fold (*white P*) and its corresponding palatopharyngeal muscle (*black P*), the uvula (*u*), the circumvallate papillae (*tiny white arrow*), the left pharyngo-epiglottic fold (*arrowhead*), the left piriform sinus (*one white dot on the left*), the mucosa overlying the cuneiform and corniculate cartilages (*tiny black arrows*), the right arytenoid muscle (*one white dot on the right*, and the cricoarytenoid muscle (*two white dots on the right*). (Reproduced with permission from Rubesin et al. 1987a, Figs. 8b, 11c)

relaxation of the UES or incoordination of pharyngeal contraction. It is also not known whether chronic gastroesophageal reflux predisposes to the development of Zenker's diverticulum. Clearly, between 65 and 95% of patients with Zenker's diverticulum have gastroesophageal reflux (Smiley et al. 1970; Delahunty et al. 1971; Rubesin and Levine 2001).

Zenker's diverticulum is usually first detected in elderly patients who complain of dysphagia, halitosis, choking, hoarseness, or regurgitation of undigested food. Zenker's diverticulum is not infrequently found in asymptomatic individuals or patients being studied for symptoms of gastroesophageal reflux disease. Change in the character of dysphagia or bloody discharge in a patient with a known Zenker's

diverticulum suggests development of a complication such as ulceration, fistula formation, or carcinoma (Nanson 1976; Shirazi et al. 1977).

Radiographically, in the frontal view, Zenker's diverticulum appears as a barium-filled sac midline below the tips of the piriform sinuses (Figs. 11, 12). In the lateral view, Zenker's diverticulum appears as a barium-filled sac posterior to a prominent pharyngoesophageal segment and the upper cervical esophagus (see Fig. 12). During swallowing, Zenker's diverticulum appears as a protrusion of the lower hypopharyngeal wall posterior to the expected luminal contour, the neck of the diverticulum originating above a "prominent" pharyngoesophageal segment. The opening of the diverticulum may be very large

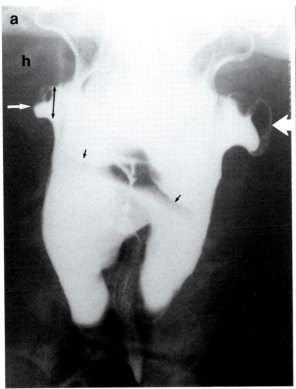
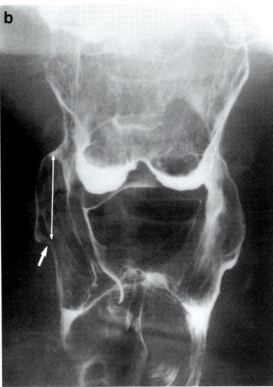

Fig. 8 Lateral pharyngeal pouches. **a** Spot radiograph obtained during drinking showing a small right (*small white arrow*) and larger left (*large white arrow*) lateral pharyngeal pouch. Note the relationship with the hyoid bone (*h*). The epiglottis (*small black arrows*) is tilting asymmetrically. Note the height of the right lateral pharyngeal pouch (*double arrow*) while the patient drinks the bolus.

b Spot radiograph obtained just after the swallow in **a** showing that the pharynx has descended to its normal resting position. The notch identifying the superior border of the thyroid cartilage is identified (*white arrow*). Note the difference in height of the thyrohyoid membrane during swallowing (*double arrow* in **a**) and at rest (*double arrow* in **b**)

during swallowing, almost 2 cm in height (Fig. 13). After the swallow has passed, barium regurgitates back into the hypopharynx, in rare cases, resulting in overflow aspiration. Any irregularity of the contour of the diverticulum suggests development of an ulcer or carcinoma (Wychulis et al. 1969).

Zenker's diverticulum should not be confused with a "pseudo-Zenker's diverticulum," barium trapped above a cricopharyngeal bar that has either opened incompletely or closed early (Fig. 14). Some pseudo-Zenker's diverticula are pouches arising at Killian's dehiscence. It is not known whether a Zenker's diverticulum can develop from a pseudo-Zenker's diverticulum. This author believes that many pseudo-Zenker's diverticula result from cricopharyngeal response to gastroesophageal reflux (Brady et al. 1995).

3.4 Killian-Jamieson Pouches and Diverticula

Killian-Jamieson diverticula protrude through the Killian-Jamieson space, a gap in the muscle of the proximal cervical esophagus. This gap is bounded superiorly by the inferior margin of the cricopharyngeal muscle, anteriorly by the inferior margin of the cricoid cartilage, and inferomedially by the suspensory ligament of the esophagus just below its origin on the posterior lamina of the cricoid cartilage (Killian 1908). These diverticula are also known as "proximal lateral cervical esophageal diverticula" or "lateral diverticula from the pharyngoesophageal junction area" (Ekberg and Nylander 1983a). Patients with Killian-Jamieson diverticula are usually asymptomatic or have symptoms caused by abnormal pharyngeal motility (Rubesin and Levine 2001).

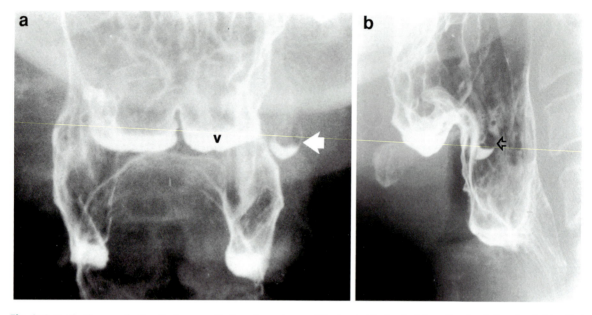

Fig. 9 Lateral pharyngeal diverticulum. **a** Spot radiograph obtained with the patient in the frontal position showing a 5-mm ovoid sac (*arrow*), partially filled with barium. Note that the diverticulum protruding from the left lateral upper hypopharyngeal wall is about at the level of the valleculae (left vallecula identified with *v*). **b** Spot radiograph obtained with the patient in the lateral position showing that the ovoid diverticulum (*arrow*) arises from the anterior portion of the lateral hypopharyngeal wall

During pharyngography, the opening of the Killian-Jamieson diverticulum lies just below the cricopharyngeal muscle (Fig. 15). The opening of the sac changes size and shape with elevation of the cervical esophagus during swallowing (see Fig. 15). The sac of the diverticulum lies lateral to the proximal cervical esophagus on frontal views and overlaps the cervical esophagus on lateral views. Killian-Jamieson diverticula are more frequently unilateral than bilateral and are usually left-sided (Fig. 16) (Rubesin and Levine 2001). Bilateral diverticula are seen in about one quarter of patients. Killian-Jamieson diverticula are smaller than Zenker's diverticula, averaging about 1.4 cm (Rubesin and Levine 2001). Regurgitation of barium from the sac into the hypopharynx is uncommon because regurgitation is prevented by the cricopharyngeal muscle. Occasionally, Killian-Jamieson diverticula and a Zenker's diverticulum are seen in the same patient (Fig. 17).

Pouches are also frequently detected at the Killian-Jamieson space. These pouches may be related to early closure of the upper cervical esophagus, a finding associated with gastroesophageal reflux. On the frontal view, pouches appear as shallow, broad-based protrusions of the lateral proximal cervical esophageal wall; these pouches are effaced during swallowing (Ekberg and Nylander 1983a).

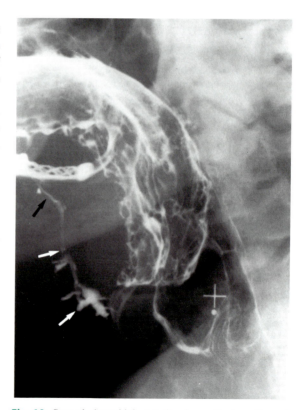

Fig. 10 Second branchial pouch sinus. Spot radiograph obtained with the patient in a steep right posterior oblique position showing an irregular barium-filled track (*arrows*) arising from the region of the right palatine fossa. (Reproduced with permission from Rubesin and Glick 1988, Fig. 23b)

Fig. 11 Small Zenker's diverticulum. **a** Spot radiograph obtained with the patient in the frontal position showing a 5-mm ovoid barium-filled sac (*arrow*) midline below the tips of the piriform sinuses. **b** Spot radiograph obtained with the patient in the lateral position showing a 4-mm barium-filled sac (*arrow*) posterior to the expected lumen of the pharyngoesophageal segment. Note that this tiny diverticulum persists after swallowing but does not extend posterior to the pharyngoesophageal segment

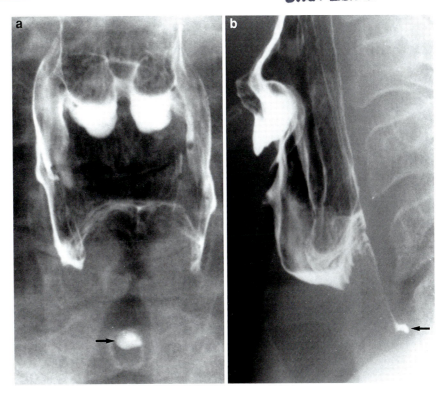

Fig. 12 Moderately large Zenker's diverticulum. **a** Spot radiograph obtained with the patient in the frontal position showing a 3-cm barium-filled sac (*arrow*) midline below the tips of the piriform sinuses. **b** Spot radiograph obtained with the patient in the lateral position showing a relatively flat, but long barium-filled sac (*large arrows*) posterior to the pharyngoesophageal segment and upper cervical esophagus (*small arrow*)

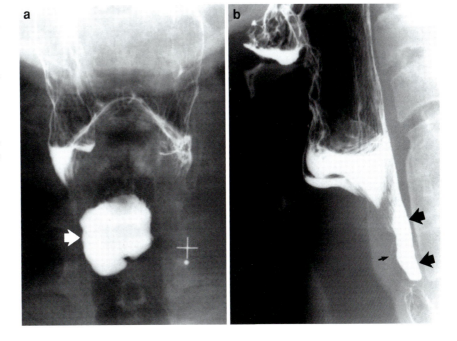

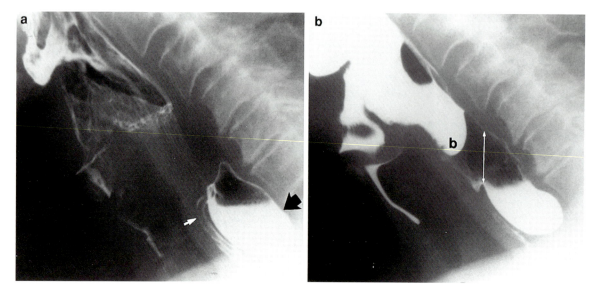

Fig. 13 Opening of a moderately large Zenker's diverticulum. **a** Spot radiograph obtained with the patient at rest and in the lateral position showing a 2 cm × 3 cm sac (*large arrow*) posterior to the pharyngoesophageal segment (*small arrow*) and upper cervical esophagus. **b** Spot radiograph obtained just as the bolus (*b*) had approached the pharyngoesophageal segment showing that the opening (*double arrow*) of the Zenker's diverticulum is very high, at least the height of one vertebral body. Barium entering the laryngeal vestibule was due to abnormal timing between the oral and pharyngeal phases of swallowing. (**b** Reproduced with permission from Rubesin 1991, Fig. 5c)

Fig. 14 Pseudo-Zenker's diverticulum. **a** Spot image obtained during swallowing showing no evidence of a diverticulum at the level of the cricoid cartilage, as identified by redundant postcricoid mucosa (*open arrow*). **b** Spot image obtained just after the swallow had passed showing barium trapped (*arrow*) above a cricopharyngeal bar that had closed early. Seconds later the pseudo-Zenker's diverticulum disappeared when the collection of barium entered the cervical esophagus

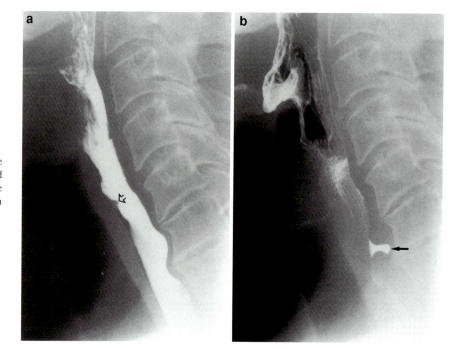

Fig. 15 Killian-Jamieson diverticula. **a** Spot radiograph obtained at the end of the swallow showing a 1.3-cm diverticulum (*thick arrow*) arising from the left lateral wall just below the level of the cricopharyngeal muscle. The neck (*double arrow*) of the diverticulum is broad during swallowing. **b** Spot radiograph obtained just after the bolus had passed showing a narrower neck (*double arrow*) of the diverticulum. **c** Spot radiograph obtained with the patient in the lateral position showing a 1.3-cm diverticulum (*large arrow*) below the level of the cricopharyngeal muscle. Part of the diverticulum lies anterior to the expected course of the pharyngoesophageal segment and upper cervical esophagus (*small arrow*). Barium in the laryngeal vestibule and proximal trachea was related to a pharyngeal motor disorder. **d** Spot radiograph obtained during swallowing demonstrating that part of the diverticulum (*white arrow*) lies anterior to the pharyngoesophageal segment. The presence of a prominent cricopharyngeal muscle (*black arrow*) demonstrates that the diverticulum lies below the cricopharyngeal muscle. (Reproduced with permission from Rubesin and Levine 2001, Fig. 1)

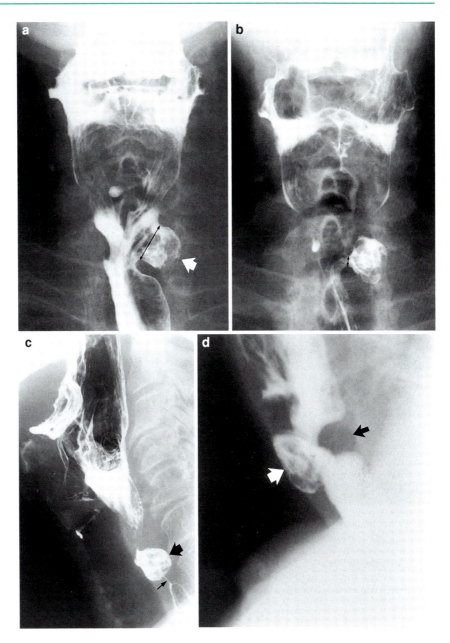

4 Inflammatory and Other Lesions

4.1 Lymphoid Hyperplasia

The normal surface of the base of the tongue has a reticular pattern created by the underlying lingual tonsil, an aggregate of 30–100 follicles extending from the circumvallate papillae to the root of the epiglottis (see Fig. 2) (Gromet et al. 1982). Hypertrophy of the lingual tonsils may occur after puberty, as a compensatory response to tonsillectomy/adenoidectomy, or as nonspecific response to allergy or repeated infection.

Hypertrophy of the lingual tonsils disrupts the normal reticular surface pattern. There are no radiographic criteria, however, to differentiate nodularity of the base of the tongue attributed to the normal

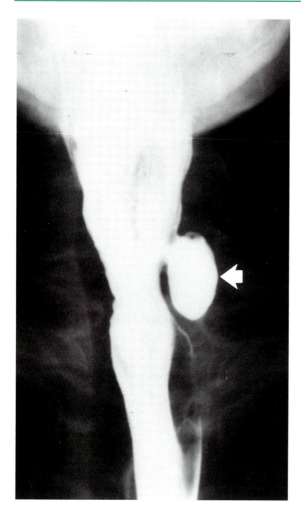

Fig. 16 Killian-Jamieson diverticulum. Spot radiograph obtained during swallowing showing a 1.5-cm barium-filled sac (*arrow*) arising from the left lateral wall near the pharyngoesophageal segment. After swallowing the orifice of the diverticulum was shown to be below the cricopharyngeal muscle (Reproduced with permission from Rubesin and Levine 2001, Fig. 2)

lingual tonsil from that of lymphoid hyperplasia. On frontal views in patients with lymphoid hyperplasia, there are large 5–7 mm, smooth-surfaced nodules carpeting the vertical surface of the tongue (Figs. 18, 19a). On the lateral view, these nodules protrude posteriorly (Fig. 19b). With severe lymphoid hyperplasia, nodules may be detected in the valleculae, on the lingual surface of the epiglottis, and in the upper hypopharynx. Although lymphoid hyperplasia can appear coarsely nodular, asymmetrically distributed, or masslike, if any asymmetric or masslike nodularity

is demonstrated radiographically, carcinoma or lymphoma should be excluded via ENT examination and/or MRI.

4.2 Acute Pharyngitis

Acute epiglottitis usually affects children between 3 and 6 years of age, but may also be seen in adults (Harris et al. 1970). Plain film diagnosis is important, as manipulation of the tongue/pharynx or barium studies may exacerbate edema and trigger acute respiratory arrest (Balfe and Heiken 1986). Smooth enlargement of the epiglottis and aryepiglottic folds allows plain film diagnosis of severe epiglottitis.

Barium studies are usually not performed in immunocompetent patients with acute sore throat. In immunocompromised patients, barium studies are used to demonstrate the presence, type, and severity of esophagitis. Thus, in patients with AIDS, a double-contrast examination may demonstrate the small ulcers of herpetic pharyngitis or the plaques of *Candida* pharyngitis (Fig. 20) (Rubesin and Glick 1988). Acute inflammatory disorders may cause laryngeal penetration due to abnormal pharyngeal elevation, epiglottic tilt, or laryngeal closure.

Videopharyngography may be performed, however, on patients with acute odynophagia or dysphagia after trauma or suspected iatrogenic trauma. A nonionic water-soluble contrast agent is given first, followed by an ionic, water-soluble contrast agent if no laryngeal penetration is seen (Fig. 21). When no perforation is demonstrated with a water-soluble contrast agent, this author prefers to give high-density barium, as this form of barium sticks to the mucosal surface and is easier to detect in the extraluminal soft tissues than thin barium.

4.3 Chronic Inflammatory Conditions

In patients with acute corrosive ingestion, water-soluble contrast agent studies may be utilized to exclude perforation of the pharynx, esophagus, or stomach. Corrosive ingestion can result in amputation of the uvula and epiglottis and diffuse ulceration. With healing and scarring, epiglottic and pharyngeal

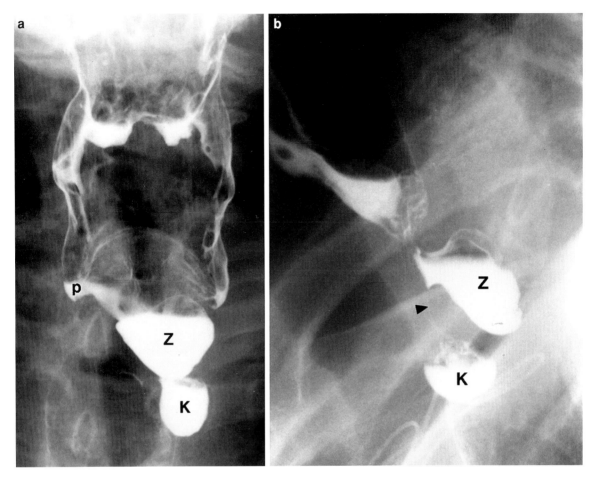

Fig. 17 Zenker's diverticulum and left lateral Killian-Jamieson diverticulum arising in same patient. **a** Spot radiograph obtained with the patient in the frontal position demonstrating a 3-cm barium-filled Zenker's diverticulum (Z) positioned slightly to the left of the midline. Barium in the right piriform sinus (p) results from reflux of barium from the Zenker's diverticulum back into the hypopharynx. A 1.6-cm left lateral, barium-filled Killian-Jamieson diverticulum (K) lies below and to the left of the Zenker's diverticulum. **b** Spot radiograph obtained with the patient in a steep right posterior oblique position showing that the Zenker's diverticulum (Z) extends posterior to the pharyngoesophageal segment (*arrowhead*). Part of the Killian-Jamieson diverticulum (K) lies anterior to the course of the proximal cervical esophagus. (Reproduced with permission from Rubesin and Levine 2001, Fig. 3)

wall deformity results in pharyngeal dysmotility (Fig. 22).

Aphthous stomatitis and oropharyngeal ulceration with subsequent scarring may be seen in Behçet's syndrome, bullous pemphigoid, epidermolysis bullosa, Reiter's syndrome, and Stevens-Johnson syndrome (Bosma et al. 1968; Kabakian and Dahmash 1978). Amputation of the uvula and tip of the epiglottis may be detected radiographically (Bosma et al. 1968).

4.4 Webs

Webs are thin folds of epithelium and lamina propria most frequently found on the anterior wall of the lower hypopharynx and proximal cervical esophagus (Clements et al. 1974). Pharyngeal and cervical esophageal webs are seen in 3–8% of patients undergoing an upper gastrointestinal examination and in up to 16% of patients on autopsy (Seaman 1967; Clements et al. 1974; Nosher et al. 1975; Ekberg

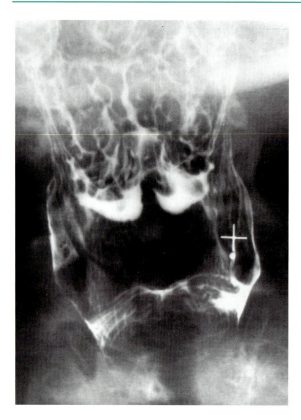

Fig. 18 Lymphoid hyperplasia, base of tongue. Frontal view showing many large, 5–7 mm nodules carpeting the surface of the base of the tongue. (Reproduced with permission from Rubesin et al. 1987a, Fig. 9c)

1981; Ekberg and Nylander 1983b). Some webs are the result of diseases that cause chronic inflammation and scarring, such as epidermolysis bullosa and benign mucous membrane pemphigoid. Webs in the valleculae or piriform sinuses may be normal variants (Ekberg et al. 1986). This author believes that some cervical esophageal webs are related to chronic gastroesophageal reflux, similar to the association of distal esophageal webs and gastroesophageal reflux disease (Weaver et al. 1984). The association of cervical esophageal webs, iron-deficiency anemia, and pharyngeal or esophageal carcinoma—the Plummer–Vinson or Patterson–Kelly syndrome—is controversial (Waldenstrom and Kjellberg 1939; Mcnab-Jones 1961).

Webs are manifested radiographically as 1–2 mm in height, shelflike radiolucent filling defects on the anterior wall of the pharyngoesophageal segment or proximal cervical esophagus. Larger webs may protrude deeply into the lumen or extend circumferentially around the wall of the cervical esophagus (Fig. 23).

Dilatation of the pharynx or cervical esophagus proximal to the web or a stream of barium spurting through the web (the "jet phenomenon") is a sign of partial obstruction and is usually seen in symptomatic patients (Shauffer et al. 1977; Taylor et al. 1990). Webs should not be confused with redundant mucosa just posterior to the cricoid cartilage or a prominent cricopharyngeal muscle (Fig. 24).

5   Tumors

5.1   Benign Tumors

A wide variety of benign tumors originate in the pharynx (Hyams et al. 1988; Bachman 1978). Retention cysts are lined by squamous epithelium and filled with desquamated debris. These cysts are the most common benign tumors of the base of the tongue (Fig. 25) and aryepiglottic folds (Fig. 26) (Bachman 1978). Ectopic thyroid tissue, thyroglossal duct cysts, granular cell tumors, and benign tumors of minor mucoserous salivary gland origin also arise in the base of the tongue. Saccular cysts of the aryepiglottic folds are the mucus-filled variant of internal laryngoceles, arising from mucous-secreting glands of the appendix of the laryngeal ventricle. Lipomas, neurofibromas, granular cell tumors, and oncocytomas rarely also be seen in the aryepiglottic folds (Mannsson et al. 1978; Patterson et al. 1981; Hyams et al. 1988). Tumors related to neurofibromatosis (von Recklinghausen's disease) typically occur in the aryepiglottic folds (Fig. 27) and arytenoid cartilages (Chang-Lo 1977). Chondromas may originate in the posterior lamina of the cricoid cartilage (Hyams and Rabuzzi 1970).

Benign pharyngeal tumors are usually sessile submucosal masses, appearing radiographically *en face* as smooth, round, sharply circumscribed protrusions (see Fig. 26) and in profile as hemispheric lines with abrupt angulation to the luminal contour (see Fig. 25). (Balfe and Heiken 1986). Pedunculated tumors such as lipoma, papilloma, and fibrovascular polyp are uncommon.

5.2   Squamous Cell Carcinoma

Squamous cell carcinomas constitute 90% of malignant pharyngeal lesions (Hyams et al. 1988; Cunningham and Catlin 1967). Multiple primary sites

Fig. 19 Lymphoid hyperplasia of palatine tonsils and the base of the tongue. **a** Frontal view demonstrating large left and right palatine tonsils (*arrows*) protruding into the oropharynx. The reticular surface of the base of the tongue is slightly prominent and the nodules are slightly enlarged. **b** Lateral view obtained while the patient sang "Eeee…" showing a slightly nodular mass (*white arrows*) in the tonsillar fossa. Several nodules (*black arrows*) protrude into the barium pooling in the valleculae. (Reproduced with permission from Rubesin 1994, Fig. 17.12)

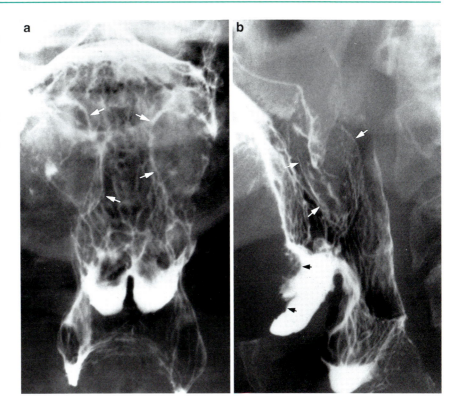

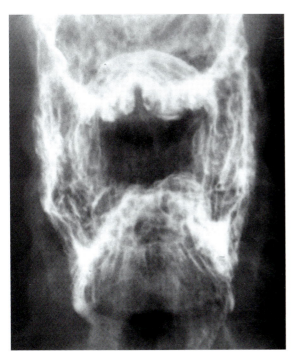

Fig. 20 *Candida* pharyngitis. Frontal view of the pharynx showing numerous small nodules etched in white by barium. The nodules carpet the pharynx. (Reproduced with permission from Rubesin 2000c, Fig. 15.14)

of squamous carcinoma are found in the oral cavity, pharynx, larynx, esophagus, and lung in more than 20% of patients (Carpenter et al. 1976). Between 1 and 20% of patients with a head and neck squamous cell carcinoma will subsequently develop an esophageal squamous cell carcinoma (Goldstein and Zornoza 1978; Thompson et al. 1978).

Squamous cell carcinoma may be initially detected in patients undergoing pharyngoesophagography for pharyngeal symptoms or a palpable neck mass. The symptoms are usually of short duration and include sore throat, dysphagia, odynophagia, choking, or coughing. Hoarseness occurs in patients with laryngeal carcinoma, supraglottic cancers, or tumors infiltrating the arytenoid cartilage and medial pharyngeal wall. Most patients are 50–70 years of age and almost all abuse alcohol and tobacco.

In patients with known pharyngeal carcinoma, pharyngoesophagography assists in planning patient workup and therapy. A pharyngogram establishes baseline motility and helps define the size, extent, and inferior border of the tumor. Barium examination can exclude a synchronous esophageal tumor or a structural disorder (Zenker's diverticulum) that may

Fig. 21 Acute perforation during endoscopy. **a** Scout radiograph showing a large amount of air (arrows) in the retropharyngeal space. The posterior wall of the pharynx (*open arrow*) is deviated anteriorly. **b** Spot radiograph obtained while the patient swallowed water-soluble contrast agent showing a small spurt of contrast agent (*arrow*) just above the cricopharyngeal muscle (*open arrow*). The contrast agent spreads in the retropharyngeal space

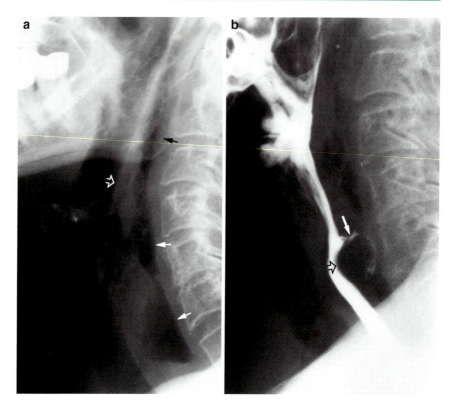

Fig. 22 Sequelae of corrosive ingestion. Twenty years prior to this examination, the patient had ingested lye. **a** Frontal view demonstrating a low and easily seen epiglottis (*white arrows*). The right piriform sinus is contracted; the left piriform sinus has a radiolucent band representing a scar (*black arrow*) crossing its lower portion. **b** Lateral view showing that the truncated epiglottis (*arrow*) is displaced posteriorly. A small amount of barium coats the anterior wall of the laryngeal vestibule. (Reproduced with permission from Rubesin 2000a, Fig. 4.20)

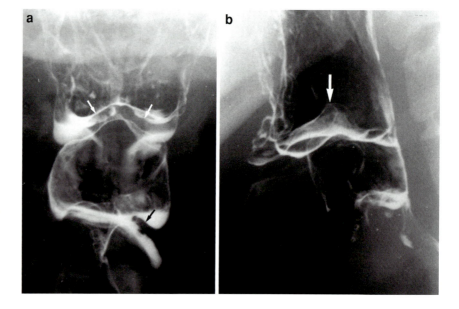

change the way endoscopy is performed or the patient is treated. Pharyngography cannot be used to screen for pharyngeal cancer, as small, flat tumors can be missed in the region of the palatine tonsils or the base of the tongue, areas of normal mucosal nodularity. Below the pharyngoesophageal fold, however, barium studies detect 95% of structural abnormalities (Semenkovich et al. 1985). Barium studies are

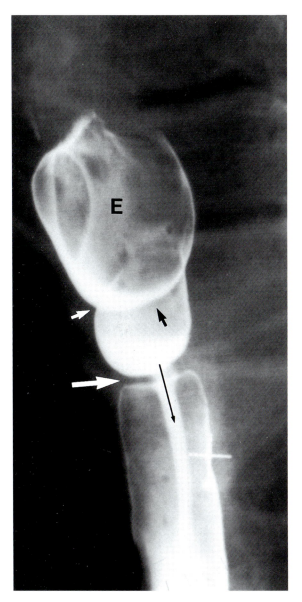

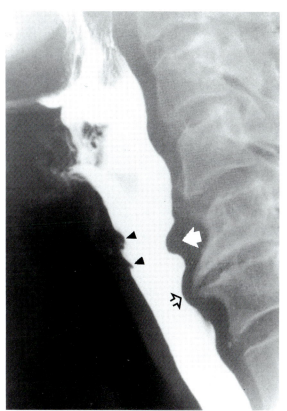

Fig. 24 Postcricoid mucosa, prominent cricopharyngeal muscle, and cervical osteophyte impression. Spot radiograph obtained while the patient was drinking demonstrating osteophytes mildly impressing the upper cervical esophagus (*open black arrow*). Also note a mildly prominent cricopharyngeal muscle (*white arrow*) and redundant mucosa posterior to the cricoid cartilage (*arrowheads*). None of these entities should be confused with cervical esophageal webs. (Reproduced with permission from Rubesin 1995, Fig. 7)

Fig. 23 Cervical esophageal webs. Spot radiograph obtained with the patient in an erect slightly right posterior oblique position showing two circumferential webs in the cervical esophagus. The upper web (*short white and black arrows*) is circumferential and only mildly compromises the lumen. The lower web (*large white arrow*) is also circumferential, but occludes more than two thirds of the luminal diameter. Partial obstruction is manifested by dilatation of the proximal cervical esophagus (*E*) and the "jet phenomenon," barium spurting (*long black arrow*) through the web. (Reproduced with permission from Rubesin 1995, Fig. 1)

especially valuable in the deep valleculae, lower hypopharynx, and pharyngoesophageal segment, areas that are difficult to visualize on endoscopy (Fig. 28).

The radiographic findings of pharyngeal cancer are similar to those for tumors elsewhere in the gastrointestinal tract (Rubesin and Glick 1988). A mass protruding intraluminally may be manifested as loss of the normal expected contour, a focal area of increased radiodensity replacing the original air of the lumen, extra barium-coated lines protruding into the pharyngeal air column (Fig. 29), or a radiolucent filling defect in the barium pool (Fig. 30) (Jing 1970; Balfe and Heiken 1986; Rubesin 2000a; Rubesin and Laufer 1991). Mucosal ulceration is manifested as shallow pools of barium. Surface irregularity is manifested as a granular, finely nodular, or lobulated surface texture (Fig. 31). Asymmetric motion may

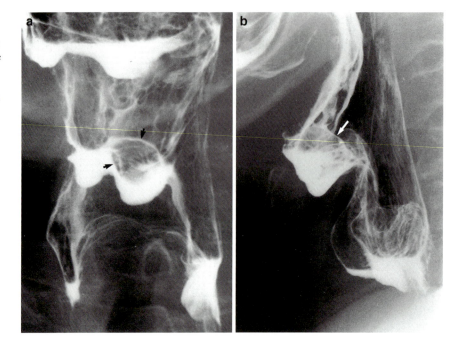

Fig. 25 Retention cyst, left vallecula. **a** Spot radiograph obtained with the patient in a slightly right posterior oblique position showing an ovoid, 1.5-cm radiolucent filling defect (*arrows*) in the barium pool of the left vallecula. **b** Lateral view showing an ovoid area of increased radiodensity (*arrow*) etched by barium

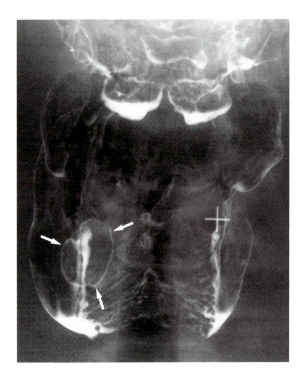

Fig. 26 Retention cyst arising in mucosa overlying the muscular process of the right arytenoid cartilage. A ring shadow (*arrows*) surrounding a 1.7 cm smooth-surfaced area of increased radiodensity is seen. This lesion had been missed on two previous endoscopies. (Reproduced with permission from Rubesin and Glick 1988, Fig. 25a)

result from fixation of structures due to infiltrating tumor (Fig. 32). Asymmetric distensibility may result from an extrinsic mass impinging on the pharynx. In some patients with pharyngeal carcinoma, a focal area of mucosal nodularity is the only radiographic finding (Figs. 33, 34).

The palatine tonsil is the most frequent site of pharyngeal squamous cell carcinoma. Exophytic tumors are easily seen in barium studies. Small infiltrative or ulcerative tumors may be missed in the normally nodular surface of the palatine tonsils. Tonsillar tumors spread to the soft palate, base of the tongue, and posterior pharyngeal wall. Cervical nodal metastases are found in half of patients (Balfe and Heiken 1986).

Squamous cell cancers of the base of the tongue often present as deeply infiltrative, advanced lesions with nodal metastases (Frazell and Lucas 1962; Strong 1979). Lymph node metastases are detected ipsilaterally or bilaterally in more than 70% of patients. Exophytic lesions protrude into the oropharyngeal air space (Jimenez 1970; Apter et al. 1984). Ulcerated lesions appear as irregular barium collections extending deep to the expected contour of the base of the tongue. Tumor spreads to the palatine tonsil, valleculae, or pharyngoepiglottic fold. Small plaquelike or ulcerative lesions may be hidden in the

Fig. 27 Neurofibroma in 27-year-old-man with known neurofibromatosis and stridor. **a** Plain radiograph of the neck obtained with the patient in the lateral position showing a large, round soft-tissue mass (*arrows*) near the aryepiglottic folds. The epiglottic tip (*e*) is identified. **b** Axial image from CT scan showing a soft-tissue mass (*m*) arising from the right aryepiglottic fold (*arrowhead*). The tip of the epiglottis (*small arrow*) is calcified. (**a** Reproduced with permission from Rubesin 1991, Fig. 1a; **b** reproduced with permission from Rubesin 1994, Fig. 17.17b)

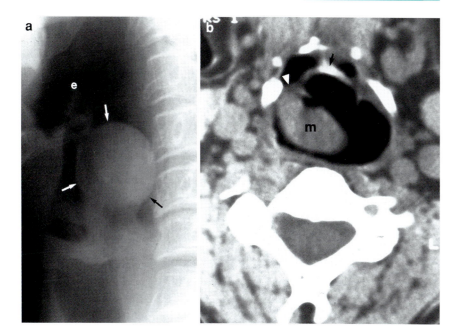

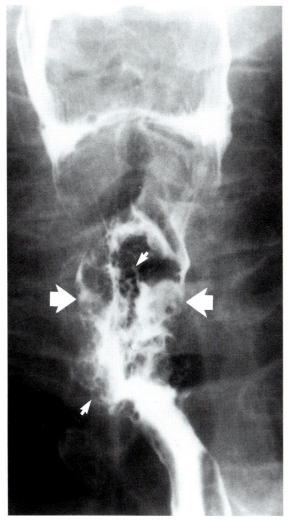

◀**Fig. 28** Carcinoma of the pharyngoesophageal segment missed on ENT endoscopy. Spot radiograph showing mucosal nodularity (representative areas of nodularity identified by *small arrows*) involving the distal hypopharynx, pharyngoesophageal segment, and upper cervical esophagus. The pharyngoesophageal segment is expanded (*large arrows*) by tumor. This patient had two ENT endoscopies within 6 months of the pharyngoesophagram

valleculae or in the recess between the tongue and tonsil.

Supraglottic carcinomas are tumors that arise in the epiglottis (see Fig. 30), aryepiglottic folds, mucosa overlying the muscular processes of the arytenoid cartilages (see Fig. 32), false vocal cords, and laryngeal ventricles. Supraglottic carcinomas spread rapidly through the rich lymphatic network of the supraglottic space. Ulcerative lesions penetrate the tongue, valleculae, and pre-epiglottic space, pharyngoepiglottic folds, and lateral pharyngeal walls (Seaman 1974). A paucity of lymphatics near the true vocal cords limits the spread of supraglottic tumors through the laryngeal ventricles into the true vocal folds. Cervical lymph node metastases are found in 30–50% of patients (Balfe and Heiken 1986; Kirchner and Owen 1977).

Piriform sinus carcinomas are bulky, exophytic lesions that spread quickly and metastasize widely. Medial wall tumors spread to the aryepiglottic fold, arytenoid and cricoid cartilages, and the paraglottic space (Jing 1970; Johnson et al. 1995). Lateral wall tumors (see Fig. 33) may invade the thyrohyoid

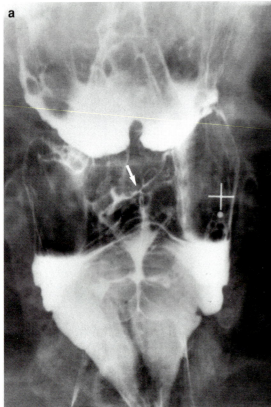

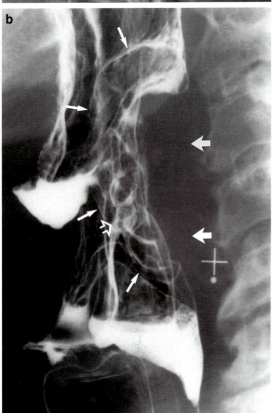

◀**Fig. 29** Radiographic findings of pharyngeal cancer and the value of obtaining multiple projections. **a** Frontal view of the pharynx showing a few barium-etched nodules in the upper hypopharynx (*arrow*). Aspirated barium coats the false and true vocal cords. There is moderate stasis in the hypopharynx. **b** Lateral view demonstrating a large mass arising from the posterior pharyngeal wall as the explanation for the subtle mucosal nodularity seen on the frontal view. The mass is manifested as loss of the normal contour and soft-tissue density partially replacing the air shadow of the lower oropharynx and upper hypopharynx (*large arrows*), barium-etched lines within the lumen (*thin arrows*), and focal mucosal nodularity (*open arrow*). Barium coating the laryngeal vestibule and upper trachea and stasis in the lower hypopharynx is the result of pharyngeal dysmotility. (Reproduced with permission from Rubesin and Glick 1988, Fig. 30a, b)

membrane, thyroid cartilage, and soft tissues of the neck, including the carotid sheath (Zbaren and Egger 1997). Lymph node metastases are found in 70–80% of patients (Balfe and Heiken 1986; Silver 1977).

Carcinomas of the posterior pharyngeal wall are typically long fungating lesions that may spread vertically into the nasopharynx or cervical esophagus. Jugular or retropharyngeal lymphatic metastases are found in 50% of patients (Carpenter et al. 1976).

Postcricoid squamous cell carcinomas are uncommon, annular, infiltrating lesions that may extend into the hypopharynx or cervical esophagus (see Fig. 28). In Scandinavia, these are the tumors that have been associated with Plummer–Vinson syndrome.

5.3   Lymphoma

Lymphomas constitute about 10% of pharyngeal malignancies (Banfi et al. 1970). Almost all pharyngeal lymphomas are non-Hodgkin's lymphoma, arising in the palatine or lingual tonsils or the adenoids. Pharyngeal involvement in Hodgkin's disease occurs in only 1–2% of patients, despite the fact that Hodgkin's disease often begins in cervical lymph nodes (Todd and Michaels 1974).

Lymphoma of the pharynx occurs in the palatine tonsils in 40-60% of patients, the nasopharynx in 18–28% of patients, and the base of the tongue in 10% of patients (Hyams et al. 1988; Al-Saleem et al. 1970). Multiple sites of involvement are seen in 25% of patients. Fifteen percent of patients have bilateral palatine tonsillar involvement (Banfi et al. 1970). Lymphomas only rarely arise in the hypopharynx.

Fig. 30 Spot radiographs versus dynamic imaging in a patient with large supraglottic carcinoma. **a** Image obtained during dynamic imaging showing lack of epiglottic tilt (*black arrow*) and probable epiglottic enlargement. Barium enters the laryngeal vestibule (*white arrow*) during swallowing, with subsequent coating of the laryngeal ventricle and trachea. **b** Spot radiograph demonstrating massive enlargement of the epiglottis (*arrows*). The epiglottic mucosa is markedly nodular. These images show how spot radiographs demonstrate morphology better than dynamic images, but dynamic images demonstrate motility. (Reproduced with permission from Rubesin 1991, Fig. 11c, d)

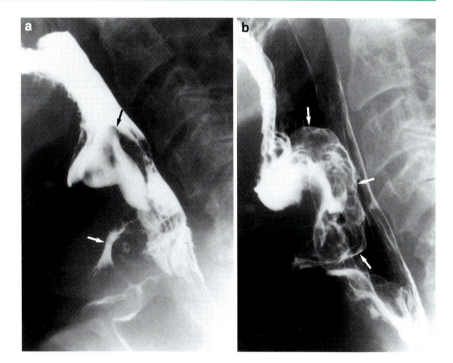

Fig. 31 Mucosal nodularity as a sign of cancer. **a** Frontal view showing diffuse narrowing of the lumen (*arrows*) of the lower hypopharynx, pharyngoesophageal segment, and upper cervical esophagus. The normal tips of the piriform sinuses are obliterated. **b** Lateral view obtained while the patient was drinking showing numerous radiolucent nodules (representative nodules identified by *arrows*) in the barium bolus. The tumor involves the base of the tongue, the anterior wall of the laryngeal vestibule, the entire glottis, and the anterior wall of the lower hypopharynx

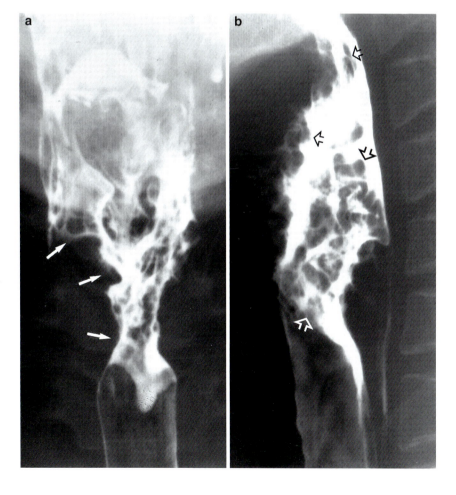

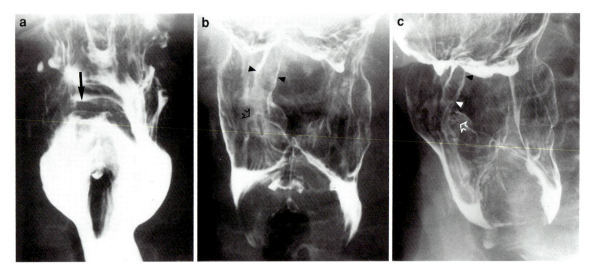

Fig. 32 Value of spot radiographs. **a** Frontal view obtained at the end of bolus passage through the pharynx showing diminished epiglottic tilt on the right (*arrow*). **b, c** Spot radiographs obtained in frontal (**b**) and slight right posterior oblique (**c**) positions showing moderate thickening of the right aryepiglottic fold (*arrowheads*), mild enlargement, and tumor nodularity involving the mucosa overlying the muscular process of the right arytenoid cartilage (*open arrow*). (Reproduced with permission from Rubesin 1991, Fig. 12a–c)

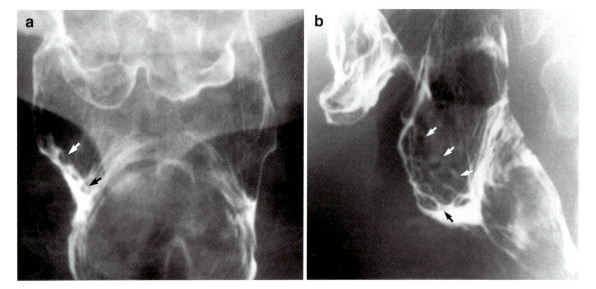

Fig. 33 Early squamous cell carcinoma manifested as tumor nodularity. **a** Frontal view showing subtle, focal nodularity (*arrows*) in the lower right piriform sinus. **b** Lateral view demonstrating a focal area of nodularity along the anterior wall of the hypopharynx (*arrows*). This 64-year-old woman had a tip of the tongue squamous cell carcinoma and was being studied to exclude an esophageal carcinoma prior to surgery. (Reproduced with permission from Levine Levine and Rubesin 1990a, Fig. 4)

At the time of initial diagnosis, the cervical lymph nodes are involved in 60% of patients, and 10% of patients have extranodal involvement.

Pharyngeal lymphomas typically appear as large, lobulated masses involving the nasopharynx, palatine tonsil (Fig. 35), base of the tongue, or a combination

Fig. 34 Recurrent squamous cell carcinoma 2 years after total laryngectomy and radiation therapy. **a** Frontal view showing large nodules (*arrows*) altering the normally smooth contour of the neopharyngeal tube. **b** Lateral view showing a mass (*arrows*) etched in white by barium just below the level of the neovalleculae. The posterior neopharyngeal wall is poorly coated by barium

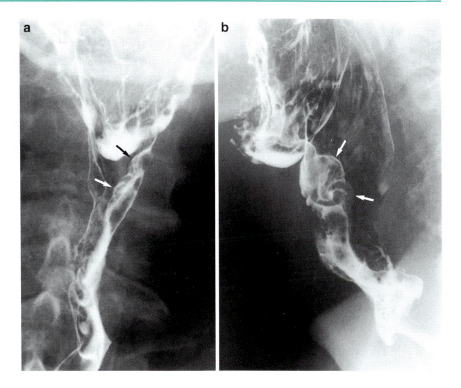

of these locations (Fig. 36) (Hyams et al. 1988; Rubesin 2000b, c). The bulging submucosal masses obliterate the normal lymphoid follicular pattern of the base of the tongue or palatine tonsil (Rubesin 2000c).

5.4 Other Malignant Tumors

The minor mucoserous salivary glands scattered deep to the epithelial layer of the pharynx give rise to tumors of diverse histologic characteristics and clinical course. Most (65–88%) minor salivary gland tumors are malignant (Spiro et al. 1973; Conley and Dingman 1974). The most frequent malignant minor salivary tumors are adenoid cystic carcinoma (35%), solid adenocarcinoma (22%) (Fig. 37), and mucoepidermoid carcinoma (16%) (Spiro et al. 1973). Most pharyngeal minor salivary tumors arise in the soft palate. Palatal salivary gland tumors spread directly to the tongue, submandibular gland, mandible, and lingual and hypoglossal nerves. Adenoid cystic carcinoma typically spreads via a perineural route. Cervical metastases are infrequent,

occurring in 23% of patients with malignant minor salivary tumors.

Synovial sarcomas of the pharynx are extremely rare (Krugman et al. 1973). These lesions are large, bulky tumors involving the larynx, pharynx, and soft tissues of the neck (Gatti et al. 1975).

Kaposi sarcoma may detected in the pharynx in patients with AIDS. Kaposi sarcoma has a wide range of radiographic appearances, including small nodules, plaquelike lesions, small submucosal masses with or without central ulceration, and larger polypoid masses (Fig. 38) (Emery et al. 1986).

The pharynx may be invaded by a variety of tumors arising in the laryngeal cartilages, most frequently the cricoid cartilage. These cartilaginous tumors include chondroma, osteochondroma, and chondrosarcoma (Huizenga and Balogh 1970). Radiographically, the lower hypopharynx and pharyngoesophageal segment is compressed by a smooth-surfaced mass arising in the posterior lamina of the cricoid cartilage. In more than 80% of patients, stippled calcification is detected centrally or peripherally (Hyams et al. 1988).

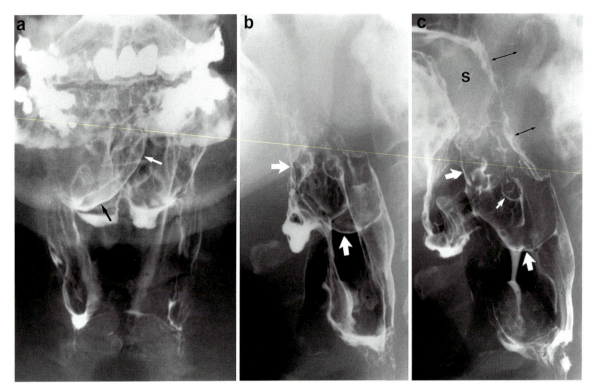

Fig. 35 Lymphoma of pharynx and the value of phonation. **a** Frontal view showing a soft-tissue mass (*arrows*) obliterating the right oropharyngeal wall. **b** Lateral view showing a soft-tissue mass (*arrows*) in the oropharynx. **c** Lateral view obtained after instillation of 1 ml barium into each naris and having the patient phonate "Eeee...." The mass (*large arrows*) has a smooth surface inferiorly and a central ring (*small arrow*) demarcating an empty ulcer. The mass is clearly separated from the base of the tongue by the patient's phonation. Tumor extension into the soft palate and posterior pharyngeal wall is manifested as enlargement and nodularity of the soft palate (*s*) and enlargement of the retropharyngeal space and nodularity of its surface (*double arrows*). (Reproduced with permission from Levine and Rubesin 1990b)

Fig. 36 Lymphoma of tongue and right palatine tonsil. **a** Frontal view showing a mass (*arrows*) manifested by increased soft-tissue density and tumor nodularity. **b** Right posterior oblique view showing tumor nodularity *en face* involving the right palatine fossa (*small arrows*) and the base of the tongue (*large arrow*)

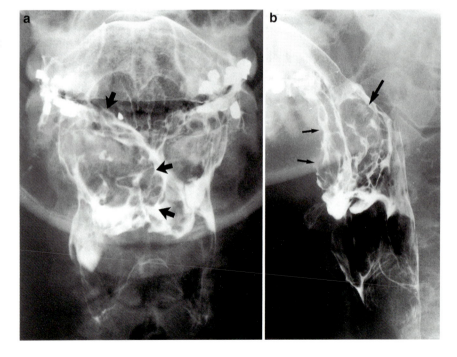

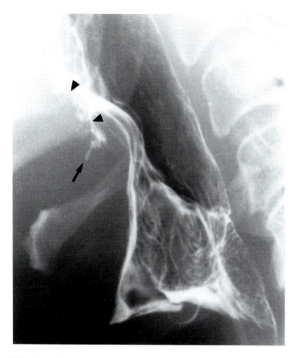

Fig. 37 Adenocarcinoma of the base of the tongue. Lateral view showing obliteration of the valleculae (*arrow*) and nodularity of the base of the tongue (*arrowheads*). Barium coating the laryngeal vestibule and ventricle resulted from absent epiglottic tilt. The tumor presumptively arose in submucosal glands in the base of the tongue. (Reproduced with permission from Rubesin 1994, Fig. 17.37)

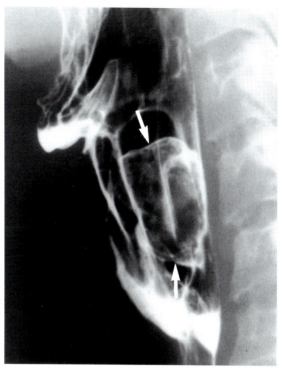

Fig. 38 Kaposi sarcoma. Lateral view showing a relatively smooth surfaced mass (*arrows*) in the air space of the upper hypopharynx. (Courtesy of Dean D.T. Maglinte, University of Indiana)

References

Al-Saleem T, Harwick R, Robbins R et al (1970) Malignant lymphomas of the pharynx. Cancer 26:1769–1778

Apter AJ, Levine MS, Glick SN (1984) Carcinomas of the base of the tongue: diagnosis using double-contrast radiography of the pharynx. Radiology 151:123–126

Bachman AL (1978) Benign non-neoplastic conditions of the larynx and pharynx. Radiol Clin North Am 16:273–290

Bachman AL, Seaman WB, Macken KL (1968) Lateral pharyngeal diverticula. Radiology 91:774–782

Balfe DM, Heiken JP (1986) Contrast evaluation of structural lesions of the pharynx. Curr Probl Diagn Radiol 15:73–160

Banfi A, Bonadonna G, Carnevali G et al (1970) Lymphoreticular sarcomas with primary involvement of Waldeyer's ring. Cancer 26:341–351

Bosma JF, Gravkowski EA, Tyrostad CW (1968) Chronic ulcerative pharyngitis. Arch Otolaryngol 87:85–96

Brady AP, Stevenson GW, Somers S (1995) Premature contraction of the cricopharyngeus: new sign of gastroesophageal reflux disease. Abdom Imaging 20:225–229

Carpenter RJ III, DeSanto LW, Devine KD et al (1976) Cancer of the hypopharynx. Arch Otolaryngol 102:716–721

Chang-Lo M (1977) Laryngeal involvement in Von Recklinghausen's disease. Laryngoscope 87:435–442

Clements JL, Cox GW, Torres WE et al (1974) Cervical esophageal webs–a roentgen-anatomic correlation. Am J Roentgenol 121:221–231

Conley J, Dingman DL (1974) Adenoid cystic carcinoma in the head and neck (cylindroma). Arch Otolaryngol 100:81–90

Cunningham MP, Catlin D (1967) Cancer of the pharyngeal wall. Cancer 20:1859–1866

Curtis DJ, Cruess DF, Crain M et al (1988) Lateral pharyngeal outpouchings: a comparison of dysphagic and asymptomatic patients. Dysphagia 2:156–161

Delahunty JE, Margulies SE, Alonso UA et al (1971) The relationship of reflux esophageal to pharyngeal pouch (Zenker's diverticulum). Laryngoscope 81:570–577

DuBrul EL (1980) Sicher's oral anatomy, 7th edn. Mosby, St. Louis, pp 319–350

Ekberg O (1981) Cervical esophageal webs in patients with dysphagia. Clin Radiol 32:633–641

Ekberg O, Nylander G (1983a) Lateral diverticula from the pharyngoesophageal junction area. Radiology 146:117–122

Ekberg O, Nylander G (1983b) Webs and web-like formations in the pharynx and cervical esophagus. Diagn Imaging 52:10–18

Ekberg O, Birch-lensen M, Lindstrom C (1986) Mucosal folds in the valleculae. Dysphagia 1:68–72

Emery CD, Wall S, Federle MP et al (1986) Pharyngeal Kaposi's sarcoma in patients with AIDS. Am J Roentgenol 147:919–922

Frazell EL, Lucas JC (1962) Cancer of the tongue: report of the management of 1554 patients. Cancer 15:1085–1099

Frieling T, Berges W, Lubke HJ et al (1988) Upper esophageal sphincter function in patients with Zenker's diverticulum. Dysphagia 3:90–92

Gatti WM, Strom CG, Orfei E (1975) Synovial sarcoma of the laryngopharynx. Arch Otolaryngol 98:53–54

Goldstein HM, Zornoza J (1978) Association of squamous cell carcinoma of the head and neck with cancer of the esophagus. Am J Roentgenol131:791–794

Gromet M, Homer MJ, Carter BL (1982) Lymphoid hyperplasia at the base of the tongue. Radiology 144:825–828

Harris RD, Berdon WE, Baker DH (1970) Roentgen diagnosis of acute epiglottis in the adult. J Can Assoc Radiol 21:270–272

Huizenga C, Balogh K (1970) Cartilaginous tumors of the larynx. Cancer 26:201–210

Hyams VJ, Rabuzzi DD (1970) Cartilaginous tumors of the larynx. Laryngoscope 80:755–767

Hyams VJ, Batsakis JG, Michaels L (1988) Tumors of the upper respiratory tract and ear. In: Atlas of tumor pathology, second series, fascicle 25. Armed Forces Institute of Pathology, Bethesda

Jimenez JR (1970) Roentgen examination of the oropharynx and oral cavity. Rad Clin North Am 8:413–424

Jing BS (1970) Roentgen examination of the larynx and hypopharynx. Radiol Clin North Am 8:361–386

Johnson JT, Bacon GW, Meyers EN, Wagner RL (1995) Medial versus lateral wall piriform sinus carcinomas: implications for management of regional lymphatics. Head Neck 16:401–405

Kabakian HA, Dahmash MS (1978) Pharyngoesophageal manifestations of epidermolysis bullosa. Clin Radiol 29:91–94

Killian G (1908) Ueber den Mund der Speiseröhre. Z Ohrenheilkd Wiesb 55:1–41

Kirchner JA, Owen JR (1977) Five hundred cancers of the larynx and piriform sinuses: results of treatment by radiation and surgery. Laryngoscope 87:1288–1303

Knuff TE, Benjamin SB, Castell DO (1982) Pharyngoesophageal (Zenker's) diverticulum: a reappraisal. Gastroenterology 82:734–736

Krugman ME, Rosin HD, Toker C (1973) Synovial sarcoma of the laryngopharynx. Arch Otolaryngol 98:53–54

Levine MS, Rubesin SE (1990a) Update on esophageal radiology. Am J Roentgenol 155:933–994

Levine MS, Rubesin SE (1990b) Radiologic investigation of dysphagia. Am J Roentgenol154:1157–1163

Lindbichler F, Raith J, Uggowitzer M, Hausegger K (1998) Aspiration resulting from lateral hypopharyngeal pouches. Am J Roentgenol170:129–132

Mannsson T, Wilske J, Kindblom L-G (1978) Lipoma of the hypopharynx: a case report and a review of the literature. J Laryngol Otol 92:1037–1043

Maran AGD, Buchanan DR (1978) Branchial cysts, sinuses and fistulae. Clin Otolaryngol 3:407–414

McNab-Jones RF (1961) The Patterson-Brown-Kelly syndrome: its relationship to iron deficiency and postcricoid carcinoma. J Laryngol Otol 71:529–561

Nanson EM (1976) Carcinoma in a long-standing pharyngeal diverticulum. Br J Surg 63:417–419

Nosher JL, Campbell WL, Seaman WB (1975) The clinical significance of cervical esophageal and hypopharyngeal webs. Radiology 117:45–47

Patterson HC, Dickerson GR, Pilch BZ et al (1981) Hamartoma of the hypopharynx. Arch Otolaryngol 107:767–772

Pernkopf E (1989) Anatomy, vol 1. Head neck, 3rd edn. Urban & Schwarzenberg, Baltimore

Perrot JW (1962) Anatomical aspects of hypopharyngeal diverticula. Aust N Z J Surg 31:307–317

Pitman RG, Fraser GM (1965) The post-cricoid impression of the esophagus. Clin Radiol 16:34–39

Rubesin SE (1991) Pharyngeal dysfunction. In: Gore RM (ed) Categorical course on gastrointestinal radiology. American College of Radiology, Reston, pp 1–9

Rubesin SE (1994) Structural abnormalities. In: Gore RM, Levine MS, Laufer I (eds) Textbook of gastrointestinal radiology. Saunders, Philadelphia, pp 244–276

Rubesin SE (1995) Oral and pharyngeal dysphagia. Gastro Clin North Am 24:331–352

Rubesin SE (2000a) Pharynx. In: Levine MS, Rubesin SE, Laufer I (eds) Double contrast gastrointestinal radiology. Saunders, Philadelphia, pp 61–89

Rubesin SE (2000b) Pharynx: normal anatomy and examination techniques. In: Gore RM, Levine MS (eds) Textbook of gastrointestinal radiology. Saunders, Philadelphia, pp 190–211

Rubesin SE (2000c) Structural abnormalities of the pharynx. In: Gore RM, Levine MS (eds) Textbook of gastrointestinal radiology. Saunders, Philadelphia, pp 227–255

Rubesin SE, Glick SN (1988) The tailored double-contrast pharyngogram. Crit Rev Diagn Imaging 28:133–179

Rubesin SE, Laufer I (1991) Pictorial review: principles of double contrast pharyngography. Dysphagia 6:170–178

Rubesin SE, Levine MS (2001) Killian-Jamieson diverticula: radiographic findings in 16 patients. Am J Roentgenol 177:85–89

Rubesin SE, Stiles TD (1997) Principles of performing a "modified barium swallow" examination. In: Balfe DM, Levine MS (eds) Categorical course in diagnostic radiology: gastrointestinal. RSNA, Oak Brook, pp 7–20

Rubesin SE, Jessurun J, Robertson D et al (1987a) Lines of the pharynx. Radiographics 7:217–237

Rubesin SE, Jones BJ, Donner MW (1987b) Contrast pharyngography: the importance of phonation. Am J Roentgenol 148:269–272

Seaman WB (1967) The significance of webs in the hypopharynx and upper esophagus. Radiology 89:32–38

Seaman WB (1974) Contrast radiography in neoplastic disease of the larynx and pharynx. Semin Roentgenol 9:301–209

Semenkovich JW, Balfe DM, Weyman PJ et al (1985) Barium pharyngography: comparison of single and double contrast technique. Am J Roentgenol 144:715–720

Shauffer IA, Phillips HE, Sequeira J (1977) The jet phenomenon: a manifestation of esophageal web. Am J Roentgenol 129:747–748

Shirazi KK, Daffner RH, Gaede JT (1977) Ulcer occurring in Zenker's diverticulum. Gastrointest Radiol 2:117–118

Silver CE (1977) Surgical management of neoplasms of the larynx, hypopharynx and cervical esophagus. Curr Probl Surg 14:2–69

Smiley TB, Caves PK, Porter DC (1970) Relationship between posterior pharyngeal pouch and hiatus hernia. Thorax 25:725–731

Spiro RH, Koss LG, Hajdu SI et al (1973) Tumors of minor salivary origin. Cancer 31:117–129

Strong EW (1979) Carcinoma of the tongue. Otolaryngol Clin North Am 12:107–114

Taylor AJ, Stewart ET, Dodds WJ (1990) The esophageal jet phenomenon revisited. Am J Roentgenol 155:289–290

Thompson WM, Oddson TA, Kelvin F et al (1978) Synchronous and metachronous squamous cell carcinoma of the head, neck and esophagus. Gastrointest Radiol 3:123–127

Todd GB, Michaels L (1974) Hodgkin's disease involving Waldeyer's lymph ring. Cancer 34:176–1768

Waldenstrom J, Kjellberg SR (1939) The roentgenological diagnosis of sideropenic dysphagia (Plummer-Vinson's syndrome). Acta Radiol 20:618–638

Weaver JW, Kaude JV, Hamlin DJ (1984) Webs of the lower esophagus: a complication of gastroesophageal reflux? Am J Roentgenol 142:289–292

Wychulis AR, Gunnulaugsson GH, Clagett OT (1969) Carcinoma arising in pharyngoesophageal diverticulum. Surgery 66:976–979

Zaino C, Jacobson HG, Lepow H et al (1967) The pharyngo-esophageal sphincter. Radiology 89:639–645

Zaino C, Jacobson HG, Lepow H et al (1970) The pharyngo-esophageal sphincter. Thomas, Springfield

Zbaren P, Egger C (1997) Growth patterns of piriform sinus carcinomas. Laryngoscope 107:511–518

Morphology of the Esophagus

Marc S. Levine and Arastoo Vossough

Contents

Abstract

Barium esophagography is an invaluable radiologic technique for detecting a host of morphologic abnormalities in the esophagus. Double-contrast barium studies are particularly well suited for diagnosing reflux esophagitis and its complications, including peptic strictures and Barrett's esophagus. Double-contrast esophagography is also useful for detecting infectious esophagitis and for differentiating the underlying causes, including Candida albicans, the herpes simplex virus, cytomegalovirus, and human immunodeficiency virus. Barium studies can also facilitate the diagnosis of drug-induced esophagitis, eosinophilic esophagitis, and other less common forms of esophagitis. In patients with dysphagia, barium esophagography is a sensitive test for detecting the two common malignant tumors of the esophagus—squamous cell carcinoma and adenocarcinoma. Finally, esophagography can be used to diagnose other morphologic abnormalities in the esophagus, including webs, rings, diverticula, varices, foreign body impactions, fistulas, and perforation. All of these conditions are discussed in the following chapter.

M. S. Levine (✉) · A. Vossough
Department of Radiology,
Hospital of the University of Pennsylvania,
3400 Spruce Street, Philadelphia, PA 19104, USA
e-mail: marc.levine@uphs.upenn.edu

1 Inflammatory Conditions

1.1 Reflux Esophagitis

Reflux esophagitis is by far the most common inflammatory disease of the esophagus. The severity of reflux esophagitis depends not only on the

O. Ekberg (ed.), *Dysphagia*, Medical Radiology. Diagnostic Imaging, DOI: 10.1007/174_2011_347,
© Springer-Verlag Berlin Heidelberg 2012

frequency and duration of reflux episodes, but also on the content of the refluxed material and the resistance of the esophageal mucosa (Pope 1994). Gastroesophageal reflux can be detected on barium studies, scintigraphy, and pH-monitoring techniques, but reflux esophagitis can only be diagnosed using esophagography or endoscopy.

Reflux esophagitis may be manifested on single-contrast barium studies by thickened folds, decreased distensibility, and marginal ulceration. However, these findings are detected only in patients with advanced disease. In contrast, double-contrast barium studies have a sensitivity approaching 90% for the diagnosis of reflux esophagitis because of the ability to detect superficial ulcers, mucosal granularity, and other findings that cannot be visualized on single-contrast studies (Creteur et al. 1983b). Conversely, prone single-contrast views permit optimal distention of the distal esophagus for demonstration of hernias, rings, or strictures that are sometimes missed on upright double-contrast views (Chen et al. 1985).

Early reflux esophagitis may be manifested on double-contrast studies by a finely nodular or granular appearance in the distal esophagus due to mucosal inflammation and edema (Fig. 1, Kressel et al. 1981). In almost all cases, this nodularity or granularity extends proximally from the gastroesophageal junction as a continuous area of disease. As the disease progresses, other patients may develop shallow ulcers and erosions that are seen as streaks or dots of barium in the distal esophagus (Fig. 2, Laufer 1982). These ulcers are sometimes associated with radiating folds or surrounding halos of edematous mucosa. Occasionally, the ulcers may be more widespread. However, ulceration in reflux esophagitis almost always involves the distal esophagus, so the presence of one or more ulcers that are confined to the upper or midesophagus should suggest another cause for the patient's disease. Others with reflux esophagitis may have a single dominant ulcer, most commonly on the posterior wall of the distal esophagus (Hu et al. 1997). It has been hypothesized that these ulcers are located posteriorly because of prolonged exposure to refluxed acid that pools posteriorly when patients sleep in the supine position (Hu et al. 1997).

Reflux esophagitis may also be manifested by thickened longitudinal folds due to inflammation and edema extending into the submucosa. These folds may have a smooth or lobulated contour, occasionally

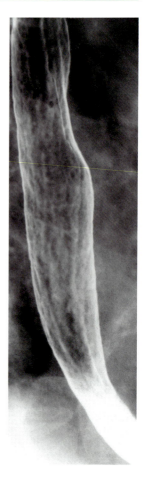

Fig. 1 Reflux esophagitis. Double-contrast view shows fine nodularity or granularity of the mucosa in the *lower* half of the thoracic esophagus. Note how this granularity extends proximally from the gastroesophageal junction as a continuous area of disease

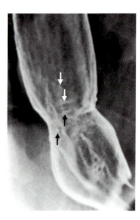

Fig. 2 Reflux esophagitis. Double-contrast view shows superficial, punctate, and linear ulcers (*arrows*) in the distal esophagus just above a hiatal hernia

mimicking the appearance of esophageal varices. Other patients with chronic reflux esophagitis have a single prominent fold that arises in the gastric fundus and extends upward into the distal esophagus as a smooth, polypoid protuberance, also known as an *inflammatory esophagogastric polyp* (Fig. 3, Bleshman et al. 1978). Because these lesions have no malignant

Fig. 3 Inflammatory esophagogastric polyp. Single-contrast view shows a prominent fold (*straight arrow*) that arises at the gastric cardia and terminates in the distal esophagus as a smooth polypoid protuberance (*curved arrow*)

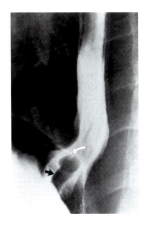

Fig. 4 Peptic stricture. Double-contrast view shows a smooth, tapered area of concentric narrowing (*arrow*) in the distal esophagus above a small hiatal hernia

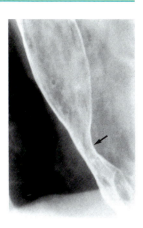

potential, endoscopy is not warranted when typical esophagogastric polyps are found on double-contrast studies.

1.1.1 Peptic Scarring and Strictures

As esophageal ulcers heal, localized flattening or puckering of the esophageal wall may occur at the site of healing. Further scarring leads to the development of circumferential strictures, also known as *peptic strictures*, which typically appear as smooth, tapered areas of concentric narrowing in the distal esophagus above a hiatal hernia (Fig. 4). However, asymmetric scarring can lead to asymmetric narrowing with focal sacculation of the wall between areas of fibrosis. Scarring from reflux esophagitis can also lead to longitudinal shortening of the distal esophagus and the development of fixed transverse folds, producing a characteristic *stepladder* appearance due to pooling of barium between the folds (Fig. 5, Levine and Goldstein 1984). These fixed transverse folds should be differentiated from the thin transverse folds (i.e., *feline esophagus*) often seen as a transient finding due to contraction of the longitudinally oriented muscularis mucosae in patients with reflux.

1.1.2 Barrett's Esophagus

Barrett's esophagus is characterized by progressive columnar metaplasia of the distal esophagus due to long-standing gastroesophageal reflux and reflux esophagitis. Although the metaplastic segment in Barrett's esophagus has been traditionally thought to extend 3 cm or more above the gastroesophageal junction, short-segment Barrett's esophagus has also been described (Yamamoto et al. 2001). Barrett's esophagus is important because it is a premalignant

Fig. 5 Mild peptic stricture with fixed transverse folds. Double-contrast view shows a mild peptic stricture in the distal esophagus with a series of incomplete transverse folds in the region of the stricture. Note how barium traps between the folds (*arrows*), producing a characteristic *stepladder* appearance

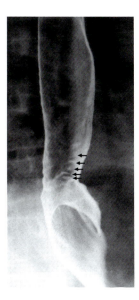

condition associated with an increased risk of developing esophageal adenocarcinoma through a sequence of progressively severe epithelial dysplasia.

The classic radiologic signs of Barrett's esophagus consist of a high stricture or ulcer associated with a hiatal hernia and reflux (Fig. 6, Levine 1994). However, strictures are actually more common in the distal esophagus in patients with this condition, so most cases do not fit the classic description of a high stricture or ulcer (Robbins et al. 1978). Another sign of Barrett's esophagus is a distinctive reticular pattern characterized by tiny barium-filled grooves resembling the areae gastricae on double-contrast studies of the stomach (Fig. 7, Levine et al. 1983). However, this reticular pattern is also found in only a small percentage of all patients with Barrett's esophagus.

Fig. 6 Barrett's esophagus. Prone single-contrast view shows a smooth, tapered stricture (*arrow*) in the midesophagus above a moderately large hiatal hernia

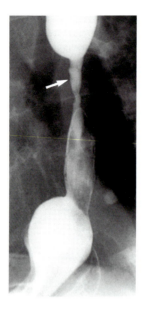

Fig. 7 Barrett's esophagus. Double-contrast view shows a tapered stricture (*arrow*) in the midesophagus. Also note a delicate reticular pattern of the mucosa in the region of the stricture in this patient with proven Barrett's esophagus

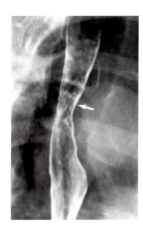

Other more common findings in Barrett's esophagus, such as reflux esophagitis and distal peptic strictures, often occur in patients with uncomplicated reflux disease. Thus, radiographic findings that are relatively specific for Barrett's esophagus are not sensitive, and findings that are more sensitive are not specific.

Some investigators have employed a novel approach for evaluating patients with reflux symptoms. These patients were classified at high risk for Barrett's esophagus if double-contrast radiographs revealed a high stricture or ulcer or a reticular pattern; at moderate risk if the radiographs revealed a distal stricture or reflux esophagitis; and at low risk if the esophagus appeared normal (Gilchrist et al. 1988). The vast majority of those classified at high risk on double-contrast barium studies were found to have

Barrett's esophagus versus only 1% classified at low risk. Thus, the major value of double-contrast esophagography in patients with reflux symptoms is its ability to stratify these individuals into various risk groups for Barrett's esophagus to determine the relative need for endoscopy and biopsy.

1.2 Infectious Esophagitis

1.2.1 *Candida* Esophagitis

Candida albicans is the most common cause of infectious esophagitis (Haulk and Sugar 1991). It most often occurs as an opportunistic infection in immunocompromised patients, particularly those with AIDS, but others may develop candidiasis as a result of local esophageal stasis due to achalasia or scleroderma (Gefter et al. 1981). It should be recognized that 50% of patients with oropharyngeal candidiasis (i.e., thrush) do not have *Candida* esophagitis, so the absence of oropharyngeal disease in no way excludes this diagnosis (Levine et al. 1987). Single-contrast barium studies have limited value in detecting esophageal candidiasis because of the superficial nature of the disease. In contrast, double-contrast barium studies have a sensitivity of nearly 90% in diagnosing *Candida* esophagitis, primarily because of the ability to demonstrate mucosal plaques (Levine et al. 1985).

Candida esophagitis usually is manifested on double-contrast studies by discrete plaque-like lesions corresponding to the characteristic white plaques seen on endoscopy (Levine et al. 1985). The plaques appear as linear or irregular filling defects that tend to be oriented longitudinally and are associated with normal intervening mucosa (Fig. 8). Patients with AIDS may develop a more fulminant form of *Candida* esophagitis characterized by a grossly irregular or *shaggy esophagus* due to coalescent plaques and pseudomembranes with trapping of barium between these lesions (Fig. 9, Levine et al. 1987). Some of the plaques may eventually slough, producing one or more deep ulcers on a background of diffuse plaque formation. Patients with scleroderma or achalasia may also develop a *foamy esophagus* due to innumerable bubbles layering out in the barium column (Fig. 10); this phenomenon presumably results from infection by a yeast form of candidiasis (Sam et al. 2000).

Fig. 8 *Candida* esophagitis. Double-contrast view shows multiple discrete plaque-like lesions in the midesophagus. Note how some of the plaques have a linear configuration. Also note how the plaques are separated by segments of normal intervening mucosa

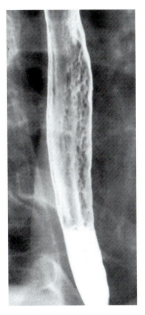

Fig. 10 *Candida* esophagitis with a *foamy esophagus*. Double-contrast view shows innumerable tiny bubbles layering out in the barium column (*arrow*) as a result of the yeast form of candidiasis. The esophagus is also dilated in this patient with underlying achalasia. It should be noted that patient did not receive an effervescent agent for this examination

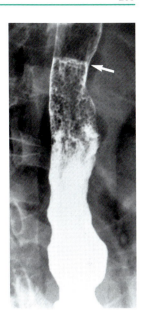

Fig. 9 Advanced *Candida* esophagitis with a *shaggy esophagus*. Double-contrast view shows a grossly irregular esophagus due to innumerable coalescent plaques and pseudomembranes with trapping of barium between the lesions. This patient had AIDS

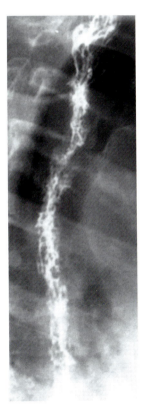

1.2.2 Herpes Esophagitis

The herpes simplex virus type I is the second most frequent cause of infectious esophagitis. Herpes esophagitis is most commonly seen in immunocompromised patients, but it occasionally may occur as an acute, self-limited disease in otherwise healthy patients who have no underlying immunologic problems (Shortsleeve and Levine 1992).

Herpes esophagitis is initially manifested by small vesicles that subsequently rupture to form discrete, punched-out ulcers on the mucosa (Levine et al. 1981). Affected individuals typically present with severe odynophagia. Although some patients may have herpetic lesions in the oropharynx, the majority are not found to have oropharyngeal disease. Moreover, some patients with oral herpes and odynophagia are found to have *Candida* esophagitis. The presence of herpetic lesions in the oropharynx therefore does not accurately predict herpes esophagitis in patients with odynophagia.

Herpes esophagitis is usually manifested on double-contrast studies by small, discrete ulcers in the upper or midesophagus (Fig. 11). The ulcers can have a punctate, stellate, or volcano-like appearance, often separated by normal intervening mucosa (Levine et al. 1981). Discrete ulcers are seen in up to 50% of patients with herpes esophagitis (Levine et al. 1988). Rarely, severe infection may be manifested by multiple ulcers and plaques, mimicking the findings of advanced *Candida* esophagitis. In the appropriate setting, however, it usually is possible to differentiate these infections on the basis of the radiographic findings without need for endoscopy (Levine et al. 1987).

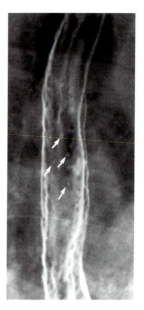

Fig. 11 Herpes esophagitis. Double-contrast view shows multiple tiny ulcers (*arrows*) in the midesophagus. Note tiny radiolucent mounds of edema surrounding the ulcers

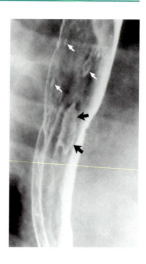

Fig. 12 HIV esophagitis. Double-contrast view shows a large *diamond*-shaped ulcer (*black arrows*) with a cluster of small satellite ulcers (*white arrows*) in the midesophagus

1.2.3 Cytomegalovirus Esophagitis

Cytomegalovirus (CMV) is another cause of infectious esophagitis associated with the development of ulcers. Affected individuals usually present with severe odynophagia and are almost always found to have AIDS. These patients may also have evidence of CMV in other organs such as the retina, liver, or colon.

CMV esophagitis is usually manifested on double-contrast barium studies by one or more giant, flat ulcers that are several centimeters or more in length (Levine et al. 1987). The ulcers may have an ovoid, elongated, or diamond-shaped configuration and are frequently surrounded by a thin radiolucent rim of edema. Because herpetic ulcers rarely become this large, the presence of one or more giant ulcers should suggest the possibility of CMV esophagitis in patients with AIDS. Nevertheless, the differential diagnosis also includes giant human immunodeficiency virus (HIV) ulcers in the esophagus (see next section). Less commonly, CMV esophagitis may be manifested by small, superficial ulcers indistinguishable from those of herpes esophagitis. CMV esophagitis is treated with potent antiviral agents such as ganciclovir that may cause bone marrow suppression. Endoscopy with biopsy specimens, brushings, and cultures from the esophagus are therefore required to confirm the presence of CMV before treating these patients.

1.2.4 Human Immunodeficiency Virus Esophagitis

HIV infection of the esophagus can lead to the development of giant ulcers indistinguishable from those caused by CMV (Levine et al. 1991b). The ulcers typically appear as ovoid or diamond-shaped collections, sometimes associated with a cluster of small satellite ulcers (Fig. 12). Affected individuals may also have palatal ulcers or a characteristic maculopapular rash on the upper half of the body. The diagnosis is confirmed by obtaining endoscopic biopsy specimens, brushings, and cultures from the esophagus to exclude CMV. Unlike CMV ulcers, these HIV-related esophageal ulcers usually respond dramatically to treatment with oral steroids. Endoscopy is therefore required in HIV-positive patients with giant esophageal ulcers to differentiate HIV from CMV, so appropriate therapy can be instituted (Sor et al. 1995).

1.3 Drug-Induced Esophagitis

Tetracycline and doxycycline are the most frequent causes of drug-induced esophagitis, but other offending agents include aspirin and other nonsteroidal anti-inflammatory drugs (NSAIDs), quinidine, potassium chloride, and alendronate. These patients typically ingest the medications with little or no water immediately before going to bed. It has therefore been postulated that prolonged contact of the esophageal mucosa with the medication causes a direct contact esophagitis. Drug-induced esophagitis usually involves the upper

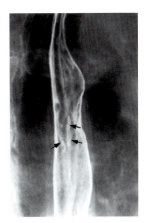

Fig. 13 Drug-induced esophagitis. Double-contrast view shows several small linear ulcers (*arrows*) in the midesophagus due to recent tetracycline ingestion

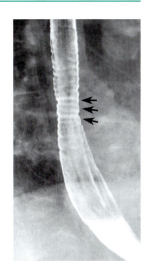

Fig. 14 EoE with a *ringed esophagus*. This patient has a smooth, tapered stricture in the lower third of the thoracic esophagus. Note multiple distinctive ring-like indentations (*arrows*) in the region of the stricture. This finding should be highly suggestive of EoE on barium studies

or middle thirds of the esophagus with sparing of the distal third (Bova et al. 1987).

The radiographic findings in drug-induced esophagitis depend on the nature of the offending medication. Tetracycline and doxycycline are associated with the development of small, superficial ulcers indistinguishable from those of herpes esophagitis (Fig. 13). In contrast, quinidine, potassium chloride, and NSAIDs may cause more severe injury, leading to the development of large ulcers and subsequent stricture formation (Creteur et al. 1983a). Alendronate may also produce extensive ulceration and strictures, but these strictures are usually confined to the distal esophagus (Ryan et al. 1998). Whatever the offending agent, a repeat esophagram usually shows marked healing of the ulcers within 7–10 days after withdrawal of the offending medication (Creteur et al. 1983a).

1.4 Eosinophilic Esophagitis

Eosinophilic esophagitis (EoE) has been recognized as an increasingly common inflammatory condition of the esophagus, occurring predominantly in young men with long-standing dysphagia and recurrent food impactions, often associated with an atopic history, asthma, and, less frequently, a peripheral eosinophilia. The diagnosis of EoE can be confirmed on endoscopic biopsy specimens showing more than 20 eosinophils per high-power field. The etiology is uncertain, but many authors believe that EoE develops as an inflammatory response to ingested food allergens in predisposed individuals. As a result, symptomatic patients often have a marked clinical response to treatment with steroids (especially inhaled steroid preparations) or elemental diets.

The diagnosis of EoE may be suggested on barium studies by the presence of segmental esophageal strictures, sometimes associated with multiple distinctive ring-like indentations, producing a *ringed esophagus* (Zimmerman et al. 2005, Fig. 14). The radiographic diagnosis can also be suggested by the development of a *small-caliber esophagus* manifested by smooth, long-segment narrowing of most or all of the thoracic esophagus (that has a mean diameter of less than 20 mm) without a discrete stricture (White et al. 2010, Fig. 15).

1.5 Radiation Esophagitis

A radiation dose of approximately 4,500–6,000 rads to the chest can cause severe injury to the esophagus (Goldstein et al. 1975). Acute radiation esophagitis usually occurs 1–3 weeks after the initiation of radiation therapy. This condition may be manifested by ulceration or, even more commonly, by a granular appearance of the mucosa and decreased distensibility due to edema and inflammation of the irradiated segment (Collazzo et al. 1997). Within several months after completion of radiation therapy, a smooth, tapered area of concentric narrowing may be seen within the radiation portal due to the development of a radiation stricture (Fig. 16). Fistula formation is another uncommon complication of chronic radiation injury (Carlyle et al. 1976).

Fig. 15 EoE with a *small-caliber esophagus*. A double-contrast esophagogram shows loss of distensibility of the entire thoracic esophagus. Note how there is diffuse luminal narrowing without a discernible stricture. This finding is characteristic of EoE on barium studies

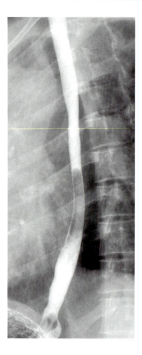

Fig. 17 Acute caustic esophagitis. A study with water-soluble contrast material shows narrowing and ulceration (*black arrow*) of the midesophagus with a small, sealed-off perforation (*white arrow*). This patient had ingested lye

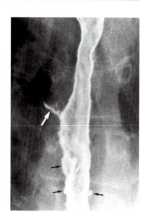

Fig. 16 Radiation stricture. A smooth, tapered stricture (*arrows*) is seen in the cervical and upper thoracic esophagus in this patient who underwent a total laryngectomy and radiation therapy for laryngeal carcinoma

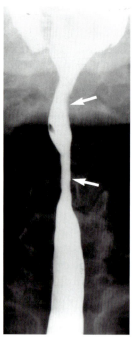

water-soluble contrast media should be used because of the risk of perforation. Such studies may reveal abnormal motility, ulceration, or even esophageal disruption (Fig. 17). If the patient survives, repeat studies may reveal marked stricture formation, typically involving a long segment of the thoracic esophagus. Patients with chronic lye strictures also have an increased risk of developing squamous cell carcinoma of the esophagus, so a new area of mucosal irregularity within a pre-existing lye stricture should raise concern about the possibility of a developing carcinoma (Appelqvist and Salmo 1980).

1.7   Other Esophagitides

Alkaline reflux esophagitis is caused by reflux of bile or pancreatic secretions into the esophagus after partial or total gastrectomy (Levine et al. 1991a). These patients may develop mucosal nodularity, ulceration, or, in severe disease, long, rapidly progressive strictures in the distal esophagus (Levine et al. 1991a). The risk of alkaline reflux esophagitis can be decreased by performing a Roux-en-Y esophagojejunostomy to prevent reflux of bile into the esophagus.

Nasogastric intubation is an unusual cause of esophagitis and stricture formation (Banfield and Hurwitz 1974). Most of these strictures develop after prolonged or repeated intubation, and they may progress rapidly after removal of the tube. It has been postulated that the strictures result from severe reflux esophagitis caused by constant reflux of acid around the tube (Graham et al. 1959). Strictures caused by nasogastric intubation tend to be long-segment

1.6   Caustic Esophagitis

Whether accidental or intentional, ingestion of lye or other caustic agents can lead to a severe form of esophagitis with ulceration, scarring, and stricture formation (Dafoe and Ross 1969). If esophagography is attempted after a patient ingests a caustic agent, strictures in the distal esophagus that progress rapidly on follow-up radiographic examinations.

Other less common causes of esophagitis include acute alcohol-induced esophagitis, Crohn's disease, chronic graft-versus-host disease, Behcet's disease, and, rarely, skin disorders involving the esophagus, such as epidermolysis bullosa dystrophica and benign mucous membrane pemphigoid.

2 Neoplasms

2.1 Benign Tumors

2.1.1 Papilloma

Squamous papillomas are the most common benign mucosal tumors in the esophagus. Histologically, these lesions consist of a central fibrovascular core with multiple digit-like projections covered by hyperplastic squamous epithelium (Miller et al. 1978). Papillomas usually appear on double-contrast esophagography as small, sessile polyps with smooth or slightly lobulated borders. Because papillomas may be difficult to distinguish radiographically from early esophageal cancer and also because of the uncertain risk of malignant degeneration, biopsy, or resection of esophageal papillomas is recommended by some investigators (Zeabart et al. 1979). Rarely, patients may have innumerable papillomas in the esophagus, a condition known as esophageal papillomatosis (Sandvik et al. 1996).

2.1.2 Adenoma

Esophageal adenomas are rare benign lesions which are almost always found to arise in metaplastic columnar epithelium associated with Barrett's esophagus (Levine et al. 1984). Because these lesions have the same potential for malignant transformation as colonic adenomas, endoscopic or surgical resection is warranted (Levine et al. 1984). Adenomas typically appear on esophagography as sessile or pedunculated polyps in the distal esophagus near the gastroesophageal junction.

2.1.3 Glycogenic Acanthosis

Glycogenic acanthosis is a benign disorder in which glycogen accumulates in the squamous epithelial cell lining of the esophagus. It is a common degenerative condition, occurring primarily in middle-aged or elderly individuals (Glick et al. 1982). Glycogenic acanthosis is manifested on double-contrast esophagography by multiple small, rounded nodules or plaques in the middle or, less commonly, distal esophagus (Glick et al. 1982). Major considerations in the differential diagnosis for these lesions include reflux and *Candida* esophagitis. However, the nodules in reflux esophagitis are more poorly defined and are usually located in the distal esophagus, whereas the plaques in *Candida* esophagitis tend to have a linear configuration and typically develop in immunocompromised patients with odynophagia. Thus, it usually is possible to differentiate these conditions on the basis of the clinical and radiographic findings.

2.1.4 Leiomyoma

Leiomyomas are the most common benign submucosal tumors in the esophagus (Goldstein et al. 1981). Unlike stromal tumors elsewhere in the gastrointestinal tract, esophageal leiomyomas almost never undergo sarcomatous degeneration, and unlike gastric leiomyomas, they almost never ulcerate (Totten et al. 1953; Glanz and Grunebaum 1977). Patients with esophageal leiomyomas are usually asymptomatic but occasionally may present with slowly progressive dysphagia (Seremetis et al. 1976).

When esophageal leiomyomas grow into the mediastinum, they can be recognized on chest radiographs by the presence of a mediastinal mass, occasionally containing punctate areas of calcification. Leiomyomas usually appear on barium studies as smooth submucosal lesions (Fig. 18) indistinguishable from other mesenchymal neoplasms such as granular cell tumors, lipomas, hemangiomas, fibromas, and neurofibromas, except that leiomyomas are more likely on empirical grounds. CT may be helpful for differentiating submucosal esophageal masses from extrinsic mediastinal tumors compressing the esophagus.

2.1.5 Fibrovascular Polyp

Fibrovascular polyps are rare, benign submucosal tumors arising from the cervical esophagus, usually at the level of the cricopharyngeus (Levine et al. 1996). Histologically, these lesions are composed of fibrous, vascular, and adipose tissue covered by normal squamous epithelium. They gradually elongate into the thoracic esophagus, forming a pedunculated mass. Some fibrovascular polyps can grow to gigantic sizes,

Fig. 18 Leiomyoma. Double-contrast view shows a smooth submucosal mass (*arrows*) in the upper thoracic esophagus

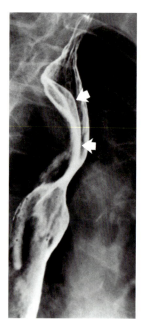

cause dysphagia or wheezing secondary to extrinsic compression of the trachea. Fibrovascular polyps usually appear on barium studies as smooth, expansile masses in the upper or midesophagus (Fig. 19), sometimes associated with a discrete pedicle that originates near the cricopharyngeus. When fibrovascular polyps contain a large amount of adipose tissue, they may be recognized by the presence of fat within the lesions on CT or MRI (Whitman and Borkowski 1989).

2.1.6 Granular Cell Tumor

Granular cell tumors arise from Schwann cells of the peripheral nervous system (Gershwind et al. 1978). Approximately 7% of granular cell tumors occur in the gastrointestinal tract, and one-third of these lesions are found in the esophagus (Johnston and Helwig 1981). Granular cell tumors usually appear on esophagography as small, round or ovoid submucosal masses that often are mistaken for leiomyomas (Rubesin et al. 1985). Most patients with granular cell tumors are asymptomatic, so these lesions usually are detected as incidental findings. However, large granular tumors that cause dysphagia may require local excision (Rubesin et al. 1985).

2.1.7 Duplication Cyst

Although duplication cysts are not true neoplasms, they are included in this section as lesions that may present as submucosal masses. Esophageal duplication cysts comprise about 20% of all duplication cysts in the gastrointestinal tract (Macpherson 1993). These cysts are developmental anomalies of the primitive foregut, often containing ectopic gastric mucosa. The cysts may or may not communicate with the esophageal lumen and usually are located in the right lower mediastinum. Most adults are asymptomatic but some may have symptoms caused by obstruction, bleeding, or infection of the cyst.

Duplication cysts sometimes can be recognized on chest radiographs by the presence of a mass in the right lower mediastinum. The cysts typically appear on barium studies as smooth submucosal masses in the esophagus. When duplication cysts communicate with the esophageal lumen, they may be recognized as tubular, branching outpouchings that fill with barium (Fig. 20). Duplication cysts usually appear as homogenous low-attenuation structures on CT and as high-signal intensity structures on T2-weighted MR images (Rafal and Markisz 1991).

2.2 Malignant Tumors

2.2.1 Esophageal Carcinoma

Esophageal carcinoma constitutes about 1% of all cancers in the United States and 7% of all gastrointestinal tumors (Livingston and Skinner 1985). Affected individuals usually develop dysphagia only after the tumor has invaded periesophageal lymphatics or other mediastinal structures. As a result, most patients have advanced lesions at the time of presentation, with overall 5-year survival rates of less than 10%. Occasionally, however, early esophageal cancer (defined as tumor limited to the mucosa or submucosa without lymphatic metastases) may be detected as a result of early onset of symptoms or screening of asymptomatic patients in high-risk groups. Unlike advanced carcinoma, early esophageal cancer is a curable lesion with 5-year survival rates as high as 95% (Levine et al. 1986). Histologically, 50% of esophageal cancers are squamous cell carcinomas and the remaining 50% are adenocarcinomas arising in Barrett's esophagus (Pera et al. 1993).

Tobacco and alcohol are the major risk factors for developing squamous carcinoma of the esophagus in the United States. Other conditions known to predispose to the development of esophageal carcinoma

Fig. 19 Giant fibrovascular polyp. A smooth, sausage-shaped mass is seen expanding in the lumen of the upper and midesophagus on three separate views (*arrow* denotes distal tip of lesion)

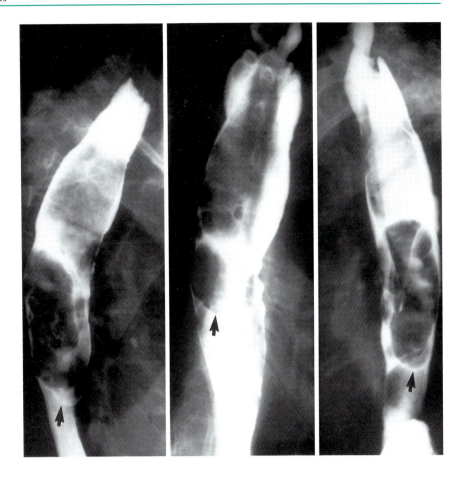

include achalasia, lye strictures, head and neck tumors, Plummer–Vinson syndrome, and tylosis (Carter and Brewer 1975; Appelqvist and Salmo 1980; Levine and Halvorsen 2000). Some authorities advocated periodic screening of patients with these conditions to detect developing cancers at the earliest possible stage.

Unlike squamous cell carcinomas, esophageal adenocarcinomas are virtually always found to arise in patients with underlying Barrett's esophagus. The reported prevalence of adenocarcinoma in patients with Barrett's esophagus is about 10% (Levine et al. 1995). Studies using incidence rather than prevalence data indicate that the relative risk of adenocarcinoma developing in patients with Barrett's esophagus is 30–40 times greater than that in the general population (Spechler et al. 1984). These adenocarcinomas evolve through a sequence of progressive epithelial dysplasia in areas of pre-existing columnar metaplasia. Many experts therefore advocate periodic endoscopic surveillance of patients with known Barrett's esophagus

Fig. 20 Communicating duplication cyst. Single-contrast view shows a tubular, branching structure (*arrows*) that communicates with the posterior wall of the midesophagus (Courtesy of Marie Latour, M.D., Philadelphia, PA)

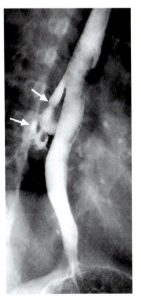

Fig. 21 Early esophageal carcinoma. Double-contrast view shows a plaque-like lesion (*black arrows*) in the midesophagus with a flat, central ulcer (*white arrows*)

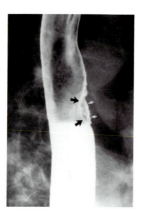

Fig. 22 Advanced infiltrating carcinoma. Single-contrast view shows an irregular segment of narrowing in midesophagus with abrupt, shelf-like proximal and distal borders (*arrows*)

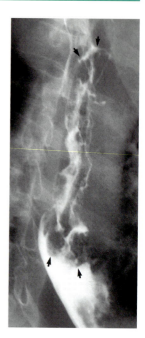

in order to detect dysplastic or carcinomatous changes at the earliest possible stage.

Double-contrast esophagography has a sensitivity of more than 95% in detecting esophageal cancer, a figure comparable to the reported endoscopic sensitivity of 95–100% when multiple brushings and biopsy specimens are obtained (Levine et al. 1997). Furthermore, endoscopy rarely finds cases of esophageal carcinoma that are missed on double-contrast studies (DiPalma et al. 1984). We therefore believe that double-contrast esophagography is a sensitive technique for detecting esophageal cancer and that endoscopy is not warranted in patients with normal findings on double-contrast studies.

Early esophageal cancers are usually small, protruded lesions less than 3.5 cm in size. These tumors may be manifested on double-contrast studies by plaque-like lesions (often containing a flat central ulcer, Fig. 21), by sessile polyps with a smooth or slightly lobulated contour, or by focal irregularity of the wall. Early adenocarcinomas in Barrett's esophagus may also be manifested by a localized area of wall flattening or irregularity within a pre-existing peptic stricture. Superficial spreading carcinoma is another form of early esophageal cancer characterized by a confluent area of nodules or plaques (Levine et al. 1986). Although these lesions may be confused with focal *Candida* esophagitis, the plaques in candidiasis tend to be discrete lesions with normal intervening mucosa, whereas the nodules in superficial spreading carcinoma tend to coalesce, producing a continuous area of disease. Although early esophageal cancers are generally thought to be small lesions, some early cancers may be relatively large intraluminal masses more than 3.5 cm in diameter (Levine et al. 1986).

Advanced esophageal carcinomas usually appear on barium studies as infiltrating, polypoid, ulcerative, or varicoid lesions. Infiltrating carcinomas are manifested by irregular luminal narrowing, nodularity, ulceration, and abrupt, often shelf-like borders (Fig. 22). Polypoid carcinomas appear as lobulated intraluminal masses. Primary ulcerative carcinomas are necrotic lesions with a giant, meniscoid ulcer surrounded by a radiolucent rim of tumor (Fig. 23, Gloyna et al. 1977). Finally, varicoid carcinomas are those in which submucosal spread of tumor produces thickened, tortuous longitudinal defects, mimicking the appearance of varices. However, varicoid tumors have a fixed configuration and relatively abrupt borders, whereas varices tend to change in size and shape at fluoroscopy. Also, varices rarely cause dysphagia because they are soft and compressible. Thus, it usually is possible to differentiate varices from varicoid tumors on clinical and radiologic criteria.

Squamous cell carcinomas and adenocarcinomas of the esophagus cannot be reliably differentiated on the basis of the radiographic findings. Nevertheless, squamous cell carcinomas tend to involve the upper or midesophagus, whereas adenocarcinomas are mainly located in the distal esophagus. Unlike squamous carcinomas, esophageal adenocarcinomas also have a marked tendency to invade the gastric cardia or fundus. In fact, 50% of all cancers involving the

Fig. 23 Primary ulcerative carcinoma. Double-contrast view shows a polypoid lesion (*large arrows*) in the midesophagus with a flat area of central ulceration (*small arrows*)

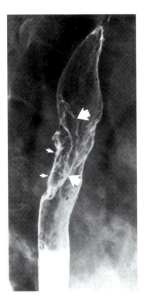

Fig. 24 Cervical esophageal webs. Lateral view of the pharynx and cervical esophagus during swallowing shows two thin, web-like indentations (*small arrows*) on the anterior wall of the cervical esophagus. Also note a rounded indentation posteriorly (*large arrow*) at the pharyngo-esophageal junction due to incomplete relaxation of the cricopharyngeus

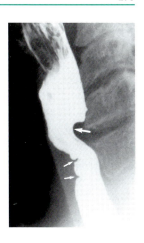

gastroesophageal junction are esophageal adenocarcinomas invading the stomach.

Esophageal carcinomas tend to metastasize to other parts of the esophagus via a network of rich submucosal lymphatic channels. These lymphatic metastases may appear as polypoid, plaque-like, or ulcerated lesions that are separated from the primary tumor by normal intervening mucosa (Glick et al. 1986). Tumor may also spread subdiaphragmatically to the gastric fundus via submucosal esophageal lymphatic vessels. These metastases to the stomach may appear as large submucosal masses, often containing central areas of ulceration.

Appropriate treatment strategies for esophageal carcinoma depend on accurate staging of the tumor. Various imaging techniques such as CT, MR, and endoscopic sonography are used for staging esophageal carcinoma (Takashima et al. 1991; Vilgrain et al. 1990). The tumor stage is assessed by evaluating the depth of esophageal wall invasion and the presence or absence of lymphatic or distant metastases.

2.2.2 Other Malignant Tumors

Non-Hodgkin's lymphoma and, rarely, Hodgkin's lymphoma may also involve the esophagus. Esophageal lymphoma may be manifested on barium studies by submucosal masses, polypoid lesions, enlarged folds, or strictures (Carnovale et al. 1977). Spindle-cell carcinoma is another rare tumor characterized by a polypoid intraluminal mass that expands the lumen of the esophagus without causing obstruction (Agha

and Keren 1985). Other malignant tumors of the esophagus include leiomyosarcoma, malignant melanoma, and Kaposi's sarcoma.

3 Webs

Webs are thin mucosal folds arising from the anterior wall of the lower hypopharynx or upper cervical esophagus. Cervical esophageal webs have been reported in 3–8% of upper gastrointestinal barium studies (Ekberg and Nylander 1983). Most patients are asymptomatic, but some may present with dysphagia. An association of cervical esophageal webs with iron-deficiency anemia and pharyngeal carcinoma has been reported in northern Europe (also known as the Plummer–Vinson or Paterson–Kelly syndrome), but this association has not been observed in the United States (Ekberg and Nylander 1983).

Webs are characterized by 1–2-mm wide, shelf-like filling defects along the anterior wall of the hypopharynx or cervical esophagus that protrude to various depths into the esophageal lumen (Fig. 24). The use of dynamic or rapid sequence imaging and large barium boluses increases the detection rate of webs. In more severe cases, webs may be associated with a jet phenomenon and proximal dilatation of the pharynx (Taylor et al. 1990).

4 Rings

Lower esophageal rings are found in 6–14% of patients who undergo esophagography, but less than 1% of patients with rings are symptomatic (Schatzki and Gary 1956). The term Schatzki ring should be reserved only for those patients with lower esophageal rings who present with dysphagia. These rings almost always occur at the gastroesophageal junction. Histologically, the superior surface of the ring is lined by stratified squamous epithelium and the inferior surface by columnar epithelium. The exact pathogenesis of Schatzki rings is uncertain but some are thought to be develop as a result of scarring from reflux esophagitis (Chen et al. 1987).

Lower esophageal rings appear on barium studies as 2–3-mm in height, web-like constrictions at the gastroesophageal junction, almost always above a hiatal hernia (see Fig. 27b). The rings can be missed if the distal esophagus is not adequately distended at fluoroscopy, so it is important to obtain prone views of the esophagus during continuous drinking of a low-density barium suspension. It has been shown that rings with a maximal luminal diameter of more than 20 mm rarely causes dysphagia, whereas rings with a maximal diameter of less than 13 mm almost always cause dysphagia (Schatzki 1963).

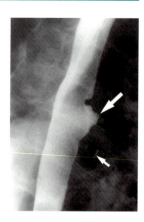

Fig. 25 Traction diverticulum. Single-contrast view shows a triangular outpouching (*upper arrow*) from the midesophagus. Note a surgical clip (*lower arrow*) in the adjacent mediastinum. The diverticulum resulted from post-surgical scarring in this region

5 Diverticula

Esophageal diverticula may be classified as *pulsion* or *traction* diverticula. The more common pulsion diverticula result from esophageal dysmotility with increased intraluminal pressures in the esophagus, whereas traction diverticula are caused by scarring in the soft tissues surrounding the esophagus. Diverticula most commonly occur in the region of the pharyngoesophageal junction (i.e., Zenker's diverticulum), midesophagus, and distal esophagus above the gastroesophageal junction (i.e., epiphrenic diverticulum).

5.1 Pulsion Diverticula

Pulsion diverticula tend to be located in the distal esophagus and are often associated with fluoroscopic or manometric evidence of esophageal dysmotility. These diverticula are usually detected as incidental findings in patients who have no esophageal symptoms. However, a large epiphrenic diverticulum adjacent to the gastroesophageal junction may fill with debris, causing dysphagia, regurgitation, or aspiration. Pulsion diverticula appear on barium studies as rounded outpouchings from the esophageal

lumen that have wide necks. They often do not empty completely when the esophagus collapses and may be associated with other radiologic findings of esophageal motor dysfunction (Levine 2000a, b).

5.2 Traction Diverticula

Traction diverticula occur in the midesophagus and are usually caused by scarring from tuberculosis or histoplasmosis involving subcarinal or perihilar lymph nodes. Traction diverticula are true diverticula containing all layers of the esophageal wall and therefore maintain their elastic recoil. As a result, they tend to empty their contents when the esophagus collapses at fluoroscopy (Levine 2000a, b). Traction diverticula often have a triangular or tented appearance caused by traction on the diverticulum by the fibrotic process in the adjacent mediastinum (Fig. 25). Thus, it often is possible to distinguish traction diverticula from pulsion diverticula on barium studies.

6 Varices

Esophageal varices can be classified as *uphill* or *downhill*. Uphill varices are caused by portal hypertension with increased pressure in the portal venous system transmitted upward via dilated esophageal collaterals to the superior vena cava. In contrast, downhill varices are caused by superior vena cava obstruction with downward flow via dilated esophageal collaterals to the portal venous system and inferior vena cava. Uphill varices are much more common than downhill varices.

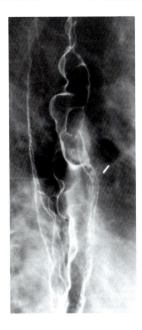

Fig. 26 Esophageal varices. Double-contrast view shows serpiginous longitudinal defects etched in white in the lower third of the esophagus due to uphill esophageal varices

6.1 Uphill Varices

Uphill esophageal varices develop as a result of portal hypertension or other causes of portal venous obstruction. Varices appear on barium studies as serpiginous or tortuous longitudinal filling defects in the distal half of the thoracic esophagus (Fig. 26). They are best seen on mucosal relief views of the collapsed esophagus using a high-density barium suspension to increase mucosal adherence (Cockerill et al. 1976). Even with proper technique, esophageal varices may be seen as a transient finding due to periodic filling and emptying of the varices with esophageal peristalsis or distention. The differential diagnosis for varices includes submucosally infiltrating esophageal carcinomas (varicoid carcinomas) and esophagitis with thickened folds due to submucosal inflammation and edema.

Esophageal varices are characterized on CT by a thickened, lobulated esophageal wall containing tubular structures that enhance markedly after intravenous administration of contrast material. Additional varices may be seen elsewhere in the abdomen at other sites of communication between the portal and systemic venous circulations. Angiography of the celiac or superior mesenteric arteries can be used to confirm the presence of extensive collateral flow and varix formation in and around the distal esophagus.

However, the need for portal venography for pre-surgical planning of portosystemic shunts has decreased with the widespread use of transjugular intrahepatic portosystemic shunting (TIPS) procedures.

6.2 Downhill Varices

The most common cause of downhill varices is bronchogenic carcinoma with mediastinal metastases and superior vena cava obstruction. Additional causes include other primary or metastatic tumors involving the mediastinum, mediastinal irradiation, sclerosing mediastinitis, substernal goiter, and central catheter-related thrombosis of the superior vena cava. Most patients with downhill varices present clinically with superior vena cava syndrome and many have melena and iron-deficiency anemia from variceal bleeding.

Downhill varices typically appear as serpiginous longitudinal filling defects which, unlike uphill esophageal varices, are confined to the upper or midesophagus. Chest radiographs or CT often reveals the underlying cause of superior vena cava obstruction. Venography may also be performed to confirm the presence of superior vena cava obstruction.

7 Foreign Body Impactions

In adults, esophageal foreign body impactions are most commonly caused by inadequately chewed pieces of meat (Nandi and Ong 1978). Most of these foreign bodies pass spontaneously into the stomach, but 10–20% require some form of therapeutic intervention. Although the risk of perforation is less than 1% during the first 24 h, this risk increases substantially after 24 h because of ischemia and pressure necrosis at the site of impaction (Barber et al. 1984). Affected individuals typically present with acute onset of dysphagia, substernal chest pain, and/or a foreign body sensation.

Contrast studies are often performed in patients with suspected food impaction to confirm the presence of obstruction and determine its level and also to rule out esophageal perforation. An impacted food bolus typically appears as a polypoid defect with an irregular meniscus superiorly (Fig. 27a). Because of the degree of obstruction, it may be difficult to assess the underlying esophagus at the time of impaction. It

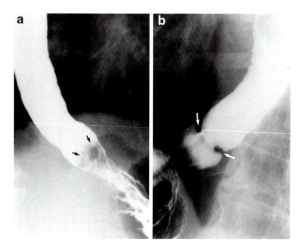

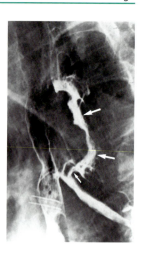

Fig. 28 Advanced esophageal carcinoma with esophagobronchial fistula. An infiltrating carcinoma (*large arrows*) is seen in the midthoracic esophagus with barium in the airway due to an esophagobronchial fistula (*small arrow*)

Fig. 27 Food impaction caused by a Schatzki ring. **a** Initial view shows a polypoid defect in the distal esophagus with an irregular meniscus superiorly (*arrows*) due to impacted meat in this region, **b** after the impaction has been relieved, a repeat view shows the underlying Schatzki ring as the cause of the impaction. Note the smooth, symmetric ring-like constriction (*arrows*) at the gastroesophageal junction above a small hiatal hernia

is therefore prudent to perform a follow-up barium study after the impaction has been relieved to determine if this impaction was caused by a pathologic area of narrowing. The most common causes are Schatzki rings (Fig. 27b) and peptic strictures. Rarely, food impactions may even result from giant thoracic osteophytes impinging on the esophagus (Underberg-Davis and Levine 1991; Levine 2000a, b).

8   Fistulas

Esophageal-airway fistulas usually result from direct invasion of the tracheobronchial tree by advanced esophageal cancer (Fig. 28). Such fistulas have been reported in 5–10% of patients with esophageal cancer, often occurring after treatment with radiation therapy (Fitzgerald et al. 1981; Little et al. 1984). Other causes of esophageal-airway fistulas include esophageal instrumentation, trauma, foreign bodies, and surgery (Vasquez et al. 1988). Affected individuals typically present with violent episodes of coughing and choking during deglutition. When an esophageal-airway fistula is suspected on clinical grounds, barium should be used instead of hyperosmolar water-soluble contrast agents which may cause severe pulmonary edema if a fistula is present.

Esophagopleural fistulas may be caused by esophageal carcinoma, radiation therapy, surgery, or instrumentation. Such patients may present with a pleural effusion, pneumothorax, or hydropneumothorax. When an esophagopleural fistula is suspected, the presence and location of the fistula can be confirmed by a study with water-soluble contrast media.

Aortoesophageal fistulas are extremely rare but are associated with a high-mortality rate. Such fistulas may be caused by a ruptured aortic aneurysm, aortic dissection, infected aortic graft, swallowed foreign body, or esophageal cancer (Baron et al. 1981, Hollander and Quick 1991). Patients with aortoesophageal fistulas may present with an initial episode of arterial hematemesis followed by a variable latent period, before experiencing massive hematemesis, exanguination, and death (Baron et al. 1981). Oral studies with water-soluble contrast agents are unlikely to show the fistula because of high aortic pressures, whereas contrast aortography may fail to show the fistula because of occlusion of the fistulous tract by thrombus (Baron et al. 1981).

9   Perforation

If untreated, perforation of the esophagus is associated with a mortality rate of nearly 100% because of a fulminant mediastinitis that occur in these patients. Early diagnosis is therefore critical. Endoscopy is the most common cause of esophageal perforation, accounting for more than 75% of cases. Other causes include foreign bodies, food impactions, penetrating and blunt trauma, and spontaneous esophageal

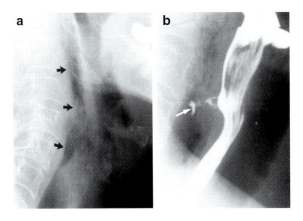

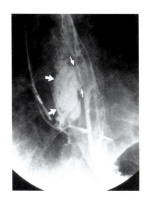

Fig. 30 Perforation of the thoracic esophagus. A study with water-soluble contrast material shows focal extravasation of contrast from the right lateral wall of the lower esophagus (*small arrows*) into a collection (*large arrows*) in the adjacent mediastinum. This perforation occurred as a complication of endoscopic dilatation

Fig. 29 Perforation of the cervical esophagus. **a** Lateral view of the neck shows mottled gas in the retropharyngeal space, **b** a subsequent study with water-soluble contrast material shows a small, sealed-off perforation (*arrow*) from the posterior aspect of the pharyngoesophageal junction. This perforation was caused by traumatic endoscopy

perforation due to a sudden, rapid increase in intra-luminal esophageal pressure (Boerhaave's syndrome).

Cervical esophageal perforation may be manifested on plain films by subcutaneous emphysema, retropharyngeal air (Fig. 29a), and pneumomediastinum. Lateral images of the neck may also show widening of the pre-vertebral space or a retropharyngeal abscess containing loculated gas and/or air–fluid levels. In contrast, thoracic esophageal perforation may be associated with pneumomediastinum, mediastinal widening, and a pleural effusion or hydropneumothorax (Parkin 1973; O'Connell 1967). In the proper setting, the presence of mediastinal gas on CT should be highly suggestive of esophageal perforation, whereas other findings such as pleural effusion or mediastinal fluid are less specific (White et al. 1993). However, CT is less reliable for determining the site of perforation.

Esophagography often is performed on patients with suspected esophageal perforation (Figs. 29b, 30). Although barium is the most sensitive contrast agent for detecting small leaks, it can potentially cause a granulomatous reaction in the mediastinum. In contrast, water-soluble agents do not incite a mediastinal reaction and are readily absorbed from the mediastinum if a leak is present. However, water-soluble contrast agents are less radiopaque than barium and can miss as many as 15–50% of esophageal perforations (Buecker et al. 1997). These agents can also

cause severe pulmonary edema if aspirated into the lungs. It is therefore recommended that the examination be repeated with high-density barium to detect subtle leaks if the initial study with water-soluble contrast media shows no evidence of perforation (Swanson et al. 2003).

References

Agha FP, Keren DF (1985) Spindle-cell squamous carcinoma of the esophagus: a tumor with biphasic morphology. AJR Am J Roentgenol 145:541–545

Appelqvist P, Salmo M (1980) Lye corrosion carcinoma of the esophagus: a review of 63 cases. Cancer 45:2655–2658

Banfield WJ, Hurwitz AL (1974) Esophageal stricture associated with nasogastric intubation. Arch Intern Med 134:1083–1086

Barber GB, Peppercorn MA, Ehrlich C et al (1984) Esophageal foreign body perforation: report of an unusual case and review of the literature. Am J Gastroenterol 79:509–511

Baron RL, Koehler RE, Gutierrez FR et al (1981) Clinical and radiographic manifestations of aortesophageal fistulas. Radiology 141:599–605

Bleshman MH, Banner MP, Johnson RC et al (1978) The inflammatory esophagogastric polyp and fold. Radiology 128:589–593

Bova JG, Dutton NE, Goldstein HM et al (1987) Medication-induced esophagitis: diagnosis by double-contrast esophagography. AJR Am J Roentgenol 148:731–732

Buecker A, Wein BB, Neuerburg JM et al (1997) Esophageal perforation: comparison of use of aqueous and barium-containing contrast media. Radiology 202:683–686

Carlyle DR, Goldstein HM, Wallace S et al (1976) Azygography in the pre-treatment evaluation of esophageal carcinoma. Br J Radiol 49:670–677

Carnovale RL, Goldstein HM, Zornoza J et al (1977) Radiologic manifestations of esophageal lymphoma. AJR Am J Roentgenol 128:751–754

Carter R, Brewer LA III (1975) Achalasia and esophageal carcinoma. Studies in early diagnosis for improved surgical management. Am J Surg 130:114–120

Chen YM, Ott DJ, Gelfand DW et al (1985) Multiphasic examination of the esophagogastric region for strictures, rings, and hiatal hernia: evaluation of the individual techniques. Gastrointest Radiol 10:311–316

Chen YM, Gelfand DW, Ott DJ et al (1987) Natural progression of the lower esophageal mucosal ring. Gastrointest Radiol 12:93–98

Cockerill EM, Miller RE, Chernish SM et al (1976) Optimal visualization of esophageal varices. Am J Roentgenol 126:512–523

Collazzo LA, Levine MS, Rubesin SE et al (1997) Acute radiation esophagitis: radiographic findings. AJR Am J Roentgenol 169:1067–1070

Creteur V, Laufer I, Kressel HY et al (1983a) Drug-induced esophagitis detected by double-contrast radiography. Radiology 147:365–368

Creteur V, Thoeni RF, Federle MP et al (1983b) The role of single and double-contrast radiography in the diagnosis of reflux esophagitis. Radiology 147:71–75

Dafoe CS, Ross CA (1969) Acute corrosive esophagitis. Thorax 24:291–294

DiPalma JA, Prechter GC, Brady CE 3rd (1984) X-ray-negative dysphagia: is endoscopy necessary? J Clin Gastroenterol 6:409–411

Ekberg O, Nylander G (1983) Webs and web-like formations in the pharynx and cervical esophagus. Diagn Imaging 52:10–18

Fitzgerald RH Jr, Bartles DM, Parker EF (1981) Tracheoesophageal fistulas secondary to carcinoma of the esophagus. J Thorac Cardiovasc Surg 82:194–197

Gefter WB, Laufer I, Edell S et al (1981) Candidiasis in the obstructed esophagus. Radiology 138:25–28

Gershwind ME, Chiat H, Addei KA et al (1978) Granular cell tumors of the esophagus. Gastrointest Radiol 2:327–330

Gilchrist AM, Levine MS, Carr RF et al (1988) Barrett's esophagus: diagnosis by double-contrast esophagography. AJR Am J Roentgenol 150:97–102

Glanz I, Grunebaum M (1977) The radiological approach to leiomyoma of the esophagus with a long-term follow-up. Clin Radiol 28:197–200

Glick SN, Teplick SK, Goldstein J et al (1982) Glycogenic acanthosis of the esophagus. AJR Am J Roentgenol 139:683–688

Glick SN, Teplick SK, Levine MS et al (1986) Gastric cardia metastasis in esophageal carcinoma. Radiology 160:627–630

Gloyna RE, Zornoza J, Goldstein HM (1977) Primary ulcerative carcinoma of the esophagus. AJR Am J Roentgenol 129:599–600

Goldstein HM, Rogers LF, Fletcher GH et al (1975) Radiological manifestations of radiation-induced injury to the normal upper gastrointestinal tract. Radiology 117:135–140

Goldstein HM, Zornoza J, Hopens T (1981) Intrinsic diseases of the adult esophagus: benign and malignant tumors. Semin Roentgenol 16:183–197

Graham J, Barnes M, Rubenstein AS (1959) The nasogastric tube as a cause of esophagitis and stricture. Am J Surg 98:116–199

Haulk AA, Sugar AM (1991) Candida esophagitis. Adv Intern Med 36:307–318

Hollander JE, Quick G (1991) Aortesophageal fistula: a comprehensive review of the literature. Am J Med 91:279–287

Hu C, Levine MS, Laufer I (1997) Solitary ulcers in reflux esophagitis: radiographic findings. Abdom Imaging 22:5–7

Johnston J, Helwig EB (1981) Granular cell tumors of the gastrointestinal tract and perianal region: a study of 74 cases. Dig Dis Sci 26:807–816

Kressel HY, Glick SN, Laufer I et al (1981) Radiologic features of esophagitis. Gastrointest Radiol 6:103–108

Laufer I (1982) Radiology of esophagitis. Radiol Clin North Am 20:687–699

Levine MS (1994) Reflux esophagitis and Barrett's esophagus. Semin Roentgenol 29:332–340

Levine MS (2000a) Infectious Esophagitis. In: Gore RM, Levine MS (eds) Textbook of gastrointestinal radiology, 2nd edn. W.B. Saunders, Philadelphia, pp 350–363

Levine MS (2000b) Miscellaneous abnormalities of the esophagus. In: Gore RM, Levine MS (eds) Textbook of gastrointestinal radiology, 2nd edn. W.B. Saunders, Philadelphia, pp 465–483

Levine MS, Goldstein HM (1984) Fixed transverse folds in the esophagus: a sign of reflux esophagitis. AJR Am J Roentgenol 143:275–278

Levine MS, Halvorsen RA (2000) Carcinoma of the esophagus. In: Gore RM, Levine MS (eds) Textbook of gastrointestinal radiology, 2nd edn. W.B. Saunders, Philadelphia, pp 403–434

Levine MS, Laufer I, Kressel HY et al (1981) Herpes esophagitis. AJR Am J Roentgenol 136:863–866

Levine MS, Kressel HY, Caroline DF et al (1983) Barrett esophagus: reticular pattern of the mucosa. Radiology 147:663–667

Levine MS, Caroline D, Thompson JJ et al (1984) Adenocarcinoma of the esophagus: relationship to Barrett mucosa. Radiology 150:305–309

Levine MS, Macones AJ Jr, Laufer I (1985) Candida esophagitis: accuracy of radiographic diagnosis. Radiology 154:581–587

Levine MS, Dillon EC, Saul SH et al (1986) Early esophageal cancer. AJR Am J Roentgenol 146:507–512

Levine MS, Woldenberg R, Herlinger H et al (1987) Opportunistic esophagitis in AIDS: radiographic diagnosis. Radiology 165:815–820

Levine MS, Loevner LA, Saul SH et al (1988) Herpes esophagitis: sensitivity of double-contrast esophagography. AJR Am J Roentgenol 151:57–62

Levine MS, Fisher AR, Rubesin SE et al (1991a) Complications after total gastrectomy and esophagojejunostomy: radiologic evaluation. AJR Am J Roentgenol 157:1189–1194

Levine MS, Loercher G, Katzka DA et al (1991b) Giant, human immunodeficiency virus-related ulcers in the esophagus. Radiology 180:323–326

Levine MS, Herman JB, Furth EE (1995) Barrett's esophagus and esophageal adenocarcinoma: the scope of the problem. Abdom Imaging 20:291–298

Levine MS, Buck JL, Pantongrag-Brown L et al (1996) Fibrovascular polyps of the esophagus: clinical, radiographic, and pathologic findings in 16 patients. AJR Am J Roentgenol 166:781–787

Levine MS, Chu P, Furth EE et al (1997) Carcinoma of the esophagus and esophagogastric junction: sensitivity of radiographic diagnosis. AJR Am J Roentgenol 168:1423–1426

Little AG, Ferguson MK, DeMeester TR et al (1984) Esophageal carcinoma with respiratory tract fistula. Cancer 53:1322–1328

Livingston EM, Skinner DB (1985) Tumors of the Esophagus. In: Berk JE (ed) Gastroenterology. W.B. Saunders, Philadelphia, pp 818–850

Macpherson RI (1993) Gastrointestinal tract duplications: clinical, pathologic, etiologic, and radiologic considerations. RadioGraphics 13:1063–1080

Miller BJ, Murphy F, Lukie BE (1978) Squamous cell papilloma of esophagus. Can J Surg 21:538–540

Nandi P, Ong GB (1978) Foreign body in the esophagus: review of 2394 cases. Br J Surg 65:5–9

O'Connell ND (1967) Spontaneous rupture of the esophagus. Am J Roentgenol Radium Ther Nucl Med 99:186–203

Parkin GJ (1973) The radiology of perforated esophagus. Clin Radiol 24:324–332

Pera M, Cameron AJ, Trastek VF et al (1993) Increasing incidence of adenocarcinoma of the esophagus and esophagogastric junction. Gastroenterology 104:510–513

Pope CE (1994) Acid-reflux disorders. N Engl J Med 331:656–660

Rafal RB, Markisz JA (1991) Magnetic resonance imaging of an esophageal duplication cyst. Am J Gastroenterol 86:1809–1811

Robbins AH, Vincent ME, Saini M et al (1978) Revised radiologic concepts of the Barrett esophagus. Gastrointest Radiol 3:377–381

Rubesin S, Herlinger H, Sigal H (1985) Granular cell tumors of the esophagus. Gastrointest Radiol 10:11–15

Ryan JM, Kelsey P, Ryan BM et al (1998) Alendronate-induced esophagitis: case report of a recently recognized form of severe esophagitis with esophageal stricture—radiographic features. Radiology 206:389–391

Sam JW, Levine MS, Rubesin SE et al (2000) The "foamy" esophagus: a radiographic sign of *Candida* esophagitis. AJR Am J Roentgenol 174:999–1002

Sandvik AK, Aase S, Kveberg KH et al (1996) Papillomatosis of the esophagus. J Clin Gastroenterol 22:35–37

Schatzki R (1963) The lower esophageal ring. Long term follow-up of symptomatic and asymptomatic rings. Am J Roentgenol 90:805

Schatzki R, Gary JE (1956) The lower esophageal ring. AJR Am J Roentgenol 75:246

Seremetis MG, Lyons WS, deGuzman VC et al (1976) Leiomyomata of the esophagus. An analysis of 838 cases. Cancer 38:2166–2177

Shortsleeve MJ, Levine MS (1992) Herpes esophagitis in otherwise healthy patients: clinical and radiographic findings. Radiology 182:859–861

Sor S, Levine MS, Kowalski TE et al (1995) Giant ulcers of the esophagus in patients with human immunodeficiency virus: clinical, radiographic, and pathologic findings. Radiology 194:447–451

Spechler SJ, Robbins AH, Rubins HB et al (1984) Adenocarcinoma and Barrett's esophagus. an overrated risk? Gastroenterology 87:927–933

Swanson JO, Levine MS, Redfern RO, Rubesin SE (2003) Usefulness of high-density barium for detection of leaks after esophagogastrectomy, total gastrectomy, and total laryngectomy. AJR Am J Roentgenol 181:415–420

Takashima S, Takeuchi N, Shiozaki H et al (1991) Carcinoma of the esophagus: CT versus MR imaging in determining resectability. AJR Am J Roentgenol 156:297–302

Taylor AJ, Stewart ET, Dodds WJ (1990) The esophageal "jet" phenomenon revisited. AJR Am J Roentgenol 155:289–290

Totten R, Stout AP, Humphreys GH (1953) Benign tumors and cysts of the esophagus. J Thorac Surg 25:606–622

Underberg-Davis S, Levine MS (1991) Giant thoracic osteophyte causing esophageal food impaction. AJR Am J Roentgenol 157:319–320

Vasquez RE, Landay M, Kilman WJ et al (1988) Benign esophagorespiratory fistulas in adults. Radiology 167:93–96

Vilgrain V, Mompoint D, Palazzo L et al (1990) Staging of esophageal carcinoma: comparison of results with endoscopic sonography and CT. AJR Am J Roentgenol 155:277–281

White CS, Templeton PA, Attar S (1993) Esophageal perforation: CT findings. AJR Am J Roentgenol 160:767–770

White SB, Levine MS, Rubesin SE et al (2010) The small-caliber esophagus: radiographic sign of idiopathic eosinophilic esophagitis. Radiology 256:127–134

Whitman GJ, Borkowski GP (1989) Giant fibrovascular polyp of the esophagus: CT and MR findings. AJR Am J Roentgenol 152:518–520

Yamamoto AJ, Levine MS, Katzka DA et al (2001) Short-segment Barrett's esophagus: findings on double-contrast esophagography in 20 patients. AJR Am J Roentgenol 176:1173–1178

Zeabart LE, Fabian J, Nord HJ (1979) Squamous papilloma of the esophagus: a report of 3 cases. Gastrointest Endosc 25:18–20

Zimmerman SL, Levine MS, Rubesin SE et al (2005) Idiopathic eosinophilic esophagitis in adults: the ringed esophagus. Radiology 236:159–165

The Pediatric Esophagus

Jane E. Benson

Contents

J. E. Benson (✉)
Russell H. Morgan Department of Radiology
and Radiological Science, The Johns Hopkins University
School of Medicine, 600 North Wolfe Street,
Baltimore, MD 21205, USA
e-mail: jbenson@jhmi.edu

Abstract

A child's feeding and swallowing problems can have anatomic and functional causes that are congenital (due to embryologic malformations), or can be acquired after birth. The anatomy of the upper GI tract is uniquely demonstrable on imaging. The radiologist is a key member of the team that diagnoses and cares for these children.

1 Introduction

Feeding one's child and watching it grow and thrive is one of the chief joys of parenting, so anything that interferes with this is likely to prompt a quick demand for medical attention. Symptoms such as vomiting, choking, irritability, and food refusal are all very distressing to both the parent and the child. However, because the gastrointestinal (GI) tract in a child, particularly a young infant, is relatively short and compact, abnormalities at the level of the pharynx, esophagus, stomach, small bowel, or even colon can result in puzzlingly similar clinical manifestations. Determining a cause for the symptoms often falls to the radiologist, who has the unique opportunity to observe the GI tract in action.

2 Imaging Methodology and Techniques: Showing Anatomy and Function for Diagnostic Efficacy

The range of procedures available to image the pediatric esophagus is the same as that available for adults, but the choice is influenced by the odds of finding certain types of pathologic abnormalities. Moreover, the application of these procedures differs from that in adults because of the unique challenge of obtaining a diagnostic examination in the pediatric patient.

2.1   Fluoroscopy

Fluoroscopy is the mainstay of esophageal examination, as it displays not only anatomy but, just as importantly, function. The area examined may be confined to the esophagus, but usually the esophagus is seen in the context of the entire upper GI tract, from the mouth to the ligament of Treitz. This examination is usually done with the child supine or in the lateral position on the fluoroscopy table. Swallows in the true lateral position are extremely important to look for contrast in the trachea and deformity or narrowing of the esophagus from the posterior or anterior aspect. True anteroposterier projections look for esophageal displacement or narrowing from the sides. Recording video clips of the fluoroscopy is extremely helpful, as abnormalities may be fleeting.

Volitional swallow and good distension of the esophagus are of paramount importance. These can only be achieved with a comfortable, cooperative patient. Infants and older children are easier to manage, whereas toddlers and young children are more apt to be frightened and less persuadable. The room should be as warm and as light as possible, and the child should be allowed to keep its clothing on; only large metallic fastenings should be removed, and the child should wear a protective gown. A pad or blanket should be put on the fluoroscopy table. The child should be allowed to hold a favorite blanket or stuffed animal. The fluoroscopy image intensifier should be introduced as a big "tent" or "house". The child should be shown how the image intensifier will get very close to it but will not touch it. Colorful stickers on the face of the image intensifier give the child something to look at. A video machine playing a children's movie or cartoon is an excellent distraction.

The choice of contrast medium can improve the chances of getting a good examination. Standard oral barium sulfate preparations have the consistency of milk, and some are sweetened with sorbitol or the like, and a very hungry infant is usually very cooperative and needs no additional persuasion. It is helpful to use the type of nipple that the infant is

familiar with, and also to enlarge the end hole slightly. With an older toddler, hiding the contrast medium in a familiar cup with a straw can be successful. Barium can be flavored with different fruit drink powders or with chocolate syrup; give the child what it chooses. Water-soluble iodinated contrast medium has a bitter taste that is more difficult to disguise, and in the concentrations often necessary for it to be seen on fluoroscopy it is not as benign as barium if it is aspirated. In postsurgical examinations when there is risk of perforation of the esophagus, however, its use may be mandated.

There are times when the child refuses to cooperate. It is helpful at this point to "triage" the clinical questions: What is the most important question to be answered? The next most important? You must do this, because structuring the examination to answer one question may take away your chance to answer another. If the examination cannot be rescheduled for another day when the child might be more hungry or better rested, then the contrast medium must be administered manually. Assistance from parents and/or technologists is necessary. Wrapping the child's legs in a sheet can often help persuade it that resistance is futile. A small syringe (5 mL for a toddler, 10 mL for an older child) is used to put aliquots of contrast medium as far back in the child's mouth as possible. At least a small amount is generally swallowed, allowing appreciation of pharyngeal function and esophageal motility. If this fails, then a small feeding tube is passed through the child's nose and into the distal esophagus. With the child in the lateral position, the radiologist pulls the tube back slowly, hand-injecting at intervals sufficient volume to distend the esophagus, until the entire esophagus is imaged. This gives a poor assessment of esophageal motility, however, and there is danger of aspiration. In addition, a "normal" study performed only with a tube will miss the abnormality associated with swallowing that can be found in up to half the patients referred for examination (Vazquez and Buonomo 1999).

Assessing gastroesophageal reflux (GER) fluoroscopically takes patience. It is best to do this at the end of the examination. The child's stomach should be full and the child should be relaxed and distracted. If the preceding part of the study has been unpleasant, the child might be allowed to feed in its parent's arms until its stomach is full, and then it should be placed again beneath the fluoroscope. Darkening the room and minimizing noise might encourage the child to fall asleep in a supine position. Videos or recorded music provides solace and distraction for the toddler. The fluoroscope should be positioned to show the esophagus, then one should image for only about 1 s out of every 7–10 s, for a total of 5 min (less than 1 min of fluoroscopy time). Significant reflux, i.e., reaching the clavicles, cervical esophagus, or pharynx, will persist long enough for it to be recorded. Crying reinforces the diaphragmatic hiatus and minimizes reflux, so assessment in an inconsolable child may have to be abandoned.

The modified barium swallow is conducted very differently. Here, the child's usual feeding position is duplicated in a chair or seat, and graded food textures are offered, opacified with contrast medium. A trained feeding therapist should be in attendance and should choose the textures to be tested, and a familiar person should do the feeding. Because of the confines of the imaging chair and the fluoroscopy image intensifier, imaging is usually done from the lateral projection only. The study is recorded on video alone. Because the child is less restrained, the radiologist must work to keep the pharynx centered in the screen.

2.2 Radiation Dose Reduction

Throughout any fluoroscopic examination, the radiologist must be constantly mindful of the accumulating radiation dose. Grids should not be used for children less than adult size. The thyroid has to be part of the field of view, but gonads, pelvic bone marrow, and the ocular lenses should be rigorously excluded by coning and shielding. Intermittent review of the recorded video may find that an abnormality has been imaged that escaped direct visualization, and that additional imaging is unnecessary. Pulsed fluoroscopy can dramatically reduce the patient dose with relatively minor image degradation (Hernandez and Goodsitt 1996). Digital fluoroscopy units have the added advantage of "last image hold," whereby the image present on the screen when the examiner stops fluoroscoping remains there and can be captured as a permanent digital image. Since the examiner can react more quickly to seeing a pathological event than the spot image device can record it, there is a better chance that it will be caught. This also avoids the dose from spot exposure technique. The use of magnification causes the fluoroscope to increase output to maintain image brightness and thereby multiplies the dose; it should be used only when absolutely necessary.

2.3 Advanced Imaging Techniques

Nuclear medicine offers a low-dose way to monitor an entire feeding and postprandial period to look for aspiration and reflux. Technetium-99 m is the isotope of choice to label a meal. The limitation is not on imaging time, but rather on patient movement during scanning: misregistration introduces an uninterpretable artifact, so sedation is sometimes necessary (del Rosario and Orenstein 1998).

CT and MRI are sometimes necessary for imaging extraesophageal structures. CT interpretation is made difficult by the lack of mediastinal fat planes and intravenously administered contrast medium is usually necessary. Scanning is quick in the newer, multidetector machines and sedation is rarely, if ever, needed. Care must be taken to adapt the scan parameters to the weight of the child and to keep the radiation dose as low as possible. MRI excels in imaging the mediastinum and its vascular structures, where cardiac and respiratory gating ensure interpretable images without administration of contrast medium. However, the long imaging time means that sedation is usually indicated.

The application of ultrasound is limited because of the location of the esophagus deep to the air-filled lungs. GER can be imaged from the epigastric region using color-Doppler ultrasonography (Jang et al. 2001). The practicality and efficacy remain to be determined, however.

3 Congenital Esophageal Abnormalities: Their Basis in Embryology

Abnormalities of the pediatric esophagus can be loosely classed as either anatomic or functional, with congenital and acquired lesions in each category. Congenital anatomic abnormalities originate in defective morphogenesis early in embryonic life (Berrocal et al. 1999; Moore 1989). Lateral tracheoesophageal folds form in the embryonic foregut during the fourth week of development. These fuse and allow the esophagus and trachea to lengthen independently. The trachea remains united with the developing pharynx cranial to the folds, through the laryngeal aditus. The esophagus is initially very short, but reaches its final length as the embryo grows.

The epithelium of the esophagus proliferates and almost obliterates the lumen; recanalization occurs during the eighth week of development. Defects in the progression of fold fusion, recanalization, or lengthening result in congenital anatomic abnormalities that the radiologist is usually called upon to characterize.

3.1   Esophageal Atresia and Tracheoesophageal Fistula

Incomplete differentiation of the presumptive trachea from the esophagus in the fourth week of embryonic development results in a spectrum of abnormalities that come to clinical attention immediately, when the infant cannot swallow oral secretions and a tube cannot be passed to the stomach. The largest group (82%) (Buonomo et al. 1998) has esophageal atresia (EA) with a distal tracheoesophageal fistula (TEF). This is visible on a plain radiograph, with an air-filled sac projecting in the neck, perhaps with a coiled tube, and air in the stomach and gut. Studies with contrast medium are not necessary and would cause aspiration. If imaging is necessary, air insufflation of the upper sac under fluoroscopy may suffice; otherwise, careful injection of a very small amount of low-osmolarity water-soluble contrast medium may delineate the needed field. The infant's head should be elevated and the contrast medium quickly removed. A few babies in this spectrum (6%) have an isolated TEF (Fig. 1). A few others not considered part of this group have a laryngeal cleft, a high defect at the level of the aditus that can be confused clinically and fluoroscopically with a TEF.

The surgeon may wish the radiologist to more extensively study a smaller group prior to surgery: the 10% that have atresia without a TEF or with a TEF from the proximal esophageal segment. These babies will have no air distally in the GI tract. The timing of the surgery may depend on the growth of the proximal and distal esophageal segments; the smaller the distance between the ends, as demonstrated by the approximation of radio-opaque catheters under fluoroscopy (Rossi et al. 1998), the more successful the repair. Postoperative follow-up must be alert for early anastomotic leaks, late anastomotic strictures, and recurrent fistulas (Cumming and Williams 1996). Pneumothorax, pneumomediastinum, or pleural

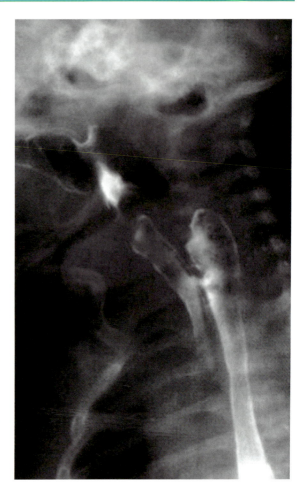

Fig. 1 Newborn male with choking and hypoxemia with feeding. Lateral view from barium swallow delineates TEF, with contrast in the trachea

effusion might be signs on plain radiographs of developing complications.

All of these infants must be screened for the skeletal, renal, anal, and cardiac anomalies that can coexist with EA–TEF in the VATER or VACTERL associations in about half of the patients (Buonomo et al. 1998). Vertebral and limb abnormalities can be diagnosed by plain radiography, whereas ultrasonography is the most efficient screen for the brain and heart. Anorectal malformations may be apparent clinically. Repair of the TEF may not relieve all respiratory symptoms; tracheomalacia almost always occurs when there is a TEF and the residual tracheal weakness may demand its own surgical intervention.

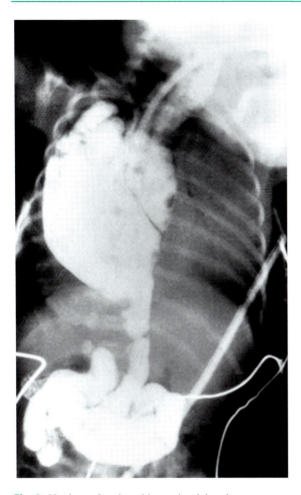

Fig. 2 Newborn female with cystic right chest mass on prenatal ultrasound. Barium fills the intrathoracic stomach and short esophagus

3.2 Other Causes of Esophageal Narrowing

If the esophagus is intact, diagnosis may be delayed until the infant begins to exhibit feeding difficulties: food refusal, slow feeding, vomiting. Again, the spectrum of possible embryologic errors gives several differential diagnostic possibilities. The esophagus may be very short, due to defective lengthening. Plain radiography and barium upper GI tract study show the stomach in the chest (Fig. 2). Defective luminal recanalization can result in webs (often in the mid esophagus, but can occur at any level) or longer-segment fibromuscular stenosis, usually in the lower third of the esophagus (del Rosario and Ohrenstein 1998). Embryonic remnants in the esophageal wall

can cause luminal narrowing. These can take the form of respiratory tract traces, such as cartilage, which will stiffen the wall and interfere with peristalsis. This can occur in conjunction with TEF and EA, and may be overlooked owing to the magnitude of these other abnormalities (Dohil and Hassall 1998).

A smoothly curving defect in the barium-filled esophagus indicates an extraluminal mass that may be intrinsic to the esophageal wall or extrinsic to the esophagus. The esophagus is the second-most common site for duplication, after the ileum (Berrocal et al. 1999). It can form a cyst lined with secretory mucosa that causes increasing symptoms as it grows. The mucosa can also be gastric in differentiation; its presentation will be due to ulceration. The location is usually in the intrathoracic esophagus. The same type of embryologic error in the respiratory tree forms bronchogenic cysts (Nobuhara et al. 1997). In their usually central location, close to the carina, they can cause respiratory symptoms that may mask feeding problems and delay diagnosis. If complicated by infection, their presence may be detected by a mediastinal air–fluid level on a plain radiograph (Hedlund et al. 1998). Leiomyomas are rare, smooth muscle tumors, and the esophagus is an unusual place for them, but they can occur. In children, they are more likely to be multiple or infiltrative than in adults. Leiomyomatosis is a very rare condition seen in about 5% of patients with Alport syndrome where widespread involvement of the esophagus and, occasionally, the tracheobronchial tree by smooth muscle proliferation leads to debilitating symptoms (Guest et al. 2000). Pericarinal adenopathy of sufficient magnitude in a small infant can compress the esophagus as well (Fig. 3).

Narrowing of the cervical esophagus has a slightly different differential list, influenced by the proximity of the branchial clefts. Cysts can form from second cleft remnants, whereas the third and fourth clefts can fistulize to the piriform sinuses. Cysts of the thyroid, thyroglossal duct, thymic remnants, or larynx can also occur. Duplication is a rare finding in this region (Wootton-Gorges et al. 2002).

Because of the complexity of embryonic morphogenic processes, multiple errors can coexist. It behooves the radiologist to recognize patterns of malformation when they occur, but not to be a slave to them. In so doing, the radiologist might reject the possibility of a certain abnormality because it does not "fit the pattern", and thereby miss a diagnosis. For example, a child with thoracic vertebral anomalies who

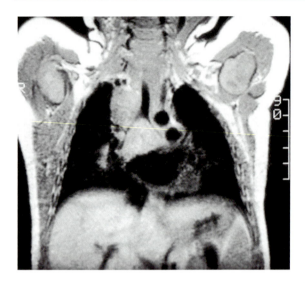

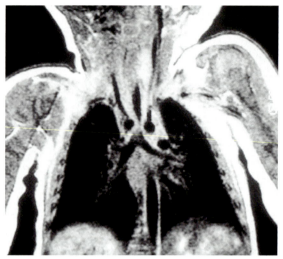

Fig. 3 Six-month-old male, 2 months after a visit from foreign relatives. Coronal MRI shows compression of mediastinal structures by pericarinal and paratracheal adenopathy. The patient was treated for tuberculosis

Fig. 4 Five-month-old male with feeding difficulty, stridor, and distorted esophagus on barium swallow. Coronal MRI shows the trachea compressed between the double aortic arches

had other VATER/VACTERL elements excluded as an infant should not be dismissed as having behavioral problems if it presents later with feeding difficulties. Rather, a search for a neuroenteric cyst or a duplication cyst should be considered, both of which can also coexist with spina bifida, hemivertebra, and fusion defects (Berrocal et al. 1999). Finding one abnormality should not stop the search for others. Case reports abound in the literature illustrating odd and unexpected assortments of allied anomalies: EA–TEF with esophageal stenosis (Newman and Bender 1997), TEF with web and duplication (Snyder et al. 1996), and anomalous origin of a bronchus from the esophagus (Lallemand et al. 1996).

3.3   Vascular Anomalies

Vascular rings and slings deserve special mention, as they can be definitively described radiologically and treatment can be planned accordingly. Like other abnormalities that narrow rather than interrupt the esophagus, these may come to clinical attention when the child's diet changes from liquid to solid. The embryonal system of parallel, interconnecting dorsal and ventral arteries normally recedes focally to leave the familiar left aortic arch and its branches. Variation in the pattern of recession can leave the fetus with

arteries that cross and impinge on mediastinal structures (Strife et al. 1998). Two entities that form anatomically complete rings that encircle the trachea and esophagus and are fairly common are the double aortic arch (Fig. 4) and the right arch with aberrant left subclavian artery and intact ductus or ligamentum (Fig. 5). These patients will present with respiratory and feeding difficulties, although when the former is thought to cause the latter, diagnosis can be delayed. Surgical treatment is usually mandated. Patients with an arch with contralateral subclavian aberrancy, such as the very common left arch with aberrant right subclavian artery, will not have respiratory symptoms if the ligamentum is broken or elongated. Although a posterior defect may be seen in the barium-filled esophagus from the aberrant vessel, surgery is not usually necessary unless the symptoms interfere with growth. Likewise, a pulmonary sling, where the left pulmonary artery passes between the trachea and esophagus on its way to the left side from its anomalous origin on the right, may distort the esophagus without compression (Fig. 6); its compressive effect on the tracheobronchial tree, however, may be profound and this can secondarily interfere with feeding (Siripornpitak et al. 1997). Where a vascular anomaly is suspected, either primarily or uncovered on a barium esophagram, MRI can definitively delineate it and show its effect on mediastinal structures; angiography is contraindicated. A contrast-enhanced CT

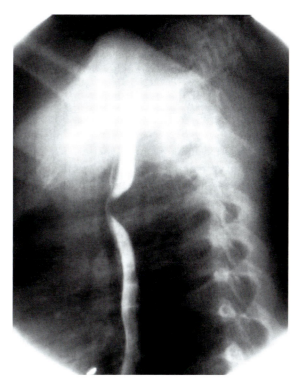

Fig. 5 Two-month-old female with wheezing and regurgitation, and right aortic arch on chest x-ray. Lateral view of barium swallow shows prominent posterior defect. MRI (not shown) confirmed vascular ring with right arch, aberrant left subclavian artery, and intact ligamentum

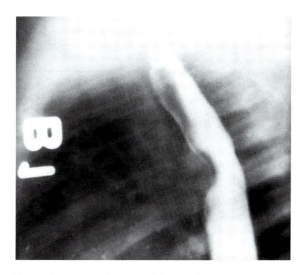

Fig. 6 One-month-old male with wheezing. Chest radiograph (not shown) was remarkable for asymmetric hyperinflation on the right. Lateral view of barium swallow shows anterior defect in the contrast column, compatible with pulmonary sling. Confirmed by MRI (not shown)

scan with 3D reconstruction can show the abnormality very well, but the radiation dose can be quite high. However, CT scanning has become so fast that sedation is almost never necessary. Thus, the radiation dose may be acceptable when the sedation needed for MRI poses a greater risk, as in a child with a narrowed airway.

4 Congenital Functional Abnormalities: The Interplay of Anatomy and Maturation

4.1 Dysphagia

Swallowing demands a certain level of central nervous system maturation and function. Musculoskeletal structures in the face and neck must act in flawless concert to safely deliver ingested food past the larynx and into the esophagus. Similar functions are brought into play to protect the airway during reflux or vomiting. Swallows can be observed in the 12-week fetus, and passage of amniotic fluid through the GI tract is essential for its growth and development. However, the oral phase of swallow requires skills that come with later fetal maturity (Derkay and Schechter 1998). The suckle behavior of premature infants is characterized by short bursts of quick jaw movements and tongue compressions. This persists in the mature infant as nonnutritive sucking, an important behavioral adjunct to successful feeding. However, premature infants cannot reliably mount the negative intraoral pressure required for extraction of fluid from the nipple and formation of a swallow bolus. Thus, an esophagram of such an infant may show fluid loss from the mouth, uncontrolled entry of fluid to the pharynx, nasopharyngeal reflux, penetration of fluid to the larynx and trachea, lack of cough response, and poor coordination of breathing and swallowing. All of these are cause for great concern when they occur in the term or near-term infant, but may prompt only watchful waiting and cautious reevaluation at a later time in a baby who could have a postconception age of 25–32 weeks at the time of the first examination. However, in both groups the finding of contrast in the trachea should be scrutinized carefully to exclude the possibility of a TEF or laryngeal cleft. Using a small, thin-walled nipple and observing swallows at the start of the examination before the patient tires help the premature infant show its best abilities.

Infants and children with central nervous system dysfunction secondary to primary brain dysplasia (due to prenatal infection or vascular events, or to chromosomal abnormality; Eicher et al. 2000) and perinatal hypoxemia or hemorrhage form a large and growing population of patients with impaired swallowing. Loss of swallow skills from head trauma, malignancy, or degenerative disorders adds these patients to this group as well. Occasionally, progressive dysphagia is the presenting symptom that leads to diagnosis (Elta et al. 1996), or it may be only one of many problems. Advances in salvage and supportive care have made the basic ability to be fed the remaining determinant of survival in this population. It is the job of the radiologist, often in tandem with a feeding therapist, to determine a patient's level of function, whether there are any anatomic impediments to safe feeding, and what food textures can be fed (Gisel et al. 1998). The esophagram is often used to elucidate the basic anatomic framework and exclude obstruction, followed by a modified barium swallow concentrating on the swallow mechanism (Mercado-Deane et al. 2001).

4.2 Gastroesophageal Reflux

GER is near-universal in infants, decreasing in frequency with growth and maturation. It still occurs in normal children as well. It becomes pathologic when associated with pain, respiratory symptoms, or dysphagia. Transient lower esophageal sphincter (LES) relaxation has been implicated in allowing reflux episodes to occur, but many factors contribute to the transition of reflux from a benign to a malignant classification (del Rosario and Orenstein 1998). One such factor is decreased esophageal clearance, from supine positioning, dysmotility, or infrequent swallowing. The presence of a nasogastric feeding tube can also impede acid clearance, although the number of reflux episodes is unchanged; a large tube can convert a nonrefluxer to a refluxer, however (Noviski et al. 1999). Straining, a favorite maneuver to provoke reflux in adults during a fluoroscopic examination, does not do the same in children, unless it happens to coincide with a transient LES relaxation (Kawahara et al. 2001). High gastric volume (due to large feeds or delayed gastric emptying) and increased osmolality in gastric contents are associated with more and

longer periods of lowered LES pressure (Salvia et al. 2001). Hiatus hernia promotes reflux because of the loss of diaphragmatic hiatal support for the LES.

The most important morbidity associated with GER is aspiration. The effects of gastric acid on the tracheobronchial tree visible on a plain radiograph may be subtle hyperinflation due to vagal-mediated bronchospasm or flagrant peribronchial inflammation, atelectasis, or pneumonia. In the child who is usually in a supine position, the upper lobes, particularly on the right, may be more involved; a child who is more erect will deposit the aspirate into the lower lobes. Even aspiration of saliva, if it occurs chronically, is far from benign. Distinguishing between salivary and gastric aspiration can be important for therapy, and in cases where GER studies fail to show expected reflux, a nuclear medicine salivagram can be useful (Cook et al. 1997).

4.3 Achalasia

Successful passage of a food bolus through the esophagus depends on sequential relaxation and closing of the upper and lower sphincters that divide the esophagus from the pharynx above and the stomach below. Achalasia of the LES is unusual in children, constituting only about 5% of the total number of cases (Buonomo et al. 1998). In older children, (mean age of onset being about 9 years) the radiologic appearance is like that in adults, with a distended, static esophagus terminating in a "beak" at the LES. In younger patients, the distension is less evident. The classic therapy is surgical myotomy; in recent years hydrostatic balloon dilatation has become popular (Upandhyaya et al. 2002). However, in all patients there is an underlying dysmotility that affects the entire esophagus, such that relief of the LES obstruction does not restore normal esophageal function. Follow-up with barium and radionuclide swallows in a series of patients showed persistent esophageal dilatation and contrast medium retention despite an open cardia (Chawda et al. 1998). Chawda et al. also indicated that radionuclide studies could substitute for barium swallows for functional follow-up, at a lower radiation dose.

Cricopharyngeal achalasia is still rarer, with scattered cases reported (de Caluwe et al. 1999). The characteristic cricopharyngeal bar (a posterior indentation in the barium column during swallow) can be seen intermittently in normal patients, but true achalasia of the upper esophageal sphincter (UES) results in obstruction to passage of the bolus, with discoordinate swallowing, cough, nasopharyngeal reflux, and aspiration. Arnold–Chiari malformation can be a cause, and should be excluded (del Rosario and Orenstein 1998). The same treatments used for LES achalasia can apply here, but in some cases conservative treatment with gavage feeding showed a slow return to normal UES function.

Special mention should be made of children with Down syndrome. They are disproportionately represented among patients with congenital GI tract abnormalities, including esophageal webs, EA–TEF, duodenal atresia, and Hirschsprung disease. They also have a high rate of esophageal dysmotility and LES achalasia, up to 30% in one study (Zárate et al. 2001).

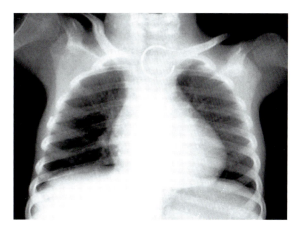

Fig. 7 Sixteen-month-old female with two-week history of food refusal. AP scout radiograph for modified barium swallow. Hoop earring is seen impacted at the thoracic inlet. Patient transferred to the endoscopy service

5   Acquired Anatomic Abnormalities: Idiopathic and Iatrogenic

5.1   Foreign Body Ingestion

The most frequent acquired abnormality among children is the ingested foreign body. The bounty of case reports in the literature attests to the child's endless ingenuity in this regard. Coins are the most frequently swallowed object (Harned et al. 1997); the local demographics will determine if the second-most-frequent items are fish bones or other metal objects such as batteries and keys (Cheng and Tam 1999; Loh et al. 2000). Diagnosis is straightforward in the case of a radio-opaque item: a lateral radiograph of the lower face and neck and an anteroposterior radiograph of the chest and abdomen to cover the entire GI tract from the nose to the anus will locate it. The lateral examination is recommended because of the young child's ability to habituate to foreign bodies in the pharynx and nasopharynx, which could be missed on chest X-ray (Fig. 7). Diagnosis of a bone ingestion is more difficult, but one study confirmed the appearance on plain radiography in 26% of cases (Cheng and Tam 1999). If the foreign body passes the UES, it will tend to impact at points where the esophageal lumen narrows: the thoracic inlet, the carina, and the LES. There is no consensus in the literature about predicting passage on the basis of

the size and location at diagnosis, but there is unanimity in the assertion that all esophageal foreign bodies should be removed within 24 h. The risk of inflammation and perforation is high and containment is poor, as the esophagus has no serosa.

The retrieval method for the foreign body depends on the institution, the kind of object, and how long it has been impacted. Coins are most frequently removed under fluoroscopy using a Foley catheter (Harned et al. 1997). Sharp, small, or multiple objects should be removed endoscopically or surgically, as should coins where the radiographic appearance suggests tracheal compression or edema, or possible perforation (pneumomediastinum, pleural effusion) (Kaye and Towbin 1996). Button batteries, such as for cameras and hearing aids, should be removed immediately as they cause chemical damage to the mucosa on contact and are a prominent cause of perforation (Samad et al. 1999).

The consequences of delayed removal are grave. High impactions at the UES can present as wheezing, cough, and vocal cord paralysis (Virgilis et al. 2001). Sharp objects such as fish bones can lacerate the mucosa, leaving hematomas (a minor complication in this series), or perforate (7% of patients), causing mediastinitis, a retropharyngeal abscess, and an aortoesophageal fistula (Loh et al. 2000). Pieces of plastic often have sharp edges and can erode and perforate (Fig. 8). The level of perforation does not necessarily determine the nature of the complication,

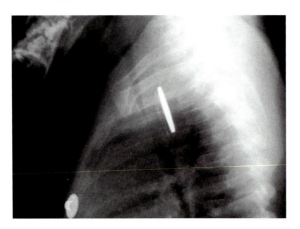

Fig. 8 Eleven-month-old female with drooling, wheezing, irritability, and food refusal. Lateral chest radiograph. Coin in the esophagus is seen on edge. Just anterior to it is the faint outline of a piece of broken plastic. The trachea is narrowed, indicating mediastinitis. This patient is not a candidate for extraction by Foley catheter because of the multiplicity, the sharp edges, and the complications

as the mediastinitis that inevitably follows can transmit infection to distant sites, such as an intervertebral disk (Fonga-Djimi et al. 1996). Because it is smooth, a coin in the esophagus can be initially asymptomatic. However with time, it too can erode and cause infection or perforation; one case report detailed a brain abscess that followed delayed extraction (Louie et al. 2000).

5.2   Iatrogenic Foreign Bodies

Nasogastric intubation is one of the most frequent hospital interventions, although inadvertent perforations rarely occur. The neonate is most frequently affected, probably because of the small diameter of the tract relative to the size of the tube, and the fact that the tube must pass through an even narrower lumen at the UES. If the UES is closed because of spasm, the tube can perforate the pharynx. Films at that point might be reminiscent of EA, with the tube curling in the neck. Air in the mediastinum, expanded retropharyngeal soft tissues, and pleural effusion will help alert the radiologist to the correct diagnosis. Cautious administration of water-soluble contrast medium may show a pseudodiverticulum or a free perforation (Sarin et al. 2000).

Thoracostomy tubes are placed to drain air or fluid from the pleural space. There is a tendency for the operator to place the tube as far medially as possible to ensure that it does not become dislodged. However, should the tube rest against mediastinal structures such as the esophagus, pressure necrosis can result (Cairns et al. 1999). When a percutaneous gastrostomy tube is changed, the internal rubber bumper is often left in the stomach to pass in the stool. Occasionally, this can cause gastric outlet obstruction. In one case, the remnant migrated into the distal esophagus and impacted, where, despite its being soft and malleable, it ulcerated the mucosa and caused scarring (Nowicki et al. 1996).

5.3   Mucosal Destruction

Widespread trauma to the esophageal mucosa can result in perforation acutely, or eventually lead to scarring and narrowing. The cause can be chemical burns, infection, or inflammation. Corrosive ingestions do the most damage when the agent is an alkali, such as drain cleaner. Burns are found most usually in the mouth, with fewer patients exhibiting pharyngeal involvement and still fewer with esophageal burns. In one series, 29% of patients had complications, and about half of these required esophageal replacement (de Jong et al. 2001). Contrast esophagram evaluation is generally delayed until after the initial inflammation subsides; if it is done earlier, it tends to underestimate the extent of damage. It is most valuable in assessing esophageal function in cases of moderate burns and gauging the extent of strictures and the results of dilatation. Immunosuppressed patients with oral candidiasis can develop candidal esophagitis. Graft-versus-host disease, a feature of the same population, can behave similarly. Where the mucosa is too friable for endoscopy, contrast medium swallow can help assess the extent of ulceration, response to therapy, and the occurrence of strictures. In advanced, invasive candidiasis cases, perforation can occur, necessitating esophageal replacement (Gaissert et al. 1999). Stevens–Johnson syndrome, or toxic epidermal necrolysis, is characterized by skin and mucosal lesions, precipitated by certain drugs or infectious agents. Oral lesions are frequent (60–80% of patients), and their severity can mask esophageal involvement. Strictures are not common sequelae, however (Lamireau et al. 2001).

Reflux esophagitis has several recognized complications. Barrett esophagus, where a specialized epithelium known to be preneoplastic is found in an esophageal segment of variable length, is found particularly in patients predisposed to severe GER: those with severe neurologic impairment who are mainly recumbent, those with chronic lung disease such as cystic fibrosis who cough and have pulmonary toilet in the head-down position, and those with primary esophageal dysmotility or hiatus hernia (Hassall 1997). Mucosal irregularity, ulceration, and narrowing can be seen in studies using contrast medium. Schatzki rings, less familiar in children than in adults, are found in a similar group of patients (Buckley et al. 1998). Esophagitis can have a predictable outcome (multiple mucosal rings), but an unusual cause: eosinophilia with food allergy, not reflux (Siafakas et al. 2000).

5.4 Miscellaneous Causes of Esophageal Dysfunction

Esophageal perforation due to blunt chest trauma is a familiar scenario for an adult in a motor vehicle accident, but is very rare in a child. Diagnosis can be delayed unless there is a high index of suspicion (Sartorelli et al. 1999). Iatrogenic perforation during stricture dilatation is more common, 21% in one series where balloon dilatation was used (Kang et al. 1998) . Anastomotic (after EA repair) and peptic strictures reacted the same way to dilatation. Another series documented fewer than that 1% perforations with bougie and olive dilators (Panieri et al. 1996). Contrast medium swallows in these series showed abnormalities ranging from mucosal disruption to frank perforation or fistula.

Nissen fundoplication is the surgical procedure of choice to control GER. It has its own complications, however, which can adversely affect the patient's ability to eat (Trinh and Benson1997). Tightening the gastro-esophageal junction is a delicate balance: tight enough to prevent reflux but loose enough to permit bolus passage. Patients who have had an EA–TEF repaired already suffer from dysmotility of the esophagus below the anastomosis. This promotes reflux and is usually the reason for the Nissen fundoplication. However, the ability to propel the bolus may then be completely compromised. Fundoplications can completely break down, but more often a large paraesophageal hernia forms that extends into the chest through the loosened hiatus. This can compress the distal esophagus still further and impede bolus passage. Many Nissen fundoplication patients are fed not by mouth but by gastrostomy tube and it is tempting, when asked to look for recurrent

reflux to explain the patient's vomiting, to only inject the tube. However, giving just a few milliliters of barium by mouth can find the possible distal esophageal obstruction and show the distended esophagus filled with secretions that the patient regurgitates.

Two final acquired complications can narrow the esophagus. In one, an arterial switch procedure puts the aorta into a position to compress the esophagus (McElhinney et al. 1998). The other represents the end stage of any of a number of diseases that cause portal hypertension (Buonomo et al. 1998). Extrahepatic portal obstruction is much more common in children. Varices form around the distal esophagus, causing vermiform defects in the margins of the contrast medium column.

6 Acquired Functional Abnormalities: The Diagnosis of Exclusion

Difficult feeding or food refusal suspected to be psychogenic in origin is a frequent reason for ordering a modified barium swallow prior to instituting behavioral therapy. There are some historical cues that can support this request: early history of prematurity or surgical procedures that interfered with the evolution of feeding skills, or bizarre dietary choices that have no logic. However, all of this chapter has attempted to show that there can be a compelling anatomic or functional abnormality to explain the symptoms, and that it is the radiologist's job to find it. History clues, such as suddenness of onset, wheezing, coughing, irritability, and taking liquids but refusing solids all point toward a physical cause. A formal upper GI tract examination should precede any modified swallow. It is a small, "low-tech" effort that can reap impressive results. Once the radiologist is satisfied that the child is normal anatomically and functionally, a psychogenic diagnosis might be entertained.

References

Berrocal T, Torres I, Gutierrez J, Prieto C, del Hoyo ML, Lamas M (1999) Congenital anomalies of the upper gastrointestinal tract. Radiographics 19:855–872

Buckley K, Buonomo C, Husain K, Nurko S (1998) Schatzki ring in children and young adults: clinical and radiologic findings. Pediatr Radiol 28:884–886

Buonomo C, Taylor GA, Share JC, Kirks DR (1998) Gastrointestinal tract. In: Kirks DR, Griscome NT (eds) Practical pediatric radiology. Lippincott-Raven, Philadelphia, pp 821–1008

Cairns PA, McClure BG, Halliday HL, McReid M (1999) Unusual site for esophageal perforation in an extremely low birth weight infant. Eur J Pediatr 158:152–153

Chawda SJ, Watura R, Adams H, Smith PM (1998) A comparison of barium swallow and erect esophageal transit scintigraphy following balloon dilation for achalasia. Dis Esophagus 11:181–188

Cheng W, Tam PKH (1999) Foreign-body ingestion in children: experience with 1,265 cases. J Pediatr Surg 34(10): 1472–1476

Cook SP, Lawless S, Mandell GA, Reilly JS (1997) The use of the salivagram in the evaluation of severe and chronic aspiration. Int J Pediatr Otorhinolaryngol 41:353–361

Cumming WA, Williams JL (1996) Neonatal gastrointestinal imaging. Clin Perinatol 23(2):387–407

de Caluwe D, Nassogne MC, Reding R, de Ville de Goyet J, Clapuyt P, Otte JB (1999) Cricopharyngeal achalasia: case reports and review of the literature. Eur J Pediatr Surg 9:109–112

de Jong AL, Macdonald R, Ein S, Forte V, Turner A (2001) Corrosive esophagitis in children: a 30-year review. Int J Pediatr Otorhinolaryngol 57:203–211

del Rosario JF, Orenstein SR (1998) Common pediatric esophageal disorders. Gastroenterologist 6(2):104–121

Derkay CS, Schechter GL (1998) Anatomy and physiology of pediatric swallowing disorders. Otolaryngol Clin North Am 31(3):397–404

Dohil R, Hassall E (1998) Esophageal stenosis in children. Gastrointest Endosc Clin N Am 8(2):369–375

Eicher PS, McDonald-McGinn DM, Fox CA, Driscoll DA, Emanuel BS, Zackia EH (2000) Dysphagia in children with a 22q11.2 deletion: Unusual pattern found on modified barium swallow. J Pediatr 137(2):158–164

Elta GH, Caldwell CA, Nostrant TT (1996) Esophageal dysphagia as the sole symptom in type 1 Chiari malformation. Dig Dis Sci 41(3):512–515

Fonga-Djimi H, Leclerc F, Martinot A, Hue V, Fourier C, Deschildre A, Flurin V (1996) Spondylodiscitis and mediastinitis after esophageal perforation owing to a swallowed radiolucent foreign body. J Pediatr Surg 31(5):698–700

Gaissert HA, Breuer CK, Weissburg A, Mermel L (1999) Surgical management of necrotizing Candida esophagitis. Ann Thorac Surg 67(1):231–233

Gisel EG, Birnbaum R, Schwartz S (1998) Feeding impairments in children: diagnosis and effective intervention. Int J Orofacial Myology 24:27–33

Guest AR, Strouse PJ, Hiew CC, Arca M (2000) Progressive esophageal leiomyomatosis with respiratory compromise. Pediatr Radiol 30:247–250

Harned RK, Strain JD, Hay TC, Douglas MR (1997) Esophageal foreign bodies: safety and efficacy of foley catheter extraction of coins. AJR Am J Roentgenol 168:443–446

Hassall E (1997) Comorbidities in childhood Barrett's esophagus. J Pediatr Gastroenterol Nutr 25:255–260

Hedlund GL, Griscome NT, Cleveland RH, Kirks DR (1998) Respiratory system. In: Kirks DR, Griscome NT (eds) Practical pediatric radiology. Lippincott-Raven, Philadelphia, pp 619–820

Hernandez RJ, Goodsitt MM (1996) Reduction of radiation dose in pediatric patients using pulsed fluoroscopy. AJR Am J Roentgenol 167:1247–1253

Jang HS, Lee JS, Lim GY, Choi BG, Choi GH, Park SH (2001) Correlation of color Doppler sonographic findings with pH measurements in gastroesophageal reflux in children. J Clin Ultrasound 29(4):212–216

Kang SG, Song HY, Lim MK, Yoon HK, Goo DE, Sung KB (1998) Esophageal rupture during balloon dilation of strictures of benign or malignant causes: prevalence and clinical importance. Radiology 209:741–746

Kawahara H, Dent J, Chir B, Davidson G, Okada A (2001) Relationship between straining, transient lower esophageal sphincter relaxation, and gastroesophageal reflux in children. Am J Gastroenterol 96(7):2019–2025

Kaye RD, Towbin RB (1996) Interventional procedures in the gastrointestinal tract in children. Radiol Clin North Am 34(4):903–917

Lallemand D, Quignodon JF, Courtel JV (1996) The anomalous origin of bronchus from the esophagus: report of three cases. Pediatr Radiol 26:179–182

Lamireau T, Leauté -Labrèze C, Le Bail B, Taieb A (2001) Esophageal involvement in Stevens-Johnson syndrome. Endoscopy 33(6):550–553

Loh KS, Tan LKS, Smith JD, Yeoh KH, Dong F (2000) Complications of foreign bodies in the esophagus. Otolaryngol Head Neck Surg 123(5):613–616

Louie JP, Osterhoudt KC, Christian CW (2000) Brain abscess following delayed endoscopic removal of an initially asymptomatic esophageal coin. Pediatr Emerg Care 16(2): 102–105

McElhinney DB, Reddy VM, Reddy GP, Higgins CB, Hanley FL (1998) Esophageal compression by aorta after arterial switch. Ann Thorac Surg 65:246–248

Mercado-Deane MG, Burton EM, Harlow SA, Glover AS, Deane DA, Guill MF, Hudson V (2001) Swallowing dysfunction in infants less than 1 year of age. Pediatr Radiol 31:423–428

Moore KL (1989) Before we are born: basic embryology and birth defects, 3rd edn. Saunders, Philadelphia, pp 159–161

Newman B, Bender TM (1997) Esophageal atresia/tracheoesophageal fistula and associated congenital esophageal stenosis. Pediatr Radiol 27:530–534

Nobuhara KK, Gorski YC, La Quaglia MP, Shamberger RC (1997) Bronchogenic cysts and esophageal duplications: common origins and treatment. J Pediatr Surg 32(10): 1408–1413

Noviski N, Yehuda YB, Serour F, Gorenstein A, Mandelberg A (1999) Does the size of nasogastric tubes affect gastroesophageal reflux in children? J Pediatr Gastroenterol Nutr 29(4):448–451

Nowicki MJ, Johnson ND, Rudolph CD (1996) Esophageal stricture caused by a retained percutaneous gastrostomy tube remnant. J Pediatr Gastroentero Nutr 22(2):208–211

Panieri E, Millar AJW, Rode H, Brown RA, Cywes S (1996) Iatrogenic esophageal perforation in children: patterns of injury, presentation, management, and outcome. J Pediatr Surg 31(7):890–895

Rossi C, Domini M, Aquino A, Persico A, Lelli-Chiesa P (1998) A simple and safe method to visualize the inferior pouch in esophageal atresia without fistula. Pediatr Surg Int 13:535–536

Salvia G, De Vizia B, Manguso F, Iula VD, Terrin G, Spadaro R, Russo G, Cucchiara S (2001) Effects of intragastric volume and osmolality on mechanisms of gastroesophageal reflux in children with gastroesophageal reflux disease. Am J Gastroenterol 96(6):1725–1732

Samad L, Ali M, Ramzi H (1999) Button battery ingestion: hazards of esophageal impaction. J Pediatr Surg 34(10):1527–1531

Sarin YK, Goel D, Mathur NB, Maria A (2000) Neonatal pharyngeal pseudo-diverticulum. Indian Pediatr 37: 1134–1137

Sartorelli KH, McBride WJ, Vane DW (1999) Perforation of the intrathoracic esophagus from blunt trauma in a child: case report and review of the literature. J Pediatr Surg 34(3):495–497

Siafakas CG, Ryan CK, Brown MR, Miller TL (2000) Multiple esophageal rings: an association with eosinophilic esophagitis. Am J Gastroenterol 95(6):1572–1575

Siripornpitak S, Reddy GP, Schwitter J, Higgins CB (1997) Pulmonary artery sling: anatomical and functional evaluation by MRI. J Comput Assist Tomogr 21(5):766–768

Snyder CL, Bickler SW, Gittes GK, Ramachandran V, Ashcraft KW (1996) Esophageal duplication cyst with esophageal web and tracheoesophageal fistula. J Pediatr Surg 31(7): 968–969

Strife JL, Bisset III GS, Burrows PE (1998) Cardiovascular system. In: Kirks DR, Griscome NT (eds) Practical pediatric radiology. Lippincott-Raven, Philadelphia, pp 511–618

Trinh TD, Benson JE (1997) Fluoroscopic diagnosis of complications after Nissen antireflux fundoplication in children. AJR Am J Roentgenol 169(4):1023–1028

Upadhyaya M, Fataar S, Sajwany MJ (2002) Achalasia of the cardia: experience with hydrostatic balloon dilation in children. Pediatr Radiol 32:409–412

Vazquez JL, Buonomo C (1999) Feeding difficulties in the first days of life: findings on upper gastrointestinal series and the role of the videofluoroscopic swallowing study. Pediatr Radiol 29:894–896

Virgilis D, Weinberger JM, Fisher D, Goldberg S, Picard E, Kerem E (2001) Vocal cord paralysis secondary to impacted esophageal foreign bodies in young children. Pediatrics 107(6):e101

Wootton-Gorges SL, Eckel GM, Poulos ND, Kappler S, Milstein JM (2002) Duplication of the cervical esophagus: a case report and review of the literature. Pediatr Radiol 32:533–535

Zárate N, Mearin F, Hidalgo A, Malagelada J-R (2001) Prospective evaluation of esophageal motor dysfunction in Down's syndrome. Am J Gastroenterol 96(6):1718–1724

Pharyngeal Manometry

Rolf Olsson

Contents

Abstract

Pharyngeal manometry is an important diagnostic tool in the evaluation of dysphagia. This chapter describes the technique and the simultaneous examination with videoradiography.

1 Introduction

Dysphagia is the subjective awareness of swallowing difficulties. A normal swallow is the smoothly coordinated transportation of a bolus from the oral cavity, through the pharynx and esophagus, into the stomach. When normal it is the combination of voluntary, automatic, and autonomic functions (Miller 1986). Abnormalities in the oral cavity, pharynx, and esophagus may hamper normal swallow, as may impairment of the neurologic control (Bosma et al. 1986; Buchholz et al. 1985; Gordon et al. 1987). Swallowing complaints are common, especially in hospitalized patients. Several studies have reported up to 30% of these populations to suffer from dysphagia (Groher and Bukatman 1986; Lindgren and Janzon 1991).

In the examination of the dysphagic patient several diagnostic modalities are available. The clinical and neurological examination is important, followed by radiographic and/or endoscopic examination for assessment of morphological changes (Dodds et al. 1990; Ekberg and Wahlgren 1985). When such examinations are ruled out, more functional investigations come into place, such as dynamic barium swallow, pH monitoring, manometry, scintigraphy, ultrasonography, and electromyography.

R. Olsson (✉)
Diagnostic Centre of Imaging and Functional Medicine,
Skåne University Hospital, 205 02 Malmö, Sweden
e-mail: rolf.olsson@med.lu.se

O. Ekberg (ed.), *Dysphagia*, Medical Radiology. Diagnostic Imaging, DOI: 10.1007/174_2011_343,
© Springer-Verlag Berlin Heidelberg 2012

Dynamic cine- and videoradiography of pharyngeal barium swallow provides morphological as well as qualitative functional information of the swallowing sequence (Ekberg 1987; Ekberg and Nylander 1982). However, dynamic barium swallow relies mainly on functional qualitative judgment, failing to quantify the results. This is, for example, the case when trying to assess pharyngeal paresis in terms of the degree of barium retention in the pharynx.

In this context, pharyngeal manometry is capable of providing a more quantitative analysis of pharyngeal muscle function in terms of intraluminal pressure registration. Concurrent barium swallow and pharyngeal manometry combines the qualitative assessment of bolus transport with quantitative registration of the contractions of the pharyngeal wall.

The previously described results obtained with combined manometry and videoradiography in the literature are promising. Recent advances in manometric technology together with computer analysis of the data have facilitated pharyngeal manometry and the combined technique has been advocated by several authors.

2   Manometry

Pressure is the force acting perpendicular to an area. Physiological pressures are usually expressed in millimeters of mercury (mm Hg). Many other pressure units are available, for example, pascals (Pa), newtons per square meter (N/m^2), and centimeters of water (cm H_2O). Manometry records intraluminal pressure activity and detects and quantifies changes in intraluminal pressures that in the pharynx are caused by contractions of the muscles of the gullet. Such intraluminal pressures can be described as either contact pressures, when the manometric sensor is in direct contact with the pharyngeal wall, or cavity pressures, when the sensor is completely surrounded by air or fluid. The latter is also called intrabolus pressure (Brasseur 1987; Brasseur and Dodds 1991).

Intraluminal esophageal manometry has been used extensively as a test of esophageal function for more than 100 years (Kronecker and Meltzer 1883). In the early history of manometry, pressures were obtained by means of static water-filled catheters within the esophagus. Around 20 years ago the development of low-compliance perfusion systems contributed to more accurate measurements of intraluminal pressure

and motility (Arndorfer et al. 1977). The continuous perfusion prevented occlusion of the sensors.

Solid-state intraluminal transducers have developed during the last decade and have further improved the manometric accuracy (Castell and Castell 1993). These sensors are located on the catheter and can be placed in the gullet, allowing direct measurement on the site of interest.

Together with the advances in computer technology, analysis and storage of manometric data have been facilitated.

3   Pharyngeal Manometry

Pharyngeal manometry is a less frequently used technique, with difficulties in pressure recording because of the rapid pharyngeal swallowing sequence, as well as the movement of the soft palate and the larynx and also the radial asymmetry of intraluminal contact pressure (Welch et al. 1979; Winans 1972). Perfused manometry is not suitable in the pharynx because of the continuous flow that will trigger swallows.

Furthermore, perfused manometry has to be performed with the subject in a supine position because of the need to calibrate the sensors at the same level. Pharyngeal manometry with the subject in an upright physiologic position, with accurate recording technique, makes solid-state manometry a prerequisite in pharyngeal manometry (Orlowski et al. 1982).

Manometric evaluation of the pharynx with solid-state manometry and computerized analysis has been described in several articles by Don Castell and his group in Philadelphia (Castell and Castell 1993; Castell et al. 1993, 1990). They have thoroughly described the difficulties in pharyngeal manometry due to the rapid contractions of the striated muscles in the pharynx and the radial asymmetry with higher pressure in the anteroposterior direction. This group has also reported normal values in pharyngeal manometry in terms of contraction and relaxation but also in timing and coordination between events during pharyngeal swallow.

We have established normal values in pharyngeal manometry with simultaneous videoradiography and fluoroscopic control of sensor positioning (Olsson et al. 1995a) (Figs. 1, 2). We included 25 nondysphagic volunteers with normal videoradiographic parameters in this study. The examination was performed with the volunteers in an upright physiologic

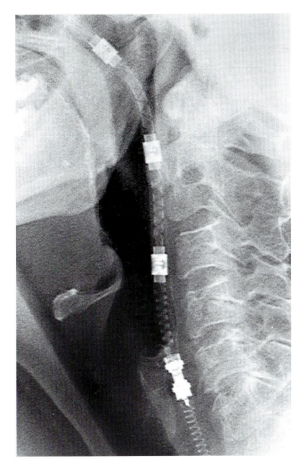

Fig. 1 Pharyngeal manometry with a solid-state manometry catheter in the pharynx. The distal sensor is positioned in the upper esophageal sphincter

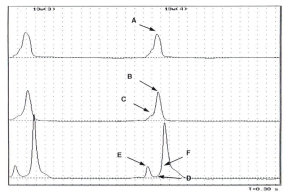

Fig. 2 A manometric tracing from a normal pharyngeal swallow. *A* pharyngeal peak pressure at the tongue-base level, *B* pharyngeal peak pressure at the level of the inferior pharyngeal constrictor, *C* intrabolus pressure, *D* upper esophageal sphincter relaxation pressure, *E,F* upper esophageal sphincter relaxation duration

caused pressures around 600 mm Hg. A standardized manometric technique is important in videomanometry and normal values as described in this study are essential in clinical use.

4 Technical Considerations in Pharyngeal Manometry

Pharyngeal pressures are usually expressed in millimeters of mercury and they are normally expressed relative to atmospheric pressure. Changes in atmospheric pressure seldom have an effect on physiological pressures, but calibration and establishing a "zero" pressure is necessary to achieve reproducible and comparative data.

In 1982 Orlowski et al. (1982) described the requirements for accurate recording of pharyngeal pressures. They studied the frequency characteristics of pharyngeal pressure complexes in normal subjects and found a recording accuracy of up to 48 Hz needed for high-fidelity recording in the pharynx. The frequency content of upper esophageal pressure has also been reported by Ask et al. (1979).

A low-compliance perfusion system has a bandwidth of approximately only 23 Hz (Ask et al. 1979). Orlowski et al. (1982) concluded that solid-state sensors are needed in pharyngeal manometry. Furthermore, the mechanical recording pens of a polygraph record only to a frequency of 20–40 Hz

position during 10-ml barium and dry swallows. The mean resting pressure in the upper esophageal sphincter was 90 ± 33 (± 2 standard deviations, SD) mm Hg. The mean residual pressure during relaxation of the upper esophageal sphincter was 7.2 ± 8.0 (± 2 SD) mm Hg during barium swallow and 3.8 ± 6.2 (± 2 SD) mm Hg during dry swallow. The mean duration of upper esophageal sphincter relaxation was 601 ± 248 (± 2 SD) ms.

The mean peristaltic contraction of the upper esophageal sphincter was 254 ± 143 (± 2 SD) mm Hg. Fourteen (56%) of the 25 volunteers had a measurable intrabolus pressure (mean 33 ± 17 mm Hg) at the level of the inferior pharyngeal constrictor.

A specific finding was discovered when the epiglottis tilts down, hitting the manometric sensor. This epiglottic tilt was identified in seven subjects (28%) and

(Stef et al. 1974). Thus, a computerized recording system is needed to faithfully register frequencies up to 48 Hz.

In upper esophageal sphincter manometry, displacement of the manometric sensor is a problem because of the movement of the anatomical structures during swallowing. The Dent sleeve (Dent 1976) is a 6-cm-long sensor developed to measure the sphincter pressure in spite of sphincter movement. The sleeve is, however, perfused and the recording accuracy is not in line with that of the solid-state technique. Another drawback with the sleeve is the risk of underestimating sphincter relaxation duration because of the oncoming peristaltic contraction at the top of the sleeve.

We have also studied the movements of the soft palate and the larynx, which are crucial in pharyngeal manometry because of the potential risk of manometry sensor dislocation (Olsson et al. 1994a). A total of 20 dysphagic patients and 20 nondysphagic volunteers were examined with simultaneous videoradiography and intraluminal pharyngeal solid-state manometry.

The movements of the manometric sensors were analyzed from lateral video recording. Two different types of catheter movement were found. The sensor in the upper esophageal sphincter could either be lifted cranially during the closure of the soft palate (type 1) or stay unaltered in the sphincter until the beginning of the laryngeal elevation and then follow the sphincter cranially during laryngeal elevation with no previous response to soft palate closure (type 2). Type 1 movement was found in eight of 20 patients but in only one of the 20 volunteers. The resting pressure of the upper esophageal sphincter was significantly higher in type 2 movement ($p = 0.004$). A total of 19 of 20 participants with a high resting pressure of the upper esophageal sphincter (above 83 mm Hg) were found to have the type 2 movement.

5   Contact and Cavity Pressures in the Pharynx

Contact pressure is defined when the manometric sensor is in direct contact with the pharyngeal wall, with direct contact force on the sensor membrane. Such contact pressure is relatively easy to define and measure, as long as the recording device is properly

calibrated and meets the previously described requirements of pharyngeal manometry (Brasseur 1987; Brasseur and Dodds 1991).

Cavity pressures are defined when the manometric sensor is completely surrounded by air or fluid. When the sensor is surrounded by air, for example, in the oropharynx, the pressure should be equal to atmospheric pressure if proper calibration is done. The pressure should then be zero (0 mm Hg).

Another cavity pressure occurs when the sensor is completely surrounded by fluid when swallowing. This pressure is called hydrodynamic pressure or synonymously intrabolus pressure. In a static fluid the pressure is the same at all levels. The pressure in a static fluid will increase with gravity, which means a pressure increase proportional to the depth of the sensor in the fluid. The density of the fluid will also affect the static intrabolus pressure.

In a fluid with flow, however, many different factors become important. This type of intrabolus pressure is very difficult to define and standardize in an exact and reproducible way. The cause of the flow will be a pressure gradient from one place to another within the fluid. The frictional resistance and the fluid acceleration are important. Furthermore, the elasticity of the walls and the viscosity of the fluid have to be considered.

The viscosity can be explained as the friction within the fluid. The units are newton seconds per square meter ($N\ s/m^2$) or centipoises (cP), where $1\ cP = 1 \times 10^{-3}\ N\ s/m^2$. The density ($kg/m^3$) of a fluid is also important.

The rheological properties of the fluid in terms of turbulent or laminar flow are also important.

In a laboratory model we have shown that the intrabolus pressure is dependent on position of the manometric sensor, degree of lumen narrowing, bolus volume, flow rate, and fluid viscosity (Olsson et al. 1994b).

We have also elucidated elevated intrabolus pressure above a cricopharyngeal narrowing in a study of 16 patients with cricopharyngeal bars compared with a control group of 16 patients without cricopharyngeal bars (Olsson and Ekberg 1995). The patients with cricopharyngeal bars showed a significantly wider upper esophageal sphincter above and below the cricopharyngeal muscle and the contraction pressure within the inferior pharyngeal constrictor was significantly weaker in patients with cricopharyngeal bars.

These findings suggested that the cricopharyngeal indentation is due to weak constrictors with out-pouching of the gullet above and below the cricopharyngeal muscle. The cricopharyngeal muscle showed no abnormalities in terms of resting pressure, relaxation, and contraction pressure. Furthermore, there was no significant difference in intrabolus pressure, neither above nor at the level of the cricopharyngeal muscle.

6 Simultaneous Examination

The combination of simultaneous videoradiography and intraluminal manometry provides fluoroscopic control of sensor positioning and allows pressure recording and analysis with respect to bolus transport. It combines movement analysis with pressure recordings.

When solid-state sensors are used, the technique can be performed with the patient in an upright, physiologic position and comfortably seated without the discomfort of swallowing in a supine position and without the discomfort of the continuous flow of perfused manometry (Fig. 3).

The history of simultaneous examinations goes back to 1995 when Fyke and Code (1955) measured pharyngeal pressure with a microtip transducer fitted on a gastric tube. They used simultaneous cineradiography, but the manometric recordings were made with a galvanometer and a polygraph. Atkinson et al. (1957) took rapid serial radiographs during pharyngeal manometry with a perfused technique. Sokol et al. (1966) reported their experience with simultaneous cineradiography and perfused intraluminal manometry of the pharynx.

Isberg et al. (1985) reported solid-state manometry with Gaeltec sensors and simultaneous cineradiography. They studied movement of the upper esophageal sphincter and the manometric device in nine healthy volunteers. They found an upward movement of the manometry catheter that correlated with the elevation of the soft palate. The pressure was recorded on a polygraph.

Mendelsohn and McConnel (1987) described a simultaneous technique with perfused manometry and McConnel et al. (1988) and also Cerenko et al. (1989) described simultaneous fluoroscopy and solid-state

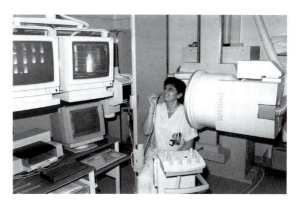

Fig. 3 Simultaneous videoradiography and solid-state intraluminal manometry during barium swallow. The pressure registration is displayed on the video screen and is also registered on the computer. The subject is comfortably seated and fluoroscopy is performed in a lateral projection

manometry. McConnel et al. called the technique "manofluorography."

Jacob et al. (1989) used solid-state manometry and simultaneous videoradiography with polygraph recording to study the upper esophageal sphincter in eight volunteers. This was a thorough study of upper esophageal sphincter opening and volume-dependent variables such as intrabolus pressure and opening duration.

In the same year, Cook et al. (1989) described the simultaneous technique in two studies involving healthy volunteers. They used solid-state sensors but a conventional eight-channel polygraph. This was a study of the upper esophageal sphincter where they concluded that upper esophageal sphincter opening involves sphincter relaxation, anterior laryngeal traction, and intrabolus pressure. They also found volume-dependent changes in upper esophageal sphincter dimensions and upper esophageal sphincter timing indicating a sensory feedback mechanism generated by the brainstem swallow centers.

The following year, Dantas et al. (1990) used the technique in six patients with cricopharyngeal bars. They found normal contact pressures in the pharynx but increased upstream intrabolus pressure. They also studied different bolus variables with this technique (Dantas et al. 1989).

A high-density barium preparation increased the intrabolus pressure as well as the upper esophageal sphincter opening duration and anterior hyoid movement. All these studies used the Gaeltec solid-state catheter but recording was with an ordinary polygraph without computerized analysis.

Shaker et al. (1992) used the perfused sleeve device concurrent with videoradiography to study the esophagoglottal closure reflex. They concluded that esophageal distension by air or balloon evokes a glottal closure mechanism, suggesting the existence of an esophagoglottal reflex.

Ren et al. (1993) used perfused manometry concurrent with videofluoroscopy in a study of intrabolus pressure and concluded that intrabolus pressure can serve as an indicator of the forces resisting peristaltic transport. They called the technique "videofluoromanometry." Ergun et al. (1993) used the simultaneous technique in eight volunteers. They argued strongly for the use of fluoroscopic sensor positioning when performing pharyngeal timing studies. They used solid-state sensors and video recording but polygraph registration without a computer. Dejaeger et al. (1994) used manofluorography to analyze swallowing in the elderly. This study used a solid-state technique and video recording but also a conventional polygraph.

In another study we examined 19 patients (12 males, seven females, mean age 47 years, range 19–69 years) with pharyngeal dysphagia but a normal barium swallow and compared them with normal volunteers (Olsson et al. 1995a, b). The patient group showed statistically significant differences for eight of ten manometric variables. We found manometric abnormalities that might contribute to dysphagia: five with high upper esophageal sphincter resting pressure, five with high upper esophageal sphincter residual pressure, three with weak pharyngeal contractions, seven with prolonged contraction/relaxation time, and seven with incoordination. The conclusion of this study was that manometry could provide additional information in the diagnosis of dysphagic patients.

We have also studied patients with penetration of barium into the larynx during swallowing (Olsson et al. 1998). Videomanometry revealed an increased frequency of manometric abnormalities in patients with penetration. There was, however, no specific finding and a multitude of abnormalities were found with no association between manometric abnormalities and the degree of barium penetration.

In patients with pharyngeal retention we found a significantly lower laryngeal elevation, indicating the importance of pharyngeal shortening in the swallowing sequence (Olsson et al. 1997).

7 Conclusion

Simultaneous videoradiography and pharyngeal solid-state manometry provides qualitative and quantitative information by assessing bolus transport and intraluminal pharyngeal pressures combined. It can be performed with the subject seated in an upright physiologic swallowing position during fluoroscopy in a gastrointestinal radiology laboratory.

Our experience is that the most complete understanding of bolus transport requires both manometric and radiographic input and that concurrent radiography and manometry will play a more prominent role in the future.

References

Arndorfer RC, Stef JJ, Dodds WJ, Linehan JH, Hogan WJ (1977) Improved infusion system for intraluminal esophageal manometry. Gastroenterology 73:23–27

Ask P, Öberg Å, Tibbling L (1979) Frequency content of esophageal peristaltic pressure. Am J Physiol 236: E296–E300

Atkinson M, Kramer P, Wyman SM, Ingelfinger FJ (1957) The dynamics of swallowing. I. Normal pharyngeal mechanisms. J Clin Invest 36:581–588

Bosma JF, Donner MW, Tanaka E, Robertson D (1986) Anatomy of the pharynx, pertinent to swallowing. Dysphagia 1:23–33

Brasseur JG (1987) A fluid mechanical perspective on esophageal bolus transport. Dysphagia 2:32–39

Brasseur JG, Dodds WJ (1991) Interpretation of intraluminal manometric measurements in terms of swallowing mechanics. Dysphagia 6:100–119

Buchholz DW, Bosma JF, Donner MW (1985) Adaptation, compensation, and decompensation of the pharyngeal swallow. Gastrointest Radiol 10:235–239

Castell JA, Castell DO (1993) Modern solid state computerized manometry of the pharyngoesophageal segment. Dysphagia 8:270–275

Castell JA, Dalton CB, Castell DO (1990) Pharyngeal and upper esophageal manometry in humans. Am J Physiol 258:G173–G178

Castell JA, Castell DO, Schultz AR, Georgeson S (1993) Effect of head position on the dynamics of the upper esophageal sphincter and pharynx. Dysphagia 8:1–6

Cerenko D, McConnel FMS, Jackson RT (1989) Quantitative assessment of pharyngeal bolus driving forces. Otolaryngol Head Neck Surg 100:57–63

Cook IJ, Dodds WJ, Dantas RO, Kern MK, Massey BT, Shaker R, Hogan WJ (1989) Timing of videofluoroscopic, manometric events, and bolus transit during the oral and pharyngeal phases of swallowing. Dysphagia 4:8–15

Dantas RO, Dodds WJ, Massey BT, Kern MK (1989) The effect of high- vs. low-density barium preparations on the quantitative features of swallowing. AJR 153:1191–1195

Dantas RO, Cook IJ, Dodds WJ, Kern MK, Lang IM, Brasseur JG (1990) Biomechanics of cricopharyngeal bars. Gastroenterology 99:1269–1274

Dejaeger E, Pelemans W, Bibau G, Ponette E (1994) Manofluorographic analysis of swallowing in the elderly. Dysphagia 9:156–161

Dent J (1976) A new technique for continuos sphincter pressure measurement. Gastroenterology 71:263–267

Dodds WJ, Logemann JA, Stewart ET (1990) Radiologic assessment of abnormal oral and pharyngeal phases of swallowing. Am J Roentgenol 154:965–974

Ekberg O (1987) Dysfunction of the pharyngo-esophageal segment in patients with normal opening of the upper esophageal sphincter: a cineradiographic study. Br J Radiol 60:637–644

Ekberg O, Nylander G (1982) Cineradiography of the pharyngeal stage of deglutition in 150 individuals without dysphagia. Br J Radiol 55:253–257

Ekberg O, Wahlgren O (1985) Dysfunction of pharyngeal swallowing. A cineradiographic investigation in 854 dysphagial patients. Acta Radiol Diagn 26:389–395

Ergun GA, Kahrilas PJ, Logemann JA (1993) Interpretation of pharyngeal manometric recordings: limitations and variability. Dis Esophagus 6:11–16

Fyke FE, Code CF (1955) Resting and deglutition pressures in the pharyngo-esophageal region. Gastroenterology 29:24–34

Gordon C, Hewer RL, Wade DT (1987) Dysphagia in acute stroke. BMJ 295:411–414

Groher ME, Bukatman R (1986) The prevalence of swallowing disorders in two teaching hospitals. Dysphagia 1:3–6

Isberg A, Nilsson ME, Schiratzki H (1985) Movement of the upper esophageal sphincter and a manometric device during deglutition. Acta Radiol Diagn 26:381–388

Jacob P, Kahrilas PJ, Logemann JA, Shah V, Ha T (1989) Upper esophageal sphincter opening and modulation during swallowing. Gastroenterology 97:1469–1478

Kronecker H, Meltzer S (1883) Der Schluckmechanismus, seine Erregung und seine Hemmung. Arch Anat Phys (Suppl) 7:328

Lindgren S, Janzon L (1991) Prevalence of swallowing complaints and clinical findings among 50–79 year-old men and women in an urban population. Dysphagia 6:187–192

McConnel FMS, Cerenko D, Jackson RT, Hersh T (1988) Clinical application of the manofluorogram. Laryngoscope 98:705–711

Mendelsohn MS, McConnel FMS (1987) Function in the pharyngoesophageal segment. Laryngoscope 97:483–489

Miller AJ (1986) Neurophysiological basis of swallowing. Dysphagia 1:91–100

Olsson R, Ekberg O (1995) Videomanometry of the pharynx in dysphagic patients with a posterior cricopharyngeal indentation. Acad Radiol 2:597–601

Olsson R, Nilsson H, Ekberg O (1994a) Pharyngeal solid state manometry catheter movement during swallowing. A simultaneous videoradiographic and manometric study in 20 dysphagic patients and 20 nondysphagic volunteers. Acad Radiol 1:339–344

Olsson R, Nilsson H, Ekberg O (1994b) An experimental manometric study simulating upper esophageal sphincter narrowing. Invest Radiol 29:630–635

Olsson R, Nilsson H, Ekberg O (1995a) Simultaneous videoradiography and pharyngeal solid state manometry in 25 nondysphagic volunteers. Dysphagia 10:36–41

Olsson R, Castell JA, Castell DO, Ekberg O (1995b) Solid-state computerized manometry improves diagnostic yield in patients with pharyngeal dysphagia: simultaneous videoradiography and manometry in dysphagia patients with normal barium swallows. Abdom Imaging 20:230–235

Olsson R, Castell J, Johnston B, Ekberg O, Castell DO (1997) Combined videomanometric identification of abnormalities related to pharyngeal retention. Acad Radiol 4:349–354

Olsson R, Castell J, Ekberg O, Castell DO (1998) Videomanometry of the pharynx in dysphagic patients with laryngeal barium penetration during swallowing. Acta Radiol 39:405–409

Orlowski J, Dodds WJ, Linehan JH, Dent J, Hogan WJ, Arndorfer RC (1982) Requirements for accurate manometric recording of pharyngeal and esophageal peristaltic pressure waves. Invest Radiol 17:567–572

Ren J, Massey BT, Dodds WJ, Kern MK, Brasseur JG, Shaker R, Harrington SS, Hogan WJ, Arndorfer RC (1993) Determinants of intrabolus pressure during esophageal peristaltic bolus transport. Am J Physiol 264:G407–G413

Shaker R, Dodds WJ, Ren J, Hogan WJ, Arndorfer RC (1992) Esophagoglottal closure reflex: a mechanism of airway protection. Gastroenterology 102:857–861

Sokol EM, Heitman P, Wolf BS, Cohen BR (1966) Simultaneous cineradiographic and manometric study of the pharynx, hypopharynx, and cervical esophagus. Gastroenterology 51:960–973

Stef JJ, Dodds WJ, Hogan WJ, Linehan JH, Stewart ET (1974) Intraluminal esophageal manometry: an analysis of variables affecting recording fidelity of peristaltic pressures. Gastroenterology 67:221–230

Welch RW, Luckmann K, Ricks PM, Drake ST, Gates GA (1979) Manometry of the normal upper esophageal sphincter and its alterations in laryngectomy. J Clin Invest 63:1036–1041

Winans CS (1972) The pharyngoesophageal closure mechanism: a manometric study. Gastroenterology 63:768–777

Esophageal Manometry and Gastroesophageal Reflux Monitoring

Karin Aksglæde, Per Thommesen, and Peter Funch-Jensen

Contents

Abstract

Manometry and gastroesophageal reflux (GER) monitoring are important tests in evaluation of patients suspected of having motility disorders and/or gastroesophageal reflux disease (GERD), but we do not recommend these as first choice investigations. If a functional, benign esophageal disease is suspected, a video-radiologic investigation based on physiological principles using bread-and-barium could often separate patients with normal manometry from patients with severe motility disorders, i.e., diffuse esophageal spasms (DES) and achalasia (Nellemann et al. 2000). Furthermore, this radiologic method could demonstrate GER in adults with a sensitivity of 52 % and a specificity of 100 %, thus reducing the number of patients referred to manometry and GER monitoring (Aksglæde et al. 1999).

1 Esophageal Manometry

Manometry is used to measure intraluminal pressure and pressure changes in the esophagus generated by contractions in the circular muscles. Esophageal manometry can be used in patients with suspected primary or secondary motility disorders. Secondary esophageal motility disorders are those occurring in patients having a generalized or systemic disease, i.e., systemic sclerosis or diabetes mellitus. Furthermore, manometry is used preoperatively before fundoplication (Kahrilas et al. 1994).

In difficult diagnostic cases an approach with combined video-radiology and manometry is often useful.

K. Aksglæde (✉) · P. Thommesen · P. Funch-Jensen
Division for Gastrointestinal Motility Disorders,
Department of Radiology, Aarhus University Hospital,
Nørrebrogade 44, Aarhus, Aarhus C 8000, Denmark
e-mail: kariaksg@rm.dk

P. Funch-Jensen
Aleris-Hamlet Hospital, and Clinical Institute,
Aarhus University, Aarhus, Aarhus C, Denmark

O. Ekberg (ed.), *Dysphagia*, Medical Radiology. Diagnostic Imaging, DOI: 10.1007/174_2012_655,
© Springer-Verlag Berlin Heidelberg 2012

1.1   Technique

Esophageal pressures are measured directly with solid-state transducers, or indirectly with external transducers connected to a water-perfused system. The solid-state system measures pressures independently of body position and requires no external water supply and pumps, thus making it advantageous in long-term investigations.

The pressure catheter used for conventional esophageal manometry contains 3–8 pressure channels spaced ≤5 cm. The catheter is introduced through a nostril and guided into the stomach, and then retracted through the lower esophageal sphincter (LES) at a rate of 0.5–1.0 cm/s ("rapid pull-through technique") to measure the resting lower esophageal sphincter pressure (LESP) in proportion to the fundic pressure. The relaxation is best measured using the "station pull-through technique", where the probe is pulled through the LES at 0.5–1.0 cm at a time until recordings become stable, and relaxation is determined by wet or dry swallows. Finally, it is placed with the distal channel 2–5 cm above the LES and a manometric study of the esophageal body is performed. Pressure amplitude, velocity, and duration of contractions are registered after dry, wet, and solid swallows. (Keren et al. 1992). Furthermore, the intra-esophageal baseline pressure can be determined during continuous swallowing. Measurement of the relaxation of the LES is not always easy, but a gradual increase in baseline pressure during swill is seen in patients with incomplete opening of the LES (Funch-Jensen et al. 2000).

A newer manometric methodology called high-resolution manometry (HRM) has been introduced recently. The catheter used contains 22–36 pressure channels spaced at ≤2 cm intervals. The catheter is passed transnasally and positioned with recording sites from hypopharynx to the stomach. The catheter remains in this position during the examination, thereby eliminating movement artifacts. Advanced analysis software displays the measurements into color pressure topographic plots, where functionality of the upper and lower sphincter and the motility in the esophagus can be investigated simultaneously and with a greater spatial solution than with conventional manometry (Fox et al. 2008; Pandolfino et al. 2008).

1.2   Manometric Findings

The manometric tracings are classified according to generally accepted criteria:

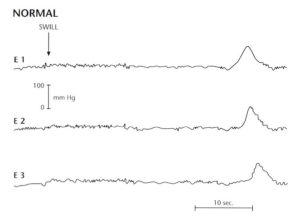

Fig. 1 Esophageal manometric recordings 15 cm (*E1*), 10 cm (*E2*), and 5 cm (*E3*) above the oral border of the lower esophageal sphincter (LES) during continuous drinking (swill) in a patient with normal LES relaxation, followed by a normal peristaltic contraction with normal amplitude and duration

1. *Normal:* Mean LESP 10–30 mm Hg, and normal swallow-induced relaxation of LES. In the body of the esophagus peristaltic pressure waves with a mean amplitude distally 30–110 mm Hg, and mean duration distally maximal 5.5 s. (Fig. 1).
2. *Achalasia:* Incomplete relaxation of LES and aperistalsis and common cavity oscillations in the esophageal body (Fig. 2).
3. *DES:* Spontaneous or simultaneous repetitive broad-based contractions intermingled with normal peristaltic waves (Fig. 3).
4. *Nutcracker esophagus:* Peristaltic waves with amplitudes of more than 200 mm Hg.
5. *Hypomotility:* Low amplitude contractions ≤ 30 mm Hg occurring peristaltically or nonperistaltically, with or without low resting LESP.
6. *Non-specific esophageal motility disorder (NSEMD):* Abnormal findings derived of classification according to the definitions above.

1.3   Clinical Interpretation

Abnormal esophageal motility can potentially cause chest pain or dysphagia, or both. Interpretation of the clinical manometric result is rather simple and limited to a few possible pathologic observations, e.g., weak or absent peristalsis, disordered peristalsis, or impaired LES relaxation.

Although manometry is sensitive in detecting esophageal motor disorders, it is often non-specific,

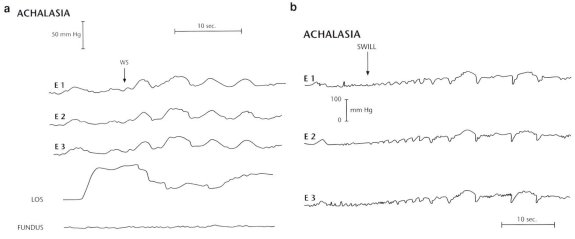

Fig. 2 a Esophageal manometric recordings 15 cm (*E1*), 10 cm (*E2*), and 5 cm (*E3*) above the oral border of the lower esophageal sphincter (*LES*) shows non-peristaltic common-cavity waves in the esophageal body during deglutition in patient with achalasia. Recording in LES shows incomplete relaxation. **b** Esophageal manometric recordings during swill show a steady increase in baseline pressure in a patient with achalasia and incomplete LES relaxation. This method can be used in patients where gastric intubations are impossible. Compare to Fig. 1

Fig. 3 The manometric signature after dry, wet, and solid swallow. Although pressure peaks are simultaneous during dry and wet swallows, the diagnosis of diffuse esophageal spasms (*DES*) is only possible after the solid bolus

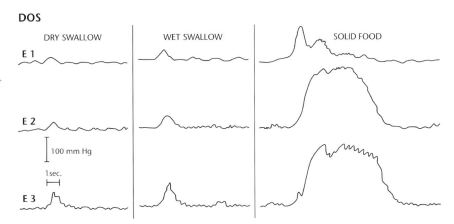

except when achalasia or DES is a suspected (Kahrilas et al. 1994; Nelleman et al. 2000).

2 Gastroesophageal Reflux Monitoring

GER monitoring can document normal or abnormal gastric content in the esophagus. Indications for prolonged monitoring include:

1. Patients with typical symptoms of gastroesophageal reflux disease (GERD) and normal endoscopy.
2. Patients with atypical symptoms of GERD (i.e., noncardiac chest pain, pulmonary symptoms, hoarseness).
3. Prior to and subsequent to anti-reflux therapy (medical or surgical).

2.1 Technique

Esophageal pH monitoring: Intraluminal pH monitoring is used to evaluate acidic gastroesophageal reflux. A widely accepted technique is a catheter-based pH recording system. The basic equipment requirements include a portable data logger for data storage, a pH electrode, a computer, and software for analysis of the pH data.

Data logger's used in esophageal ambulatory pH studies are lightweight, battery-powered units that can be worn by the patient on a waist belt or shoulder straps. The data logger also has an event marker that can be activated by the patient during the study to indicate the timing of symptoms, meals, and recumbency (sleep). The patient can also record these events on a diary card.

24-h pH MONITORING

Compressed 24-hour pH Graph

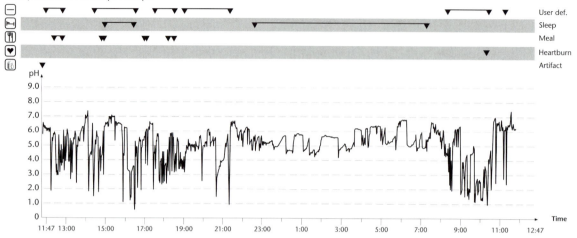

Period Table

Item		Total	Upright	Supine	Meal	PostP	NONE	HrtBrn
Duration of period	(HH:MM)	24:00	13:52	10:08	01:21	09:07	08:28	00:04
Number of acid refluxes	(#)	139	136	4	22	85	96	1
Number of long acid refluxes	(#)	6	5	1	0	5	6	0
Longest acid reflux	(min)	31	31	20	1	31	31	4
Total time pH below 4.00	(min)	165	144	21	8	130	139	4
Fraction time pH below 4.00	**(%)**	**11.5**	**17.3**	**3.5**	**9.3**	**23.7**	**27.4**	**100.0**
Symptom Index	(%)	n/a	n/a	n/a	n/a	n/a	83.3	100.0

DeMeester score
Total score= 39.5 DeMeester normals: <14.72 (95th percentile)

Fig. 4 Compressed 24 h pH graph and period table. Fraction time of pH below 4 is accentuated

The probes are usually 2–4 mm in diameter, composed of antimony, ISFET (Ion Sensitive Field Effect Transistor), or glass. Each probe consists of single or multiple channels which can be customized for the individual laboratories.

The pH probe is passed through a nostril into the stomach to verify an acidic pH, and then positioned 5 cm above the superior margin of the gastro-esophageal junction (GEJ), identified by manometry or radiography (Aksglæde et al. 1999, 2003a, b). This probe positioning avoids possible probe displacement into the stomach due to swallow-induced esophageal shortening, which is not fully compensated by concomitant electrode oscillation during eating and talking (Aksglæde et al. 2003a, b).

The length of the study should be at least 16 h, thus allowing assessment of at least two post-prandial periods and overnight supine position.

Recent technical advance has been incorporation of an antimony electrode into a wireless capsule, which can be placed transorally in the esophagus. The capsule sends data via radiofrequency telemetry to an external receiver. Endoscopy has to be performed prior to capsule placement to avoid severe esophagitis and strictures, which are among the contraindications for the use of the wireless capsule. The wireless pH system routinely records for 48 h.

Esophageal Impedance Measurements. Impedance measurement is based on measurements of changes in the electrical impedance. Air yields an increase in impedance, liquid results in a drop in impedance. Often a thin probe 2–4 mm in diameter is used to measure pH 5 cm above the LES, and impedance 3, 5, 7, 9, 15, and 17 cm above the LES. This combined multichannel impedance and pH monitoring can evaluate all types of GER (liquid, gas, mixed, acid, and nonacid), and furthermore, the duration and proximal extent of a reflux event can be evaluated. (Hirano et al. 2007; Sifrim et al. 2008).

2.2 Diet and Drugs While Performing the Study

Discontinuing prokinetic agents, drugs that neutralize acids, and drugs that have an influence on the LESP 24–48 h prior to an examination is recommended. Proton pump inhibitors must be discontinued at least 72 h prior to examination due to the accumulation of the drug in parietal cell canaliculi and the irreversible nature of proton pump inhibition. During the examination the patient can eat a normal diet excluding acid food and beverage, and physical activity need not be restricted.

2.3 Evaluation of GER Monitoring

Acid GER episodes are defined as periods with pH $\leq$ 4. To obtain a global assessment, several parameters are often used: The percentage of time pH $\leq$ 4 for the whole investigation time (reflux index), percentage of time pH $\leq$ 4 in the supine and upright periods, the number of reflux episodes, number of episodes lasting more than 5 min, and the longest reflux episode.

Johnson and DeMeester (1986) devised a scoring system based on these six parameters to calculate the degree in which reflux patterns differ between individuals (Fig. 4). However, in order to discriminate between physiological and pathological GER in adults, the most useful parameter is the reflux index, with normal values varying from 3.9 to 7.2 % (Kahrilas and Quigley 1996). We have adopted reflux index <5 % as the upper normal limit when using the cathter-based system. Some studies have reported a value of 5.3 % as the upper value using the wireless system, which may be a consequence of a better tolerability with less restriction in daily activities.

The amount of impedance liquid reflux episodes are considered abnormal when they exceed 73 episodes/24 h. Manual differentiation between liquid reflux episodes, gas reflux, and swallows are still necessary and rather time-consuming. (Hirano et al. 2007).

References

Aksglæde K, Funch-Jensen P, Thommesen P (1999) Radiological demonstration of gastroesophageal reflux. Diagnostic value of barium and bread studies compared with 24 h pH monitoring. Acta Radiol 40:652–655

Aksglæde K, Funch-Jensen P, Thommesen P (2003a) Which is the better method for location of the gastro-esophageal junction: radiography or manometry? Acta Radiol 44:121–126

Aksglæde K, Funch-Jensen P, Thommesen P (2003b) Intraoesophageal pH probe movement during eating and talking. A video-radiographic study. Acta Radiol 44:131–135

Fox MR, Bredenoord AJ (2008) Oesophageal high-resolution manometry: moving from research into clinical practice. Gut 57:405–423

Funch-Jensen P, Aksglæde K, Thommesen P (2000) A new method for the detection of incomplete lower esophageal sphincter relaxation in patients with achalasia. Scand J Gastroenterol 35:349–352

Hirano I, Richter JE (2007) The Practice Parameters Committee of the American College of Gastroenterology. Am J Gastroenterol 102:668–685

Johnson LF, DeMeester TR (1986) Development of the 24 h intraesophageal pH monitoring composite scoring system. J Clin Gastroenterol 8(1):52–58

Kahrilas PJ, Quigley EMM (1996) Clinical esophageal pH recording: a technical review for practice guideline development. Gastroenterology 110:1982–1996

Kahrilas PJ, Clouse RE, Hogan WJ (1994) An American Gastroenterological Association medical position statement on the clinical use of esophageal manometry. Gastroenterology 107:1865–1884

Keren S, Argaman E, Golan M (1992) Solid swallowing vs. water swallowing: manometric study of dysphagia. Dig Dis Sci 37(4):603–608

Nellemann H, Aksglæde K, Funch-Jensen P, Thommesen P (2000) Bread and barium: diagnostic value in patients with suspected primary esophageal motility disorders. Acta Radiol 41:145–150

Pandolfino JE, Gosh SK, Rice J, Clarke JO, Kwiatek MA, Kahrilas PJ (2008) Classifying esophageal motility by pressure topography characteristics: a study of 400 patients and 75 controls. Am J Gastroenterol 108:27–37

Sifrim D, Fornari F (2008) Esophageal impedance-pH monitoring. Dig Liver Dis 40:161–166

Impedance Planimetry

Johannes Lenglinger

Contents

J. Lenglinger (✉)
Motility Laboratory, Department of Surgery,
Medical University of Vienna, Vienna, Austria
e-mail: johannes.lenglinger@meduniwien.ac.at

Abstract

Impedance planimetry is an imaging technique that displays the distensibility of hollow viscera. Inside a bag filled with a conductive solution multiple impedance tracings between pairs of electrodes are converted to estimate cross sectional areas. With simultaneous measurement of intrabag pressure distensibility (smallest cross sectional area vs. intrabag pressure) is calculated. Impedance planimetry measurements characterize biomechanical properties of the esophagogastric junction, the esophageal body and the pharyngoesophageal sphincter. In healthy volunteers distensibility of the esophagogastric junction was lowest at the diaphragmatic hiatus and cross sectional areas of 38, 94, and 264 mm2 at distension volumes of 20, 30 and 40 ml were reported. Distension of the esophageal body resulted in a cylindrical bag configuration up to a plateau of 400 mm2 in most subjects. In patients with achalasia distensibility of the esophagogastric junction was reduced even when sphincter pressure was in the normal range. In patients with eosinophilic esophagitis distensibility was decreased at the esophagogastric junction and in the tubular esophagus. By contrast, in subjects with gastro-esophageal reflux disease the diameter of the esophagogastric junction was larger at any given intrabag pressure than in controls. In clinical practice impedance planimetry of the esophagus serves as a diagnostic test for the work-up of dysphagia, especially if structural or mucosal lesions are absent and peristalsis of the esophageal body is preserved. Impedance planimetry can be performed during or immediately after surgical or endoscopic procedures and is therefore a valuable tool for the ad hoc assessment of the effects of therapeutic interventions.

O. Ekberg (ed.), *Dysphagia*, Medical Radiology. Diagnostic Imaging, DOI: 10.1007/174_2012_640,
© Springer-Verlag Berlin Heidelberg 2012

1   Introduction

Impedance planimetry is an imaging technique that is able to assess the distensibility of organs in the alimentary tract. Tonic and phasic muscular contractions as well as wall compliance determine the dimensions of hollow viscera and the movement of contents within them. In areas with a narrow lumen, i.e. the esophagus, the antroduodenal segment and the anorectum, motility can be studied by manometry. However, the correlation of pressure measurements with symptoms and radiological transit studies is poor in many disease states because only muscular tone and contractions can be studied by manometry. Impedance planimetry combines an estimation of cross sectional areas with pressure readings and thus characterizes biomechanical properties of the organ wall. In the clinical setting this new imaging tool is currently used for the evaluation of dysphagia and as monitoring instrument during antireflux surgery and cardiomyotomy.

2   Technical Principles of Impedance Planimetry

Impedance planimetry is an examination technique that uses measurements of AC voltage to estimate cross-sectional areas of a liquid conductor contained in a cylindrical bag. An array of ring electrodes mounted on the catheter segment inside the bag delineates the measurement area. The outermost electrodes are connected to a low voltage AC current source. Via infusion ports near the ends, the bag is gradually filled with a saline solution. Voltage measurements are made between pairs of electrodes. Since electrical current, the conductivity of the fluid and the distance between the electrodes are constants, impedance (the resistance to AC current flow) is proportional to the cross-sectional area of the conductor, i.e., the liquid column. Impedance measurements are converted to diameter estimations and a dynamic image of the bag geometry is created and displayed on a screen in real time at 10 frames per second. Simultaneously, a solid-state pressure transducer monitors intra-bag pressure. Currently an impedance planimetry system is commercially available as Endo-FLIP® (Endolumenal Functional Lumen Imaging Probe). A central unit with a display and a motor syringe is connected to a disposable catheter equipped with a bag that comprises 16 impedance tracings over a measurement area of 8 cm in length. (Fig. 1).

Main applications of impedance planimetry are the assessment of esophago-gastric junction and esophageal body distensibility as these regions are easily accessible by catheter and have a narrow lumen. In practice, an initial distension is performed in a calibration tube. Thereafter, the catheter is inserted transnasally or via the instrumentation channel of the endoscope and it is advanced until the center of the measurement bag is in the region of interest. By convention, distensibility at rest is assessed with filling volumes of 10 to 50 ml in 10 ml increments over 30 s, respectively. The smallest cross-sectional area in the region of interest and the corresponding distensibility index (cross-sectional area vs. intrabag pressure) are parameters used to characterize distensibility (Kwiatek et al. 2010a).

3   Impedance Planimetry of the Esophagus

The esophagus is a muscular tube of 20–25 cm in length that transports ingesta from the pharynx into the stomach. Sphincter at the proximal and distal ends of the organ contribute to the regulation of in- and outflow. The high-pressure zone at the esophago-gastric junction is crucial for the protection against reflux of gastric contents into the esophagus. Esophageal transport function and gastro-esophageal reflux activity are determined by organ geometry, muscular tone and relaxation at the sphincter regions, peristalsis and wall compliance. At present, impedance planimetry is the most useful imaging technique to measure biomechanical wall properties. The application of this technique in the clinical work-up of esophageal disorders is the subject of this chapter.

4   Impedance Planimetry of the Esophagus in Healthy Volunteers

In healthy subjects the high-pressure zone at the esophago-gastric junction is to the most part located in and below the diaphragmatic hiatus. Resting pressure is highest at the hiatus. Conversely, the lumen at this location assumes an hourglass-shape with volumetric distension and the hiatus is the least distensible area. The cross-sectional areas and intrabag pressure increase with filling volume with a tendency towards a higher distensibility index at higher volumes. Median values of the smallest cross-sectional areas were

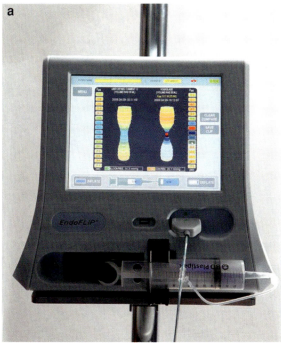

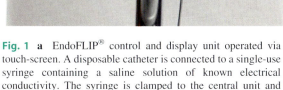

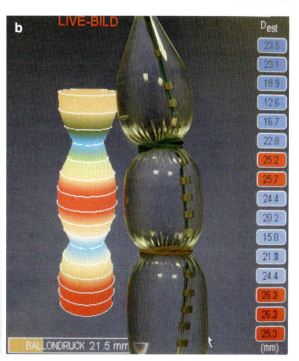

Fig. 1 **a** EndoFLIP® control and display unit operated via touch-screen. A disposable catheter is connected to a single-use syringe containing a saline solution of known electrical conductivity. The syringe is clamped to the central unit and motor-controlled. **b** The EndoFLIP® catheter with the measurement bag filled and narrowed by two rubber bands, held in front of the corresponding image on the screen

reported to be 38, 94, and 264 mm^2 at distension volumes of 20, 30 and 40 ml, respectively (Kwiatek et al. 2010a). In the esophageal body, the tubular form of the organ is reflected by a cylindrical configuration of the measurement bag. In most subjects, distension reaches a plateau at a cross-sectional area of approximately 400 mm^2 (Kwiatek et al. 2011). Distensibility of the pharyngo-esophageal sphincter has been studied in a small group of healthy volunteers with ramp distensions up to 20 ml. At rest, a median diameter of 4.9 mm at 31 mm Hg pressure was encountered. During dry swallows, diameter increased to 9.2 mm (Regan et al. 2012). Fig. 2.

5 Impedance Planimetry for Investigation of Dysphagia

In patients with swallowing disorders, impedance planimetry is used to characterize the mechanical properties of the esophageal wall and to localize areas of reduced distensibility that affect bolus transport.

A clinically useful distinction between esophageal versus oropharyngeal dysphagia is commonly made by symptom profile. Esophageal dysphagia is characterized by the sensation of failed or incomplete bolus transport after unimpaired deglutition, possibly associated with retrosternal pressure or regurgitation of non-acidified food remnants and mucus. More severely, a bolus may be impacted in the esophagus and require acute endoscopic intervention. Diagnostic workup of esophageal dysphagia begins with esophago-gastroscopy and an esophagogram to exclude tumors and to assess organ geometry and mucosal integrity. Esophagitis, a hiatal hernia or structural lesions such as diverticula, webs or rings may be encountered and be responsible for the swallowing disorder. If no structural lesion is found, symptoms persist despite adequate treatment or if esophageal surgery is considered, further investigation by a motility study and reflux monitoring is indicated. Sphincter pressures and esophageal body motility can be assessed by manometry. Ineffective motility, characterized by weak peristalsis, may be identified as

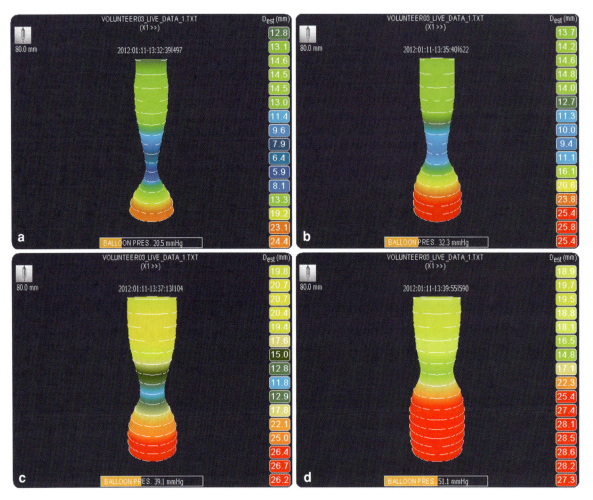

Fig. 2 Distensibility of the esophago-gastric junction in a healthy volunteer at volumes of 20-**a**, 30-**b**, 40-**c** and 50 ml **d**. Diameter values calculated from the 16 impedance tracings are listed in the column at the right side. Intrabag pressure is displayed below the image

a cause of dysphagia. This condition is frequently associated with gastro-esophageal reflux disease and less commonly with scleroderma or mixed connective tissue disease. An impairment of swallow-induced relaxation and aperistalsis of the esophageal body is a diagnostic for achalasia. In early stages of this disease, dilatation of the tubular esophagus may not be visible by endoscopy or video-fluoroscopy. Impedance planimetry yields clinically important information in this disease. Distensibility of the esophago-gastric junction in achalasia patients is reduced compared to healthy subjects, even if lower esophageal sphincter pressure is within the normal range (Rohof et al. 2012). Treatment by dilatation or cardiomyotomy aims to reduce outflow obstruction at the level of the lower esophageal sphincter. The success

of treatment, measured by esophageal emptying in a timed barium esophagram and the Eckardt dysphagia score is significantly correlated with an increase in esophago-gastric junction distensibility, but not measurements of lower esophageal sphincter pressure (Rohof et al. 2012).

A discrepancy between measures of bolus transport and motility should be investigated by impedance planimetry. Bolus retention in the esophagus—despite normal peristalsis—raises the suspicion of discrete fibrotic lesions or reduced wall compliance not detectable by standard esophagram and endoscopy. Eosinophilic esophagitis, a chronic, immune/antigen-mediated esophageal disease characterized clinically by symptoms related to esophageal dysfunction and histologically by eosinophil-predominant inflammation may be

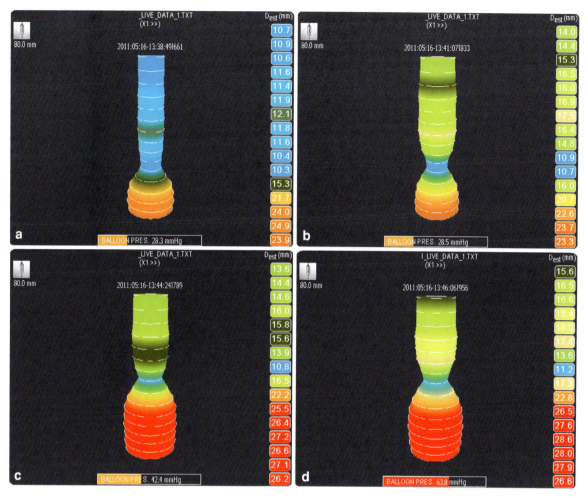

Fig. 3 Distensibility of the esophago-gastric junction in a patient with eosinophilic esophagitis. There is only a minimal increase of the smallest cross-sectional area with higher filling volumes. Intrabag pressure rises, however, resulting in a low distensibility at volumes of 40- and 50 ml, respectively

the underlying cause. Diagnosis is made by a combination of clinical and histopathologic features. Symptoms in adult patients are mainly dysphagia, food impaction and chest pain. Multiple biopsies from the proximal and distal esophagus should be evaluated, and a minimum of 15 eosinophil granulozytes per high power field in at least a biopsy sample is a diagnostic criterion. Distribution of lesions may be patchy and eosinophil microabscesses are often seen. Eosinophilic esophagitis is associated with esophageal remodelling, endoscopically characterized by fixed or transient rings, longitudinal furrows, diffuse esophageal narrowing and whitish exudates (Liacouras et al. 2011). A lower compliance of the esophago-gastric junction and the distal esophageal body compared to healthy controls has been reported in an impedance planimetry study of patients with

eosinophilic esophagitis (Kwiatek et al. 2011). Eosinophilic esophagitis is managed by topical corticosteroid therapy and exclusion of foods that a patient has an allergic reaction to. In addition, balloon dilatation of esophageal strictures may be required. The clinical role of impedance planimetry in the workup of eosinophilic esophagitis is less a purely diagnostic test as findings are not exclusive to this condition. More importantly, EndoFLIP® procedures can be performed to monitor the success of balloon dilatation during a treatment session. Fig. 3.

Attention should be paid to the progression of the distensibility index with increasing bag volume. In healthy subjects, in patients with hypertensive lower esophageal sphincter, and possibly achalasia, distensibility tends to increase with filling volume of the

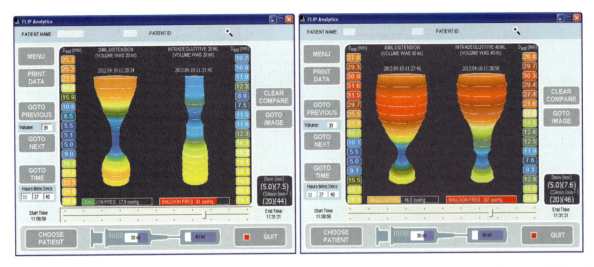

Fig. 4 Distensibility of the pharyngo-esophageal junction in a patient with graft-vs.-host disease after bone marrow transplantation for acute myeloid leukemia. A high-grade stenosis of the pharyngo-esophageal junction and dilatation of the valleculae was seen in video-fluoroscopy. Distension with 20 ml bag volume is displayed in 4a, while a filling volume of 40 ml was applied in 4b. The images depict distensibility at rest (left) and during deglutition (right). The smallest diameter at rest was 5 mm for both volumes. Deglutition resulted in a narrowing of the pharynx and a rise of intrabag pressure, but the smallest diameter remained below 8 mm, respectively. This is indicative of a highly rigid stenosis

measurement bag. In contrast, in conditions characterized by localized fibrosis—as in the case of a Schatzki ring, eosinophilic esophagitis or peptic stenosis—the distensibility index may be normal or high at low volumes and decreases after a plateau of the cross-sectional area is reached. This consideration applies to post-fundoplication dysphagia as well. In the case of a tight fundic wrap, a similar degree of low distensibility is seen over a length of several centimeters with increasing bag volume. In contrast, if the hiatal closure is too narrow, the area of narrowing shortens with increasing filling and the distensibility index decreases.

Few data exist about the application of impedance planimetry in the study of the pharyngo-esophageal sphincter (Regan et al. 2012). To ascertain that the airway is not compressed, maximal filling volume of the measurement bag was limited to 20 ml in this study. At rest, the pharyngo-esophageal sphincter was not distended beyond the minimum diameter of 4.8 mm that the EndoFLIP® system can measure. During deglutition, a maximal diameter of 9.2 mm for dry swallows and 7.7 mm for 5 ml water swallows at a bag volume of 20 ml was recorded, respectively. It was also demonstrated that maneuvers such as head turn and supraglottic swallow yield higher opening diameters. However, the reported opening diameters of the pharyngo-esophageal junction during swallowing are surprisingly low with respect to bolus size at meals. Higher filling volumes were not investigated because of concerns that airway patency might be compromised and because of poor tolerability of the EndoFLIP® bag at this location. A similar maximal diameter was described in a case report about a patient with a high-grade pharyngo-esophageal stenosis after bone marrow transplantation and graft-versus-host disease (Scharitzer et al. 2012). Fig. 4.

6 Impedance Planimetry in Patients with Gastro-Esophageal Reflux Disease

Gastro-esophageal reflux develops when the reflux of gastric contents into the esophagus causes troublesome symptoms and/or complications. The diaphragmatic crura and the intrinsic lower esophageal sphincter form an antireflux barrier. Transient lower esophageal relaxations are the main mechanism for reflux episodes. These vagally mediated drops of pressure at the esophago-gastric junction mainly occur in the postprandial period and are induced by distension of the gastric fundus (Schoeman et al. 1995). If esophago-gastric junction anatomy is

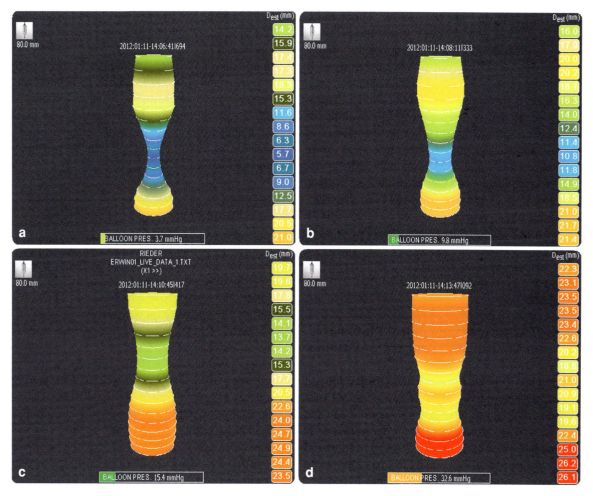

Fig. 5 Distensibility of the esophago-gastric junction in a patient with gastro-esophageal reflux disease. The smallest cross-sectional area increases with bag volume. The bag almost acquires a cylindrical shape with 50 ml volume. Intrabag pressure increases by a small extent only

disrupted and a hiatal hernia is present, a significant proportion of reflux episodes may occur by other mechanisms such as straining, deep inhalation or swallow-induced sphincter relaxation (van Herwaarden et al. 2000). In an impedance planimetry study of healthy controls versus subjects with symptomatic gastro-esophageal reflux disease, the hiatal diameter increased with increasing distention volume in both groups. However, distension pressure was consistently lower in the group of reflux patients than in control subjects at 20-, 30-, and 40-ml bag volumes. At any given intrabag pressure, the opening of the esophago-gastric junction was wider in reflux patients (Kwiatek et al. 2010a). It can be deducted from these findings that compliance of the esophago-gastric junction may become a therapeutic target to prevent excessive reflux. Fig. 5.

7 Application of Impedance Planimetry During Therapeutic Interventions

Antireflux surgery and gastric sleeve resection for the treatment of morbid obesity are sometimes complicated by postoperative dysphagia. Bougies have been used with inconsistent success to calibrate hiatal closure and the fundic wrap. The application of impedance planimetry during these operations may be a promising approach. With this technique, surgery can be tailored so that the desired endoluminal diameter is maintained at a low distension pressure. The use of EndoFLIP® as a "smart bougie" during antireflux surgery is currently investigated as recently reported (Perretta et al. 2011). Intra-abdominal pressure induced by pneumoperitoneum during laparoscopic surgery has an impact on the distensibility of the esophago-gastric junction, while the effects of general anesthesia and muscle relaxation were reported to be minimal (Nathanson et al. 2012).

Impedance planimetry during sessions of balloon dilatation of esophageal strictures or of the esophagogastric junction in achalasia may be useful as well. In contrast to radiological transit studies, this investigation can be performed with the patient still under anesthesia and repeat treatments are possible in the same session if a satisfactory effect has not been achieved.

8   The role of Impedance Planimetry in Clinical Management of Patients

If symptoms of possible esophageal origin develop in a patient, organ morphology and the state of the mucosal lining are of principal interest. Video-fluoroscopy and endoscopy cover these aspects to a large extent. If mucosal integrity is preserved, and tumors or structural lesions are excluded, functional disorders have to be considered. Manometry and intraluminal impedance monitoring are sophisticated tools to assess muscular function and bolus clearance. Compliance of the organ wall becomes the center of interest if transport function is impaired despite adequate peristalsis. Impedance planimetry has a diagnostic role in the clinical work-up of esophageal dysphagia. At present, it is the only diagnostic tool available for clinical routine to examine mechanical wall properties in vivo. As such, it complements endoscopy, video-fluoroscopy and manometry. The response of the esophageal wall to different distension volumes yields information on whether dysfunction is due to muscular versus connective tissue components. The effect of deglutition on distensibility of the sphincteric regions and the esophageal body has yet to be studied by impedance planimetry.

A role of impedance planimetry in the clinical work-up of patients complaining of heartburn or regurgitation has not been established so far. However, if dysphagia is present in addition to typical reflux symptoms, esophageal manometry and an EndoFLIP® procedure may help to distinguish between reflux-associated hypomotility and the presence of a fibrotic ring as cause of the swallowing disorder.

In addition, impedance planimetry is successfully used to tailor and monitor therapeutic procedures such as fundoplication for treatment of gastro-esophageal reflux disease as well as cardiomyotomy and pneumatic dilatations for achalasia. In these applications it is superior to radiology since it can be performed during anesthesia.

9   Summary

Impedance planimetry is an imaging technique to characterize distensibility of hollow viscera that has recently become available for clinical application.

Small sets of normative data have been published regarding distensibility measurements of the esophago-gastric junction, the esophageal body and the pharyngo-esophageal junction.

Esophageal dysphagia is the main application of impedance planimetry for clinical purposes at present. In patients with achalasia or eosinophilic esophagitis, distensibility of the esophago-gastric junction is reduced compared to healthy controls.

Impedance planimetry is indicated if bolus transport through the esophagus is impaired despite normal motility and preserved mucosal integrity. Decreasing distensibility of the esophago-gastric junction with increasing distension volume is indicative of local fibrosis.

In patients with gastro-esophageal reflux disease, esophago-gastric-junction distensibility is increased compared to healthy subjects.

Impedance planimetry is used for tailoring of surgical procedures at the esophago-gastric junction and for ad hoc monitoring of the effects of endoscopic interventions.

References

Kwiatek MA, Pandolfino JE, Hirano I, Kahrilas PJ (2010a) Esophagogastric junction distensibility assessed with an endoscopic functional luminal imaging probe (EndoFLIP). Gastrointest Endosc 72:272–278

Kwiatek MA, Kahrilas K, Soper NJ, Bulsiewicz WJ, McMahon BP, Gregersen H, Pandolfino JE (2010b) Esophagogastric junction distensibility after fundoplication assessed with a novel functional luminal imaging probe. J Gastrointest Surg 14:268–276

Kwiatek MA, Hirano I, Kahrilas PJ, Rothe J, Luger D, Pandolfino JE (2011) Mechanical properties of the esophagus in eosinophilic esophagitis. Gastroenterol 140:82–90

Liacouras CA, Furuta GT, Hirano I, Atkins D, Attwood SE, Bonis PA, Burks AW, Chehade M, Collins MH, Dellon ES, Dohil R, Falk GW, Gonsalves N, Gupta SK, Katzka DA, Lucendo AJ, Markowitz JE, Noel RJ, Odze RD, Putnam PE, Richter JE, Romero Y, Ruchelli E, Sampson HA, Schoepfer A, Shaheen NJ, Sicherer SH, Spechler S, Spergel JM, Straumann A, Wershil BK, Rothenberg ME, Aceves SS (2011) Eosinophilic esophagitis: updated consensus recommendations for children and adults. J Allergy Clin Immunol 128:3–20

Nathanson LK, Brunott N, Cavallucci D (2012) Adult esophagogastric junction distensibility during general anesthesia assessed with an endoscopic functional luminal imaging probe (EndoFLIP®). Surg Endosc 26:1051–1055

Perretta S, Dallemagne B, McMahon B, D'Agostino J, Marescaux J (2011) Video. Improving functional esophageal surgery with a "smart" bougie: Endoflip. Surg Endosc 25:3109

Regan J, Walshe M, Rommel N, McMahon BP (2012) A new evaluation of the upper esophageal sphincter using the functional lumen imaging probe: a preliminary report. Dis Esophagus. doi:10.1111/j.1442-2050.2012.01331.x

Rohof WO, Hirsch DP, Kessing BF, Boeckxstaens GE (2012) Efficacy of Treatment for Patients with Achalasia Depends on the Distensibility of the Esophagogastric Junction. Gastroenterology May 2. [Epub ahead of print]

Scharitzer M, Denk-Linert D (2012). Case 28. Difficult evaluation and treatment of an upper esophageal stenosis. http://www.hon.ch/cgi-bin/OESO/myOESO.pl?selogguer

Schoeman MN, Tippett MD, Akkermans LM, Dent J, Holloway RH (1995) Mechanisms of gastroesophageal reflux in ambulant healthy human subjects. Gastroenterol 108:83–91

van Herwaarden MA, Samsom M, Smout AJ (2000). Excess gastroesophageal reflux in patients with hiatus hernia is caused by mechanisms other than transient LES relaxations. Gastroenterology;119:1439–1446

Radiologic Evaluation of Esophageal Function

Wolfgang Schima, Edith Eisenhuber, and Christiane Kulinna-Cosentini

Contents

W. Schima (✉)
Department of Radiology,
Krankenhaus Goettlicher Heiland,
Dornbacher Strasse 20–28,
1170 Vienna, Austria
e-mail: wolfgang.schima@khgh.at;
wolfgang.schima@meduniwien.ac.at

E. Eisenhuber
Krankenhaus Goettlicher Heiland,
Dornbacher Strasse 20–28, 1170 Vienna, Austria

C. Kulinna-Cosentini
Department of Radiology, Medical University of Vienna,
Währinger Gürtel 18–20, 1090 Vienna, Austria

Abstract

In patients with dysphagia, radiographic studies evaluate both esophageal morphology and esophageal function. Videofluoroscopy accurately diagnoses achalasia, diffuse esophageal spasm, and PSS (scleroderma). Videofluoroscopy is less sensitive for the study of nonspecific motor disorders and gastroesophageal reflux. When accuracy, costs, availability, and patient acceptance are considered (Parkman et al. Dig Dis Sci 41:1355–1368, 1996), videofluoroscopy should be the initial diagnostic test for patients with esophageal dysphagia.

1 Introduction

Radiologic assessment of the esophagus is an essential part of the diagnostic workup of patients with deglutition disorders. The radiologic examination comprises two parts: single- and double-contrast examinations to assess the morphology of the esophagus and the esophagogastric junction, which may reveal signs of esophagitis, tumor, strictures, or rings. Radiologic evaluation of the esophagus would be incomplete without assessing esophageal function. Attempts to diagnose esophageal motor dysfunction, such as achalasia, were undertaken in the early days of single-contrast barium radiology (Hurst and Rake 1930). The development of cinefluoroscopy and videofluoroscopy has significantly improved the ability to study the motor function of the pharynx and esophagus in detail. The pharyngeal and esophageal transport of liquid and solid boluses can be studied in real time and in slow motion. Although slow motion analysis is more crucial for the assessment of pharyngeal function, video recording of esophageal bolus transport is also essential for a thorough analysis of the esophagus. Subtle abnormalities of motor function may go undetected during real-time observation of swallowing.

2 Normal Function of the Esophagus and the Lower Esophageal Sphincter

The esophagus is a tubular muscular structure, measuring approximately 23 cm in length (Li et al. 1994), which comprises outer longitudinal and inner circular muscle fibers. The proximal part of the esophagus consists of striated muscle fibers, whereas the distal part is composed of smooth muscle. The level of the transition zone between striated and smooth muscle is highly variable, with only the proximal 4 cm of the esophagus always composed of striated muscle. This dual structure of the esophageal musculature comprising striated muscle and smooth muscle fibers is significant in diseases that selectively affect either striated or smooth muscle. At the distal end of the esophagus, the tubular esophagus widens to the vestibular esophagus.

The lower esophageal sphincter between the vestibular esophagus and the stomach measures 3–5 cm in length. The lower esophageal sphincter corresponds to the high-pressure zone at the esophagogastric junction seen during esophageal manometry (Cohen 1979).

2.1 Primary and Secondary Peristalsis

Swallowing of a bolus triggers a primary peristaltic contraction wave in 95–96% of patients (Richter et al.

1987), and this propagates with a velocity of 2–3.5 cm/s. Manometric studies have revealed that the lower esophageal sphincter has a resting pressure. Upon swallowing, the sphincter relaxes some seconds after triggering of swallowing. Radiologically, the lower esophageal sphincter is pushed open by the bolus arriving at the gastroesophageal junction (Dodds 1977). Immediately after bolus passage, the sphincter recontracts (Dodds 1977). The amplitude and propagation velocity of primary peristalsis are modulated by bolus consistency, volume, and temperature (Dooley et al. 1988). If there is residual bolus in the esophagus or if there is a gastroesophageal reflux, a secondary peristaltic contraction wave can be triggered by the volume remaining in the esophagus to clear the esophagus. Both primary and secondary esophageal contractions are peristaltic and considered normal.

2.2 Nonpropulsive (or Tertiary) Contractions

Nonpropulsive (or tertiary) contractions may also be seen in the esophagus during videofluoroscopy or manometry. They result in segmental muscular contractions, which do not propagate to the distal esophagus. They may occur simultaneously at multiple sites and they may be repetitive. They occur spontaneously or may be triggered by swallowing or other stimuli, such as acoustic emissions (Stacher et al. 1979). In young adults, these nonpropulsive contractions are rarely seen upon swallowing (Richter et al. 1987). The prevalence and severity of nonpropulsive contractions increase with age (Grishaw et al. 1996). Most often, they are signs of abnormal esophageal function.

2.3 Radiologic Evaluation of Esophageal Motor Function

Radiologic evaluation of esophageal function always includes assessment of the esophageal body as well as the pharyngoesophageal and lower esophageal sphincters. In contrast to the assessment of pharyngeal function, esophageal peristalsis can be assessed in real time. However, videotaping of a study is helpful to allow repeated analysis of bolus transport that would demonstrate subtle abnormalities. Esophageal function should be assessed in all patients who suffer from dysphagia or globus sensation when they are referred for a videofluoroscopic study. One must be careful in patients with clinically suspected aspiration. The study should always be initiated with an examination of pharyngeal function. If there is only laryngeal penetration or minimal aspiration of the contrast material, the examiner can proceed to assess esophageal function. In general, the use of intravenously administered glucagon or Buscopan® should be avoided. Glucagon and Buscopan can alter the esophageal bolus transit and produce relaxation of the gastroesophageal sphincter, resulting in spontaneous gastroesophageal reflux (Anvari et al. 1989). For esophageal motor function studies, low-density barium (approximately 100% g/v) should be used. Barium at this consistency flows easily and is radio-opaque enough to provide good contrast in the esophagus. Since it is known that bolus viscosity alters peristalsis, thick high-density barium or barium paste should not be used. In the case of aspiration, a limited study of esophageal function with iodinated, nonionic contrast material may be considered.

For assessment of esophageal peristalsis, the observation of "single swallows" is essential. Repetitive swallowing inhibits the propagation of esophageal peristalsis (Meyer et al. 1981), a phenomenon, which is referred to as "deglutitive inhibition." If the patient swallows repeatedly within 5–10 s, every new peristaltic contraction generated by swallowing will inhibit the preceding peristaltic contraction. Radiologically, this may be misinterpreted as impaired peristalsis or nonpropulsive contractions. After the end of a series of repeated swallows, a large contraction wave will "clear" the esophagus. Therefore, the size of the bolus administered is critical for assessment of esophageal peristalsis: we routinely use a bolus size of 10 ml of barium to ensure that the patient swallows only once. In contrast, rapid repetitive swallows maximally distend the esophagus for morphologic evaluation (e.g., the search for Schatzki rings).

Esophageal peristalsis is assessed with the patient in the upright and in the prone oblique position. Usually, swallows in the prone oblique position provide more information, because gravity does not support bolus transit. The peristaltic contraction wave occludes the esophageal lumen, giving the bolus tail

typically an inverted-V shape (Fig. 1). It propels the complete bolus through the esophagus into the stomach. The proximal escape of a small amount of barium is not considered abnormal (Schima et al. 1992). Swallows in the upright position are sometimes of value because they may reveal subtle motor abnormalities not seen in the prone oblique position (Sears et al. 1989). In the upright position, bolus transit through the esophagus is normally rapid. The persistence of an air–fluid level ("support level") is indicative of the presence of a disordered motor function or a stenosis (Schober et al. 1993).

The use of up to ten swallows per patient during videofluoroscopy has been shown to be more sensitive for the detection of subtle motor abnormalities (Hewson et al. 1990); however, in clinical practice, the number of swallows observed must be limited because of radiation exposure, practicability, and patient comfort. Therefore, our routine examination protocol includes the observation of one bolus with the patient in the upright position and three boluses with the patient in the prone oblique position. The diagnostic value of videofluoroscopic studies can be increased by using solid barium-soaked marshmallows or globules, tablets, or rice (Aksglaede et al. 1992; Schwickert et al. 1993; Ott et al. 1991; Hannig et al. 1990).

3 Examination Technique

1. Upright position, left posterior oblique: The patient takes a bolus of low-density barium and is asked to swallow only once. The left posterior oblique position is preferred to avoid superposition of the esophagus by the spine and to provide better visualization of the gastroesophageal segment (Schima et al. 1995).
2. After the table has been tilted, the patient is turned to a prone oblique position. The patient takes a bolus with a straw. Up to three swallows are recorded. Imaging is centered on the tail of the bolus to look for proximal escape and stasis of the barium.
3. Assessment of the gastroesophageal reflux: Reflux may or may not occur spontaneously during the examination. There are also provocative tests to elicit gastroesophageal reflux, including placing

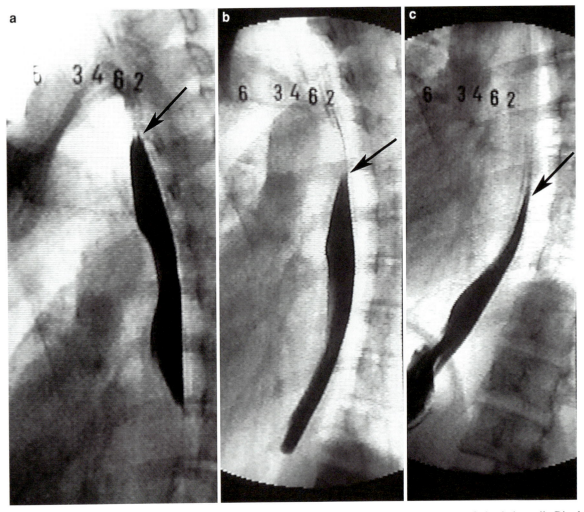

Fig. 1 a–c Normal esophageal motility. The patient is placed in the prone oblique position. There is a peristaltic contraction wave, which occludes the esophageal lumen, resulting in the typical inverted-V shape (*arrows*) of the bolus tail. Distal propagation of the bolus is shown

the patient in the Trendelenburg position, the water-siphon test, the Valsalva maneuver, and turning of the patient (Stewart 1981). We use only the latter two tests, which are more physiological than the former two. If reflux is noted during the examination, spot-film or video recording should be used to document it. With the invention of picture archiving and communication systems (PACS), an attractive alternative to storage of examination data on videotapes or DVDs has emerged. "Videoflurososcopic" examinations can now stored directly in a PACS, which allows easy retrieval of prior examinations for comparison.

4. Solid bolus with the patient in the upright position: If the patient suffers from dysphagia for solids and the examination with liquid barium does not reveal the cause, a solid bolus (barium-soaked cookies, marshmallows, tablets, etc.) may be used. Transit of solid food may be slow in some individuals. There is no standardized reference value for evaluation of solid food transit (Pouderoux et al. 1999). The best indicator for the presence of a significant stenosis (i.e., a Schatzki ring or a malignant stricture) or a motor abnormality is the induction of the typical symptoms of "food sticking in the throat" by a retained solid bolus.

5. Double-contrast and mucosal relief films of the esophagus and the lower esophageal sphincter (see the chapter on esophageal morphology).

4 Esophageal Motility Disorders

Esophageal motor disorders can be divided into two major categories. Primary motor disorders occur independent of other diseases and include achalasia, diffuse esophageal spasm, nonspecific esophageal motor disorders, and nutcracker esophagus. Secondary motor disorders include a long list of motor abnormalities seen in conjunction with other diseases (Table 1). Classification of motor disorders is based on manometric findings. Diagnosis of a secondary motor abnormality requires, in addition, the diagnosis of an extraesophageal disorder known to affect the esophagus. Esophageal motility disorders present with the nonspecific symptom of dysphagia or chest pain. Although the clinical presentation may be the same in patients with different motor abnormalities, it is important to characterize the abnormality precisely. The optimal therapy is based on the specific knowledge of a manometric abnormality and may differ considerably between different groups. However, esophageal manometry is not widely available and in most cases is not the first diagnostic test in patients with dysphagia. In these patients, either endoscopy or barium radiography is recommended in many institutions and countries (Tscholakoff et al. 2011; The Royal College of Radiologists 2007). Radiographic assessment, in particular videofluoroscopic recording, has been shown to be very useful in detecting and reliably characterizing esophageal motor abnormalities (Ott et al. 1987, 1990; Schima et al. 1992).

5 Primary Motor Disorders

5.1 Achalasia

Achalasia is the most widely known esophageal motor disorder. It is characterized by aperistalsis in the esophageal body and incomplete relaxation of the lower esophageal sphincter upon swallowing (Stacher et al. 1994; Richter 2001). The cause is not exactly known, but histopathologic lesions have been found in the dorsal motor nuclei of the brainstem, the vagal

Table 1 Classification of esophageal motility disorders

Primary motility disorders

Achalasia

Diffuse esophageal spasm

Nutcracker esophagus

Esophageal atresia

Nonspecific esophageal motor disorders

Secondary motility disorders

Connective tissue diseases

  Progressive systemic sclerosis

  Dermatomyositis

  Polymyositis

  Mixed connective tissue disease

  Lupus erythematosus

Endocrine disease

  Diabetes mellitus

  Myxoedema

  Hyperthyroidism

Metabolic disorders

  Alcohol-induced

  Amyloidosis

Infectious disorders

  Chagas disease

  Candida

  Herpes

Chemical

  Gastroesophageal reflux

  Caustic agents

Muscular disorders

  Myasthenia gravis

  Muscle dystrophy

Neurologic diseases

  Parkinson disease

  Guillain–Barré syndrome

  Poliomyelitis

  Amyotrophic lateral sclerosis

  Multiple sclerosis

Immunologic

  Chronic graft-versus-host disease

  Eosinophilic esophagitis

Iatrogenic

  Medication (anticholinergic agents, benzodiazepines, barbiturates, etc.)

  Radiation

  Postvagotomy

branches, and the myenteric plexus of the esophagus. The primary region of damage is the esophageal myenteric plexus (Auerbach's plexus), including patchy inflammatory response, loss of ganglionic cells, and some myenteric neurofibrosis (Richter 2010). Diagnosis of achalasia should be suspected when patients present with a long history of slowly progressive dysphagia for solids and liquids. Regurgitation of saliva and food immediately after swallowing (in contrast to gastroesophageal reflux) is common. Achalasia may also present as (noncardiac) chest pain. Some patients complain of heartburn, despite the fact that incomplete opening of the lower esophageal sphincter is one of the key features of achalasia (Spechler et al. 1995). Esophageal manometry is the gold standard for the diagnosis of achalasia. The resting pressure of the lower esophageal sphincter is either normal or high, and there is incomplete relaxation of the sphincter upon swallowing. Aperistalsis is present in the esophageal body. Contractions are simultaneous and sometimes even of high amplitude (so-called vigorous achalasia) (Goldenberg et al. 1991).

Videofluoroscopy is the best initial diagnostic test (Richter 2010). Radiologically, there is a typical appearance of esophageal dilatation with beaklike narrowing of the lower esophageal sphincter (Meshkinpour et al. 1992; Francis and Katzka 2010). Early in the disease, the esophagus has a normal diameter (Fig. 2). With progression of the disease, the esophagus becomes dilated and retains food and saliva (Fig. 3). In advanced cases, esophageal dilatation may be severe (so-called sigmoid esophagus) (Fig. 4) (Schima et al. 1993). Barium radiography has a low sensitivity in detecting achalasia, as alterations in esophageal morphology are present in advanced cases only. The radiologic staging system for achalasia according to Brombart (1980) is based on the grade of esophageal dilatation (less than 4 cm, 4–6 cm, more than 6 cm in diameter), which explains the low sensitivity of single-contrast upper gastrointestinal tract studies.

Multiphasic radiographic evaluations including fluoroscopic assessment of esophageal motility shows a support level of contrast material due to slowed esophageal transit. This sign hints at the presence of either a motor abnormality or a distal stenosis (Fig. 2). The sensitivity of radiologic studies (either barium radiography or videofluoroscopy) for the detection of achalasia has been reported to be 58–95% (Howard et al. 1992; Ott et al. 1987; Schima et al. 1992, 1998). With videofluoroscopy, diagnosis is based not only on morphologic alterations of the esophagus, but also on assessment of functional abnormalities. Videofluoroscopy may reveal incomplete lower esophageal sphincter opening with delayed transit into the stomach. The feature of a transient support level of barium with the patient in the upright position can be explained by variations in examination technique and patient populations. As described, the diagnosis is much more difficult to make in patients with early stages of the disease when esophageal dilatation is not yet present.

Several studies have reported a relation between achalasia and esophageal carcinoma. Patients with long-standing achalasia are at increased risk of carcinoma. The exact cause is unknown, but chronic stasis of food and saliva has been suggested. The reported incidences range from 1.7 to 20% (Meijssen et al. 1992). In a large prospective trial, the risk of patients with achalasia developing cancer was found to be increased 33-fold, for a total of 3.4 cancers per 1,000 patients per year. Close follow-up of patients with achalasia is therefore strongly recommended (Meijssen et al. 1992).

5.2 Pseudoachalasia (Malignancy-Induced Achalasia)

Malignancies involving the gastroesophageal junction can result in a clinical syndrome, pseudoachalasia, that mimics idiopathic achalasia. Pseudoachalasia is most often caused by adenocarcinoma of the fundus invading the distal esophagus. Other causes are squamous carcinoma of the distal esophagus with predominantly submucosal spread (Park et al. 2010) and hematogenous metastatic disease of the gastroesophageal junction (Dodds et al. 1986; Parkman and Cohen 1993; Kahrilas et al. 1987; Paulsen et al. 2010). Conventional esophageal manometry may not differentiate between idiopathic achalasia and pseudoachalasia. However, the correct diagnosis can be determined in most cases by the clinical history and the radiologic features. The mean duration of dysphagia is much shorter in patients with malignant pseudoachalasia than in patients with idiopathic achalasia (1.9 months vs. 4.5 years) (Woodfield et al.

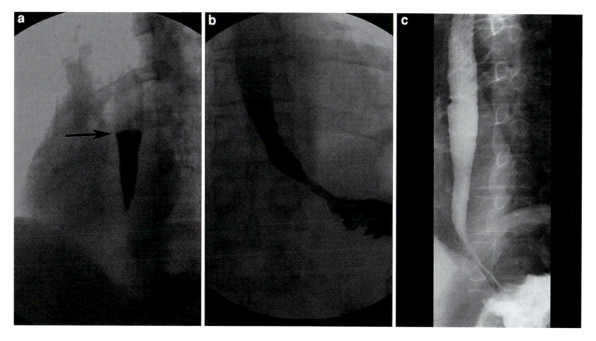

Fig. 2 Achalasia—early stage. **a** Videofluoroscopy with the patient in the upright position reveals a support level of contrast material indicative of delayed transit (*arrow*). The esophagus is not dilated. **b** With the patient in the supine position narrowing of the gastroesophageal junction is evident. **c** Radiography confirms narrowing of the gastroesophageal junction. Subsequently, manometry revealed achalasia

Fig. 3 Advanced achalasia. Barium radiography reveals moderate esophageal dilatation with retention of barium and secretions. There is the typical beaklike narrowing of the lower esophageal sphincter

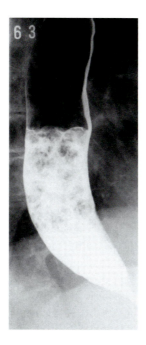

Fig. 4 Long-standing achalasia. In this patient with a 36-year history of untreated achalasia, there is massive dilatation of the esophagus, which nearly fills the right hemithorax. (From Schima et al. 1993)

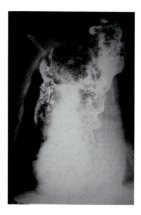

2000) and there is pronounced weight loss over time in malignancy-induced achalasia (Reynolds and Parkman 1989; Tremble 1959). Radiologically, the narrowed segment is longer in pseudoachalasia (4.4 vs. 1.9 cm) and reveals nodularity and abrupt proximal borders rather than a beaklike narrowing (Fig. 5) (Woodfield et al. 2000). The muscle-relaxing effect of amyl nitrite inhalation can be used to help make the correct diagnosis during barium radiography. After administration, there is relaxation of the lower esophageal sphincter, with a subsequent opening of 2 mm or more in sphincter diameter (Dodds et al. 1986). In pseudoachalasia with tumor infiltration, the

Fig. 5 Pseudoachalasia due
to adenocarcinoma of the
cardia. Barium radiography
reveals moderate esophageal
dilatation similar to that seen
in achalasia. However,
narrowing of the
gastroesophageal junction
does not appear beaklike.
It is more irregular (*arrow*)

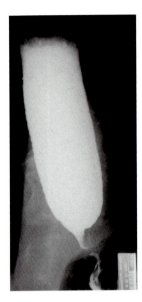

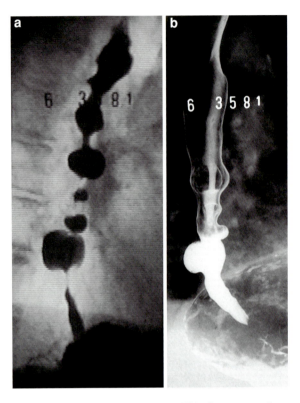

Fig. 6 Diffuse esophageal spasm. **a** Videofluoroscopy shows
severe nonpropulsive contractions, which give the esophagus a
corkscrew appearance. **b** Barium radiography shows partial
relaxation of these transient contractions. There is formation of
pseudodiverticulum-like sacculations between the contractions

sphincter is unaffected by amyl nitrite. Computed
tomography (CT) is also helpful in differentiating the
two syndromes. Circumferential thickening of the
lower esophageal sphincter of less than 10 mm is
indicative of idiopathic achalasia, whereas pseudoachalasia patients have CT findings of marked or
asymmetric wall thickening or a mass (Carter et al.
1997). When pseudoachalasia is suspected on the
basis of clinical history and radiologic features, negative endoscopic or biopsy findings should be viewed
with caution (Tremble 1959). Repeated biopsies,
endoscopic ultrasonography, or even surgical exploration may finally lead to the diagnosis of malignancy-induced pseudoachalasia.

5.3 Diffuse Esophageal Spasm

The incidence of diffuse esophageal spasm is much
lower than that of achalasia. Diffuse esophageal
spasm is characterized by substernal chest pain, dysphagia, and the manometric evidence of simultaneous
nonpropulsive contractions on more than 20% of
swallows with intermittent peristaltic contractions,
with a minimum amplitude of 30 mmHg (Richter and
Castell 1984; Konturek and Lembo 2008; Grübel
et al. 2008). It has been found that even "normal"
peristaltic contractions of diffuse esophageal spasm
patients are more rapidly propagated than normal
swallows of a control group (Krieger-Grübel et al.

2010). Differentiation between diffuse spasm and
vigorous achalasia is based on the presence of normal
relaxation of the lower sphincter in the former.
However, diffuse esophageal spasm may evolve into
vigorous achalasia or classic achalasia over time
(Hannig and Wuttge-Hannig 1987).

The classic radiologic features of diffuse spasm are
the presence of severe nonpropulsive contractions
causing esophageal curling or a "corkscrew" or
"rosary bead" appearance (Chen et al. 1989) (Fig. 6).
In two large studies by Ott et al. (1987, 1990) the
correct diagnosis of diffuse spasm was made radiologically in 55–71% of patients. Incomplete or absent
peristalsis and nonpropulsive contractions are present
in 71–76% of patients (Chen et al. 1989). However,
radiologic findings are often nonspecific and do not
allow the diagnosis of diffuse esophageal spasm to be
made; therefore, patients with otherwise unexplained
chest pain and radiologic evidence of a nonspecific
esophageal contraction abnormality should be

referred for manometry. On CT, diffuse esophageal spasm may appear as smooth circumferential wall thickening of the lower esophagus in 21% of patients (Goldberg et al. 2008) and should be included in the differential diagnosis of esophageal wall thickening.

5.4 Nutcracker Esophagus

As more patients with noncardiac chest pain were studied manometrically, an abnormality clearly different from diffuse spasm was recognized in 1979 (Benjamin et al. 1979). In the so-called nutcracker esophagus, primary peristalsis is preserved, but there are peristaltic contractions of high amplitude and long duration. The diagnosis of nutcracker esophagus is made by manometry.

It is known that approximately 20% of patients admitted to cardiac care units show no abnormality in a detailed cardiac workup (Bassotti et al. 1998). In a large percentage of these patients with noncardiac chest pain, nutcracker esophagus or diffuse esophageal spasms are present.

Radiologically, the diagnosis is difficult to make, because peristalsis is preserved. Chobanian et al. (1986) found nonspecific abnormalities of esophageal bolus transit in 36% of patients. These findings were confirmed in a study by Ott et al. (1990): in a series of 170 patients suffering from chest pain, nutcracker esophagus was even more prevalent than diffuse esophageal spasm, but a specific radiologic diagnosis could not be made in any of the patients.

The patho-physiological of nutcracker esophagus remains unclear. The transition of nutcracker esophagus into achalsia has been shown, suggesting that both diseases lie within the same part of a spectrum of motor disorders (Konturek and Lembo 2008).

5.5 Esophageal Atresia

In infants with esophageal atresia, Vogt's classification is based on the presence and location of an esophagotracheal fistula (Hasse 1968). After esophageal repair, swallowing difficulties are common. The most common source of postoperative dysphagia is the presence of strictures; however, esophageal dysfunction is also common (Auringer and Sumner 1994). There is absence of swallow-induced primary peristalsis, and secondary peristaltic contractions have lower amplitudes than those seen in normal infants (Daum and Keuerleber 1969).

5.6 Nonspecific Esophageal Motor Disorders

By far the most common esophageal motor disorders are nonspecific contraction abnormalities. They may be idiopathic (primary) or secondary to a variety of extraesophageal diseases (Table 1). Manometrically, contraction waves with multiple peaks, peristaltic waves with decreased amplitude, and isolated simultaneous or spontaneous contractions may be found (Gelfand and Botoman 1987). These contraction abnormalities do not fit into one of the aforementioned categories of specific motor disorders.

Radiologically, incomplete or absent peristalsis and nonpropulsive contractions can be seen. The sensitivity of radiographic studies is only 46–73%, because intermittent contraction abnormalities may elude radiographic detection (Ott et al. 1987; Schima et al. 1992). Clinically, it is important to search for underlying diseases, such as diabetes, alcoholism, eosinophilic esophagitis, and progressive systemic sclerosis (PSS), which may cause esophageal motility disorders (secondary motility disorders). In these cases, therapy is directed at the underlying disorder. Especially eosinophilic esophagitis may mimic all categories of motor disorders, including nutcracker esophagus and vigorous achalasia (Hejazi et al. 2010). Appropriate treatment may reverse motor abnormalities to the normal state.

5.7 Presbyesophagus

Soergel et al. (1964) reported a high incidence of esophageal motor abnormalities in elderly individuals, for which they coined the term "presbyesophagus." In their study on nonagenarians, nonpropulsive contractions were prevalent in ten of 15 patients. However, the existence of such a clinical entity has been much disputed. In another study (Hollis and Castell 1974), esophageal peristalsis was not found to be abnormal in elderly healthy individuals. It has been suggested that the increased prevalence of esophageal motor abnormalities is likely a function of an

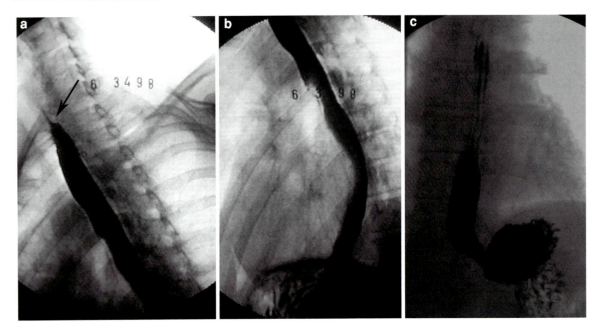

Fig. 7 Progressive systemic sclerosis: early stage. **a** Videofluoroscopy with the patient in the prone oblique position shows normal peristaltic contraction in the proximal, striated muscle part of the esophagus. **b** The peristaltic wave subsides in the middle third of the esophagus with massive retention of barium, indicative of hypomotility. **c** There is no evidence of narrowing of the gastroesophageal junction. Together with the clinical history, this is typical of esophageal involvement in progressive systemic sclerosis

increased prevalence of underlying diseases, such as diabetes and neuromuscular disorders, which can affect esophageal motility (Ekberg and Feinberg 1991; Price and Castell 1978). It is most important in elderly individuals with newly developed dysphagia to rule out the presence of a tumor or a stricture before making the diagnosis of a motor disorder.

6 Secondary Motility Disorders

6.1 Progressive Systemic Sclerosis and Other Connective Tissue Diseases

Esophageal dysmotility is a well-known feature of PSS (or scleroderma) (Campbell and Schultz 1986) and other connective tissue diseases. PSS often affects the gastrointestinal tract, especially the esophagus and the small bowel, resulting in fibrosis and atrophy of smooth muscle. Esophageal involvement in PSS where the smooth muscle segment is affected results in hypomotility of the distal esophagus with absence of peristalsis and a patulous lower esophageal

sphincter. Gastroesophageal reflux is common because of the incompetent sphincter, and refluxed acidic gastric contents are not readily cleared from the esophagus by secondary peristalsis. Esophageal symptoms, especially heartburn and dysphagia, are common in PSS. Such symptoms are found in up to 50% of patients (Sprung and Gibb 1985).

In the early stages of esophageal involvement, there is weak peristalsis in the distal esophagus (Montesi et al. 1991). Radiographically, the esophagus may be air-distended for a prolonged period after swallowing, without exhibiting the typical swallowing-induced collapse of the lumen due to a peristaltic contraction. In the prone oblique position, hypomotility is present in the distal esophagus with retention of barium (Fig. 7). With more advanced disease, esophageal dilatation and a patulous lower esophageal sphincter are apparent (Fig. 8). With the patient in the prone oblique position, complete aperistalsis with severe retention of barium (and saliva) will be found. Oropharyngeal dysfunction, including pharyngeal retention and aspiration, is found in 26% of patients (Montesi et al. 1991). Patients with an oropharyngeal disorder have a higher incidence of PSS-related pulmonary disease.

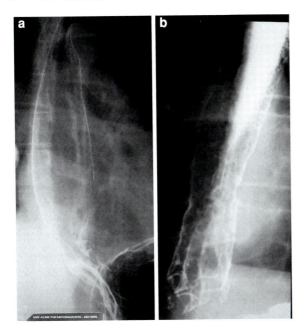

Fig. 8 Progressive systemic sclerosis: advanced disease. **a** Barium radiography demonstrates esophageal dilatation and a widely patent gastroesophageal junction (*arrows*). **b** In another patient, there is obvious distal fold thickening indicative of reflux esophagitis. Barium radiography also shows a slight peptic stricture in the distal esophagus (*arrow*)

As esophageal dysmotility progresses, gastroesophageal reflux and its sequelae will predominate. Severe reflux esophagitis, strictures, and Barrett esophagus develops (Fig. 8). In the early advanced stages of the disease, differentiation between PSS and achalasia can be made with a high level of certainty. Although aperistalsis and esophageal dilatation are present in both diseases, the shape of the gastroesophageal junction is markedly different. However, the development of distal peptic strictures in PSS may be confusing, although these strictures almost never have the bird-beak-like appearance seen in achalasia. PSS patients with severe reflux esophagitis are at increased risk of developing Barrett esophagus and, subsequently, adenocarcinoma (Sprung and Gibb 1985). Although barium radiography and videofluoroscopy are very sensitive (67–100%) for the detection of motor dysfunction in PSS (Campbell and Schultz 1986; Schima et al. 1992), these tests are not very accurate in the detection of peptic complications. For this reason, close endoscopic surveillance of PSS patients with reflux esophagitis and peptic strictures is recommended.

Esophageal dysmotility has also been reported to occur in patients with dermatomyositis/polymyositis and mixed connective tissue disease. Radiographic findings are nonspecific, including low-amplitude peristalsis, aperistalsis, and delayed esophageal emptying on scintigraphy (Marshall et al. 1990; Horowitz et al. 1986).

6.2 Diabetes Mellitus

Esophageal symptoms are common in patients with diabetes, and the likelihood of dysphagia is more than threefold higher than in nondiabetic controls (Bytzer et al. 2001). Esophageal motor dysfunction has been demonstrated, characterized by weak peristalsis and increased frequency of nonpropulsive contractions (Hollis et al. 1977; Holloway et al. 1999). Not surprisingly, a relation between the presence of esophageal dysmotility and diabetic neuropathy has also been reported (Mandelstam et al. 1969; Hollis et al. 1977). It has been suggested that autonomic neuropathy of the vagal nerve supplying the esophagus plays a major role in the development of diabetic dysmotility (Holloway et al. 1999). Radiographically, weak peristalsis or nonpropulsive contractions can be observed (Borgström et al. 1988).

6.3 Chagas Disease

Chagas disease (South American trypanosomiasis) is caused by infection with the protozoon *Trypanosoma cruzi* (Dantas et al. 1999). In the chronic phase, the disease most often involves the heart, esophagus, and colon, causing cardiomegaly, megaesophagus, and megacolon. Chagas disease and achalasia share the same histopathologic lesion and the loss of ganglion cells within the esophageal myenteric plexus (Dantas et al. 2001), which are destroyed by the infectious organism in Chagas disease. The clinical and radiological appearance of achalasia and Chagas disease may be identical (Fig. 9). Manometry may help to differentiate the two by identifying a higher resting pressure of the lower esophageal sphincter pressure in Chagas disease. The geographic origin of the patient may also provide a clue to the right diagnosis, and proof of Chagas disease is based on serologic testing.

Fig. 9 Megaesophagus in a
14-year-old boy with Chagas
disease. Barium radiography
reveals esophageal dilation
with tapering of the sphincter
indistinguishable from
idiopathic achalasia.
(Courtesy of Roberto Dantas,
Ribeirão Preto, Brazil)

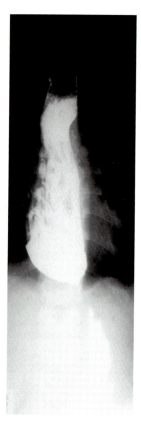

6.4   Other Secondary Motility Disorders

There are a variety of other diseases and clinical conditions that may affect the esophagus and cause a secondary motility disorder (Table 1), including amyloidosis (Rubinow et al. 1983; Lefkowitz et al. 1989; Burakoff et al. 1985), alcoholism (Grande et al. 1996), myxedema (Wright and Penner 1981), hyperthyroidism, parkinsonism (Leopold and Kagel 1997), graft-versus-host disease (Schima et al. 1994), Sjögren syndrome (Kjellén et al. 1986; Palma et al. 1994), and eosinophilic esophagitis (Hejazi et al. 2010). In all these diseases, except PSS and Chagas disease, which have a typical radiographic appearance, nonspecific esophageal function abnormalities have been found. Therefore, in all patients with an otherwise unexplained dysphagia and a nonspecific esophageal contraction abnormality, the search should be directed toward the detection of and therapy for an underlying disease.

7   Esophageal Diverticula Associated with Motility Disorders

Esophageal diverticula are included in this chapter because they are associated with an esophageal motility disorder in the vast majority of cases. Classification is based in the location: Zenker's diverticulum above the pharyngoesophageal sphincter (i.e., a pharyngeal diverticulum that will not be covered in this chapter), midesophageal diverticulum just inferior to the level of the aortic arch, and epiphrenic diverticulum just above the diaphragm.

7.1   Midesophageal Diverticula

In the past, midesophageal diverticula were widely considered to be traction-type diverticula of no clinical significance (Schmidt et al. 1991). Recently, this view has been questioned by some studies, which have shown that these diverticula resemble more the pulsion-type diverticula (Borrie and Wilson 1980; Evander et al. 1986). Kaye (1974) reported on associated esophageal motor disorders found by manometry. In a series of 12 patients, diffuse spasms and nonspecific contraction abnormalities were the most common findings.

On the basis of radiographic findings, Rivkin et al. (1984) pointed out that midesophageal diverticula are likely of the pulsion type. The pear-shaped configuration of most diverticula and their movement on swallowing resembles the appearance of Zenker's and epiphrenic diverticula. In our study including 30 patients with 33 midesophageal diverticula, 80% were diagnosed as propulsion-type diverticula on the basis of radiographic findings. Diverticula were classified as pulsion-type when they were pear-shaped, when the size and shape changed during bolus passage, and when there was upward and downward movement of the diverticulum of at least 2 cm upon swallowing (Fig. 10) (Schima et al. 1997). In this study, 88% of patients with a pulsion diverticulum suffered from an esophageal motor disorder, and six of 20 patients (30%) were diagnosed as having achalasia as evidenced by videofluoroscopy and manometry (Schima et al. 1997). In conclusion, midesophageal diverticula in symptomatic patients are primarily of the pulsion type and tend to be associated with esophageal motor disorders.

Fig. 10 Midesophageal propulsion diverticulum in a patient with nonspecific motor disorder. **a** The spot film of the esophagus taken during deglutition is normal. **b** Another spot film taken approximately 2 s later shows outpouching of a propulsion diverticulum in the midesophagus (*arrow*). A nonspecific motor disorder was found by videofluoroscopy

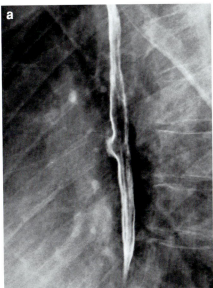
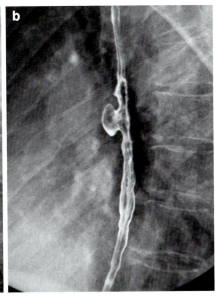

7.2 Epiphrenic Diverticula

Epiphrenic diverticula are generally associated with and probably caused by an underlying esophageal motor dysfunction. Approximately two thirds of patients will have specific motor disorders, with achalasia the most common (Bruggeman and Seaman 1973; Debas et al. 1980) (Fig. 11). The high percentage of motor abnormalities in association with epiphrenic diverticula determines the therapeutic and especially the surgical approach. Patients should always be referred for manometry to search for a curable manometric disorder before surgical resection of a "symptomatic" midesophageal diverticulum (Fig. 10). In these cases, diverticulectomy alone carries the risk of postoperative suture breakdown and predisposes the patient to recurrence of the diverticulum (Rivkin et al. 1984). Myotomy of the lower esophageal sphincter is now a routine part of the operation (Evander et al. 1986).

8 Gastroesophageal Reflux Disease and Esophageal Function

The term "Gastroesophageal reflux disease" (GERD) covers the entire spectrum of clinical conditions and histologic esophageal alterations that result from gastroesophageal reflux (Dodds 1988). GERD is by far the most common cause of esophagitis in the general population. In the last 15–20 years, our knowledge of the cause and pathogenesis of gastroesophageal reflux and the development of esophagitis has considerably broadened. The pathogenesis is multifactorial and the factors believed to be important include (1) inadequate antireflux mechanisms, (2) chemical consistency of refluxed material, (3) esophageal clearance of refluxed material, (4) esophageal mucosal resistance, and (5) volume of gastric contents and efficacy of gastric emptying (Dodds et al. 1981; Dodds 1988).

8.1 Hiatal Hernia and Reflux

In the past, the finding of a hiatal hernia was considered the most important predisposing factor for the development of reflux. The exact prevalence of hiatal hernia in the general population remains unknown, largely because of the differences in examination techniques and diagnostic criteria (Fransson et al. 1989; Ott et al. 1985; Kahrilas et al. 1999). The relationship between the presence of a hiatal hernia and reflux disease remains controversial. Several studies have found that a hiatal hernia is much more common in patients with symptomatic reflux or

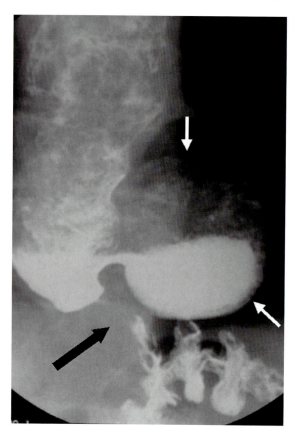

Fig. 11 Giant epiphrenic diverticulum in a patient with achalasia. Barium radiography demonstrates massive esophageal dilatation and a severe narrowing of the gastroesophageal junction, indicative of achalasia (*black arrow*). Videofluoroscopy showed there was only a minimal transient opening of the sphincter, with passage of only small amounts of barium. There is a giant epiphrenic diverticulum (*white arrows*) located above the sphincter

abnormal findings on pH testing than in patients without reflux disease (prevalence, 80–94 vs. 59–60%) (Chen et al. 1992; Ott et al. 1985). Moreover, the presence of a hiatal hernia reduces lower esophageal sphincter pressure, which may increase the susceptibility to reflux events (Kahrilas et al. 1999). However, severe reflux esophagitis can also be found in patients without hiatal hernia (Kaul et al. 1986). Thus hiatal hernia is a nonspecific radiologic finding with a poor predictive value: the presence of a hiatal hernia does not predict the presence of GERD (Ott et al. 1995). Conversely, the absence of a hiatal hernia does not exclude severe reflux esophagitis (Kaul et al. 1986).

8.2   Gastroesophageal Reflux and Esophageal Function

Effective esophageal peristalsis is a prerequisite for appropriate esophageal clearance of refluxed gastric contents. In normal subjects, a secondary peristaltic contraction is triggered by gastric contents refluxed into the esophagus, which rapidly clears the esophagus of the irritating agent. In patients with GERD, abnormalities of esophageal function are a common finding (Stein et al. 1990; Schoeman and Holloway 1995). Motor function deteriorates with increasing severity of mucosal injury (Fibbe et al. 2001). Swallow-induced primary peristalsis is impaired in GERD patients. It has also been shown that patients with GERD exhibit a defect in the triggering of secondary peristalsis (Schoeman and Holloway 1995). Instillation of water boluses or distension of the esophagus by air frequently fails to elicit a peristaltic contraction in reflux patients.

Interestingly, Timmer et al. (1994) demonstrated that impairment of esophageal peristalsis remained unchanged after healing of esophagitis (Howard et al. 1994). Likewise, esophageal motility did not recover after fundoplication despite significant improvement in clinical symptoms and endoscopic signs of esophagitis (Fibbe et al. 2001). These results can be interpreted in two ways: first, deterioration of esophageal motility is irreversible in GERD; or, second, esophageal motility dysfunction is a preexisting factor in the pathogenesis of reflux disease (Timmer et al. 1994). The lack of improvement of esophageal motility with healing of esophagitis explains the high recurrence of esophagitis (50%) at 2 months after discontinuation of omeprazole therapy (Howard et al. 1994). These facts support the hypothesis that dysmotility is rather induced by irreversible inflammatory changes of the esophagus. However, a conclusive answer to this question will require a large prospective study of reflux patients with normal motility to determine whether motility deteriorates over time.

Both the barium swallow and radionuclide transit studies are useful in detecting motor disorders in GERD patients. Abnormalities seen in GERD include weak or even absent primary peristalsis and nonperistaltic contractions (Ott 1994). Clearance of barium that has refluxed from the stomach can also be

Fig. 12 Gastroesophageal reflux and reflux esophagitis. **a** In this patient with severe heartburn, there is spontaneous reflux of liquid barium and a barium tablet in the right lateral position. **b** Double-contrast esophagram showing signs of severe reflux esophagitis in the distal esophagus with linear ulcerations (*arrow*)

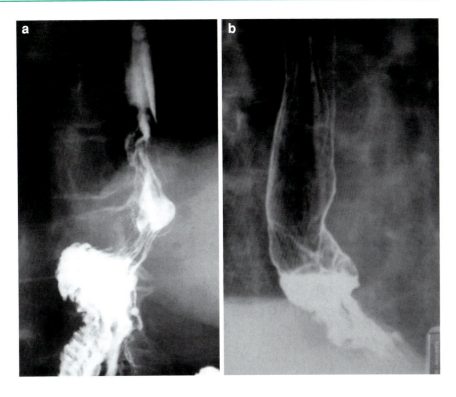

assessed with the patient in the recumbent position. Presently, 24-h pH monitoring is the gold standard in the detection and quantitation of gastroesophageal reflux (Thompson et al. 1994). However, abnormal results from 24-h pH monitoring do not necessarily mean that the patient has clinical symptoms or endoscopic signs of esophagitis, and vice versa. The results of several studies evaluating the role of radiology in patients with GERD have been disappointing (Chen et al. 1992; Kaul et al. 1986; Johnston et al. 1996). A major reason for the poor performance of radiology is that there is only limited time for fluoroscopic observation of barium. A meta-analysis of nine studies on radiographic detection of gastroesophageal reflux revealed an average sensitivity of 39% (Ott 1994). In a study by Thompson et al. (1994) the diagnostic yield of spontaneous and provoked gastroesophageal reflux during barium radiography was assessed. The detection of spontaneous reflux revealed a sensitivity of 26% and a specificity of 94%. Using provocative tests, including cough/Valsalva maneuver, rolling, and the water-siphon test, increased the sensitivity of radiography to 31, 44, and 70%, respectively. However, with increasing sensitivity the specificity dropped to 74%. Thus, prolonged

observation and the use of provocative maneuvers increases the sensitivity of barium radiography in the detection of reflux (Fig. 12). The absence of a reflux episode during fluoroscopy does not exclude the presence of GERD. Radiologic studies are not accurate enough to be used as a screening test in GERD patients: However, they may help to discover complications of GERD and to define the anatomy of the gastroesophageal junction in patients who are candidates for antireflux surgery.

9 Dynamic Magnetic Resonance Imaging To Assess Esophageal Motor Function

To avoid exposure to ionizing radiation, dynamic magnetic resonance (MR) imaging protocols have been developed for assessing esophageal function and the gastroesophageal junction. Boluses of buttermilk or other test meals spiked with gadolinium chelates and ferric ammonium citrate have been used as contrast materials (Kulinna-Cosentini et al. 2007; Manabe et al. 2009; Curcic et al. 2010). Steady-state free-precession MR pulse sequences (B-FFE, Philips) with parallel

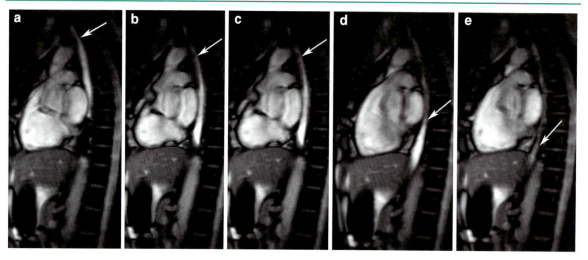

Fig. 13 Dynamic magnetic resonance imaging (sagittal view) at a frame rate of one per second using a bolus of buttermilk spiked with gadolinium shows normal esophageal peristalsis. There is distal propagation of the peristaltic contraction wave (*arrows*)

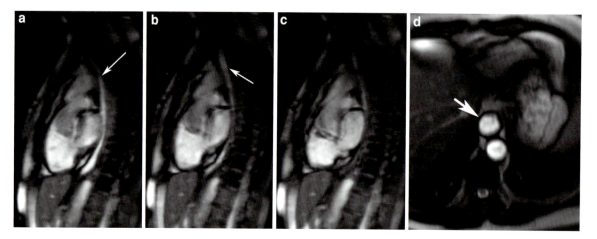

Fig. 14 Dynamic magnetic resonance imaging of gastroesophageal reflux and hiatal hernia. Sagittal view showing (**a**), (**b**) proximal propagation of the bolus in the esophagus (*arrows*) and (**c**) delayed clearance of the esophagus. **d** Axial view showing a hiatal hernia (*arrow*) anterior to the aorta

imaging allow a time resolution of one image per second, enough to assess esophageal function and the gastroesophageal region. Dynamic MR imaging can reliably depict normal peristaltic contractions as well as gastroesophageal reflux (Figs. 13, 14), as evidenced by manometry (Curcic et al. 2010). Another advantage is the lack of radiation, which allows repeated acquisitions to assess swallowing function. However, this technique is not without limitations. The time resolution is inferior to that of videofluoroscopy. Moreover, swallowing in the recumbent position is not physiologic, and the reflux of small volumes may escape detection (Manabe et al. 2009). Dynamic MR imaging

of esophageal function is still a research tool, but it may provide new insights into esophageal function, which we could not obtain with fluoroscopy.

References

Aksglaede K, Funch-Jensen P, Vestergaard H, Thommesen P (1992) Diagnosis of esophageal motor disorders: a prospective study comparing barium swallow, food barium mixture, and continuous swallows with manometry. Gastrointest Radiol 17:1–4

Anvari M, Richards D, Dent J, Waterfall WE, Stevenson GW (1989) The effect of glucagon on esophageal peristalsis and clearance. Gastrointest Radiol 14:100–102

Auringer ST, Sumner E (1994) Pediatric upper gastrointestinal tract. Radiol Clin North Am 32:1051–1066

Bassotti G, Fiorella S, Germani U, Roselli P, Bataglia E, Morelli A (1998) The nutcracker esophagus: a late diagnostic yield notwithstanding chest pain and dysphagia. Dysphagia 13:213–217

Benjamin SB, Gerhardt DC, Castell DO (1979) High amplitude, peristaltic esophageal contractions associated with chest pain and/or dysphagia. Gastroenterology 77:478–483

Borgström PS, Olsson R, Sundkvist G, Ekberg O (1988) Pharyngeal and esophageal function in patients with diabetes mellitus and swallowing complaints. Br J Radiol 61:817–821

Borrie J, Wilson RLK (1980) Esophageal diverticula: principles of management and appraisal of classification. Thorax 35:759–767

Brombart MM (1980) Radiologie des Verdauungstraktes. Thieme, Stuttgart, pp 244–245

Bruggeman LL, Seaman WB (1973) Epiphrenic diverticula: an analysis of 80 cases. Am J Roentgenol 119:266–276

Burakoff R, Rubinow A, Cohen AS (1985) Esophageal manometry in familial amyloid polyneuropathy. Am J Med 79:85–89

Bytzer P, Talley NJ, Leemon M, Young LJ, Jones MP, Horowitz M (2001) Prevalence of gastrointestinal symptoms associated with diabetes mellitus. Arch Intern Med 161:1989–1996

Campbell WL, Schultz JC (1986) Specificity and sensitivity of esophageal motor abnormality in systemic sclerosis (scleroderma) and related diseases: a cineradiographic study. Gastrointest Radiol 11:218–222

Carter M, Deckmann RC, Smith RC, Burrell MI, Traube M (1997) Differentiation of achalasia from pseudoachalasia by computed tomography. Am J Gastoenterol 92:624–628

Chen YM, Ott DJ, Hewson EG et al (1989) Diffuse esophageal spasm: radiographic and manometric correlation. Radiology 170:807–810

Chen MYM, Ott DJ, Sinclair JW, Wu WC, Gelfand DW (1992) Gastroesophageal reflux disease: correlation of esophageal pH testing and radiographic findings. Radiology 185:483–486

Chobanian SJ, Curtis DJ, Benjamin SB, Cattau EL (1986) Radiology of the nutcracker esophagus. J Clin Gastroenterol 8:230–232

Cohen S (1979) Motor disorders of the esophagus. N Engl J Med 301:184–192

Curcic J, Fox M, Kaufman E et al (2010) Gastroesophageal junction: structure and function as assessed by using MR imaging. Radiology 257:115–124

Dantas RO, Deghaide NHS, Donadi EA (1999) Esophageal manometric and radiologic findings in asymptomatic subjects with Chagas disease. J Clin Gastroenterol 28:245–248

Dantas RO, Deghaide NHS, Donadi EA (2001) Esophageal motility of patients with Chagas disease and idiopathic achalasia. Dig Dis Sci 46:1200–1206

Daum R, Keuerleber M (1969) Spätfunktion der intrathorakalen Speiseröhre nach operierter Ösophagusatresie. Kinderchir 7:49–60

Debas HT, Payne WS, Cameron AJ, Carlson HC (1980) Physiopathology of lower esophageal diverticulum and its implication for treatment. Surg Gynecol Obstet 151:593–600

Dodds WJ (1977) Current concepts of esophageal motor function: clinical implications for radiology. Am J Roentgenol 128:549–561

Dodds WJ (1988) The pathogenesis of gastroesophageal reflux disease. Am J Roentgenol 151:49–56

Dodds WJ, Hogan WJ, Helm JF, Dent J (1981) Pathogenesis of reflux esophagitis. Gastroenterology 81:376–394

Dodds WJ, Stewart ET, Kishk SM, Kahrilas PJ, Hogan WJ (1986) Radiologic amyl nitrite test for distinguishing pseudoachalasia from idiopathic achalasia. Am J Roentgenol 146:21–23

Dooley CP, Schlossmacher B, Valenzuela JE (1988) Effects of alterations in bolus viscosity of esophageal peristalsis in humans. Am J Physiol 254:G8–G11

Ekberg O, Feinberg MJ (1991) Altered swallowing function in elderly patients without dysphagia: radiologic findings in 56 patients. Am J Roentgenol 156:1181–1184

Evander A, Little AG, Ferguson MK, Skinner DB (1986) Diverticula of the mid- and lower esophagus: pathogenesis and surgical management. World J Surg 10:820–828

Fibbe C, Layer P, Keller J, Strate U, Emmermann A, Zornig C (2001) Esophageal motility in reflux disease before and after fundoplication: a prospective, randomized, clinical and manometric study. Gastroenterology 121:5–14

Francis DL, Katzka DA (2010) Achalasia: update on the disease and its treatment. Gastroenterology 139:369–374

Fransson S-G, Sökjer H, Johansson K-E, Tibbling L (1989) Radiologic diagnosis of gastro-esophageal reflux. Acta Radiol 30:187–192

Gelfand MD, Botoman AV (1987) Esophageal motility disorders: a clinical overview. Am J Gastroenterol 82:181–187

Goldenberg SP, Burrell M, Fette GG, Vos C, Traube M (1991) Classic and vigorous achalasia: a comparison of manometric, radiographic, and clinical findings. Gastroenterology 101:743–748

Goldberg MF, Levine MS, Torigian DA (2008) Diffuse esophageal spasm: CT findings in seven patients. Am J Roentgenol 191:758–763

Grande L, Monforte R, Ros E et al (1996) High amplitude contractions in the middle third of the esophagus: a manometric marker of chronic alcoholism? Gut 38:655–662

Grishaw EK, Ott DJ, Frederick MG, Gelfand DW, Chen MYM (1996) Functional abnormalities of the esophagus: a prospective analysis of radiographic findings relative to age and symptoms. Am J Roentgenol 167:719–723

Grübel C, Borovicka J, Schwizer W, Fox M, Hebbard G (2008) Diffuse esophageal spasm. Am J Gastroenterol 103:450–457

Hannig C, Wuttge-Hannig A (1987) Röntgendiagnostik von Motilitätsstörungen des Pharynx und Ösophagus. Leber Magen Darm 1:7–17

Hannig C, Wuttge-Hannig A, Daschner H, Baum S, Güntner G (1990) Bariumsulfat–Gelatinekugeln zur Diagnostik spezieller pharyngoösophagealer Fragestellungen. Rontgenpraxis 43:15–19

Hasse W (1968) Ösophagusatresie. Thoraxchir 16:432–438

Hejazi RA, Reddymasu SC, Sostarich S, McCallum RW (2010) Disturbances of esophageal motility in eosinophilic esophagitis: a case series. Dysphagia 25:231–237

Hewson EG, Ott DJ, Dalton CB, Chen YM, Wu WC, Richter JE (1990) Manometry and radiology: complementary studies in the assessment of esophageal motility disorders. Gastroenterology 98:626–632

Hollis JB, Castell DO (1974) Esophageal function in elderly men: a new look at "presbyesophagus". Ann Intern Med 80: 371–374

Hollis JB, Castell DO, Braddom RL (1977) Esophageal function in diabetes mellitus and its relationship to peripheral neuropathy. Gastroenterology 73:1098–1102

Holloway RH, Tippett MD, Horowitz M, Maddox AF, Moten J, Russo A (1999) Relationship between esophageal motility and transit in patients with type I diabetes mellitus. Am J Gastroenterol 94:3150–3157

Horowitz M, McNeil JD, Maddern GJ, Collins PJ, Shearman DJC (1986) Abnormalities of gastric and esophageal emptying in polymyositis and dermatomyositis. Gastroenterology 90:434–439

Howard PJ, Maher L, Pryde A, Cameron EWJ, Heading RC (1992) Five years prospective study of the incidence, clinical features, and diagnosis of achalasia in Edinburgh. Gut 33:1011–1015

Howard JM, Reynolds RPE, Frei JV et al (1994) Macrosopic healing of esophagitis does not improve esophageal motility. Dig Dis Sci 39:648–654

Hurst AF, Rake GW (1930) Achalasia of the cardia. Q J Med 23:491–509

Johnston BT, Troshinsky MB, Castell JA, Castell DO (1996) Comparison of barium radiology with esophageal pH monitoring in the diagnosis of gastroesophageal reflux disease. Am J Gastroenterol 91:1181–1185

Kahrilas PJ, Kishk SM, Helm JF, Dodds WJ, Harig JM, Hogan WJ (1987) Comparison of achalasia and pseudoachalasia. Am J Med 82:439–446

Kahrilas PJ, Lin S, Chen J, Manka M (1999) The effect of hiatus hernia on gastro-esophageal junction pressure. Gut 44:476–482

Kaul B, Petersen H, Myrvold HE, Grette K, Røysland P, Halvorsen T (1986) Hiatus hernia in gastroesophageal reflux disease. Scand J Gastroenterol 21:31–34

Kaye MD (1974) Esophageal motor dysfunction in patients with diverticula of the mid-thoracic esophagus. Thorax 29:666–672

Kjellén G, Fransson SG, Lindström F, Sökjer H, Tibbling L (1986) Esophageal function, radiography, and dysphagia in Sjögren's syndrome. Dig Dis Sci 31:225–229

Konturek T, Lembo A (2008) Spasm, nutcracker, and IEM: real or manometry findings? J Clin Gastroenterol 42:647–651

Krieger-Grübel C, Hiscock R, Nandurkar S, Heddle R, Hebbard G (2010) Physiology of diffuse esophageal spasm (DES)–when normal swallows are not normal. Neurogastroenterol Motil 22:1056–e279

Kulinna-Cosentini C, Schima W, Cosentini EP (2007) Dynamic MR imaging of the gastroesophageal junction in healthy volunteers during bolus passage. J Magn Reson Imaging 25:749–754

Lefkowitz JR, Brand DL, Schuffler MD, Brugge WR (1989) Amyloidosis mimics achalasia's effect on lower esophageal sphincter. Dig Dis Sci 34:630–635

Leopold NA, Kagel MC (1997) Pharyngo-esophageal dysphagia in Parkinson's disease. Dysphagia 12:11–18

Li Q, Castell JA, Castell DO (1994) Manometric determination of esophageal length. Am J Gastroenterol 89:722–725

Manabe T, Kawamitsu H, Higashino T, Shirasaka D, Aoyama N, Sugimura K (2009) Observation of gastro-esophageal reflux by MRI: a feasibility study. Abdom Imaging 34:419–423

Mandelstam P, Siegel CI, Lieber A, Siegel M (1969) The swallowing disorder in patients with diabetic neuropathy-gastroenteropathy. Gastroenterology 56:1–12

Marshall JB, Kretschmar DC, Winship DC, Winn D, Treadwell EL, Sharp GC (1990) Gastrointestinal manifestations of mixed connective tissue disease. Gastroenterology 98:1232–1238

Meijssen MAC, Tilanus HW, van Blankenstein M, Hop WCJ, Ong GL (1992) Achalasia complicated by esophageal squamous cell carcinoma: a prospective study in 195 patients. Gut 33:155–158

Meshkinpour H, Kaye L, Elias A, Glick ME (1992) Manometric and radiologic correlations in achalasia. Am J Gastroenterol 87:1567–1570

Meyer GW, Gerhardt DC, Castell DO (1981) Human esophageal response to rapid swallowing: muscle refractory period or neural inhibition? Am J Physiol 241:G129–G136

Montesi A, Pesaresi A, Cavalli ML, Ripa G, Candela M, Gabrielli A (1991) Oropharyngeal and eophageal function in scleroderma. Dysphagia 6:219–223

Ott DJ (1994) Gastroesophageal reflux disease. Radiol Clin North Am 32:1147–1166

Ott DJ, Gelfand DW, Chen YM, Wu WC, Munitz HA (1985) Predictive relationship of hiatal hernia to reflux esophagitis. Gastrointest Radiol 10:317–320

Ott DJ, Richter JE, Chen MY, Wu WC, Gelfand DW, Castell DO (1987) Esophageal radiography and manometry: correlation in 172 patients with dysphagia. Am J Roentgenol 149:307–311

Ott DJ, Abernethy WB, Chen MYM, Wu WC, Gelfand DW (1990) Radiologic evaluation of esophageal motility: results in 170 patients with chest pain. Am J Roentgenol 155:983–985

Ott DJ, Kelley TF, Chen MYM et al (1991) Evaluation of the esophagus with a marshmallow bolus: clarifying the cause of dysphagia. Gastrointest Radiol 16:1–4

Ott DJ, Glauser SJ, Ledbetter MS, Chen MYM, Koufman JA, Gelfand DW (1995) Association of hiatal hernia and gastroesophageal reflux: correlation between presence and size of hiatal hernia and 24-h pH monitoring of the esophagus. Am J Roentgenol 165:557–559

Palma R, Freire A, Freitas J et al (1994) Esophageal motility disorders in patients with Sjögren's syndrome. Dig Dis Sci 39:758–761

Parkman HP, Cohen S (1993) Malignancy-induced secondary achalasia. Dysphagia 8:292–296

Parkman HP, Maurer AH, Caroline DF, Miller DL, Krevsky B, Fisher RS (1996) Optimal evaluation of patients with nonobstructive dysphagia. Manometry, scintigraphy, or videesophagography? Dig Dis Sci 41:1355–1368

Park JH, Park DI, Kim HJ et al (2010) An unusual case of submucosal invasion of esophageal squamous cell carcinoma mistaken as primary achalasia. J Neurogastroenterol Motil 16:194–198

Paulsen JM, Aragon GC, Ali MA, Brody FJ, Borum ML (2010) Pseudoachalasia secondary to metastatic breast carcinoma. Dig Dis Sci 55:1179–1181

Pouderoux P, Shi G, Tatum RP, Kahrilas PJ (1999) Esophageal solid bolus transit: studies using concurrent videofluoroscopy and manometry. Am J Gastroenterol 94:1458–1463

Price S, Castell DO (1978) Esophageal mythology. J Am Med Assoc 240:44–46

Reynolds JC, Parkman HP (1989) Achalasia. Gastroenterol Clin North Am 18:223–255

Richter JE (2001) Esophageal motility disorders. Lancet 358:823–828

Richter JE (2010) Achalasia—an update. J Neurogastroenterol Motil 16:232–242

Richter JE, Castell DO (1984) Diffuse esophageal spasm. Ann Intern Med 100:242–245

Richter JE, Wu WC, Johns DN et al (1987) Esophageal manometry in 95 healthy adult volunteers: variability of pressures with age and frequency of "abnormal" contractions. Dig Dis Sci 32:583–592

Rivkin L, Bremner CG, Bremner CH (1984) Pathophysiology of mid-esophageal and epiphrenic diverticula of the esophagus. S Afr Med J 66:127–129

Rubinow A, Burakoff R, Cohen AS, Harris LD (1983) Esophageal manometry in systemic amyloidosis. Am J Med 75:951–956

Schima W, Stacher P, Pokieser P et al (1992) Esophageal motor disorders: videofluoroscopic and manometric evaluation–prospective study in 88 symptomatic patients. Radiology 185:487–491

Schima W, Sterz F, Pokieser P (1993) Syncope after eating. N Engl J Med 328:1572

Schima W, Pokieser P, Forstinger C et al (1994) Videofluoroscopy of the pharynx and esophagus in chronic graft-versus-host disease. Abdom Imaging 19:191–194

Schima W, Pokieser P, Schober E (1995) Funktionsstörungen des Ösophagus: Radiologische Funktionsdiagnostik. Radiologe 35:693–702

Schima W, Schober E, Stacher G et al (1997) Association of midesophageal diverticula with esophageal motor disorders: videofluoroscopy and manometry. Acta Radiol 38:108–114

Schima W, Ryan JM, Harisinghani M et al (1998) Radiographic detection of achalasia: diagnostic accuracy of videofluoroscopy. Clin Radiol 53:372–375

Schmidt R, Weidemann H, Bücherl ES (1991) Ösophagusdivertikel. Klinik und Therapie. Zentralbl Chir 116:89–93

Schober E, Schima W, Stacher G, Pokieser P, Uranitsch K, Tscholakoff D (1993) Yield of a sustained barium "support level" upon video-fluoroscopy in the diagnosis of esophageal motor disorders (abstract). In: 8th European Congress of Radiology, scientific programme and abstracts, p 112

Schoeman MN, Holloway RH (1995) Integrity and characteristics of secondary esophageal peristalsis in patients with gastro-esophageal reflux disease. Gut 36:499–504

Schwickert HC, Schadmand-Fischer S, Klose P, Staritz M, Ueberschaer B, Thelen M (1993) Motilitätsstörungen des Ösophagus–Diagnostik mit dem Reisbreischluck. Fortschr Rontgenstr 159:511–517

Sears V, Castell J, Castell D (1989) "Abnormal" motility during upright and solid swallows in normal volunteers (abstract). Gastroenterology 96:A693

Soergel K, Zboralske FF, Amberg JR (1964) Presbyesophagus: esophageal motility in nonagenarians. J Clin Invest 43:1472–1479

Spechler SJ, Souza RF, Rosenberg SJ, Ruben RA, Goyal RK (1995) Heartburn in patients with achalasia. Gut 37:305–308

Sprung DJ, Gibb SP (1985) Dysplastic Barrett's esophagus in scleroderma. Am J Gastroenterol 80:518–522

Stacher G, Schmierer G, Landgraf M (1979) Tertiary esophageal contractions evoked by acoustic stimuli. Gastroenterology 77:49–54

Stacher G, Schima W, Bergmann H et al (1994) Sensitivity of radionuclide bolus transport and videofluoroscopic studies compared with manometry in the detection of achalasia. Am J Gastroenterol 89:1484–1488

Stein HJ, Eypasch EP, DeMeester TR, Smyrk TC, Attwood SEA (1990) Circadian esophageal motor function in patients with gastroesophageal reflux disease. Surgery 108:769–778

Stewart ET (1981) Radiographic evaluation of the esophagus and its motor disorders. Med Clin N Am 65:1173–1194

The Royal College of Radiologists (2007) Making the best use of a clinical radiology services: referral guidelines, 6th edn. Royal College of Radiologists, London, p 85

Thompson JK, Koehler RE, Richter JE (1994) Detection of gastroesophageal reflux: value of barium studies compared with 24-h pH monitoring. Am J Roentgenol 162:621–626

Timmer R, Breumelhof R, Nadorp JHSM, Smout AJPM (1994) Esophageal motility and gastro-esophageal reflux before and after healing of reflux esophagitis. A study using 24-h ambulatory pH and pressure monitoring. Gut 35:1519–1522

Tremble GE (1959) The clinical significance of a lump in the throat. Arch Otolaryngol 70:157–165

Tscholakoff D, Frühwald F, Kainberger F, Wicke K (2011) Orientierungshilfe radiologie: anleitung zum optimalen klinischen einsatz der radiologie, 4th edn. Verlagshaus der Ärzte, Vienna, p 79

Woodfield CA, Levine MS, Rubesin SE, Langlotz CP, Laufer I (2000) Diagnosis of primary versus secondary achalasia: reassessment of clinical and radiographic criteria. Am J Roentgenol 175:727–731

Wright RA, Penner DB (1981) Myxedema and upper esophageal dysmotility. Dig Dis Sci 26:376–377

Neuroimaging in Patients with Dysphagia

Kasim Abul-Kasim

Contents

Abstract

With increasing availability of computed tomography (CT) and magnetic resonance imaging (MRI), patients with dysphagia are nowadays often investigated with these modalities in order to localize a possible site of injury causing dysphagia. However, these radiological modalities often reveal some abnormalities especially in elderly patients and the correlation of these findings with clinical symptoms needs therefore a good knowledge about the anatomy of different structures involved in swallowing. Beside description of these different anatomical structures and the most common pathological conditions that cause dysphagia, this chapter is also enriched with illustrative radiological images, often at the axial plane that radiologists are familiar with.

1 Neuroanatomy of Swallowing

Different structures in the central nervous system (CNS) are responsible for coordination of the three sequential phases of swallowing, namely, the oral, the pharyngeal, and the esophageal phases. There are sensory and motor structures in the CNS that play an important role in swallowing. The three most important locations that are involved in processing information related to swallowing are the cerebral cortex, the medulla oblongata, and the cranial nerves and their nuclei located in different parts of the brain stem.

The sensory nerves and cranial nerve nuclei involved in swallowing are as follows (Figs. 1, 2):

K. Abul-Kasim (✉)
Faculty of Medicine, Diagnostic Centre
for Imaging and Functional Medicine,
Skåne University Hospital, Malmö, Sweden
e-mail: kasim.abul-kasim@med.lu.se

K. Abul-Kasim
Lund University, Malmö, Sweden

O. Ekberg (ed.), *Dysphagia*, Medical Radiology. Diagnostic Imaging, DOI: 10.1007/174_2011_489,
© Springer-Verlag Berlin Heidelberg 2012

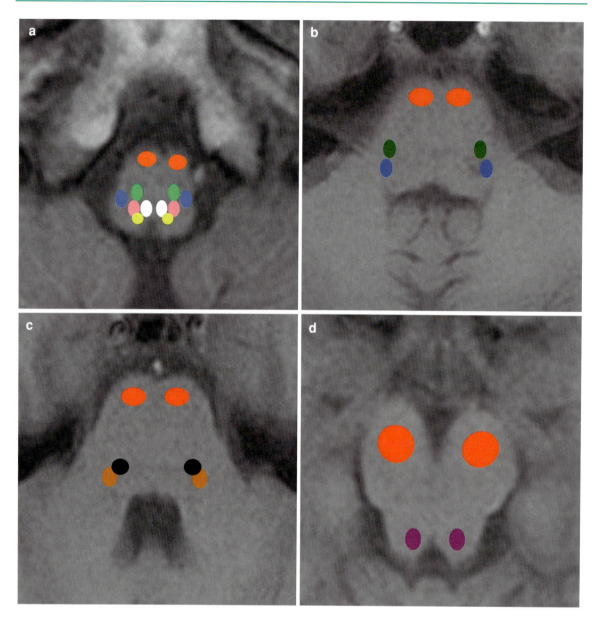

Fig. 1 Axial T1-weighted magnetic resonance imaging (MRI) showing the location of cranial nerve nuclei in the brain stem that are involved in the swallowing process. **a** At the level of the medulla oblongata: corticospinal tract (pyramidal tract) in *red*, ambiguous nucleus in *green*, spinal nucleus of trigeminal nerve in *blue*, dorsal nucleus of vagus nerve in *pink*, hypoglossal nerve nucleus in *white*, and solitary nucleus/solitary tract in *yellow*. **b** At the level of the lower pons: corticospinal tract (pyramidal tract) in *red*, facial nerve nucleus in *green*, and spinal nucleus of trigeminal nerve in *blue*. **c** At the level of the upper pons: corticospinal tract (pyramidal tract) in *red*, motor nucleus of trigeminal nerve in *black*, and sensory nucleus of trigeminal nerve in *brown*. **d** At the level of the mesencephalon: corticospinal tract (pyramidal tract) in *red* and mesencephalic nucleus of trigeminal nerve in *purple*

1. Trigeminal nerve (V): the main sensory nucleus, the mesencephalic nucleus, and the spinal nucleus extending in the spinal cord.
2. Facial nerve (VII).
3. Glossopharyngeal nerve (IX).
4. Vagus nerve (X).

The motor nerves and cranial nerve nuclei involved in swallowing are as follows (Figs. 1, 2, 3):
1. Motor nucleus of trigeminal nerve.
2. Motor nucleus of facial nerve.

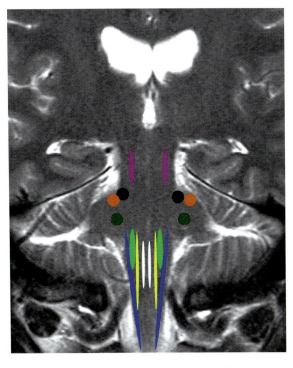

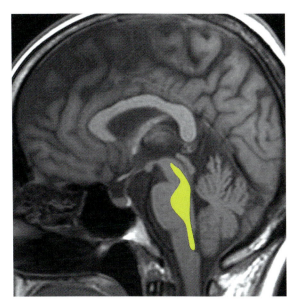

Fig. 3 Sagittal T1-weighted MRI showing the distribution of the reticular formation of the brain stem (marked in *yellow*)

Fig. 2 Coronal T2-weighted MRI showing the distribution of different cranial nerve nuclei in the brain stem: The *lower part* (medulla oblongata): spinal nucleus of trigeminal nerve in *blue*, ambiguous nucleus in *light green*, solitary nucleus/solitary tract in *yellow*, and hypoglossal nerve nucleus in *white*. The *middle part* (pons): facial nerve nucleus in *dark green*, motor nucleus of trigeminal nerve in *black*, and sensory nucleus of trigeminal nerve in *brown*. The *upper part* (mesencephalon): mesencephalic nucleus of trigeminal nerve in *purple*

3. Ambiguous nucleus of the vagus and glossopharyngeal nerves.
4. Dorsal motor nucleus of the vagus nerve.
5. Hypoglossal nerve nucleus (XII).
6. Solitary nucleus and solitary tract with contribution from glossopharyngeal, vagus, and hypoglossal nerves.
7. Reticular formation representing an interconnecting pathway between the motor nuclei of the trigeminal, facial, and hypoglossal nerves and the ambiguous nucleus.

The supratentorial structures involved in swallowing are as follows (Daniels and Foundas 1997; Miller 1999; Fig. 4):

1. Premotor cortex (Brodmann's area 6) located anterior to the primary motor cortex.
2. The primary motor cortical representation of swallowing is located at the level of the frontoparietal operculum at the lower part of the precentral gyrus (M1, Brodmann's area 4).
3. The primary somatosensory cortical representation of swallowing is located at the level of the frontoparietal operculum at the lower part of the postcentral gyrus (S1, Brodmann's areas 3, 2, and 1).
4. Anterior part of the insular cortex.

Generally, esophageal cortical representation is located cranial to the pharyngeal cortical representation; the latter is located cranial to the oral cortical representation (Hamdy et al. 1996). Swallowing centers are usually present bilaterally but one center, independent of the language-dominant hemisphere, is usually larger than the other one (Barrit and Smithard 2009). The fibers connecting the supratentorial motor areas involved in swallowing to the brain stem constitute the corticobulbar tracts. The cerebellum is usually involved in modulating the movements required to accomplish the swallowing.

2 Neurological Disorders Causing Dysphagia

Many neurological disorders can cause dysphagia. Neurological causes of dysphagia can be classified simply into degenerative and nondegenerative disorders (Daniels 2006). Stroke is the most common cause

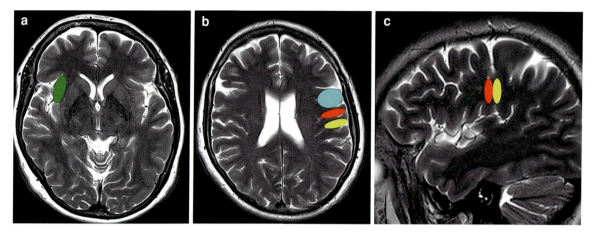

Fig. 4 a, b Axial T2-weighted images and **c** sagittal T2-weighted image showing the anterior part of the insular cortex (marked in *green* in **a**), primary sensory cortical representation (marked in *yellow* in **b** and **c**), primary motor cortical representation (marked in *red* in **b** and **c**), and premotor cortex (marked in *blue* in **b**) at the level of the frontoparietal operculum. The cortical representation is usually present on both sides

of the nondegenerative type of dysphagia, followed by trauma. Among other causes are multiple sclerosis (MS), cerebral palsy, brain tumors, and iatrogenic lesions (following cervical spine surgery, carotid artery surgery, and head and neck surgery). Degenerative disorders include different types of dementia, movement disorders, e.g., Parkinson's disease, Huntington's disease, Wilson's disease, progressive supranuclear palsy, and pontocerebellar atrophy. Amyotrophic lateral sclerosis (ALS) is a progressive and eventually fatal disorder affecting both the upper and the lower motor neurons involving predominantly the corticobulbar or corticospinal tracts. Limb weakness and spasticity is the dominating feature of the disease, whereas dysphagia and dysarthria are among the most common features of the bulbar palsy associated with ALS. Other causes of dysphagia include myasthenia gravis and different types of myopathy, e.g., dermatomyositis and myotonic dystrophy.

The workup of patients with dysphagia is based on a thorough medical history and clinical examination. Videofluoroscopy is the method of choice to study the dynamics of swallowing. Fiber endoscopic evaluation of swallowing may also be used.

The course and the prognosis of dysphagia differ widely depending on the cause of dysphagia. Dysphagia in stroke, traumatic brain injury, and following neck surgery has an acute presentation but in many patients is reversible, with spontaneous recovery or successive improvement. However, radiological abnormalities of swallowing may still be evident even in patients receiving an oral diet months after the stroke (Logemann et al. 1999). Dysphagia in other neurological disorders such as MS and ALS is progressive. In ALS the progression of dysphagia is usually rapid, whereas dysphagia among patients with MS is slowly progressive.

3 Neuroimaging in Dysphagia

Neuroimaging is usually included in the workup of patients with dysphagia following stroke and trauma and is usually performed before videofluoroscopy. Neuroimaging is also routine in patients with MS, brain tumors, and Wilson's disease suffering from dysphagia. Although the diagnosis of conditions such as dementia and Parkinson's disease is not primarily radiological, in the last 20 years the different radiological modalities have been increasingly used during the course of events of these diseases as well. Computed tomography (CT) is the method of choice in the workup of acute supratentorial stroke and trauma, whereas magnetic resonance imaging (MRI) is preferred in infratentorial stroke, MS, and degenerative disorders. CT is cheaper, less time-consuming (both in performing and in evaluating the examination), and more widely available than MRI. The disadvantages of CT are the radiation exposure and the lower sensitivity in detecting lesions in the brain stem, where

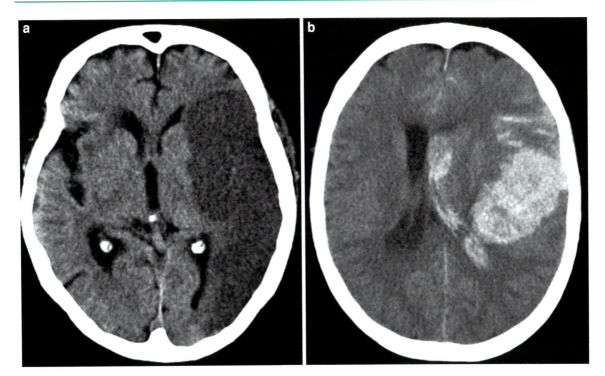

Fig. 5 Axial computed tomography images of two different patients. **a** A large cerebral infarct (*dark area*) involving the whole left middle cerebral artery territory. The patient complained of aphasia, hemianopia, right-sided hemiplegia, and sensory loss. **b** A large cerebral hemorrhage in the left frontal and parietal lobes with blood in the subarachnoid space and the left lateral ventricle. The patient complained of aphasia and sensory and motor deficit. The hemorrhage affects the cortical representation of the face and the tongue, resulting in swallowing difficulties primarily due to impairment of the oral phase of swallowing. Both patients needed long-standing tube feeding

different cranial nerve nuclei involved in the swallowing are located. MRI provides more detailed anatomical and morphological information than CT especially in pathological conditions of the skull base and posterior cranial fossa, including the brain stem. In the last decade new MRI modalities have been introduced enabling functional evaluation of different CNS structures involved in swallowing using functional MRI. Structural evaluation of different tracts involved in the swallowing connecting the motor cortex with swallowing centers of the brain stem is now possible by using diffusion tensor imaging and tractography.

4 Dysphagia Following Stroke

Stroke affects 2,000 people per million worldwide each year (Thorvaldsen et al. 1995); 80–85% of strokes are ischemic and 15–20% are hemorrhagic. Up to 35–50% of patients with stroke develop dysphagia (Paciaroni et al. 2004; Gordon et al. 1987). In a systematic review of published literature concerning dysphagia after stroke, the incidence of stroke was about 50% using clinical testing and about 75% using instrumental testing. Dysphagia tends to be less severe compared with brain stem stroke (Martino et al. 2005). Among patients with middle cerebral artery ischemic stroke, the size of the infarct plays a more important role than the location of the ischemic injury (Paciaroni et al. 2004; Fig. 5). Cortical and subcortical supratentorial lacunar infarcts as well as brain stem infarcts may result in dysphagia (Fig. 6). Cerebral infarctions affect all three phases of swallowing with subsequently increased risk of aspiration of liquid or solid food and development of pneumonia, which is one of the life-threatening complications of stroke (Miller 1999). Cerebral infarctions may be classified as either large-vessel infarcts or small-vessel infarcts. Patients with large-vessel infarcts affecting the middle cerebral artery territory present with hemiplegia, sensory loss, aphasia, neglect, and

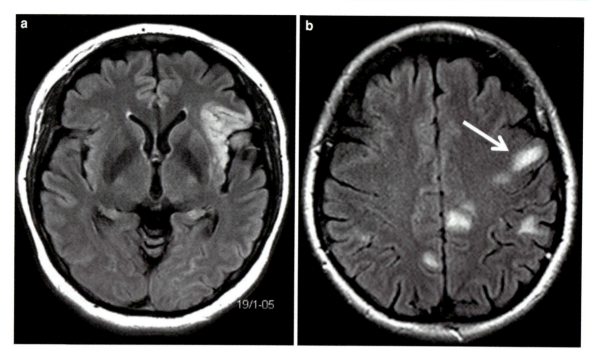

Fig. 6 Axial T2 fluid-attenuated inversion recovery (FLAIR) MRI of two different patients. **a** A small infarct affecting the frontal lobe operculum responsible for speech and the anterior part of the insular cortex. The patient had complained of expressive aphasia and swallowing difficulties. **b** Multiple lacunar cortical and subcortical infarcts. The infarct marked with an *arrow* affects the precentral gyrus

visual disturbance (hemianopia). Patients with bilateral infarcts involving the frontoparietal operculum develop severe dysphagia (Foix–Chavany–Marie syndrome). The clinical presentation of large-vessel infarcts affecting the brain stem differs depending on the structures affected, often with evidence of involvement of different cranial nerves, dysarthria, dysphagia, syncope, and ataxia as well as motor and sensory deficit (Fig. 7). Large-vessel infarcts affecting the middle cerebral artery territory induce dysphagia by affecting the cortical structures responsible for the processing of the swallowing, whereas large-vessel infarcts affecting the vertebrobasilar circulation result in infarcts affecting different cranial nerve nuclei and fibers as well as the reticular formation and solitary tract. There are several vascular syndromes affecting different parts of the brain stem and medulla oblongata that can potentially result in dysphagia. One specific syndrome is Wallenberg's syndrome (posterolateral medullary syndrome). Patients with this syndrome present with Horner's syndrome (ptosis, mitosis, and anhydrosis of the ipsilateral side of the face), sensory loss of temperature, and pain in the ipsilateral side of the face and in the contralateral side

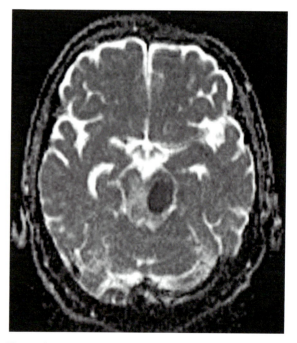

Fig. 7 Apparent diffusion coefficient of magnetic resonance diffusion showing a large infarct of the left side of the upper pons and mesencephalon (*dark area* of restricted diffusion indicating acute infarction). Among other neurological deficits, the patient complained of dysphagia due to affection of cranial nerve nuclei, primarily those of the trigeminal nerve

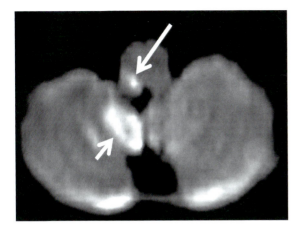

Fig. 8 MRI diffusion showing a small infarct (*bright lesion* marked with a *long arrow*) in the right posterolateral part of the medulla oblongata. The patient presented with symptoms and signs consistent with Wallenberg's syndrome. Dysphagia was primarily caused by involvement of the solitary tract. The image shows also a larger infarct in the right adjacent part of the cerebellum (marked with a *short arrow*)

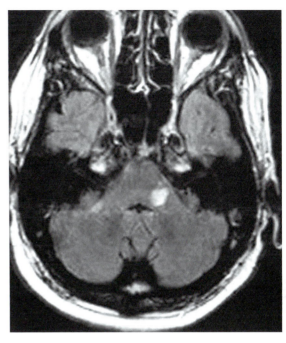

Fig. 10 Axial T2 FLAIR MRI showing a small bright lesion in the lateral dorsal pons. Dysphagia in this case was due to involvement of motor and sensory nuclei of the trigeminal nerve

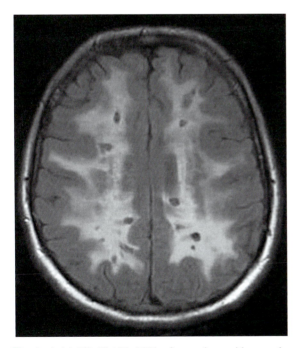

Fig. 9 Axial T2 FLAIR MRI of a patient with vascular dementia with widespread signal abnormalities in the white matter (confluent *bright area*) and multiple small infarcts (*black lesions*). The patient had hypertension, cognitive impairment, and dysphagia

In the acute phase of the stroke, CT is the method of choice to detect early signs of large-vessel infarcts and cerebral hemorrhage. When the CT findings are normal on admission of the patient and when the patient complains of dysphagia and/or the presence of other neurological deficits, MRI is usually performed to visualize small supratentorial cortical and subcortical infarcts as well as brain stem infarcts that have failed to be detected by CT. Special attention should be paid to small infarcts in the medulla oblongata, brain stem, anterior insula, lateral portion of the precentral gyrus, posterior portion of the inferior frontal gyrus, basal ganglia, and internal capsule. MRI enables detection of small infarcts and helps to determine their age by demonstrating restricted diffusion on diffusion-weighted images in the acute phase of ischemia and showing contrast enhancement in the subacute stage. Evidence of chronic ischemic changes in the white matter of the brain stem or the supratentorial white matter as in cases of vascular dementia may explain the occurrence of dysphagia among these patients (Fig. 9).

of the extremities. Dysphagia is always present due to involvement of the solitary tract (vagus and glossopharyngeal nerve nuclei) (Fig. 8).

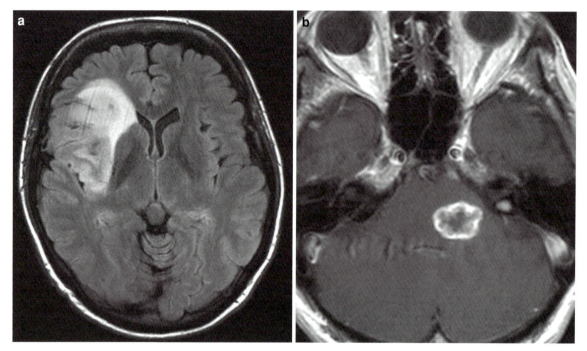

Fig. 11 Axial T2 FLAIR and postcontrast T1-weighted MRI, respectively. **a** A large glial tumor (histopathologically proven to be grade II astrocytoma) in the right frontal lobe in a patient with epilepsy, and slowly progressive speech and swallowing difficulties. **b** Contrast-enhanced tumor in the left side of the pons in a patient with right-sided sensory loss and dysphagia due to involvement of the lateral spinothalamic tract and trigeminal and facial nerve nuclei

5 Other Neurological Disorders Causing Dysphagia

In trauma, CT is the method of choice as it can detect brain contusions, hemorrhages, and brain swelling. However, small cortical and subcortical hemorrhages, brain stem hemorrhages, and nonhemorrhagic lesions that usually occur in patients with deep axonal injury are not commonly to detected by CT. These patients usually have dysphagia, and the establishment of this diagnosis by performing MRI is essential from a therapeutic and prognostic point of view.

MS is believed to be an autoimmune disease resulting in inflammation of the myelin sheaths around the axons of the brain and spinal cord with subsequent demyelination, damage, and scarring of the affected brain tissue. MS often affects young adults, is more common in women than in men, and has a prevalence ranging between 2 and 150 per 100,000 individuals (Rosati 2001). The clinical presentation of MS differs depending on the site of the MS lesions. Optic neuritis is a common clinical

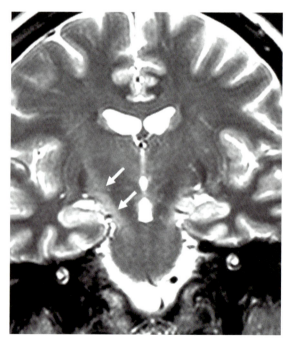

Fig. 12 Coronal T2-weighted MRI of a patient with amyotrophic lateral sclerosis showing high signal intensity along the corticospinal tract (*arrows*)

presentation and in many patients is the presenting feature. MS has the predilection to affect the brain stem, the cerebellar peduncles, the corpus callosum, and the periventricular white matter (Fig. 10). However, at least one subcortical lesion should be present to establish the diagnosis according to McDonald's four radiological criteria for the diagnosis of MS. Lesions affecting the brain stem and the subcortical white matter may produce dysphagia in patients with MS. In advanced and late-stage MS, dysphagia and the requirement of tube feeding are not uncommon. In patients with MS, MRI is the method of choice to establish the diagnosis, help the clinicoradiological correlation, and depict lesions with ongoing activity by showing restricted diffusion and/or contrast enhancement. Patients with MS might exhibit plenty of lesions in their white matter, and MRI helps to detect lesions that are responsible for the symptoms, including dysphagia.

In patients with brain tumors, both CT and MRI are suitable methods in the workup of these diseases, although MRI is more sensitive to show the accurate extent of the tumor (Fig. 11), the perifocal edema, or to detect subtle contrast enhancement that might affect regions responsible for swallowing not depicted by CT.

MRI is also the method of choice in the workup of diseases such as ALS (showing increased signal along the corticospinal tract; Fig. 12), Wilson's disease (showing bilateral symmetrical low T1 signal and high T2 signal in basal ganglia, especially putamen), and pontocerebellar atrophy.

References

Barritt AW, Smithard DG (2009) Role of cerebral cortex plasticity in the recovery of swallowing function following dysphagic stroke. Dysphagia 24:83–90

Daniels SK (2006) Neurological disorders affecting oral, pharyngeal swallowing. Part 1 oral cavity, pharynx and esophagus. GI Motil Online. doi: 10.1038/gimo34

Daniels SK, Foundas AL (1997) The role of the insular cortex in dysphagia. Dysphagia 12:146–156

Gordon C, Hewer RL, Wade DT (1987) Dysphagia in acute stroke. Br Med J 295:411–414

Hamdy S, Aziz Q, Rothwell JC, Singh KD, Barlow J, Hughes DG, Tallis RC, Thompson DG (1996) The cortical topography of human swallowing musculature in health and disease. Nat Med 2:1217–1224

Logemann JA, Veis S, Rademaker AW, Huang CW (1999) Early recovery of swallowing post-CVA. Paper presented at the eighth annual meeting of the Dysphagia Research Society, Burlington, VT

Martino R, Foley N, Bhogal S, Diamant N, Speechley M, Teasell R (2005) Dysphagia after stroke: incidence, diagnosis, and pulmonary complications. Stroke 36:2756–2763

Miller AJ (1999) The neuroscientific principles of swallowing and dysphagia. Singular, San Diego

Paciaroni M, Mazzotta G, Corea F, Caso V, Venti M, Milia P, Silvestrelli G, Palmerini F, Parnetti L, Gallai V (2004) Dysphagia following stroke. Eur Neurol 51: 162–167

Rosati G (2001) The prevalence of multiple sclerosis in the world: an update. Neurol Sci 22:117–139

Thorvaldsen P, Asplund K, Kuulasmaa K, Rajakangas AM, Schroll M (1995) Stroke incidence, case fatality, and mortality in the WHO MONICA project. World Health Organization monitoring trends and determinants in cardiovascular disease. Stroke 26:361–367

Cross-Sectional Imaging of the Oesophagus Using CT and PET/Techniques

Ahmed Ba-Ssalamah, Barbara J. Fueger, and Wolfgang Schima

Contents

A. Ba-Ssalamah (✉) · B. J. Fueger
Department of Radiology,
Medical University of Vienna, Vienna, Austria
e-mail: ahmed.ba-ssalamah@meduniwien.ac.at

W. Schima
Department of Radiology, KH Göttlicher Heiland, KH der
Barmherzigen Schwestern Wien,
and Sankt Josef-Krankenhaus, Vienna, Austria

Abstract

Multidetector computed tomograpy (MDCT) is the most frequent imaging modality in the diagnostic work-up of oncologic diseases of the abdomen. Although CT has been used for preoperative evaluation of oesophageal cancer, the major role of CT has been the depiction of lymph nodes, distant metastases, or both, rather than the evaluation of the local status of oesophageal cancer. The sensitivity of conventional or helical CT protocols for the localization of oesophageal cancer, especially early stage cancer, is not satisfactory. This may be attributed to the fact that conventional or helical CT cannot offer optimal conspicuity of oesophageal cancers against the normal oesophageal wall, or because the oesophagus is too long to be imaged entirely using thin slices during a single breath-hold on conventional or helical CT scans, especially in the absence of lumen distension, since inadequately distended hollow viscera on CT may hide small lesions and may even mimic pseudolesions. Thus, optimal distension of the oesophagus and stomach is important to overcome this limitation. The combination of the MDCT technique with thin slice sections and the possibility to obtain high-quality, isotropic, multi-planar reconstructions and the water filling, or the application of gas-producing effervescent granules to distend the stomach and the oesophagus are important factors that may increase the efficacy of CT for local staging of oesophageal cancer. Using this technique is not only useful for a complete preoperative staging of oesophageal malignancies according to TNM classification but

O. Ekberg (ed.), *Dysphagia*, Medical Radiology. Diagnostic Imaging, DOI: 10.1007/174_2012_656,
© Springer-Verlag Berlin Heidelberg 2012

also clinically relevant for evaluation of a broad spectrum of inflammatory and traumatic diseases. The introduction of FDG PET in combination with MDCT resulted in further optimizing the diagnostic work-up of oesophageal cancer and other malignant diseases rendering this technique to be the modality of choice depending on its availability. In this book chapter we review the value of the hydro-MDCT technique and hydro-FDG-PET-CT technique in the diagnostic work-up of oesophageal diseases.

resulted in further optimising the diagnostic work-up of oesophageal cancer (Flamen et al. 2000; Kobori et al. 1999). Therefore, it can be expected that PET/hydro-MDCT will further increase the sensitivity and accuracy in patients with oesophageal cancer for the initial diagnosis, stratifying patients in the proper therapeutic options, monitoring during neoadjuvant chemotherapy and for search of possible recurrence after treatment (Sharma et al. 2011; Jeganathan et al. 2011; Bradley et al. 2012; Krause et al. 2009). Therefore, FDG-PET/Hydro-MDCT can be considered as the primary modality of choice if available.

1   Introduction

Cross-sectional imaging of the oesophagus is challenging due to its pathoanatomical morphology. The oesophagus is a long tube, and poorly distensible, with a close relationship to many vital organs. These factors make the detection and staging of oesophageal cancer difficult using the cross-sectional modalities. In addition, the lack of a serosal layer of the oesophagus facilitates the spread of the tumour into surrounding organs (Ludeman and Shepherd 2005). Furthermore, the first symptom of oesophageal cancer is often dysphagia, which is a late manifestation, and, at that point, a direct invasion of some vital organs is almost always present, which renders these patients inoperable (Smithers et al. 2010).

Using the multi-detector computer tomography (MDCT) technology covering a large anatomic volume with thin collimation, imaging of the entire oesophagus in a single breath hold becomes possible with high quality multiplanar reformation and three-dimensional visualisation (Panebianco et al. 2006; Ba-Ssalamah et al. 2009). Adequate distension of the oesophagus and stomach, using water and effervescent granulate as a negative contrast agent, is a prerequisite for assessing the oesophageal wall and gastrooesophageal junction (Ba-Ssalamah et al. 2009, 2003). Proper contrast material injection techniques (Mani et al. 2001) enhance further the differentiation of pathologic tissue from normal mucosa. Compared to endosonography, multi-detector CT is able to demonstrate not only the immediate vicinity of the oesophagus but also the infiltration of the adjacent organs and the involvement of lymph node regions or distant metastases (Choi et al. 2010). The introduction of FDG-PET in combination with MDCT

2   CT and PET/CT Technique

CT examinations of oesophagus should be performed on at least a 16-detector row CT with a 0.5 s tube rotation. To acquire a near-isotropic data set, primary sub millimetre (0.75–0.63 mm) thin collimation raw data should be performed (Ba-Ssalamah et al. 2009). For diagnostic viewing, reconstructions of 3–4 mm thick axial sections directly from the scanning raw data using the multiplanar reformation function of the scanner console can be obtained. In addition, routinely coronal and sagittal reformation (with 3−5 mm slice thickness) along the entire oesophagus and the stomach are performed (Panebianco et al. 2006; Ba-Ssalamah et al. 2003). Contrast material injection for the oesophagus and stomach is timed in a manner that ensures capture of the arterial phase for imaging of the oesophageal and gastric mucosa and evaluation of possible associated hypervascular focal liver lesions (Mani et al. 2001; Umeoka et al. 2010; Prokop 2005). An additional portal venous phase examination of the whole abdomen is performed for complete staging purposes as well. In this protocol, the scanning range includes the cervical region, chest, and the whole abdomen.

For preparation either for hydro-MDCT as well as for fused FDG-PET/hydro-MDCT, patients are instructed to fast for at least 4−6 h prior to the examination (Ba-Ssalamah et al. 2003). Additionally, in case of combined FDG-PET/hydro-MDCT blood glucose levels are measured before the injection of the FDG tracer (Skehan et al. 2000; Haley et al. 2009). The scanning starts after a resting period of at least 45 min post injection of the tracer (Kobori et al. 1999; Weber et al. 2001). During this time period, patients are encouraged to drink 1.0–1.5 l of tap water in order to distend the stomach and oesophagus. Hydro-MDCT scanning starts immediately after the ingestion of the last portion of tap water (250 ml) and effervescent gas producing granules. Adequate distension of the oesophagus and stomach, using water and effervescent granulate as a negative contrast agent, is a prerequisite for assessing the wall of these organs (Ba-Ssalamah et al. 2009; Ulla et al. 2010; Ba-Ssalamah et al. 2011).

In case of simultaneous FDG-PET/hydro-MDCT examinations, the patient remains on the examination table for both scans. Emission PET-scans last between 3 and 5 min per bed position depending on the body weight (Halpern et al. 2004; Nagaki et al. 2011; Talanow and Shrikanthan 2010). Scans are corrected for decay, scatter and randoms. There are various reconstruction algorithms for PET images. The most popular algorithm, ordered subset expected maximisation (OSEM), use CT-derived attenuation correction (Boellaard et al. 2001; Kontaxakis et al. 2002) Axial and coronal reformatted scans of iodine contrast-enhanced hydro-MDCT are performed to match the PET section thickness. The examination of hydro-MDCT and fused FDG-PET is performed in the supine position from the top of the head to the mid-thigh.

The use of FDG-PET yields physiologic information that provides a means for diagnosing cancer based on altered tissue metabolism enabling co-registration of both anatomic and functional information obtained by Hydro-MDCT (Bar-Shalom et al. 2005; Rampin et al. 2005). FDG-PET takes advantage of the principle that biochemical changes often precede or are more specific than the structural changes associated with any given disease process (Luketich et al. 1997; Hsu et al. 2009). Therefore, fused FDG-PET/MDCT offers the potential to show early oesophageal cancer or small lymph node metastases before any structural abnormality is detectable, or to exclude the presence of tumour in an anatomically altered structure. The tumour uptake of FDG, measured as the maximal standardised uptake value (SUVmax) in FDG-PET, even provides a quantitative estimate of tumour aggressiveness (Cerfolio and Bryant 2006).

Recent studies demonstrate that FDG-PET can be used not only for pretreatment staging, but also for the assessment of treatment response, detection of recurrence, and prediction of survival in patients with adenocarcinoma of the oesophagus (Hsu et al. 2009; Cerfolio and Bryant 2006). FDG-PET/CT more accurately shows the extent of disease than do other imaging methods, and this frequently leads to a radical change in patient management.

3   Oesophageal Cancer

Oesophageal cancer is one of deadliest cancers worldwide and is the sixth leading cause of death from malignancies (Edwards et al. 2002). Recent advances in the diagnosis, staging and treatment of this neoplastic condition have led to small but significant improvements in survival. The lifetime risk of developing this cancer is 0.8 % for men and 0.3 % for women. The risk increases with age, the mean age at diagnosis is 67 years (Edwards et al. 2002; Daly et al. 2000). More than 90 % of oesophageal cancers are either squamous cell carcinomas or adenocarcinomas (Edwards et al. 2002). Rarely, carcinomas of other histologic types, including melanomas, gastrointestinal stroma tumours, carcinoids and lymphomas, may develop in the oesophagus as well (Barr 2011). Smoking is associated with an increased risk of both squamous cell carcinoma and adenocarcinoma of the oesophagus (Wu et al. 2001; Brown et al. 2001). Individuals with recurrent symptoms of reflux have an eightfold increase in risk for oesophageal adenocarcinoma (Lagergren et al. 1999). Barrett's oesophagus develops in approximately 5–8 % of patients with gastrooesophageal reflux disease (Csikos et al. 1985). The relatively low incidence of oesophageal cancer, the absence of early symptoms, and the rarity of a hereditary cause of the disease (Romero et al. 2002) make prevention, surveillance, and evaluation-based screening untenable except in certain high-risk areas (Lagergren et al. 2000) of the world. Patients who are found to have Barrett's oesophagus, however, may be candidates for regular endoscopic surveillance (Yang et al. 2002).

Over the past 25 years, the nature of oesophageal cancer has changed from primarily a squamous cell neoplasm involving the mid-thoracic oesophagus in 50 % of patients, to adenocarcinoma of the gastro oesophageal junction in nearly two thirds of cases (Daly et al. 2000; Siewert et al. 2001; Parfitt et al. 2006). Once cancer develops, it may spread rapidly. Only 2 % of T1 cancers, but 38–60 % of T2 cancers are

Fig. 1 Hydro-MDCT of the oesophagus in coronal (**a**) and sagittal (**b**) reformations to follow the course of the oesophagus, demonstrating the normal wall thickening of the oesophagus (≤3mm) and homogeneous enhancement (*arrows*). *Note* On the sagittal reformation, the physiologic angulation caused by the aortic arch with pseudothickening (partial volume) of the oesophageal wall (*arrowhead*)

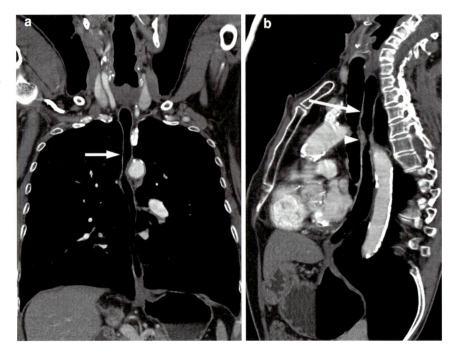

associated with extension of the disease to lymph nodes (Siewert et al. 2001; Stein et al. 2005). Therefore an accurate local staging in terms of (T staging) has a great impact on the therapeutic management (Ba-Ssalamah et al. 2011). At the time of the diagnosis of oesophageal cancer, more than 50 % of patients have either locally unresectable tumours or radiographically detectable metastases (Pennathur and Luketich 2008). Thus, hydro-MDCT and even better combined PET/hydro-MDCT (if available) helps to obtain an accurate staging and consequently to choose the most appropriate treatment option for those patients in a single examination (Wolf et al. 2011).

4 CT, PET/CT Imaging of the Oesophagus

4.1 Tumour Detection and Classification

From a morphological point-of-view, oesophageal carcinoma may manifest as a focal area of mural thickening with or without ulceration, as a flat or polypoid lesion, or as generalised mural thickening.

Since the thickness of individual layers of the normal oesophageal wall cannot be determined using CT with certainty because of the variable distensibility of

its lumen, we use 3 mm as the upper limit of normal (Fig. 1); any increase beyond this is considered abnormal. Therefore, the following criteria, taken from the literature (Umeoka et al. 2010; Halvorsen and Thompson 1984; Moss et al. 1981; Lea et al. 1984; Picus et al. 1983; Quint et al. 1985; Thompson and Halvorsen 1994) and recently modified by Ba-Ssalamah et al. (Ba-Ssalamah et al. 2011), are used to determine the CT-T stage, according to the TNM classification (pT) adapted by the AJCC 7th edition (Greene et al. 2002; Sobin and Wittekind 2002; Rice et al. 2010).

T1: Focal or circumferential wall thickening of >3 and ≤10 mm and/or intense enhancement of the oesophageal wall, without stenosis. The outer borders of the tumour are smooth (Fig. 2).

T2: Focal, polypoid, or diffuse circumferential thickening of the oesophageal wall >10 and ≤15 mm, with the possible presence of a mild stenosis. The outer borders of the tumour are either smooth or show stranding for less than one-third of the tumour extension (Fig. 3).

T3: Tumour appears symmetric or asymmetric, markedly diffuse or circumferential wall thickening of ≥15 mm, with mild to severe stenosis, and marked stranding for over one-third of the tumour extension, or extensive blurring of the outer border (Fig. 4).

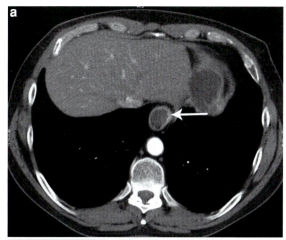

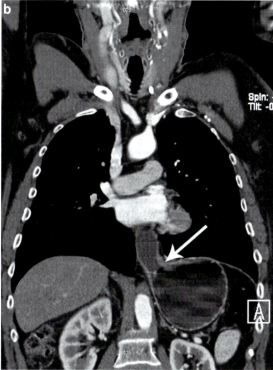

Fig. 2 Hydro-MDCT of the oesophagus in axial (**a**) and coronal (**b**) reformations shows a small focal polypoid lesion in the distal third of the oesophagus, with homogeneous enhancement in terms of the T1 tumour (*arrows*). The outer borders are smooth

T4: Tumour shows invasion into one of the adjacent structures, such as the pericardium, the diaphragm, the pleura (T4a), the tracheobronchial tree, or the aorta and spine (T4b), using the criteria described in the literature (Thompson and Halvorsen 1994) (Fig. 5).

These structures may be invaded by contiguous tumour spread. However, it is often difficult to distinguish infiltration into these adjacent organs (T4) from a broad contact without infiltration. Evaluation for direct invasion by oesophageal cancer into adjacent vital structures by CT is based on two criteria: mass effect and loss of fat planes. When the trachea or bronchial wall is indented or displaced away from the spine by a tumour mass, then mass effect is present and invasion is presumed (Lagergren et al. 2000). Coronal or sagittal reformatted images are best suited for this purpose and seem to be helpful. The cardia is directly involved by carcinoma of the distal oesophagus in about 60 % of patients according to the Siewert classification (AEG I-III) (Fig 6) (Siewert 2007). The depiction of the anatomic location of the tumour and assessment of the degree of cardia involvement is crucial for the surgical strategy. This is a key factor to define gastric fundus involvement, since the stomach is the organ usually used as the first choice for reconstruction after esophagectomy.

In case of using fused FDG-PET/hydro-MDCT, tracer uptake is markedly helpful in the detection of even a small primary tumour and may be better in the estimation of its local staging and response to therapy (Fig 7).

The sensitivity of FDG-PET for detecting primary oesophageal tumours has been reported to be 91–95 % in prospective studies (Lowe et al. 2005; Meyers et al. 2007) reported that 75 patients with oesophageal cancer PET correctly assessed T stage in 43 %, understaged in 29 % and overstaged in 29 %. Since PET scanners have a limited spatial resolution of about 5–8 mm, lesions smaller than 1 cm might not be detected, however, the combination of PET/CT and hydro technique may improve its efficiency.

N Staging. Lymphatic spread is found in 74–88 % of patients with oesophageal carcinoma because of the abundant lymphatic vessels in the oesophagus (Siewert 2007). The frequency of lymphatic metastases is related to the T local staging including the size and depth of penetration of the tumour (Stein et al. 2005). The extensive mediastinal lymphatic drainage of the oesophagus, which communicates with abdominal and cervical collateral vessels, is responsible for the findings of mediastinal, supraclavicular, celiac lymph node metastases in at least 75 % of patients (Thompson et al. 1983). According to the American Joint Committee on Cancer (Suga et al.

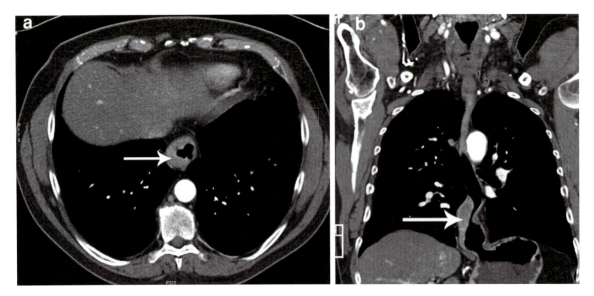

Fig. 3 Hydro-MDCT of the oesophagus in axial (**a**) and coronal (**b**) reformations shows a circumferential wall thickening 10 mm in depth in the middle third of the oesophagus, with homogeneous enhancement and smooth outer borders in terms of the T2 tumour (*arrows*)

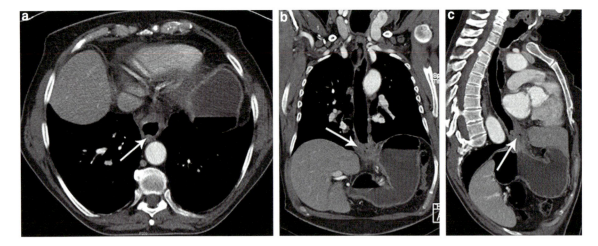

Fig. 4 Hydro-MDCT of the oesophagus in axial (**a**), coronal (**b**), and sagittal (**c**) reformations shows a markedly diffuse oesophageal wall thickening 18 mm in depth in the distal third of the oesophagus, with inhomogeneous enhancement and blurred outer borders in terms of the T3 tumour (*arrows*)

2005), N staging depends on the presence of positive locoregional or perioesophageal lymph nodes (affected lymph nodes) (Fig. 8). The N staging is explained according to the 7th edition (AJCC Cancer Staging Manual, 7th edition) as following:

- N0 no regional lymph node metastasis.
- N1 1–2 positive regional lymph nodes.
- N2 3–6 positive regional lymph nodes.
- N3 ≥ 7 positive regional lymph nodes.

Lymph node assessment for metastatic spread remains a challenge, even with PET/MDCT. However, improved evaluation appears possible if both morphology including size and shape, contrast enhancement pattern as well as tracer uptake of lymph nodes are used (Blom et al. 2011; Okada et al. 2009). On CT perioesophageal lymph nodes are considered positive if they are ≥6 mm in diameter, rounded in shape, and show marked or inhomogenous contrast

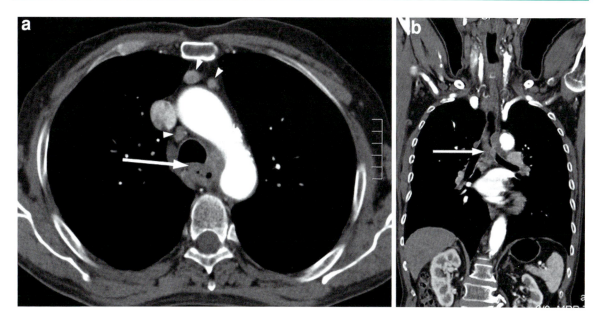

Fig. 5 Hydro-MDCT of the oesophagus in axial (**a**), and coronal (**b**), reformations shows a huge mass with inhomogeneous enhancement in the mediastinum arising from the oesophageal wall, with infiltration of the trachea (**a**, *arrow*), in terms of the T4 tumour, note the enlarged pathologic lymph node as stage N2 (**a**, *arrowheads*)

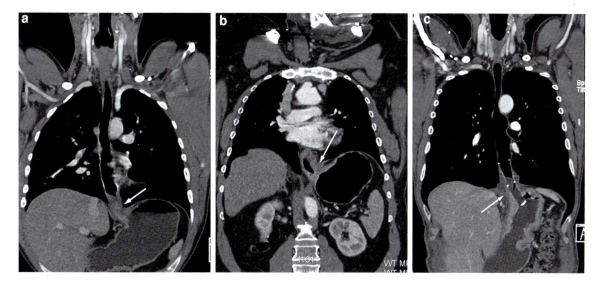

Fig. 6 Hydro-MDCT of the oesophagus in coronal reformations showing examples of large cancer in the lower third of the oesophagus at the gastroesophageal junction, with AEG I (**a**), AEG II (**b**), and AEG III (**c**). The differentiation between distal oesophageal cancer and gastric cancer located in the cardia is difficult in some cases

enhancement (Ba-Ssalamah et al. 2003). In case of FDG-PET there is no established SUV cutoff for lymph node metastases, although single institutions have their own cutoffs (Yu et al. 2011; Kato et al. 2009). However, in general, lymph nodes are considered involved if they show an FDG uptake that is higher than the background. A meta-analysis of 12 studies ($n = 490$) examined the diagnostic accuracy of FDG-PET in preoperative staging of oesophageal cancer and reported sensitivity and specificity for detecting locoregional lymph node involvement of 51 and 84 %, respectively (van Westreenen et al. 2004).

Fig. 7 FDG-PET/CT of a
patient with oesophageal
cancer in axial and coronal
reformations. The area of the
untreated tumour shows
intense FDG uptake (**a**, **b**,
arrows). After treatment no
FDG uptake is appreciated
(**c**, **d**, *arrows*).
Histopathological work-up
after resection confirmed
no viable tumour tissue

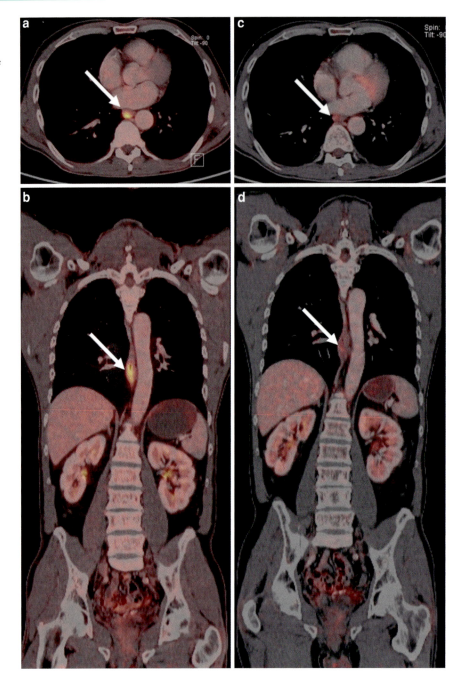

M Staging. Hematogenous metastases from oesoph-ageal carcinoma most commonly involve the liver because the oesophagus is drained by the portal vein (Fig. 8). Other less common sites of hematogenous spread include the lungs, adrenal glands, kidneys, bones, and brain. Lymph node involvement outside a perio-esophageal location is considered M1 disease (Nomura et al. 2012). Advanced distal cancers can develop peritoneal metastases (Fig. 9).

FDG-PET is most helpful in distinguishing potentially resectable, locally advanced disease (T3-4, N0, M0) from distant disease (M1). In prospective studies M1 disease was detected by FDG-PET and missed by CT (with or without EUS) in 5–7 % of

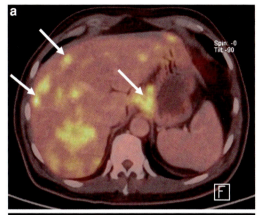
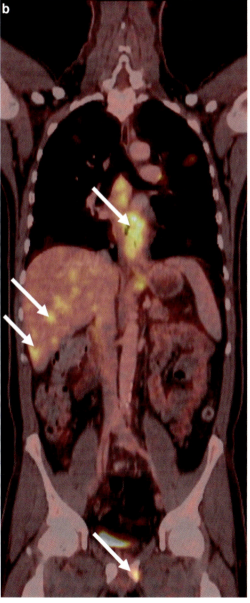

Fig. 8 FDG-PET/CT of a patient with distal oesophageal cancer in axial and coronal reformations. There is an intense FDG uptake in the area of primary tumour as well as in the liver and left pubic bone indicating distant metastases (**a**, **b**, *arrows*)

cases (Meyers et al. 2007; Heeren et al. 2004). M1 disease was detected by FDG-PET and missed by CT in 6–15 % of patients (Flamen et al. 2000; Meyers et al. 2007; Heeren et al. 2004).

4.2 Follow-Up After Oesophagectomy

Tumour recurrence of oesophageal cancer can be divided into locoregional recurrence and distant metastatic disease. The rate of recurrence of oesophageal cancer even after curative surgery was found to be high in most reports (AJCC 2009). In the detection of tumour recurrence, the selected imaging modalities are important in many regards. First of all, the imaging modality must be suitable and cost-effective, and able to detect the pathology in the early stages. After oesophagectomy and gastric excision, the anatomy of the posterior mediastinum is markedly changed. This makes assessment of possible local tumour recurrence difficult. Wall thickening or adjacent mass and suspicious lymph nodes are highly predictive for recurrent disease (AJCC 2009). Hydro technique in combination with FDG-PET/MDCT is again the modality of choice in early detection of recurrent tumour (Guo et al. 2007).

4.2.1 CT Findings

Locoregional recurrent oesophageal tumour is well demonstrated by CT. A smooth or spiculated area of extrinsic mass effect on the mediastinal border can be visualised by CT. Furthermore, MDCT with multiplanar reformations is accurate in detecting masses after oesophageal surgery and superior for distant metastatic disease, and can accurately delineate the neoesophagus and its surroundings (Fig. 10). However, differentiating between fibrosis and tumour tissue at CT is based on indirect signs and may be difficult or even impossible in some cases. FDG-PET/MDCT can overcome this limitation (Sun et al. 2009; Carlisle et al. 1993; Tunaci 2002). Early postoperative cases with possible inflammatory reactions or early post-radiation changes, in particular, must be interpreted with caution.

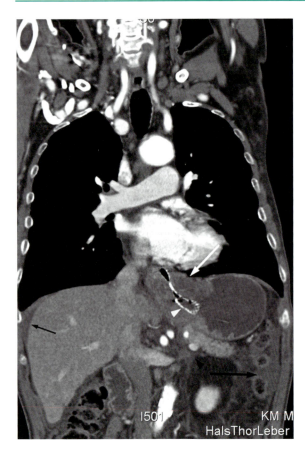

Fig. 9 Hydro-MDCT of the oesophagus in coronal reformations shows a distal oesophageal cancer (*white arrow*) with marked ascites (*small black arrow*), and diffuse stranding of the mesenteric root (*black arrowhead*) indicative of peritoneal carcinomatosis (*large black arrow*). Note the oesophageal stent (*white arrowhead*)

5   Other Oesophageal Malignancies

5.1   Oesophageal Lymphoma

The oesophagus is the alimentary organ least commonly involved with lymphoma, therefore lymphoma of the oesophagus is rare. Any histologic variety of lymphoma may affect the oesophagus (Mendelson and Fermoyle 2005). To diagnose primary oesophageal lymphoma, the following criteria have been proposed: (a) predominantly oesophageal involvement with only regional lymph node involvement; (b) no definite enlargement of mediastinal lymph nodes; (c) no involvement of liver and spleen; and (d) no superficial lymphadenopathy (Kaplan 2004).

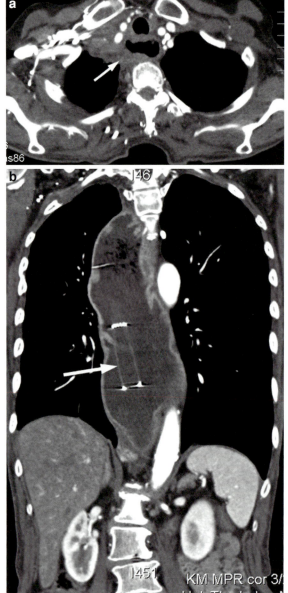

Fig. 10 Hydro-MDCT of the oesophagus in axial (**a**) and coronal (**b**) reformations in a patient with a clinical history of oesophageal cancer and esophagectomy and gastric transposition. We can detect a recurrence demonstrated as a solid mass with inhomogeneous enhancement at the anastomosis site (*right side cervical*, **a**, *arrow*). Note the stent dislocation (**b**, *arrow*)

5.1.1   CT and PET/CT Findings

CT may demonstrate a homogeneously enhancing mass with irregular borders or sharply delineated, pronounced, polypoid wall thickening in any part of the oesophagus (Fig. 11), with or without associated lymphadenopathy. Lymphoma may infiltrate the

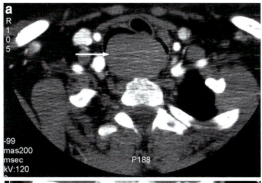

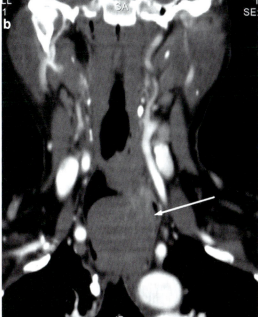

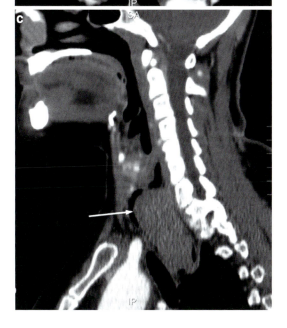

◄Fig. 11 Hydro-MDCT of the oesophagus in (**a**), coronal (**b**), and sagittal (**c**) reformations in a patient with surgically proven lymphoma shows a large polypoid mass in the cervical oesophagus (*arrows*) without infiltration the oesophageal wall

entire oesophagus diffusely. While splenic involvement is suggestive of lymphoma, hepatic metastases are characteristic of oesophageal cancer. There is no specific CT finding for oesophageal lymphoma. PET/CT scans can also be used in staging patients with primary oesophageal lymphoma, as well as for monitoring these tumours after therapy (Suga et al. 2009). However, the availability of FDG/PET and, in particular, FDG-PET/CT, is still limited and expensive.

5.2 Leiomyoma and GIST

Leiomyoma accounts for 60–70 % of all benign oesophageal neoplasms and is the most common benign tumour of the oesophagus, while rare in the remaining gastrointestinal tract (Hatch et al. 2000; Seremetis and Lyons 1976; Simmang et al. 1989). The tumour is present more often in male patients (2:1) at a median age of 30–35 years. Usually, leiomyomas are between two and eight cm in diameter. They are multiple in less than 3 % of cases. More than half of the patients with oesophageal leiomyoma are asymptomatic. Typical complaints are either dysphagia or substernal chest pain due to obstruction of oesophageal bolus transit. Gastrointestinal stromal tumours (GISTs) are the most common nonepithelial tumours of the gastrointestinal tract, although they are rare in the oesophagus (Monges et al. 2010).

5.2.1 CT Findings

Enhanced CT scans reveal a smooth or lobulated tumour margin, with either iso or homogeneously low attenuation. Leiomyoma and GIST may appear as a well-circumscribed, intensely enhancing mass or may be a sessile (Fig. 12), pedunculated, polypoidal, exophytic intraluminal solid mass, sometimes with secondary ulceration. Leiomyomas are the only tumours that may contain calcification (Fig. 13). Absence of infiltration of the oesophageal wall or the absence of the typical circumferential growth pattern enables differentiation from oesophageal cancer. GISTs may not change in size or may even enlarge during therapy, but show a decrease in CT attenuation values (Hounsfield

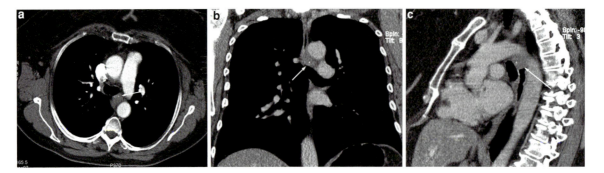

Fig. 12 Hydro-MDCT of the oesophagus in axial (**a**), coronal (**b**) and sagittal (**c**) reformations in a patient with leiomyoma, demonstrated as a small soft tissue mass with slight calcifications in thoracic area of the oesophagus (*arrows*)

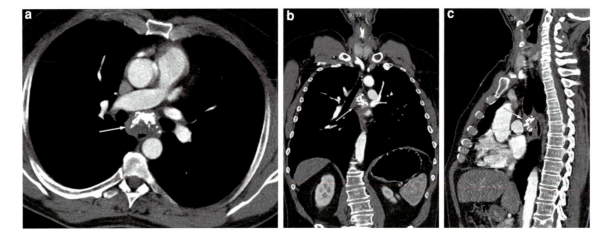

Fig. 13 Hydro-MDCT of the oesophagus in axial (**a**), coronal (**b**) and sagittal (**c**) reformations in a patient with biopsy-proven leiomyoma, demonstrated as a large tumour-like mass with marked calcifications invading the oesophagus in the thoracic area (*arrows*)

units, HU) (Choi et al. 2004). PET/CT is able to show early effects in patients undergoing treatment. Functional imaging proved significantly more accurate than CT alone when assessing GIST response to therapy. Combined PET/CT imaging is, therefore, a valuable diagnostic tool for the primary diagnosis of GISTs or for the assessment of therapeutic response (Suga et al. 2009; Antoch et al. 2004).

5.3 Fibrovascular Polyps

Fibrovascular polyps of the oesophagus are rare benign tumours, comprising about 1 % of all benign oesophageal tumours. However they are the most common intraluminal benign tumours of the oesophagus (Sargent and Hood 2006). Giant fibrovascular polyps are defined as polyps larger than 5 cm in maximum diameter. Even though they are benign, they may be lethal due to either bleeding or, rarely, asphyxiation if a large polyp is regurgitated. Patients commonly present with dysphagia or hematemesis.

5.3.1 CT Findings

The polyps may not be well visualised on endoscopy and imaging plays a vital role in aiding diagnosis as well as providing important information for preoperative planning, such as the location of the pedicle, the vascularity of the polyp and the tissue elements of the mass. These polyps contain predominantly fibrovascular and fatty tissue, which gives them their typical CT appearance of a pedunculated intraluminal mass of fat density, which expands the oesophagus (Ascenti et al. 1999).

5.4 Oesophageal Fistula

Oesophageal fistulas can be classified according to their anatomic relationship into oesophageal-airway, oesophago-pleural, aorto-oesophageal and oesophago-pericardial fistulas. Oesophageal-airway fistulas can be either congenital (so-called tracheo-oesophageal fistulas) or acquired. The development of an oesophageal–airway fistula is a life-threatening complication of oesophageal cancer or secondary to oesophageal trauma, infection, or radiochemotherapy. Initial symptoms most often include cough, aspiration and fever, frequently culminating in pneumonia. More than half such fistulas involve the trachea; alternatively, a connection with the left or right main or lower lobe bronchus may be formed. Patients with oesophageal-airway fistulas are treated with covered stents to seal off the leak. CT may be necessary to localise the fistula and to aid in treatment planning. CT can also be used to detect pleuro-plumonary or mediastinal inflammatory reactions to oesophageal fistulae (Peyrin-Biroulet et al. 2006; Liu et al. 2006).

5.4.1 CT Findings

CT can demonstrate a fistulous connection between the oesophagus and the tracheobronchial system, pleura, pericardium, or mediastinal fat if the fistulous tract is of sufficient size and contains air or oral contrast medium. Oral administration of dilute iodine contrast material (contrast material: water 1:100) can help to delineate the fistula. CT can also detect perifocal reactions in the form of empyema, pneumonia, or mediastinitis (Fig. 14).

5.5 Oesophageal Perforation

Oesophageal injuries include penetrating injuries, blunt traumatic perforation, iatrogenic perforation as well as spontaneous perforation due to a sudden rise in intraluminal pressure during vomiting (so-called Boerhaave syndrome). Most often, oesophageal perforation occurs during endoscopic investigation of malignant disease and presents a difficult problem. Oesophageal diseases, such as strictures, achalasia, and tumours, predispose the oesophagus to perforation. Oesophageal perforation is associated with high mortality, and postoperative leaks

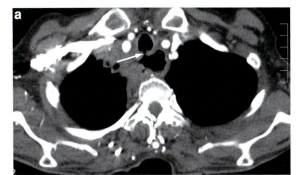
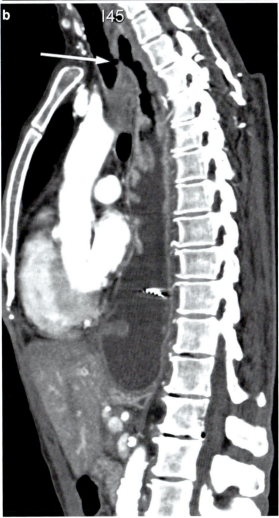

Fig. 14 Hydro-MDCT of the oesophagus in axial (**a**) and sagittal (**b**) reformations in a patient with a clinical history of oesophageal cancer with symptoms suspicious for fistula, due to continuous coughing and recurrent pneumonia, shows a fistula tract between the tumour and the trachea (*arrows*)

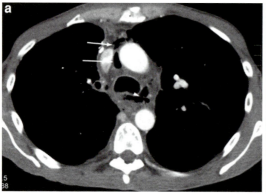
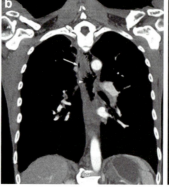
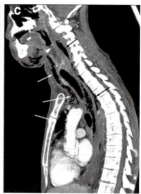

Fig. 15 Hydro-MDCT of the oesophagus in axial (**a**), coronal (**b**), and sagittal (**c**) reformations in a patient with oesophageal perforation after dilation of tumour stenosis. CT scan shows pneumomediastinum, and air bubbles in the mediastinum (**a**, **b**, *arrows*), as well as a tissue defect of the oesophageal wall (*arrows*), and extensive soft tissue emphysema in the cervical region (**c**)

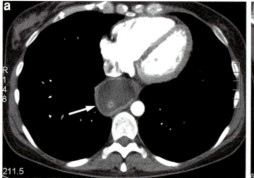
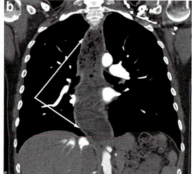
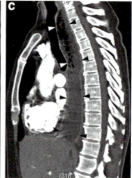

Fig. 16 Hydro-MDCT of the oesophagus in a patient with primary achalasia shows a marked diffuse dilatation of the entire oesophagus, which is filled with fluid and food without wall thickening and malignancy (*arrows*)

occur frequently after primary surgical repair (Chao et al. 2005). Early and accurate diagnosis of oesophageal perforation is critical, because the consequences of missed oesophageal injury are devastating, with potential progression to fulminate mediastinitis and septic shock. Delay in treatment beyond 24 h after onset may adversely affect prognosis. Contrast studies are the method of choice to demonstrate oesophageal rupture. CT has been increasingly used for the diagnosis of oesophageal injuries (LeBlang and Nunez 1999).

5.5.1 CT Findings

Radiographic detection of oesophageal injuries relies on the presence of indirect radiological signs, including subcutaneous or muscular, thoracic or cervical emphysema, a widened mediastinum, pneumomediastinum, pneumopericardium, left-sided pneumothorax, pleural effusion, an abnormal course of a nasogastric tube when it is inserted, and a left lower lobe atelectasis. CT can also display subtle signs such as localised oesophageal wall thickening, mucosal hyperemia, mucosal dissection, and oesophageal hematoma, as well as oedema (De Lutio di Castelguidone et al. 2005). CT also allows the visualisation of very small collections of mediastinal air in cases with small tears (Fig. 15).

6   Other Conditions

6.1   Achalasia

Achalasia is a primary rare motor disorder of the oesophagus, with an incidence of about 1/100,000. Symptoms usually become manifest in early adult age, but even children may be affected. Achalasia is

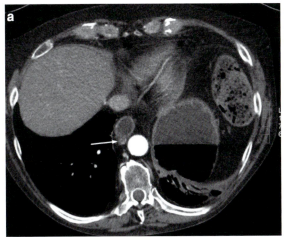

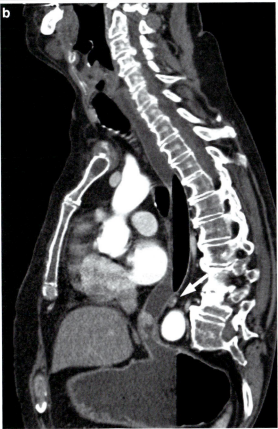

Fig. 17 Hydro-MDCT of the oesophagus in axial (**a**), and sagittal (**b**) reformations shows a small, circumscribed bulge at the gastroesophageal junction, representing a small diverticulum (arrow)

characterised by incomplete relaxation of the lower oesophageal sphincter (LES) on swallowing and aperistalsis of the oesophageal body (Gelfand and

Botoman 1987). In 1947, Ogilvie recognised the syndrome of neoplastic involvement of the distal oesophagus that mimicked idiopathic achalasia, with submucosal infiltration of the lower oesophagus and cardia by carcinoma, which is now commonly referred to as pseudoachalasia (Carter et al. 1997). Therefore, CT can be helpful in differentiating between achalasia and the pseudoachalasia of malignancy. Usually endoscopy and biopsy are used to detect tumour spread in pseudoachalasia. However, CT may be used in suspect cases, when submucosal tumour growth escaped endoscopic detection. Moreover, CT may delineate the presence of other tumour manifestations (Carter et al. 1997).

6.1.1 CT Findings

CT shows uniform dilatation that affects a long segment of the oesophagus, with no wall thickening and with normal-appearing boundary surfaces and mediastinal fat. The oesophagus narrows abruptly at the oesophagogastric junction with no evidence of an intramural or extrinsic obstructive lesion (Fig. 16). In contrast to a stricture, the oesophageal wall is not thinned at the site of the narrowing, and the wall is not thickened as it is with the oesophageal tumour or oesophagitis. Most pseudoachalasia patients have CT findings of oesophageal dilation, more marked and/or asymmetric wall thickening, or mass. In this group, asymmetric or marked thickening (>10mm) indicates pseudoachalasia.

6.2   Diverticula

Oesophageal diverticula are divided into the pulsion or traction type. The two predominant locations of oesophageal diverticula are the mid-oesophagus (at the level of the tracheal bifurcation) and the distal oesophagus (so-called epiphrenic diverticula). Diverticula are incidental findings at CT (Pearlberg et al. 1983).

6.2.1 CT Findings

Diverticula appear as an air-, water- or contrast-filled bulge. Mid-oesophageal and epiphrenic diverticula are better visualised on coronal or sagittal (Fig. 17). reformations on hydro-MDCT. The most frequent location is posteroinferior to the cricoid cartilage, the so-called Zenker diverticulum, which actually is a pharyngeal diverticulum (Fig. 18).

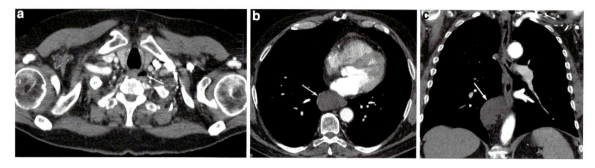

Fig. 18 Hydro-MDCT of the oesophagus in axial (**a**, **b**), and coronal (**c**) reformations in a patient with a small Zenker's diverticulum, lateroposterior to the upper oesophagus filled with air (**a**, *arrow*), and a duplication cyst, which appears as a smoothly marginated homogeneous mass with water-equivalent attenuation in the lower oesophagus (**b**, **c**, *arrows*)

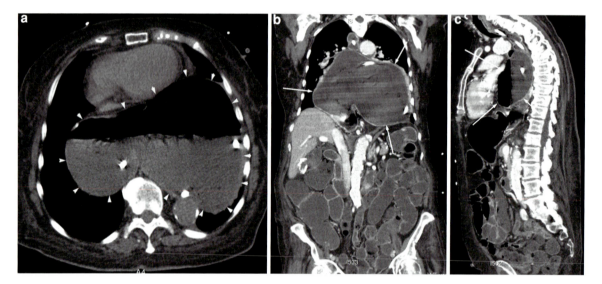

Fig. 19 Hydro-MDCT of the oesophagus in axial (**a**), coronal (**b**), and sagittal (**c**) reformations shows a large paraesophageal hernia with so-called "upside down stomach," which is an extreme form in which all of the stomach has herniated into the thoracic cavity and no portions of the stomach can be detected below the diaphragm (*arrows* and *arrowheads*)

6.3 Duplication Cyst

Duplication cysts of the oesophagus are rare congenital anomalies that may be noted incidentally on conventional chest radiographs as an indeterminate mediastinal mass and require further investigation by CT (Kuhlman et al. 1985).

6.3.1 CT Findings

Duplication cysts are smoothly marginated, homogeneous masses with water-equivalent attenuation that most commonly occur in the lower oesophagus (60 %). They are intimately related to the oesophagus but rarely communicate with it. The cyst may have a paraoesophageal or intramural location (Fig. 18).

6.4 Hiatal Hernia

Oesophageal hiatal hernias comprise two types: sliding axial hernia and paraoesophageal hernia (Eren and Ciris 2005). Sliding hiatal hernia is a displacement of the upper stomach with the cardioesophageal junction upward into the posterior mediastinum. In the paraoesophageal type, all or part of the stomach herniates into the thorax with an undisplaced gastrooesophageal

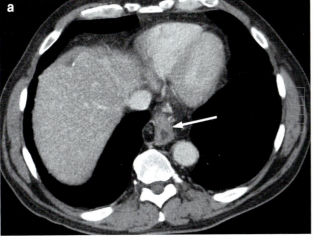
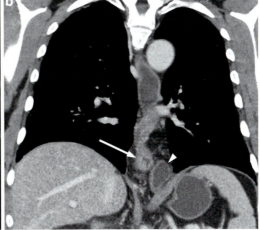

Fig. 20 Hydro-MDCT of the oesophagus in coronal reformation shows a small axial herniation of the stomach that has resulting in a small retrocardiac mass, and the cardia is displaced into the thoracic cavity (*arrowheads*). The gastroesophageal junction and distal oesophagus show marked wall thickening due to reflux oesophagitis (*arrow*)

junction. Haemorrhage, incarceration, obstruction, and strangulation of the stomach and intestine are the most common complications.

6.4.1 CT Findings

Axial herniation of the stomach results in a large retrocardiac mass and the cardia is displaced into the thoracic cavity. With CT, the demonstration of gastric folds is frequent and pathognomonic. A good distension of the stomach and oesophagus is very helpful in the differential diagnosis. A paraoesophageal hernia is associated with fixation of the gastric cardia and portions of the stomach herniated alongside the oesophagus. "Upside down stomach" is an extreme form of hernia, in which all of the stomach has herniated into the thoracic cavity and no portions of the stomach can be detected below the diaphragm (Fig. 19).

6.5 Oesophagitis

Inflammation of the oesophagus is not an indication for CT. Oesophagitis may be noted incidentally during the course of a CT staging examination or follow-up (Berkovich et al. 2000). High-grade oesophagitis manifests in 33–41 % of patients with malignancies, who are treated with concurrent chemo-radiotherapy. Painful oesophagitis decreases the nutritional status of

patients and can lead to treatment interruptions, which in turn adversely affects survival.

6.5.1 CT Findings

The inflamed oesophageal mucosa shows uniform, circumferential wall thickening that usually involves a relatively long oesophageal segment. Inflammatory and neoplastic wall changes cannot be reliably distinguished based on CT morphology. Short segments of ulcerative wall thickening are more suggestive of a malignant lesion, while longer segments are more consistent with an inflammatory process. The most common CT findings are a thickened oesophageal wall and a target sign. Although endoscopy is a more sensitive modality for detecting this condition, the CT finding of a relatively long segment of circumferential oesophageal wall thickening, with or without a target sign, should suggest the diagnosis of oesophagitis in the proper clinical setting (Fig. 20).

6.6 Oesophageal Varices

Varices of the oesophagus are mainly caused by portal hypertension. In this case gastric varices communicate with the oesophageal and perioesophageal veins, which are drained via the azygos/hemiazygos venous system to the superior vena cava (Balthazar et al. 1987).

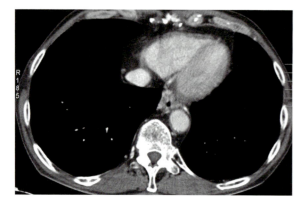

Fig. 21 Hydro-MDCT of the oesophagus in the axial reformation (venous phase) views in a patient with oesophageal varices, which appear as brightly enhancing dot-like structures within the oesophageal wall (*arrows*)

6.6.1 CT Findings

Oesophageal varices are best visualised in the portal venous phase or in the delayed phase after administration of contrast material. Oesophageal varices present as intraluminal (intramural, submucous) tubular, often dot-like structures that show marked pooling of intravenous contrast medium (Fig. 21). Paraoesophageal varices are often larger and have a more serpiginous structure. CT criteria for oesophageal varices are defined more specifically as nodular or tubular enhancing lesions within the oesophageal wall that contact the intraluminal surface, thus distinguishing oesophageal from paraoesophageal varices. While oesophageal varices can be appreciated easily by endoscopy, paraoesophageal varices are only seen on CT or endoscopic sonography (Fig. 22).

6.7 Dysphagia Lusoria and Aortic Disease

Aberrations in the course of the aortic arch or supraaortic branches can displace or compress the proximal oesophagus, leading to dysphagia. The most frequent cause is an anomalous right subclavian artery that arises from the descending aorta as a fourth supraaortic branch and passes behind the oesophagus that rarely cause dysphagia (dysphagia lusoria) (Fig. 23). Other causes are a duplicated aortic arch or an aortic aneurysm. In cases of an anomalous right subclavian artery its aortic origin may be wide due to

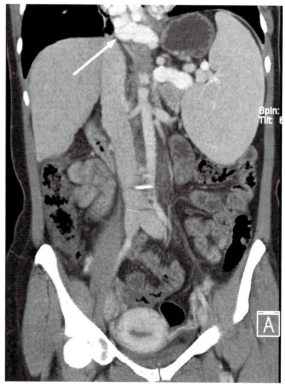

Fig. 22 Hydro-MDCT of the oesophagus in the coronal view in a patient with paraoesophageal varices, which appear as brightly enhancing tortuous veins adjacent to the oesophageal wall (arrow)

a congenital aortic diverticulum (Kommerell's diverticulum), (Fig. 24) in this case dysphagia is more likely due to compression of the oesophagus (Keum et al. 2006). CT angiography has already replaced invasive DSA in the evaluation of thoracic vascular anomalies and has become the diagnostic procedure of first choice.

6.7.1 CT Findings

Contrast-enhanced MDCT allows the diagnosis of the variants of the aortic arch very easily. The aberrant right subclavian artery, or dysphagia lusoria, demonstrates a typical pattern on contrast-enhanced MDCT and is more easily diagnosed using multiplanar reconstructions. It arises more posteriorly than normal, and runs behind the oesophagus (Fig. 23). An aortic diverticulum appears as a circumscribed asymmetric aneurysm like protrusion from wide funnel-shaped origin of the subclavian artery in the distal aortic arch (Fig. 24).

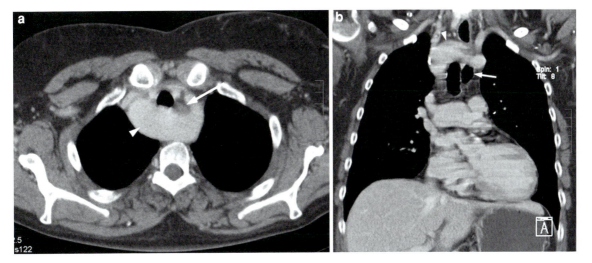

Fig. 23 Hydro-MDCT of the oesophagus in axial (**a**), and coronal (**b**) reformations shows an abberrant right subclavian artery (*arrowhead*) that courses more posteriorly to the compressed oesophagus (*arrow in a*), indicative of dysphagia lusoria. Note the non-compressed oesophagus distally (*arrow b*)

Fig. 24 Hydro-MDCT of the oesophagus in axial (**a**) and sagittal (**b**) reformations shows a right-sided aortic arch with retro-oesopahgeal left subclavian artery (lusoria type) arising from an aortic diverticulum of Kommerell (*arrowhead*), which must not confused with an aneurysm of the origin of the subclavian artery. The oesophagus is compressed (*arrow*)

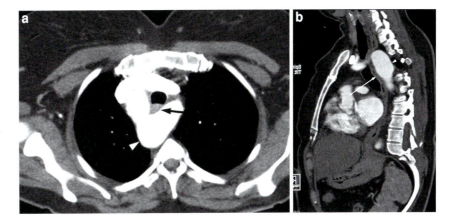

7 Clinical Value of Multi-Detector CT

Hydro-MDCT especially in combination with FDG-PET is particularly useful in the evaluation and initial staging of patients with oesophageal carcinoma as well as for treatment planning and assessing tumour response to therapy. At present, CT or FDG-PET/CT plays a major role as a triage tool to aid in choosing the appropriate treatment for patients with oesophageal cancer. FDG-PET/CT may help distinguish between surgical candidates with limited disease and possible curative surgery or patients who need preoperative chemoradiation for downstaging, and patients who need only palliative therapy in advanced cases with distant metastases. Thus, the pre-surgical assessment of patients with oesophageal cancer with surgical exploration prior to the decision about further therapeutic procedures can be avoided. If CT or PET/CT depending on availability shows definitive advanced disease with extended tumour spread, pre-surgical chemotherapy is used to downstage the tumour. After completion of chemotherapy, restaging of the tumour will be performed. If there is a positive response to chemotherapy, curative surgical therapy will be attempted. Therefore, preoperative staging of oesophageal cancer appears to be, by far, the most important indication for FDG-PET/CT of the oesophagus. In addition, multi-detector CT plays an important role in the evaluation of postoperative complications and detection of tumour recurrence following oesophagectomy. MDCT can determine the presence, location, and severity of oesophageal perforations. Furthermore, Hydro-MDCT is an evolving method for the assessment of other intra- and extraluminal processes of the oesophageal wall.

References

AJCC (2009) Cancer staging, 7th edn. Springer, New York

Antoch G, Kanja J, Bauer S et al (2004) Comparison of PET, CT, and dual-modality PET/CT imaging for monitoring of imatinib (STI571) therapy in patients with gastrointestinal stromal tumors. J Nucl Med 45(3):357–365

Ascenti G, Racchiusa S, Mazziotti S, Bottari M, Scribano E (1999) Giant fibrovascular polyp of the esophagus: CT and MR findings. Abdom Imaging 24(2):109–110

Balthazar EJ, Naidich DP, Megibow AJ, Lefleur RS (1987) CT evaluation of esophageal varices. Am J Roentgenol 148(1): 131–135

Barr H (2011) Gastrointestinal cancer: current screening strategies. Recent Results Cancer Res 185:149–157

Bar-Shalom R, Guralnik L, Tsalic M et al (2005) The additional value of PET/CT over PET in FDG imaging of oesophageal cancer. Eur J Nucl Med Mol Imaging 32(8):918–924

Ba-Ssalamah A, Prokop M, Uffmann M, Pokieser P, Teleky B, Lechner G (2003) Dedicated multidetector CT of the stomach: spectrum of diseases. Radiographics 23(3):625–644

Ba-Ssalamah A, Zacherl J, Noebauer-Huhmann IM et al (2009) Dedicated multi-detector CT of the esophagus: spectrum of diseases. Abdom Imaging 34(1):3–18

Ba-Ssalamah A, Matzek W, Baroud S et al (2011) Accuracy of hydro-multidetector row CT in the local T staging of oesophageal cancer compared to postoperative histopathological results. Eur Radiol 21(11):2326–2335

Berkovich GY, Levine MS, Miller WT Jr (2000) CT findings in patients with esophagitis. Am J Roentgenol 175(5): 1431–1434

Blom RL, Vliegen RF, Schreurs WM, et al (2011) External ultrasonography of the neck does not add diagnostic value to integrated positron emission tomography-computed tomography (PET-CT) scanning in the diagnosis of cervical lymph node metastases in patients with esophageal carcinoma. Dis Esophagus

Boellaard R, van Lingen A, Lammertsma AA (2001) Experimental and clinical evaluation of iterative reconstruction (OSEM) in dynamic PET: quantitative characteristics and effects on kinetic modeling. J Nucl Med 42(5):808–817

Bradley J, Bae K, Choi N, et al. (2012) A phase II comparative study of gross tumor volume definition with or without PET/CT fusion in dosimetric planning for Non-Small-Cell Lung Cancer (NSCLC): Primary analysis of radiation therapy oncology group (RTOG) 0515. Int J Radiat Oncol Biol Phys 82(1):435–441 e1

Brown LM, Hoover R, Silverman D et al (2001) Excess incidence of squamous cell esophageal cancer among US black men: role of social class and other risk factors. Am J Epidemiol 153(2):114–122

Carlisle JG, Quint LE, Francis IR, Orringer MB, Smick JF, Gross BH (1993) Recurrent esophageal carcinoma: CT evaluation after esophagectomy. Radiology 189(1):271–275

Carter M, Deckmann RC, Smith RC, Burrell MI, Traube M (1997) Differentiation of achalasia from pseudoachalasia by computed tomography. Am J Gastroenterol 92(4):624–628

Cerfolio RJ, Bryant AS (2006) Maximum standardized uptake values on positron emission tomography of esophageal cancer predicts stage, tumor biology, and survival. Ann thorac surg 82(2):391–394 Discussion 4–5

Chao YK, Liu YH, Ko PJ et al (2005) Treatment of esophageal perforation in a referral center in taiwan. Surg Today 35(10):828–832

Choi H, Charnsangavej C, de Castro Faria S et al (2004) CT evaluation of the response of gastrointestinal stromal tumors after imatinib mesylate treatment: a quantitative analysis correlated with FDG PET findings. Am J Roentgenol 183(6):1619–1628

Choi J, Kim SG, Kim JS, Jung HC, Song IS (2010) Comparison of endoscopic ultrasonography (EUS), positron emission tomography (PET), and computed tomography (CT) in the preoperative locoregional staging of resectable esophageal cancer. Surg Endosc 24(6):1380–1386

Csikos M, Horvath O, Petri A, Petri I, Imre J (1985) Late malignant transformation of chronic corrosive oesophageal strictures. Langenbecks Arch Chir 365(4):231–238

Daly JM, Fry WA, Little AG et al (2000) Esophageal cancer: results of an American College of Surgeons patient care evaluation study. J Am Coll Surg 190(5):562–572 discussion 72–3

De Lutio di Castelguidone E, Pinto A, Merola S, Stavolo C, Romano L (2005) Role of spiral and multislice computed tomography in the evaluation of traumatic and spontaneous oesophageal perforation our experience. Radiol Med (Torino) 109(3):252–259

Edwards BK, Howe HL, Ries LA et al (2002) Annual report to the nation on the status of cancer, 1973–1999, featuring implications of age and aging on U.S. cancer burden. Cancer 94(10):2766–2792

Eren S, Ciris F (2005) Diaphragmatic hernia: diagnostic approaches with review of the literature. Eur J Radiol 54(3):448–459

Flamen P, Lerut A, Van Cutsem E et al (2000) Utility of positron emission tomography for the staging of patients with potentially operable esophageal carcinoma. J Clin Oncol 18(18):3202–3210

Gelfand MD, Botoman VA (1987) Esophageal motility disorders: a clinical overview. Am J Gastroenterol 82(3):181–187

Greene FL, Page DL, Flemming ID, Fritz A, Balch CM, Haller DG (2002) American joint committe on cancer: AJCC cancer staging manual., 6th edn. Springer, New York

Guo H, Zhu H, Xi Y et al (2007) Diagnostic and prognostic value of 18F-FDG PET/CT for patients with suspected recurrence from squamous cell carcinoma of the esophagus. J Nucl Med 48(8):1251–1258

Haley M, Konski A, Li T et al (2009) Influence of diabetes on the interpretation of PET scans in patients with esophageal cancer. Gastrointest Cancer Res 3(4):149–152

Halpern BS, Dahlbom M, Quon A et al (2004) Impact of patient weight and emission scan duration on PET/CT image quality and lesion detectability. J Nucl Med 45(5):797–801

Halvorsen RA, Thompson WM (1984) Computed tomographic evaluation of esophageal carcinoma. Semin Oncol 11(2):113–126

Hatch GF 3rd, Wertheimer-Hatch L, Hatch KF et al (2000) Tumors of the esophagus. World J Surg 24(4):401–411

Heeren PA, Jager PL, Bongaerts F, van Dullemen H, Sluiter W, Plukker JT (2004) Detection of distant metastases in esophageal cancer with (18)F-FDG PET. J Nucl Med 45(6):980–987

Hsu WH, Hsu PK, Wang SJ et al (2009) Positron emission tomography-computed tomography in predicting locoregional invasion in esophageal squamous cell carcinoma. Ann thorac surg 87(5):1564–1568

Jeganathan R, McGuigan J, Campbell F, Lynch T (2011) Does pre-operative estimation of oesophageal tumour metabolic length using 18F-fluorodeoxyglucose PET/CT images compare with surgical pathology length? Eur J Nucl Med Mol Imaging 38(4):656–662

Kaplan KJ (2004) Primary esophageal lymphoma: a diagnostic challenge. South Med J 97(4):331–332

Kato H, Nakajima M, Sohda M et al (2009) The clinical application of (18)F-fluorodeoxyglucose positron emission tomography to predict survival in patients with operable esophageal cancer. Cancer 115(14):3196–3203

Keum B, Kim YS, Jeen YT et al (2006) Dysphagia lusoria assessed by 3-dimensional CT. Gastrointest Endosc 64(2):268–269

Kobori O, Kirihara Y, Kosaka N, Hara T (1999) Positron emission tomography of esophageal carcinoma using (11)C-choline and (18)F-fluorodeoxyglucose: a novel method of preoperative lymph node staging. Cancer 86(9):1638–1648

Kontaxakis G, Strauss LG, Thireou T et al (2002) Iterative image reconstruction for clinical PET using ordered subsets, median root prior, and a web-based interface. Mol Imaging Biol. 4(3):219–231

Krause BJ, Herrmann K, Wieder H, zum Buschenfelde CM (2009) 18F-FDG PET and 18F-FDG PET/CT for assessing response to therapy in esophageal cancer. J Nucl Med 50(Suppl 1):89S–96S

Kuhlman JE, Fishman EK, Wang KP, Siegelman SS (1985) Esophageal duplication cyst: CT and transesophageal needle aspiration. Am J Roentgenol 145(3):531–532

Lagergren J, Bergstrom R, Lindgren A, Nyren O (1999) Symptomatic gastroesophageal reflux as a risk factor for esophageal adenocarcinoma. N Engl J Med 340(11):825–831

Lagergren J, Ye W, Lindgren A, Nyren O (2000) Heredity and risk of cancer of the esophagus and gastric cardia. Cancer Epidemiol Biomarkers Prev 9(7):757–760

Lea JWt, Prager RL, Bender HW Jr (1984) The questionable role of computed tomography in preoperative staging of esophageal cancer. Ann Thorac Surg 38(5):479–481

LeBlang SD, Nunez DB Jr (1999) Helical CT of cervical spine and soft tissue injuries of the neck. Radiol Clin North Am 37(3):515–532, v-vi

Liu PS, Levine MS, Torigian DA (2006) Esophagopleural fistula secondary to esophageal wall ballooning and thinning after pneumonectomy: findings on chest CT and esophagography. Am J Roentgenol 186(6):1627–1629

Lowe VJ, Booya F, Fletcher JG et al (2005) Comparison of positron emission tomography, computed tomography, and endoscopic ultrasound in the initial staging of patients with esophageal cancer. Mol Imaging Biol 7(6):422–430

Ludeman L, Shepherd NA (2005) Serosal involvement in gastrointestinal cancer: its assessment and significance. Histopathology 47(2):123–131

Luketich JD, Schauer PR, Meltzer CC et al (1997) Role of positron emission tomography in staging esophageal cancer. Ann Thorac Surg 64(3):765–769

Mani NB, Suri S, Gupta S, Wig JD (2001) Two-phase dynamic contrast-enhanced computed tomography with water-filling method for staging of gastric carcinoma. Clin Imaging 25(1):38–43

Mendelson RM, Fermoyle S (2005) Primary gastrointestinal lymphomas: a radiological-pathological review. Part 1: Stomach, oesophagus and colon. Australas Radiol 49(5):353–364

Meyers BF, Downey RJ, Decker PA et al (2007) The utility of positron emission tomography in staging of potentially operable carcinoma of the thoracic esophagus: results of the American college of surgeons oncology group Z0060 trial. J Thorac Cardiovasc Surg 133(3):738–745

Monges G, Bisot-Locard S, Blay JY et al (2010) The estimated incidence of gastrointestinal stromal tumors in France. Results of PROGIST study conducted among pathologists. Bull Cancer 97(3):E16–E22

Moss AA, Schnyder P, Thoeni RF, Margulis AR (1981) Esophageal carcinoma: pretherapy staging by computed tomography. Am J Roentgenol 136(6):1051–1056

Nagaki A, Onoguchi M, Matsutomo N (2011) Patient weight-based acquisition protocols to optimize (18)F-FDG PET/CT image quality. J Nucl Med Technol 39(2):72–76

Nomura M, Shitara K, Kodaira T et al (2012) Prognostic impact of the 6th and 7th American joint committee on cancer TNM staging systems on esophageal cancer patients treated with chemoradiotherapy. Int J Radiat Oncol Biol Phys 82(2):946–952

Okada M, Murakami T, Kumano S et al (2009) Integrated FDG-PET/CT compared with intravenous contrast-enhanced CT for evaluation of metastatic regional lymph nodes in patients with resectable early stage esophageal cancer. Ann Nucl Med 23(1):73–80

Panebianco V, Grazhdani H, Iafrate F et al (2006) 3D CT protocol in the assessment of the esophageal neoplastic lesions: can it improve TNM staging? Eur Radiol 16(2):414–421

Parfitt JR, Miladinovic Z, Driman DK (2006) Increasing incidence of adenocarcinoma of the gastroesophageal junction and distal stomach in Canada—an epidemiological study from 1964–2002. Can J Gastroenterol 20(4):271–276

Pearlberg JL, Sandler MA, Madrazo BL (1983) Computed tomographic features of esophageal intramural pseudodiverticulosis. Radiology 147(1):189–190

Pennathur A, Luketich JD (2008) Resection for esophageal cancer: strategies for optimal management. Ann Thorac Surg 85(2):S751–S756

Peyrin-Biroulet L, Bronowicki JP, Bigard MA, Regent D, Walter S, Platini C (2006) Contribution of computed tomography with oral media contrast to the diagnosis of esophago-pericardial fistula. Clin Imaging 30(5):347–349

Picus D, Balfe DM, Koehler RE, Roper CL, Owen JW (1983) Computed tomography in the staging of esophageal carcinoma. Radiol 146(2):433–438

Prokop M (2005) New challenges in MDCT. Eur Radiol 15(Suppl 5):E35–E45

Quint LE, Glazer GM, Orringer MB, Gross BH (1985) Esophageal carcinoma: CT findings. Radiol 155(1):171–175

Rampin L, Nanni C, Fanti S, Rubello D (2005) Value of PET-CT fusion imaging in avoiding potential pitfalls in the interpretation of 18F-FDG accumulation in the distal oesophagus. Eur J Nucl Med Mol Imaging. 32(8):990–992

Rice TW, Blackstone EH, Rusch VW (2010) A cancer staging primer: esophagus and esophagogastric junction. J Thorac Cardiovasc Surg 139(3):527–529

Romero Y, Cameron AJ, Schaid DJ et al (2002) Barrett's esophagus: prevalence in symptomatic relatives. Am J Gastroenterol 97(5):1127–1132

Sargent RL, Hood IC (2006) Asphyxiation caused by giant fibrovascular polyp of the esophagus. Arch Pathol Lab Med 130(5):725–727

Seremetis MG, Lyons WS, deGuzman VC, Peabody JW Jr (1976) Leiomyomata of the esophagus. An analysis of 838 cases. Cancer 38(5):2166–2177

Sharma NK, Silverman JS, Li T et al (2011) Decreased posttreatment SUV on PET scan is associated with improved local control in medically inoperable esophageal cancer. Gastrointest Cancer Res 4(3):84–89

Siewert J R (2007) [Esophageal carcinoma]. Chirurg 78(5):475–484

Siewert JR, Stein HJ, Feith M, Bruecher BL, Bartels H, Fink U (2001) Histologic tumor type is an independent prognostic parameter in esophageal cancer: lessons from more than 1,000 consecutive resections at a single center in the Western world. Ann Surg 234(3):360–367 discussion 8–9

Simmang CL, Reed K, Rosenthal D (1989) Leiomyomas of the gastrointestinal tract. Mil Med 154(1):45–47

Skehan SJ, Brown AL, Thompson M, Young JE, Coates G, Nahmias C (2000) Imaging features of primary and recurrent esophageal cancer at FDG PET. Radiographics 20(3):713–723

Smithers BM, Fahey PP, Corish T et al (2010) Symptoms, investigations and management of patients with cancer of the oesophagus and gastro-oesophageal junction in Australia. Med J Aust 193(10):572–577

Sobin LH, Wittekind CL (2002) TNM classification of malignant tumors, 6th edn. Wiley, New York

Stein HJ, Feith M, Bruecher BL, Naehrig J, Sarbia M, Siewert JR (2005) Early esophageal cancer: pattern of lymphatic spread and prognostic factors for long-term survival after surgical resection. Ann Surg 242(4):566–573, discussion 73–5

Suga K, Shimizu K, Kawakami Y et al (2005) Lymphatic drainage from esophagogastric tract: feasibility of endoscopic CT lymphography for direct visualization of pathways. Radiol 237(3):952–960

Suga K, Yasuhiko K, Hiyama A, Takeda K, Matsunaga N (2009) F-18 FDG PET/CT findings in a patient with bilateral orbital and gastric mucosa-associated lymphoid tissue lymphomas. Clin Nucl Med 34(9):589–593

Sun L, Su XH, Guan YS et al (2009) Clinical usefulness of 18F-FDG PET/CT in the restaging of esophageal cancer after surgical resection and radiotherapy. World J Gastroenterol 15(15):1836–1842

Talanow R, Shrikanthan S (2010) Imaging protocols for 18F-FDG PET/CT in overweight patients: limitations. J Nucl Med 51(4):662 (author reply)

Thompson WM, Halvorsen RA Jr (1994) Staging esophageal carcinoma II: CT and MRI. Semin Oncol 21(4):447–452

Thompson WM, Halvorsen RA, Foster WL Jr, Williford ME, Postlethwait RW, Korobkin M (1983) Computed tomography for staging esophageal and gastroesophageal cancer: reevaluation. Am J Roentgenol 141(5):951–958

Tunaci A (2002) Postoperative imaging of gastrointestinal tract cancers. Eur J Radiol 42(3):224–230

Ulla M, Cavadas D, Munoz I, Beskow A, Seehaus A, Garcia-Monaco R (2010) Esophageal cancer: pneumo-64-MDCT. Abdom Imaging 35(4):383–389

Umeoka S, Koyama T, Watanabe G et al (2010) Preoperative local staging of esophageal carcinoma using dual-phase contrast-enhanced imaging with multi-detector row computed tomography: value of the arterial phase images. J Comput Assist Tomogr 34(3):406–412

van Westreenen HL, Westerterp M, Bossuyt PM et al (2004) Systematic review of the staging performance of 18F-fluorodeoxyglucose positron emission tomography in esophageal cancer. J Clin Oncol 22(18):3805–3812

Weber WA, Ott K, Becker K et al (2001) Prediction of response to preoperative chemotherapy in adenocarcinomas of the esophagogastric junction by metabolic imaging. J Clin Oncol 19(12):3058–3065

Wolf MC, Stahl M, Krause BJ et al (2011) Curative treatment of oesophageal carcinoma: current options and future developments. Radiat Oncol 6:55

Wu AH, Wan P, Bernstein L (2001) A multiethnic population-based study of smoking, alcohol and body size and risk of adenocarcinomas of the stomach and esophagus (United States). Cancer Causes Control 12(8):721–732

Yang H, Berner A, Mei Q et al (2002) Cytologic screening for esophageal cancer in a high-risk population in Anyang county. China. Acta Cytol 46(3):445–452

Yu W, Fu XL, Zhang YJ, Xiang JQ, Shen L, Chang JY (2011) A prospective evaluation of staging and target volume definition of lymph nodes by 18FDG PET/CT in patients with squamous cell carcinoma of thoracic esophagus. Int J Radiat Oncol Biol Phys 81(5):e759–e765

Endoscopy of the Pharynx and Esophagus

Doris-Maria Denk-Linnert and Rainer Schöfl

Contents

Abstract

Endoscopy of the pharynx and esophagus contributes to the diagnostic work-up of the patients with pharyngeal and esophageal disorders. Dysphagia is one of the main symptoms. In many cases, endoscopy has emerged as "first-line" examination. In addition to the endoscopic visualization of the (aero)-digestive tract, biopsies allow histological diagnosis, and therapeutic manipulations can be performed. However, radiography, especially videofluoroscopy, remains indispensable. A main focus of diagnostic interest is the differential diagnosis between structural diseases and functional disorders. In order to meet the diagnostic and therapeutic requirements an interdisciplinary approach is necessary. Among others, otorhinolaryngologists, gastroenterologists, radiologists and surgeons cooperate in the patient management.

1 Introduction

The pharynx and esophagus belong to the upper digestive tract; their morphology and function enable normal swallowing. Dysphagia is one of the main symptoms in patients with pharyngeal and esophageal disorders. Diagnostics need to consider the entire swallowing sequence from the oral cavity to the stomach. However, there is a close relationship between diseases of the pharynx, larynx and esophagus: gastrointestinal disorders, e.g., reflux disease, may show extraesophageal manifestations in the pharynx and larynx, and in case of tumors in the upper aerodigestive tract or esophagus, additional simultaneous tumors necessitating early diagnosis may appear.

D.-M. Denk-Linnert (✉)
Department of Otorhinolaryngology,
Section of Phoniatrics, Vienna Medical School,
Medical University of Vienna, Währinger Gürtel 18–20,
1090 Vienna, Austria
e-mail: doris-maria.denk-linnert@meduniwien.ac.at

R. Schöfl
4th Department of Internal Medicine, Hospital of the
Elisabethinen, Fadingerstraße 1, 4020 Linz, Austria

O. Ekberg (ed.), *Dysphagia*, Medical Radiology. Diagnostic Imaging, DOI: 10.1007/174_2012_634,
© Springer-Verlag Berlin Heidelberg 2012

For diagnostic evaluation, endoscopy has emerged as the "first-line" examination. Technical progress has improved the quality of endoscopic imaging and enabled clinically routine video documentation. In addition to the endoscopic visualization of the aerodigestive tract, biopsies, recently assisted by molecular diagnostics such as PCR (polymerase chain reaction), allow histological diagnosis. A wide variety of therapeutic manipulations, such as ballon dilatation, mucosal resections or stenting, can be performed. Together with radiology, endoscopy has become indispensable in the management of diseases of the pharynx and esophagus. A main focus of diagnostic interest is the differential diagnosis between structural diseases and functional disorders. For therapeutic decision-making, it is of utmost importance to prove or exclude malignancy and aspiration.

Patients with pharyngeal and esophageal diseases will often cross specialty lines. About 80 % of patients with esophageal disorders present first to an otolaryngologist because they suffer from head and neck symptoms, such as dysphagia, cough or globus sensation. Whereas otolaryngology deals with laryngo-pharyngeal disorders, the management of esophageal diseases falls more appropriately within the realm of gastroenterology (which deals with the whole intestine), as well as thoracic surgery. This interdisciplinary approach is discussed in this chapter.

Endoscopy and radiology are not the only instrumental methods in the diagnostic armamentarium. In addition, depending on the patient's symptoms and endoscopic or radiologic findings, further examinations may be needed for conclusive analysis of the pharynx and esophagus. For example, manometry, manofluorography, (impedance/) pH-metry, scintigraphy for quantification of the pharyngo-esophageal transport, or electromyography provide valuable information.

It is the aim of this chapter to describe the endoscopic examination of the upper aerodigestive tract and examples of typical findings, and in it, advantages and limitations of endoscopy are demonstrated. Moreover, the role of endoscopy within the diagnostic work-up of dysphagic patients and future aspects will be discussed.

2   Endoscopy of the Pharynx and Larynx

A critical area for deglutition without aspiration is crossing of the airway and digestive tract, which is localized in the hypopharynx. Apart from their role in

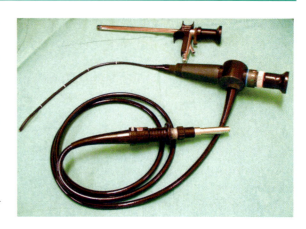

Fig. 1 Rigid telescope and flexible rhinolaryngoscope

deglutition, pharyngeal structures are part of the vocal tract, which is responsible for articulation and resonance. Therefore, the pharynx and larynx, as part of the upper aerodigestive tract, have to be evaluated in context by the otolaryngologist. With the mirror examination, the ability to adequately visualize the pharynx and larynx may be limited. Therefore, endoscopy has become a clinical routine.

Candidates for endoscopy of the pharynx and larynx are patients presenting with symptoms of respiratory and swallowing diseases, such as dysphagia, aspiration, regurgitation, odynophagia and dysphonia (hoarseness). Before endoscopy is carried out, a history is taken and a mirror examination of ears, nose, mouth, pharynx and larynx is performed.

The indirect endoscopy of the pharynx and larynx shows their inner surfaces via optical instruments, either transorally, with rigid endoscopes (telescopes), or transnasally, with flexible endoscopes. Video documentation should be obtained whenever possible.

2.1   Indirect Rigid Endoscopy of the Hypopharynx and Larynx

Rigid 70 and 90° telescopes (Fig. 1) are used to evaluate the hypopharynx and larynx indirectly. They provide a magnified view in high resolution, allow videotaping for documentation, and can be used in association with stroboscopy to evaluate vocal fold vibrations. In addition, indirect rigid endoscopy enables the performance of office-based laryngeal surgical procedures under topical anesthesia (such as biopsies and indirect phonosurgery for voice improvement in selected cases).

For endoscopy, the patient sits in an upright position, with his tongue protruding, and the examiner gently inserts the objective end of the telescope posteriorly over the base of the tongue until the hypopharynx and larynx are seen. The unphysiological patient condition with the tongue protruded allows only the examination of "hi"-phonation, but not the direct observation of articulation and swallowing. In cases of gag reflex, local anesthesia can facilitate the examination. The observer examines morphology (e.g., signs of inflammation, tumor) and function (respiratory and phonatory vocal fold mobility, pooling/aspiration of saliva).

2.2 Flexible (Video-)Endoscopy of the Pharynx and Larynx

Transnasal flexible nasopharyngolaryngoscopy is a common procedure among otorhinolaryngologists for assessing nasal, velopharyngeal and laryngeal pathology. Moreover, it is used for the evaluation of oropharyngeal swallowing and as a treatment tool in biofeedback therapy of voice and swallowing disorders.

The flexible rhinolaryngoscope consists of an objective lens at the distal end of the insertion portion of the endoscope. The diameter of the insertion tube of the scope is kept as small as possible (3–4 mm). A xenon or halogen light source is used. With a chip camera, the image is viewed on a monitor and recorded on a digital recorder.

The videoendoscopic technique is a clinical standard for esophagogastroscopes. Recently, technical progress has made video-rhinolaryngoscopes with a small diameter (about 3.2 mm outer diameter) possible for transnasal insertion (Kawaida et al. 2002). The image transfer is not performed via the fibers, but with a chip camera at the tip of the endoscope. This technique provides better optical resolution and digital signal modulation.

The flexible nasopharyngolaryngoscope is inserted through the nasal passage; a topical anesthesia (e.g. anesthetic and decongestant spray) can be applied beforehand. The examination begins with the visualization of the nasal fossa, the epipharynx and velum, and velopharyngeal competence and closure are tested. Then the endoscope is passed down to just above the epiglottis, where the larynx and hypopharynx can be seen (panoramic view). The base of the tongue, position and morphology of the epiglottis, configuration of the posterior pharyngeal wall, vallecular spaces, piriform sinuses, arytenoids and vocal folds are investigated. After that, the scope is moved further down to just above the vocal folds for detailed inspection (larynx view). Signs of inflammation, mucosal abnormalities, mass lesions and vocal fold mobility can easily be observed. If local anesthesia was administered to reduce the cough reflex, the glottic level can possibly be passed for inspection of the subglottic region and trachea.

Flexible endoscopy is also appropriate for patients who cannot be examined by mirror or rigid endoscopy because of a strong gag reflex, and for patients who are not able to cooperate, e.g., pediatric or emergency patients. The main advantage is that the flexible endoscope can be left in position during phonation, articulation and swallowing, therefore it is used for evaluation of functions. As a limitation, it has to be pointed out that the image quality of flexible endoscopy does not reach that of rigid endoscopy. Whenever videostroboscopy is performed, the method of choice is rigid endoscopy.

Our experience with more than 5,000 endoscopies shows that flexible endoscopy is a procedure without major complications. However, vasovagal reaction, laryngospasm or epistaxis are described in the literature. Therefore, all emergency measurements for managing such complications must be available.

2.3 Examples of Typical Findings

Normal Hypopharynx and Larynx. The base of the tongue, posterior pharyngeal wall, piriform sinus and supraglottis are covered by intact epithelium; the vocal folds present in a white color due to the non-keratinizing squamous epithelium. Both vocal folds move symmetrically between the respiration and phonation positions. No pooling of saliva or food is seen.

Hypopharynx Carcinoma. Foreign tissue and perhaps ulceration is seen in the hypopharynx (posterior pharyngeal wall, piriform sinus or postcricoid region). Due to tumor infiltration, vocal fold motility may be disturbed. Figure 2 shows an exophytic tumor mass in the left piriform sinus, reaching the postcricoid wall. Due to tumor infiltration, the left vocal fold is paralyzed. The patient's symptoms included dysphonia, dyspnea and long-lasting, slowly progressing dysphagia.

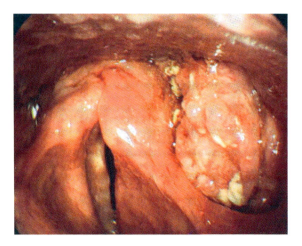

Fig. 2 Hypopharynx carcinoma tumor mass in the left pyriform sinus (indirect rigid hypopharyngolaryngoscopy [From Becker et al. (1983)]

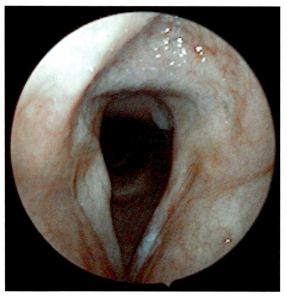

Fig. 4 Leukoplakia of the left vocal fold (flexible hypopharyngolaryngoscopy)

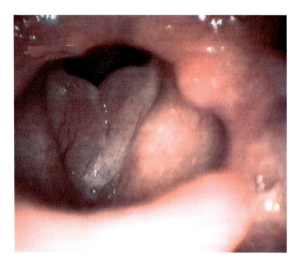

Fig. 3 Reinke's edema (rigid hypopharyngolaryngoscopy)

Reflux Laryngitis. Gastroesophageal/pharyngeal reflux disease can lead to a laryngitis that is not always limited to the posterior larynx. Possible morphological findings are reddening of the arytenoids, hypertrophy in the posterior commissure, contact granuloma of the vocal process, or glottic/subglottic stenosis.

Reinke's Edema. This type of chronic laryngitis frequently occurs in smokers, in patients with vocal abuse or with endocrinological dysfunctions (e.g., menopause, hypothyroidism). It presents with edematous, thickened vocal folds and vasectasias (Fig. 3). The voice typically sounds low and frequently hoarse.

Leukoplakia of the Vocal Folds (Fig. 4, left vocal fold). The epithelium has a white coating, and distinction from malignancy can only be made histologically. Stroboscopy helps judge whether the process is infiltrating or not, but cannot replace histology. If the vocal fold does not vibrate in stroboscopy, an infiltrating process is present, and urgent microlaryngoscopy with biopsy for histological examination is indicated.

Unilateral Vocal Fold Paralysis. The paralyzed vocal fold is in fixed position (median, paramedian, intermediate or lateral), and the arytenoid may be dislocated anteriorly. During phonation, depending on the position of the vocal fold, glottic closure is incomplete. Stroboscopy may be of some prognostic value: the presence of the mucosal wave is a good prognostic sign. Figure 5 shows a left-sided vocal fold paresis in paramedian position.

2.4   Flexible Endoscopic Evaluation of Swallowing (with Sensory Testing)

The flexible endoscopic evaluation of swallowing (FEES), also called videoendoscopic swallowing study (VESS), was introduced by Langmore et al. (1988) and Bastian (1991). This dynamic diagnostic method allows an evaluation of the oropharyngeal

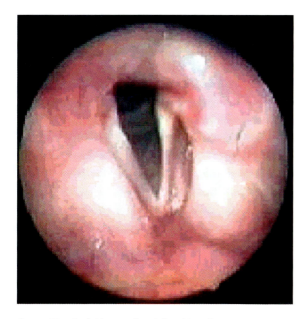

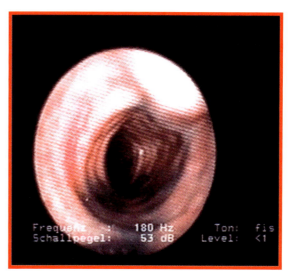

Fig. 6 Aspirate in the trachea—flexible endoscopy via tracheostoma

Fig. 5 Vocal fold paresis, left side (flexible hypopharyngolaryngoscopy)

swallow and has become a routine otorhinolaryngological/phoniatric procedure. It aims at defining the individual swallowing profile of the patient, which enables adequate treatment planning and recommendation for feeding. FEES is considered to be more than a screening procedure and does not only identify dysphagia and aspiration, but reveals the pathophysiology of the swallowing disorder.

Flexible endoscopic evaluation of swallowing with sensory testing (FEESST) is the combination of FEES with laryngopharyngeal sensory testing and was first described by Aviv et al. (1998, 2002). The quantitative testing of sensory thresholds is performed by endoscopically delivered standardized air puffs to the mucosa, innervated by the superior laryngeal nerve to elicit the laryngeal adductor reflex.

According to the modified barium swallow, FEES(ST) is performed as a tailored examination (Bigenzahn and Denk 1999; Denk and Bigenzahn 2005; Schröter-Morasch 1999; Schröter-Morasch et al. 1999; Langmore 2001): colored food in various consistencies is used, depending on the history and clinical findings. Suction must be available in case of aspiration. Before endoscopy, the patient has to be observed during the clinical examination, and neurological symptoms or disorders of speech, language or voice have to be noted.

The patient is in an upright position with the head slightly down to facilitate swallowing function.

Generally, no local anesthetic spray is used, in order not to impair pharyngolaryngeal sensibility. If needed, only cotton balls with a local anesthetic and decongestant are positioned into the nose before endoscopy. The flexible rhinopharyngolaryngoscope is introduced transnasally into the oro- and hypopharynx and is left in place during deglutition. Digital recording allows an analysis in slow motion and discussion of the findings in the interdisciplinary management team.

The endoscopic examination consists of two parts: non-swallowing and swallowing assessment. In the "non-swallowing assessment," anatomy and function are investigated. The mobility of the vocal folds, the occurrence of hyperkinetic movements, pooling/aspiration of saliva, cough reflex (elicited by gently touching the glottis with the tip of the endoscope) and the possibility of intentional (voluntary) throat-clearing are tested. The velum, pharynx and larynx are observed not only during respiration, but also during phonation, breathhold maneuvers, throat-clearing, and coughing to test intentional and reflexive mobility. The second part of the procedure comprises the swallowing assessment, i.e., "dry swallow" with saliva and "food swallows" with measured quantities of food and liquids of different consistencies, dyed with blue food coloring, according to a standardized protocol. The endoscope is positioned in the panoramic view above the tip of the epiglottis. In tracheostomized patients, endoscopy via the tracheostoma is also performed (Fig. 6).

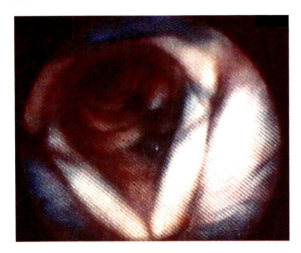

Fig. 7 Aspiration (flexible hypopharyngolaryngoscopy) [From Bigenzahn and Denk (1999)]

Swallowing function is evaluated with regard to saliva pooling, triggering of the swallowing reflex, leaking, penetration, retention, aspiration, cough reflex, and regurgitation. Hypopharyngeal regurgitation leads to suspicion of a hypopharyngeal/esophageal stenosis or Zenker's diverticulum. Aspiration before and after the swallow can be viewed, whereas aspiration during the swallow cannot be seen directly. Also, the amount of aspiration cannot be judged securely (only in patients without cough reflex or tracheostomy). The ability to effectively clear the throat of retention and aspirated material is tested. Finally, compensatory postures, swallowing techniques and various food consistencies are evaluated in order to establish an individually tailored treatment program. Moreover, flexible endoscopy has proved to be a treatment tool for visual biofeedback training in functional swallowing therapy (Denk and Kaider 1997), and it's combination with other diagnostic procedures may be useful. In addition, commercially available "workstations" will eventually comprise sonography, electromyography or other diagnostic methods. Figure 7 shows a static image of aspiration. Colored liquid is pouring down the subglottic region into the trachea.

2.4.1 Advantages and Limitations

The following *limitations* of FEES have to be taken into account:

- There is no direct visualization of the bolus on it's entire path from mouth to stomach as offered by videofluoroscopy.

- Laryngeal closure (due to of epiglottic tilting) and aspiration during the swallow cannot be examined directly. The view during the swallow is obscured because pharyngeal mucosa and the bolus touch the tip of the endoscope.

- Larynx/hyoid elevation and upper esophageal sphincter function are not shown. Diseases of the pharyngoesophageal segment and esophagus can only be indirectly presumed in the case of pharyngeal residue and/or pharyngeal regurgitation.

- Routinely, esophagoscopy is not part of the examination. Some authors propose using a longer flexible endoscope to routinely evaluate the esophagus during FEES (Herrmann 1998), especially when transnasal esophagoscopy is performed (Tong et al. 2012).

The influence of the endoscope as a foreign body during swallowing has not yet been evaluated exactly.

On the contrary, there are many *advantages* to FEES:

- The direct visualization of the upper-aerodigestive tract reveals even subtle morphological or functional findings.

- It is a non-invasive procedure without any radiation exposure, repeatable as often as necessary, and available also as a bedside examination, e.g., in the intensive care unit (ICU).

- Regular food, not barium, is used.

2.4.2 Comparison of FEES(ST) and Videofluoroscopy

The only methods for visualization of aspiration are videofluoroscopy (VFS) and FEES(ST). VFS enables watching the bolus on its entire way from the oral cavity to the stomach, and it was the first instrumental procedure for the assessment of dysphagia (Logemann 1993, 1998; Jones and Donner 1991; Ekberg and Olsson 1997). FEES(ST) shows the upper aerodigestive tract directly. Especially with regard to cost effectiveness, the question arises as to which method is best for the evaluation of dysphagia. The literature and our own studies show that these dynamic methods are not alternative, but rather complementary procedures (Schima and Denk 1998). Both are valuable, and each procedure has it's place in the clinical setting. A study by Aviv (2000) could show that the outcome of dysphagia management with regard to pneumonia incidence was the same using videofluoroscopy and FEES(ST). Comparing the findings of FEES(ST) and VFS, there is widespread agreement with regard to aspiration and retention. Due to the limitations of

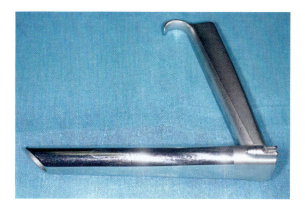

Fig. 8 Laryngoscope according to Kleinsasser for direct microlaryngoscopy

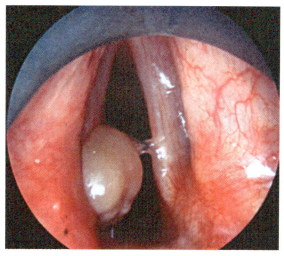

Fig. 9 Granuloma of the left vocal process (direct microlaryngoscopic view, tubeless jet ventilation)

FEES(ST) mentioned above, VFS remains indispensable ("gold standard") for the evaluation of the complete upper digestive tract in a single examination. FEES(ST) is the method of choice for the first-line examination, follow-up examinations, for seriously ill patients in the intensive care unit, and for the evaluation of compensatory maneuvers.

2.5 Direct Endoscopy of the Pharynx and Larynx

Direct rigid endoscopy of the pharynx and larynx, which was developed by Kleinsasser (1968) ("laryngeal suspension microlaryngoscopy"), does not only allow microscopic evaluation of the pharynx and larynx, but also surgical therapies (phonosurgery with the aim of voice improvement, cold steel, and laser surgery). The procedure is carried out under general anesthesia. Various laryngoscopes are available in different sizes and types, e.g. from Kleinsasser (1968) (Fig. 8). The patient lies in the supine position, and after protecting the teeth, the laryngoscope is inserted to the level of the vocal folds while the hypopharynx and supraglottis are being inspected. Then the laryngoscope is held by a laryngoscope holder that rests either on a table over or directly on the patient's chest. The microscope is then positioned.

Recently developed ventilation techniques have led to the possibility of tubeless jet ventilation to avoid intubation (Aloy et al. 1991). This method improves the operative conditions for the surgeon by providing more space for manipulation and better visibility (Fig. 9). Moreover, it is also suited for laryngeal laser surgery, thus avoiding flammable tubes, and for endoscopic surgery of stenoses.

2.5.1 Examples of Typical Findings

Vocal Fold Granuloma. Figure 9 shows the microlaryngoscopical view of a typical vocal fold granuloma, which is located on the vocal process. It may occur after intubation (intubation granuloma) or is often associated with reflux disease (contact granuloma). Additional risk factors for development of a contact granuloma are functional voice disorders and psychogenic factors. For therapy, conservative treatment with proton pump inhibitors and logopaedic voice therapy can be tried. If the pathology persists or if a histological diagnosis is necessary, microlaryngoscopic surgery is performed.

Zenker's Diverticulum. As an alternative to the external approach with resection of a Zenker's diverticulum, endoscopic laser surgery may be performed. In Fig. 10, the party wall between the esophagus and Zenker's diverticulum is seen when endoscopically exposed before laser surgery.

Laryngeal Carcinoma. An irregular mucosal surface or a tumor mass may be observed in the supraglottic (Fig. 11), glottic or subglottic area. Vocal fold motility may be impaired. Depending on the tumor size, the airway may be compromised.

Recurrent Respiratory Papillomatosis (Fig 12). Papillomas are present both at the glottic level (bilaterally), the left supraglottis region and the posterior commissure.

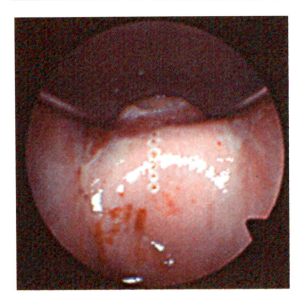

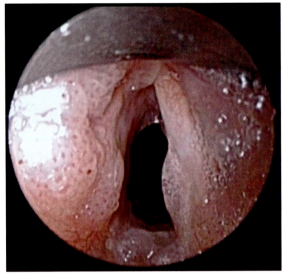

Fig. 10 Zenker's diverticulum (direct hypopharyngoscopic view), intraoperative view on a party wall between the esophagus and Zenker's diverticulum. The laser marking for the planned laser resection can be seen

Fig. 12 Recurrent respiratory papillomatosis of the larynx (direct microlaryngoscopy). Papillomas are seen at the glottis level bilaterally and the left supraglottic region (ventricular fold)

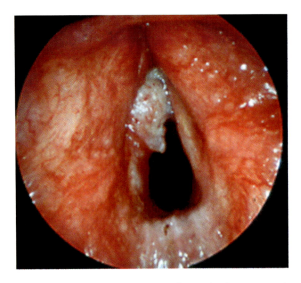

Fig. 11 Carcinoma of the larynx (direct microlaryngoscopy). The tumor mass is seen on the vocal folds

filtered blue light of a xenon short arc lamp and processed by a CCD camera system. During microlaryngoscopy, the use of autofluorescence can improve the early detection of laryngeal cancer and its precursor lesions (Malzahn et al. 2002).

Contact Endoscopy. Contact endoscopy tries to improve the assessment of benign, pre-malignant and malignant pathologies of the larynx during microlaryngoscopy. The aim is to make epithelial cells visible, as in gynecology. After staining the tissue with methylene blue, the magnifications obtained with contact endoscopy (60× and 150×) enable observation of the epithelial cells and their characteristics (Andrea et al. 1995). However, it does not replace biopsy sampling (Warnecke et al. 2010).

3-D Endoscopy. For scientific purposes, 3-D endoscopic techniques were used in microlaryngeal surgery using tubeless jet ventilation (Schragl et al. 1995). This technique has not yet become clinically routine.

2.5.2 Recent Developments and Future Aspects

Among the new technologies designed to enhance information during endoscopy are:

Autofluorescence Endoscopy. The aim of this development is to enhance endoscopic information during microlaryngoscopy. Autofluorescence is induced by the

3 Endoscopy of the Esophagus

Endoscopy of the esophagus as part of endoscopic evaluation of the upper gastrointestinal tract is one of the most frequent procedures performed in Western health care systems (Owings and Kozak 1998). The aim of esophagoscopy is diagnosis, differential diagnosis and follow-up of esophageal diseases. Moreover, endoscopy supports further diagnostic procedures, such as endosonography, and enables therapeutic interventions. Two forms of esophagoscopy are in use: rigid and flexible endoscopy. Gastroenterologists and surgeons are accustomed to using flexible gastroscopes to perform total esophagogastroduodenoscopy, whereas otorhinolaryngologists prefer rigid instruments.

3.1 Symptoms of Esophageal Diseases

As the esophagus provides transport of the bolus in the esophageal phase of swallowing, diseases of the esophagus bring about symptoms related to swallowing function. No single symptom is typical of a specific disorder. The localization of symptoms by the patient is unreliable. Patients who suffer from esophageal diseases (Table 1) may report the following symptoms (see also "Saliva and the Control of Its Secretion"):

- *Dysphagia*. In the case of esophageal stenosis (e.g., esophageal carcinoma) or functional motility disorders (e.g. achalasia of the lower esophageal sphincter), the bolus transport is disturbed and causes the feeling of a stopping of the bolus passage, especially for solid food. The dysphagia symptom needs the analysis of all the four phases of deglutition (oral preparatory, oral, pharyngeal, and esophageal phase), since oropharyngeal and esophageal dysphagia may influence each other or occur in combination. Malignancy correlates with rather fast progression of dysphagia, benign strictures with slowly progressive dysphagia, whereas functional disorders such as achalasia like to vary severity of symptoms over time. Grading of dysphagia can assist indication and quality measurement of treatment (see Table 2).
- *Regurgitation*. Reflux of swallowed bolus material from the esophagus to the pharynx and mouth due to retrograde esophageal motility, stenosing esophageal diseases, or retained material (e.g. in Zenker's diverticulum).
- *Odynophagia*. Painful swallow.
- *Globus sensation* (globus pharyngeus) Globus sensation often derives from gastro-esophageal reflux disease. Other possible underlying causes that have to be considered for differential diagnosis are not only diverticula, webs, and rings, but also

Table 1 Esophageal diseases [modified from Seiden in Parparella et al. (1991)]

Motility disorders

Primary disorders
    Achalasia
    Diffuse esophageal spasm

Nutcracker esophagus

Non-specific dysfunction (hypertensive lower esophageal sphincter, diminished amplitude of esophageal peristalsis)

Secondary disorders
    Scleroderma and other connective tissue disorders
    Diabetes mellitus
    Alcoholism
    Central nervous system disorders
    Presbyesophagus
    Chagas' disease

Structural disorders
    Extrinsic compression
    Webs, rings
    Diverticula
    Stricture due to reflux esophagitis
    Ingestion of caustic substances
    Hiatal hernia
    Varices

Foreign bodies
    Benign tumors
    Malign tumors

Congenital disorders
    Atresias
    Tracheoesophageal fistulas
    Duplications
    Dysphagia lusoria
    Achalasia

Table 2 Grading of dysphagia

0 = able to eat normal diet/no dysphagia.
1 = able to swallow some solid foods
2 = able to swallow only semi-solid foods
3 = able to swallow liquids only
4 = unable to swallow anything/total dysphagia
(Knyrim et al. 1993 N Engl J Med)

thyroid gland diseases, cervical spine syndrome or functional voice disorders.

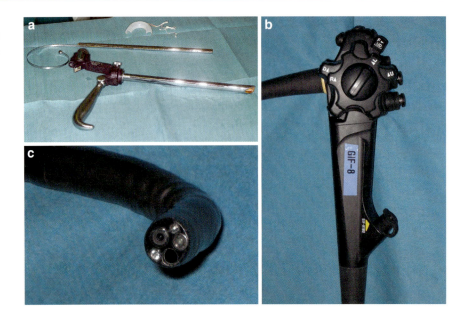

Fig. 13 a Rigid esophagoscope. **b, c** Flexible gastroscope; control part (**b**), tip (**c**)

- *Heartburn, retrocardiac chest pain.* These symptoms occur in gastro-esophageal reflux disease, as well as in esophageal carcinoma, esophageal spasms or esophagitis of other etiologies. In approximately 40 % of patients suffering from reflux disease, the typical symptom of heartburn is lacking. Exclusion of ischemic heart disease, pericarditis, aortic dilatation and pleuritis is mandatory.
- *Cough* of unknown etiology. Cough may be due to aspiration or occur in esophageal reflux disease.
- *Gastrointestinal bleeding.* Bleeding from the mouth without source in the nose, mouth, pharynx or larynx or overt/occult blood in the stool necessitates urgent esophagogastroduodenoscopy.

If one of these symptoms is present, endoscopy of the esophagus is indicated.

Esophagoscopy is appropriate in (suspected) foreign body ingestion or as part of gastroduodenoscopy.

3.2 Rigid Esophagoscopy (Rigid Hypopharyngoesophagoscopy)

Traditionally, rigid (open tube) esophagoscopy is the method of choice for otorhinolaryngologists to remove foreign bodies located in the pharyngoesophageal segment or cervical esophagus and to perform tumor staging (panendoscopy) in patients with primary malignancies in the head and neck to exclude/diagnose

simultaneous additional malignancies (Dhooge et al. 1996). The incidence of simultaneous esophageal malignancies is about 8.4 % (Dammer et al. 1999).

Rigid esophagoscopy is usually performed under general anesthesia after informed consent. The patient lies on his back, with the neck flexed and the head extended. The open-tube esophagoscope (Fig. 13a) is inserted after protection of the teeth. Behind the arytenoids, the esophageal entrance is passed. The esophagoscope has to be advanced gently to avoid perforation. It is not possible to visualize the gastric mucosa safely with an open esophagoscope in all cases. If evaluation of the distal esophagus is needed, an esophagoscope with air insufflation can be used.

Risks include tooth damage, luxation of the arytenoids, bleeding, and perforation of the hypopharynx or esophagus with consecutive mediastinitis or peritonitis. The complication rate is under 1 % (Schmidt et al. 1998).

3.3 Flexible Esophagoscopy

Esophagoscopy is performed for the diagnosis of esophageal diseases, follow-up, additional diagnostic procedures, and for therapeutic measurements (hemostasis, dilatation, stenting, argon plasma coagulation, endoscopic mucosal resection, endoscopic submucosal dissection).

Today, fiber endoscopes have been completely replaced by video endoscopes with CCD cameras (charge coupled device) at the tip. This facilitates additional techniques such as zooming, enhancement of contrast and improvement of resolution (e.g. high-definition technology, endomicroscopy). A channel in these endoscopes allows other instruments (forceps, brush, snare, injection needle, dilatation balloon) to be passed through in order to take tissue samples, remove polyps, inject varices, dilate strictures, etc. The length of the esophagogastroscope (Fig. 13b, c) is about 100–120 cm, with a diameter of about 5–14 mm, depending on it's purpose (ultra-thin stricture endoscope, therapeutic instruments with extra-thick channels). It has become standard to record the examination on a video/DVD recorder or file images in an electronic processing system for documentation. Flexible endoscopy of the esophagus is usually performed on an outpatient basis with local anesthesia, using a spray containing benzocaine or tetracaine hydrochloride. The patient, who has been fasting for 6–8 h prior to endoscopy, is offered intravenous sedation (e.g., with midazolam or propofol). He is placed in the left lateral decubitus position. After a hollow mouthpiece is introduced, the lubricated endoscope is inserted under visual control. In the case of pathological or unclear findings in the hypopharynx or larynx, the patient is referred to the otorhinolaryngologist. The instrument is advanced until the tip of the endoscope reaches the gastro-esophageal junction (approximately 40 cm from the incisors). For examination of the stomach and duodenum (flexible esophagoduodenoscopy), the tip is further advanced through the cardia, and the different portions of the stomach (cardia, fundus, corpus with greater and lesser curvature, antrum) are inspected. Afterwards, the tip is passed through the pylorus, into the duodenal bulb and the descending part of the duodenum.

The examination evaluates the lumen, wall, contents, peristalsis, and appearance of the mucosal surface and it looks at or excludes flat, protruded, or excavated lesions. If indicated, biopsies and brushing for histological, cytological and bacteriological examinations are performed.

Large clinical studies report an incidence of moderate or severe complications in 0.1–0.2 %, with mortality between 1 in 100,000 and 1 in 5,000, depending on the severity and urgency of underlying diseases and the proportion of therapeutic procedures. The complications that may occur are perforation,

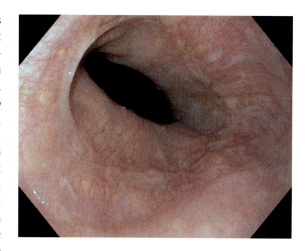

Fig. 14 Esophagogastric junction without pathology

bleeding, cardiopulmonary complications, aspiration, side effects of premedication, and infection.

3.3.1 Examples of Typical Findings

Normal esophagus. The esophageal mucosa (non-keratinizing stratified squamous epithelium) appears pale, whereas the gastric mucosa is reddish (columnar epithelium). The transition between these two types of epithelium (esophagogastric junction) should be very visible. Because of it's saw-toothed pattern, it is called the Z line (Fig. 14).

Reflux esophagitis. Among the many patients with reflux symptoms, endoscopy can define the subgroup of those with reflux esophagitis characterized by reddening, erosions, ulceration or stricture at and above the Z line. A grading of reflux esophagitis can be given with the Savary and Miller (1977), MUSE (metaplasia, ulcer, stricture, erosions), or Los Angeles Classification. According to the grading by Savary and Miller (1977), four or five subgroups are described:

Grade 1, singular erosions; Grade 2, confluent erosions; Grade 3, esophagus covered by circular erosions; Grade 4, complications with peptic stricture, with or without signs of inflammation, or ulceration; Grade 5, Barrett's esophagus. Figure 15 shows a reflux esophagitis Grade 2, Fig. 16 a peptic stricture due to acid reflux.

Barrett's Esophagus. Due to long-lasting peptic reflux, the squamocolumnar junction in the distal

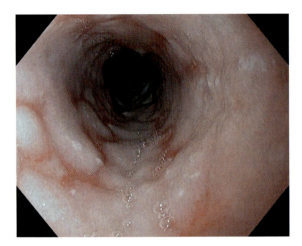

Fig. 15 Reflux esophagitis (grade 2 according to Savary and Miller)

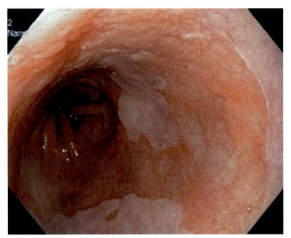

Fig. 17 Metaplasia due to chronic reflux (Barrett's esophagus)

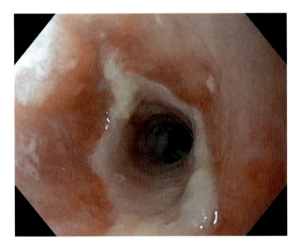

Fig. 16 Peptic stenosis in the distal esophagus

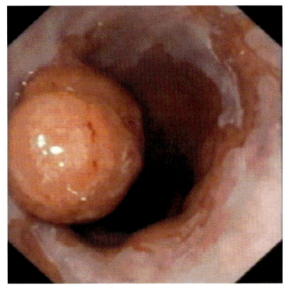

Fig. 18 Early adenocarcinoma in Barrett's esophagus

esophagus moves upwards and the squamous epithelium is replaced by a specialized columnar epithelium with intestinal metaplasia. It's extent is described by the Prague classification, with "C" for circumferential extent and "M" for the maximal longitudinal extent of Barrett's esophagus in centimeters. Barrett's metaplasia (Fig. 17) is a well-known risk factor for the development of dysplasia and adenocarcinoma (Fig. 18, early adenocarcinoma in Barrett's esophagus). Endoscopically, metaplastic gastric mucosa is recognized in the esophagus because of it's salmon-red appearance. Therefore, follow-up examinations with biopsies are necessary. For improving the diagnostic yield, chromoendoscopy with acetic acid (Fig. 19) or indigocarmine, optical filter technology

(NBI) or digital image reprocessing should be added to the routine procedure.

Esophageal carcinoma. Endoscopy shows early cancer (Fig. 20) or a polypoid or ulcerated mass or infiltration that can obstruct the esophageal lumen (Fig. 21). Multiple biopsies are taken for histological diagnosis. The incidence of adenocarcinomas derived from Barrett's esophagus has increased dramatically in the USA and Europe, whereas the alcohol and tobacco-associated squamous cell carcinoma has become less frequent. High-grade dysplasia and early cancer limited to the mucosa or superficial submucosa

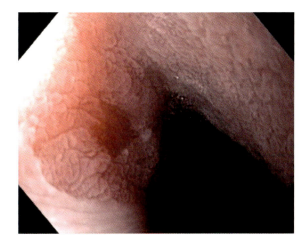

Fig. 19 Barrett's esophagus with high-grade dysplasia, chromoendoscopy with acetic acid

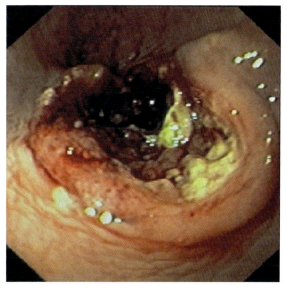

Fig. 21 Advanced ulcerated squamous cell carcinoma of the distal esophagus

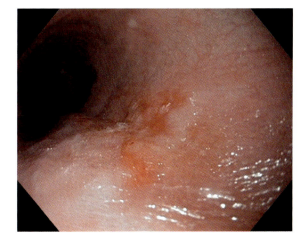

Fig. 20 Early squamous cell carcinoma of the mid-esophagus

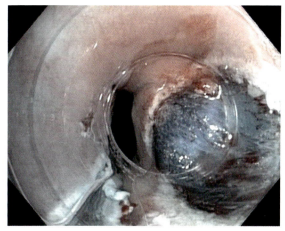

Fig. 22 Endoscopic mucosal resection

can now be removed endoscopically by endoscopic mucosal resection (EMR- Fig. 22) or endoscopic submucosal dissection (ESD). Photodynamic therapy and radiofrequency ablation can assist in curative treatment of these pre-malignant and early malignant states. In the case of a symptomatic tumor stricture, a balloon dilatation or bougienage can be performed (Fig. 23) and a metal stent positioned as part of a multimodal therapy or a palliative approach (Fig. 24).

Varices: In portal hypertension, collaterals are found preferably in the distal esophagus. The blue, more or less prominent strings can be ligated endoscopically with rubber bands or injected with glue to treat or prevent bleeding (Fig. 25).

Schatzki Ring. Endoscopy reveals a stricturing membrane in the distal esophagus. It may cause dysphagia, especially concerning solid food, and give rise to an impacted foreign body. For therapy, dilatation or thermal ablation during endoscopy is performed.

Soor esophagitis. A white cover or single white spots (Fig. 26) are seen on the esophageal wall; they can be removed with forceps, but not with rinsing. Brush cytology easily depicts *Candida* during microscopic examination.

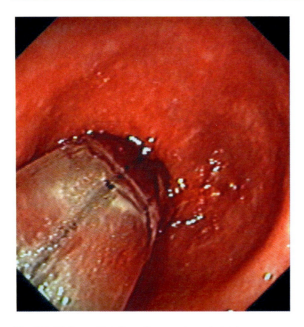

Fig. 23 Balloon dilatation of an esophageal stricture

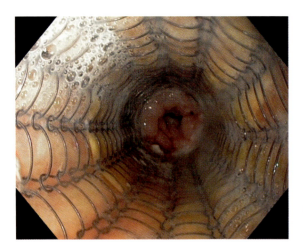

Fig. 24 Metallic stent for palliation of obstructing tumor

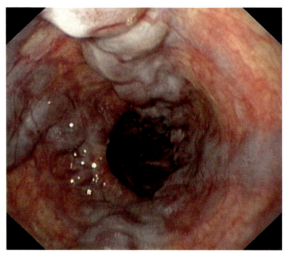

Fig. 25 Esophageal varices

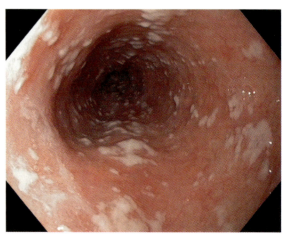

Fig. 26 Soor esophagitis

Viral esophagitis. In immunocompromized patients, viral infections (e.g., herpes simplex, cytomegalovirus) can lead to inflammation of the esophagus with scattered ulcers. Biopsies prove the diagnosis by histologic, immunochemical or molecular evidence (Fig. 27)..

Eosinophilic esophagitis. This is an allergic inflammation of the esophageal wall, histologically characterized by infiltrating eosinophilic granulocytes. Ridges, furrows, or rings, as well as white exudates may be seen in the esophagus. Topical steroids are a preferred treatment. (Fig. 28).

Esophageal web. Esophageal webs may be due to reflux disease, iron deficiency anemia (Plummer Vinson syndrome) or idiopathy. They are either destroyed when passing the endoscope or removed with dilatation or bougienage.

Achalasia. Achalasia is a neuromuscular disorder of the esophagus that is characterized by a delayed esophageal emptying due to inadequate esophageal peristalsis and a non-relaxing, hypertensive lower esophageal sphincter. The diagnostic method of choice is videofluoroscopy and manometry, but endoscopy is necessary to rule out other causes of dysphagia. It shows a dilated esophagus, weak non-propulsive esophageal peristalsis, and retention of secretion and food. Endoscopic ultrasound reveals a

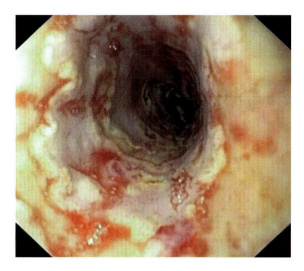

Fig. 27 Herpetic esophagitis with severe ulcerations in an immunocompromised patient

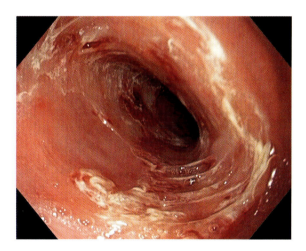

Fig. 28 Eosinophilic esophagitis

thickened hypertrophic muscle layer of the esophagogastric sphincter. Endoscopy can also be used for therapeutic purposes, as pneumatic dilatation or botulinum toxin injection. POEM (peroral endoscopic myotomy), a newly emerging endoscopic technique, becomes an alternative to the classical surgical Heller myotomy.

3.3.2 Endoscopic Ultrasound

The combined endoscopic and sonographic evaluation of the esophagus (endoscopic ultrasound, EUS) allows the identification of the different layers of the esophageal wall and contributes to the staging of esophageal tumors and locoregional nodal involvement (Tio 1998; Bergman and Fockens 1999; Richards et al. 2000; Wakelin et al. 2002). EUS proved to have a better accuracy in staging, especially in T1 and T2 tumors, than computed tomography (Ziegler et al. 1988; Tio 1998). High-frequency EUS has been performed in early esophageal cancer to select patients for local endoscopic treatment.

EUS is a valuable tool to differentiate and further define submucosal tumors and extrinsic compression. Adding fine needle aspiration to EUS substantially improves the detection of malignancies in mediastinal processes or tumors of the esophagus wall.

3.4 Rigid Versus Flexible Esophagoscopy

Both methods are less competing than complementing each other (Hörmann and Schmidt 1998): flexible equipment provides better imaging and allows air insufflation for distension, whereas rigid endoscopes facilitate instrumentation. Traditionally, otorhinolaryngology focuses on rigid hypopharyngoesophagoscopy for removing foreign bodies and for panendoscopy in patients with malignant tumors in the upper aerodigestive tract to reveal additional simultaneous malignancies. Gastroenterology uses the flexible endoscope not only for the endoscopic evaluation of the esophagus, but also of the stomach and duodenum (esophagogastroduodenoscopy, EGD). The indication for rigid or flexible endoscopy depends on the individual case and the experience of the surgeon (Schmidt et al. 2010).

Rigid esophagoscopy is superior to flexible endoscopy in the evaluation of the hypopharynx and cervical esophagus. The skill and experience of the examiner remains of utmost importance (Monnier and Lang 1997). Flexible esophagoscopy does not allow a distinct examination of the upper esophageal sphincter region. In case of suspected malignancy in this region, rigid endoscopy should be performed. As foreign bodies are found to be lodged mostly in the proximal esophagus, rigid endoscopy is an adequate procedure for the management of (suspected) foreign body ingestion (Alberty et al. 2001). Due to a higher perforation risk in the distal portion of the esophagus with rigid esophagoscopy, foreign bodies in that part are often removed by flexible endoscopy.

3.5   Recent Developments and Future Prospects

The development of ultra-thin esophagogastroscopes with an outer diameter of 5–6 mm allows the transnasal insertion of the endoscope, which may give rise to a greater acceptability and less discomfort for the patient (transnasal esophagogastroscopy). *Chromoendoscopy* has become a valuable adjunct to flexible endoscopy in oncological indications. It remains uncertain whether new technologies, such as *zoom endoscopy, spectroscopy, optical coherence tomography, endocytoscopy* or *confocal laser microscopy*, will become clinical routine. For sure, molecular pathological analysis of specimens will be of great clinical importance in the future.

4   Role of Endoscopy in the Diagnostic Work-up of Dysphagic Patients

Differential diagnosis of dysphagia is based on endoscopy and histopathological findings of biopsies, radiography, manometry and (impedance/) pH-metry. Radiology and endoscopy are both standard procedures that complement each other. Esophagoscopy is routinely performed to search for malignancy or to extract a foreign body. It is a method of first choice and capable of performing the differential diagnosis between structural or functional disorders. For motility disorders, videofluoroscopy, endoscopic ultrasound, manometry or (impedance/) pH-metry should be performed.

The advantage of radiographic studies is the identification of esophagotracheal fistulas, diverticula, atresia and hiatal/paraesophageal hernia. For radiological evaluation of dysphagia, the dynamic method of videofluoroscopy is regarded as the gold standard. However, subtle morphological changes are not radiographically visible.

The diagnostic indications for esophagoscopy are a matter of discussion: Should endoscopy be performed primarily or not? Because of direct visualization, endoscopy is best for assessing mucosal integrity, inflammation and malignancies. Furthermore, it enables biopsies to be taken for histological examination. Therefore, endoscopic follow-up is indicated in many diseases, e.g. Barrett's epithelium or achalasia.

In the last few years, gastrointestinal endoscopy has gradually replaced gastrointestinal radiography as the initial diagnostic study for the majority of patients with suspected gastrointestinal pathology. Technical developments (advances in lighting, imaging and flexibility) have improved the sensitivity and specificity and have made it a widely used examination technique.

5   Conclusion

Endoscopy of the hypopharynx and esophagus contributes to the diagnostic work-up of the dysphagic patient. In many cases, it is the method of choice. However, radiography, especially videofluoroscopy, remains indispensable. For the future, the technical progress will stimulate and enable new endoscopic and radiographic developments. It aims at the highest possible quality of diagnosis and optimal patient acceptability.

References

Alberty J, Müller C, Stoll W (2001) Is the rigid hypopharyngo-esophagoscopy for suspected body impaction still up to date? Laryngo Rhino Otol 80:682–686

Aloy A, Schachner M, Cancura W (1991) Tubeless translaryngeal superimposed jet ventilation. Eur Arch Otorhinolaryngol 248(8):475–478

Andrea M, Dias O, Santos A (1995) Contact endoscopy during microlaryngeal surgery. A new technique for endoscopic examination of the larynx. Ann Otol Rhinol Laryngol 104:333–339

Aviv JE (2000) Prospective, randomized outcome study of endoscopy versus modified barium swallow in patients with dysphagia. Laryngoscope 110(4):563–574

Aviv JE, Kim T, Sacco RL, Kaplan S, Goodhart K, Diamond B, Close LG (1998) FEESST: a new bedside endoscopic test of the motor and sensory components of swallowing. Ann Otol Rhinol Laryngol 107:378–387

Aviv JE, Spitzer J, Cohen M, Ma G, Belafsky P, Close LG (2002) Laryngeal adductor reflex and pharyngeal squeeze as predictors of laryngeal penetration and aspiration. Laryngoscope 112(2):338–341

Bastian RW (1991) Videoendoscopic evaluation of patients with dysphagia: an adjunct to the modified barium swallow. Otolaryngol Head Neck Surg 104(3):339–350

Becker W, Naumann HH, Pfaltz CR (1983) Atlas der Hals-Nasen-Ohrenkrankheiten, 2nd edn. Thieme, Stuttgart

Bergman JJ, Fockens P (1999) Endoscopic ultrasonography in patients with gastro-esophageal cancer. Eur J Ultrasound 10(2–3):127–138

Bigenzahn W, Denk D-M (1999) Oropharyngeale Dysphagien. Ätiologie, Klinik, Diagnostik und Therapie von Schluckstörungen. Thieme, Stuttgart

Dammer R, Bonkowski V, Kutz R, Friesenecker J, Schüsselbauer T (1999) Early diagnosis of additional tumors at diagnosis of primary oral carcinoma using panendoscopy. Mund Kiefer Gesichtschir 3:61–66

Denk DM, Bigenzahn W (2005) Management oropharyngealer Dysphagien. Eine Standortbestimmmung [Management of oropharyngeal dysphagia. Current status]. HNO 53(7):661–672

Denk D-M, Kaider A (1997) Videoendoscopic biofeedback: a simple method to improve the efficacy of swallowing rehabilitation of patients after head and neck surgery. Otorhinolaryngol 59: 100–105

Dhooge IJ, De Vos M, Albers FW, Van Cauwenberge PB (1996) Panendoscopy as a screening procedure for simultaneous primary tumors in head and neck cancer. Eur Arch Otorhinolaryngol 253(6):319–324

Ekberg O, Olsson R (1997) Dynamic radiology of swallowing disorders. Endoscopy 29(6):439–446

Herrmann I (1998) Advanced course in Videopanendoscopy, vol 32. Fortbildungsveranstaltung für HNO-Ärzte, Hannover

Hörmann K, Schmidt H (1998) Flexible endosopy in ENT practice. HNO 46:654–659

Jones B, Donner MW (1991) The tailored examination. In: Jones B, Donner MW (eds) Normal and abnormal swallowing: imaging in diagnosis and therapy. Springer, Berlin, pp 33–50

Kawaida M, Fukuda H, Kohno N (2002) Digital image processing of laryngeal lesions by electronic videoendoscopy. Laryngoscope 112:559–564

Kleinsasser O (1968) Mikrolaryngoskopie und endolaryngeale Mikrochirurgie. Technik und typische Befunde, Schattauer

Knyrim K, Wagner HJ, Bethge N, Keymling M, Vakil N (1993) A controlled trial of an expansile metal stent for palliation of esophageal obstruction due to inoperable cancer. N Engl J Med. 28, 329(18):1302–1307

Langmore SE (2001) Endoscopic evaluation and treatment of swallowing disorders. Thieme, Stuttgart

Langmore SE, Schatz K, Olsen N (1988) Fiberoptic endoscopic examination of swallowing safety: a new procedure. Dysphagia 2(4):216–219

Logemann J (1993) Manual for the videofluorographic study of swallowing, 2nd edn. Pro-ed, Texas

Logemann JA (1998) Evaluation and treatment of swallowing disorders. Pro-ed, Austin

Malzahn K, Dreyer T, Glanz H, Arens Ch (2002) Autofluorescence endoscopy in the diagnosis of early laryngeal cancer and its precursor lesions. Laryngoscope 112:488–493

Monnier P, Lang FJ (1997) Current position of endoscopy in otorhinolaryngology. HNO 45(11):886–887

Owings MF, Kozak LJ (1998) Ambulatory and inpatient procedure in the United States. Vital Health Stat US-DHSS 139:1–13

Parparella MM, Shumrick DA, Gluckmann JL, Meyerhoff WL (1991) Otolaryngology. Head and Neck, vol 3. WB Saunders Company, Philadelphia

Richards DG, Brown TH, Manson JM (2000) Endoscopic ultrasound in the staging of tumour of the esophagus and gastroesophageal junction. Ann R Coll Surg Engl 82(5):311–317

Savary M, Miller G (1977) Der Ösophagus. Lehrbuch und endoskopischer Atlas, Gassmann, Solothurn

Schima W, Denk D-M (1998) Videofluoroscopic and videoendoscopic studies: complementary methods for assessment of dysphagia. Proceedings, EGDG, Vienna

Schmidt H, Hormann K, Stasche N, Steiner W (1998) Tracheobronchoscopy and esophagoscopy in otorhinolaryngology. An assessment of current status. HNO 46(7):643–650

Schmidt H, Hormann K, Stasche N, Steiner W (2010) ENT-recommendations for esophagoscopy. Laryngo-Rhino Otol 89:540–543

Schragl E, Bigenzahn W, Donner A, Gradwohl I, Aloy A (1995) Laryngeal surgery with 3-D technique. Early results with the jet-laryngoscope in superimposed high-frequency jet ventilation. Anaesthesist 44(1):48–53

Schröter-Morasch H (1999) Klinische Untersuchung des Oropharynx und videoendoskopische Untersuchung der Schluckfunktion. In: Bartolome G (Hrsg) Schluckstörungen. Diagnostik und Rehabilitation vol 2. Aufl., Urban & Fischer, München-Jena, New York, pp 111–140

Schröter-Morasch H, Bartolome G, Troppmann N, Ziegler W (1999) Values and limitations of pharyngolaryngoscopy (transnasal, transoral) in patients with dysphagia. Folia Phoniatr Logop 51(4–5):172–182

Tio TL (1998) Endosonography in gastroenterology. Springer, Heidelberg

Tong MC, Gao H, Lin JS, Ng LK, Sang Chan H, Kwan Ng S. (2012) One-stop evaluation of globus pharyngeus symptoms with transnasal esophagoscopy and swallowing function test. J Otolaryngol Head Neck Surg 41(1):46–50

Wakelin SJ, Deans C, Crofts TJ, Allan PL, Plevris JN, Paterson-Brown S (2002) A comparison of computerised tomography, laparoscopic ultrasound and endoscopic ultrasound in the properative staging of osophago-gastric carcinoma. Eur J Radiol 41(2):161–167

Warnecke A, Averbeck T, Leinung M, Soudah B, Wenzel GI, Kreipe HH, Lenarz T, Stöver T (2010) Contact endoscopy for the evaluation of the pharyngeal and laryngeal mucosa. Laryngoscope 120(2):253–258

Ziegler K, Sanft C, Semsch B, Friedrich M, Gregor M, Riecken EO (1988) Endosonography is superior to computed tomography in staging tumors of the esophagus and the cardia. Gastroenterology 94:A267

Part IV
Treatment

The Therapeutic Swallowing Study

Margareta Bülow and Bonnie Martin-Harris

Contents

M. Bülow (✉)
Neurological Department and Diagnostic Centre
of Imaging and Functional Medicine,
Skåne University Hospital, 205 02 Malmö, Sweden
e-mail: margareta.bulow@med.lu.se

B. Martin-Harris
MUSC Evelyn Trammell Institute
for Voice and Swallowing Disorders,
Otolaryngology Head and Neck Surgery,
Medical University of South Carolina,
Charleston, SC, USA

Abstract

Videoradiography is one of the most frequently used instrumental techniques to assess oral and pharyngeal swallowing dysfunction. A therapeutic swallowing study should always be performed in collaboration between a trained speech/language pathologist and a radiologist. Focus during the examination is the oral and pharyngeal phases of deglutition. The swallowing function is tested with various bolus volumes and textures. Implementation of trial therapeutic strategies is another important component of the examination. The study is recorded on a dynamic medium making it possible to analyse structural movements in relation to constant flow after the examination. After the examination the SLP and the radiologist document a collaborative report.

1 Introduction

In the selection of an instrumental procedure to assess oral and pharyngeal swallowing dysfunction, videoradiography is considered the gold standard and is one of the most frequently used techniques (Donner 1988; Jones and Donner 1989; Ekberg 1990, 1992; Dodds et al. 1990a, b; Bingjie et al. 2010). The choice of instrumental technique has to be based on what the clinician wants to know to be able to make adequate decisions regarding therapeutic strategies. The video-fluoroscopic swallowing study is also referred to as the modified barium swallow study and has been shown to have high clinical yield (Martin-Harris et al. 2000; Gates et al. 2006, Martin-Harris and Jones 2008).

O. Ekberg (ed.), *Dysphagia*, Medical Radiology. Diagnostic Imaging, DOI: 10.1007/174_2011_351,
© Springer-Verlag Berlin Heidelberg 2012

Because of the therapeutic implications of the swallowing study, as well as the therapeutic approaches that can be applied and tested during the examination, the study will be described as "the therapeutic swallowing study" in this chapter. The therapeutic swallowing study permits observation of upper aerodigestive tract function as the patient swallows various volumes and textures of different radiopaque materials (Logemann 1986) and requires specialized training for accurate and reliable implementation and interpretation of test results (Logemann et al. 2000).

The study can be recorded on a dynamic medium such as videotape or computer disk, making it possible to analyse structural movements in relation to contrast flow in slow motion and frame by frame. However, nowadays digital radiography i.e. different high-resolution videofluoroscopic recording devices, is used in most radiology departments. The examination can be transmitted digitally to an electronic picture archiving and communication system to provide rapid retrieval and analyses of the entire swallowing sequence. The availability is excellent and easy to handle and any pathophysiological feature can be analysed in detail related to the flow of different given textures. For example, disordered timing and coordination of structural movement, and the presence, degree, timing and cause of aspiration can be documented.

The therapeutic swallowing study is a dynamic procedure that examines the mechanical passage of food and liquid from the mouth to the stomach. However, in most studies the focus lies on oral and pharyngeal phases of deglutition. Comprehensive examination includes the observation of oral bolus manipulation, lingual motility efficiency of mastication, timing of pharyngeal swallow initiation, soft palate elevation and retraction, tongue base retraction, pharyngeal contraction, superior and anterior hyolaryngeal movement, epiglottic inversion and extent and duration of pharyngo-oesophageal segment opening (Martin-Harris et al. 2000) (Fig. 1).

In a study from 2008, the aim was to test reliability, content, construction, and external validity of a new modified barium swallow study tool, MBSImp. The authors found that: "The MBSImp demonstrated clinical practicality, favourable inter- and intrarater reliability following standardized training, content, and external validity" (Martin Harris et al. 2008). Voluntary acceptance of universal standards for modified barium swallow protocol administration and interpretation is, however, of importance.

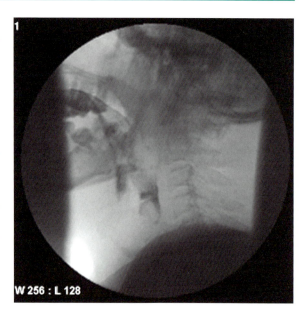

Fig. 1 Pharyngeal dysfunction

Various therapeutic strategies, such as postural techniques, manoeuvres and techniques improving oral sensory awareness can be systematically applied and tested and their effect on function can be observed (Ekberg 1986; Logemann et al. 1989; Martin et al. 1993; Martin 1994; Bülow et al. 2001). Different materials are given to the patient to identify optimal food and liquid textures that facilitate a safe and efficient oral intake.

Clinical experience and research findings provide evidence that aspiration, and more importantly the cause of aspiration, can be missed during observations made from test swallows included in a clinical or bedside examination. Studies have shown that clinicians do not consistently identify the presence of aspiration during clinical examinations. The sensitivity and specificity of the bedside examination in the detection of aspiration and in predicting patient outcome warrants further study. Furthermore, it has been reported that 50–60% of patients who aspirate do not cough (Linden and Siebens 1983; Splaingard et al. 1988; De Pippo et al. 1992; Nathadwarawala et al. 1992, 1994; Zenner et al. 1995). Despite its limitations, the bedside or non-instrumental examination provides important information regarding signs and symptoms of potential swallowing disorders and the need for further instrumental examination, impressions regarding the patient's language and cognitive status, propensity of the patient for fatigue during eating and drinking, and a realistic picture of the patient's eating and drinking patterns.

2 How To Perform the Study

In the radiology department at Skåne University Hospital, Malmö, Sweden, we have had almost 20 years' experience with a swallowing assessment team that includes collaboration between a speech/language pathologist and a radiologist in the performance and analysis of the therapeutic swallowing study. The speech/language pathologist has her own schedule at the laboratory (Fig. 2) and schedules her own patients. The teamwork of the two specialists provides rapid and adequate information about current swallowing dysfunction and management recommendations to the referring clinician, patient and caregivers.

The swallowing recording equipment includes:
- Philips MultiDiagnost Eleva.
- Digital technique.
- Picture archiving and communication system
- Microphone.

Other equipment used is the KayPENTAX 7245C, a swallowing workstation mostly used in swallowing research

The patient is given controlled food and liquid textures that are mixed with contrast material, resulting in a simulated diet but one that is dense enough to allow X-ray visualization. Typically, barium sulphate is used and allows for optimal visualization of bolus passage through the alimentary tract (Murray 1999). However, the sensory properties of food may be affected by adding barium sulphate (Ekberg et al. 2009). In another study, the importance of rheologically matched test materials is discussed (Groher et al. 2006).

The procedure is most often performed with the patient seated in an upright position. If the individual is unable to assume and maintain a seating position, adaptive seating devices can be employed. If these devices are not available, the patient may be placed on the fluoroscopic table and the examination is performed with the patient lying down. The patient's head and trunk can then be raised to a semiupright position. The individual can also be positioned seated in his or her own wheelchair if there is adequate distance between the floor and fluoroscopic tube to permit oropharyngeal and cervical oesophageal viewing.

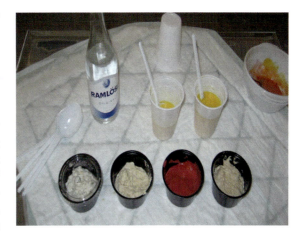

Fig. 2 The laboratory

The study typically begins with the subject in lateral view, the optimal position for visualizing penetration or aspiration of material into the laryngeal vestibule before, during and after swallowing. In lateral view, the profile contours of the soft palate, base of the tongue, posterior pharyngeal wall, epiglottis, aryepiglottic folds, anterior hypopharyngeal wall and the region of the cricopharyngeal muscle or pharyngo-oesophageal segment can be assessed. Following swallowing assessment in the lateral view, the patient is positioned in a frontal view, permitting assessment regarding asymmetric contours, the surface of the base of the tongue, median and lateral glossoepiglottic folds, tonsillar fossa, valleculae and hypopharynx.

In our experience, the amount of radiation during the study is low, 2–5 mSv (absorbed dose), which is about one eighth of the amount in a colon examination. The average radiation exposure time is 2–3 min. Radiation doses in videofluoroscopic swallow studies were studied in a study from the UK from 2007. Zammit-Maempel et al. (2007) concluded that videofluoroscopy can be performed using a minimal radiation dose. Their data are based on the largest number of videofluoroscopic swallowing studies published to date.

It is critical that caregivers, nurses (e.g. depending on the medical status of the patient) and/or family members observe the study either at the time of the examination or at a later viewing of the recorded examination. This provides the opportunity to educate the caregivers in the nature of the patient's swallowing problem, and the necessary precautions and management strategies that must be applied to ensure airway protection and efficient oral intake.

3   Routines During the Study

The swallowing therapist
- Decides how the procedure will be performed on the basis of observations of the patient during the bedside examination. The volumes and textures of contrast materials used in the study should be tailored to meet the particular needs of the patient on the basis of his or her clinical swallowing presentation.
- Selects and prepares contrast materials (mixing, measured volumes, order).
- Prepares the patient for the examination.
- Provides instructions and administers contrast materials.
- Systematically applies trial therapeutic strategies based on the observed nature of the swallowing disorder.
- Documents a collaborative report with the radiologist that includes recommendations for non-oral intake, appropriate food/liquid textures and bolus volumes, and necessary therapeutic strategies such as compensatory postures, manoeuvres and exercises.
- Completes the swallowing protocol during the procedure.

   The radiologist
- Operates the fluoroscopic equipment and observes anatomic abnormalities.
- Documents a collaborative report with the swallowing therapist.

   The assistant nurse
- Prepares the fluoroscopy suite for the study.
- Prepares the appropriate test material.
- Completes the registration and operates the videotape recorder.
- Assists the patient before and after the study.
- Completes the swallowing protocol during the procedure.

4   Test Material

Every procedure is individually adapted to the patient, even if the same routines are used. If there is a suspicion of aspiration and/or it is not known for sure whether the patient will initiate a pharyngeal swallow,

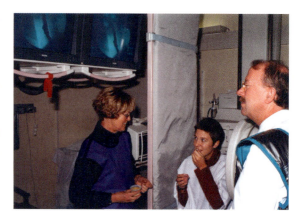

Fig. 3 Test material

the procedure starts with 2 or 3 ml of water-soluble contrast material either as thin or thickened liquid. The patient may not be exposed to any risks of aspiration pneumonia.

The normal procedure consists of material (Fig. 3) with the following consistencies:
- Pudding.
- Timbale (smooth consistency).
- Sorbet.
- Paté (corny consistency).
- Chopped solid material: either meat or vegetables in sauce.
- Thickened liquid.
- Carbonated liquid.
- Thin liquid.

When mastication is tested, some sort of crisp bread covered with barium paste can be used.

Every test material is, if possible, given twice in various amounts from 3 to 5 to 10 ml or more. However, depending on the severity of the swallowing impairment and the degree of aspiration, water-soluble contrast material may be used. The patients may be fed by the assistant nurse but may also feed themselves, giving important information about their habitual eating and drinking behaviours. For example, patients suffering from right hemispheric damage often take excessive amounts of solids and liquids during mealtime. This is important behaviour to identify and modify. Studies showing typical bolus volume during thin liquid swallows indicate that the average volume habitually ingested is 21.3–29.3 ml

Table 1 Recipe of material for the therapeutic swallowing study

1 portion of solid bolus consists of 45 g product and 15 g E-Z-HD barium sulphate for suspension and gives 60 g ready-mixed material (0.5 dl)

1 portion of thickened liquid consists of 100 g product and 30 g E-Z-HD barium sulphate for suspension and gives 130 g ready-mixed material (1 dl)

1 portion of thin liquid consists of E-Z-HD barium sulphate for suspension 40% w/w

1 portion of carbonated liquid consists of E-Z-HD barium sulphate for suspension 40% w/w mixed with sodium bicarbonate (Samarin®) (4g). This material of this consistency must be swallowed immediately after it has been prepared, otherwise the gas will disappear

by males and 13.6–20.4 ml by females (Adnerhill et al. 1989). If the patient wishes, or if he or she reports symptoms with only very specific food or liquid items, he or she may bring material to the examination, where it will be mixed with barium contrast material and tested.

The test material we use is prepared in the hospital kitchen even though it is nowadays possible to buy ready-made test meals from the food industry. Our test material is prepared according to our recipe (Table 1) and the radiology department provides the kitchen with barium sulphate. The test materials are prepared from ordinary food, familiar to the patients and easy to recognize, even though the sensory properties of the test food may be affected by adding barium sulphate. However, we have learned from clinical experience from thousands of examinations that it is possible to analyse the nature of the actual dysfunction and to decide on most appropriate therapeutic strategies, and thereby guide the patient to a safe nutrition. When the material comes to the radiology department in small cans, 0.5 dl for a solid bolus and 1 dl for liquids, it is placed in a freezer. Before every assessment the assistant nurse takes the material from the freezer in time for the study. Every patient gets his or her individual combination of test material depending on the nature of the swallowing problem.

5 Protocol I: Therapeutic Videoradiographic Swallowing Examination

The protocol is given in Table 2.

6 Protocol II: Therapeutic Videoradiographic Swallowing Examination

The protocol is given in Table 3.

7 Swallowing Management

Upon completion of the therapeutic swallowing study, the swallowing therapist has identified the nature and severity of the swallowing disorder, made recommendations for oral versus non-oral intake, and designs an individual treatment plan directed towards specific swallowing functional outcome goals. Every applied treatment strategy must be based on a sound rationale according to the nature of the swallowing problem and the physical and cognitive status of the patient. In a systematic review from 2010, Speyer et al. (2010) found that there still are many questions remaining regarding the effect of different therapeutic strategies in oropharyngeal dysphagia performed by speech/language therapists. Also, other studies have concluded that further research is necessary to evaluate the effectiveness of dysphagia treatment (Ashford et al. 2009; McCabe et al. 2009).

Strategies may include postural techniques, sensory improvement techniques, swallowing manoeuvres, isometric exercises applied to the muscle groups of the tongue and suprahyoid musculature, and bolus volume and texture modification. Combinations of different management strategies are often used (Bülow et al. 1999; Bodèn et al. 2006; Carnaby et al. 2006; Logemann 2008; Pauloski 2008).

Table 2 Protocol for therapeutic videoradiographic swallowing examination

Therapeutic videoradiographic swallowing study

Date:_____ Examination no:

Name:_____Person number:

Actual status:_____

Nutrition: Oral 100% 50% 25% Non-oral: Nasogastric tube Percutaneous endoscopic gastrostomy (PEG) Infusion

Actual diet: Solid bolus: Liquids:

	1 ml 2 ml 3 ml	5 ml 10 ml	15 ml 20 ml	Independent Has to be fed Syringe	Oral dysfunction	Delayed pharyngeal swallow	Absent pharyngeal swallow	Pharyngeal retention Mild Moderate Severe	Penetration Subepiglottic Supraglottic Tracheal
Solids (smooth consistency)									
Sorbet									
Timbale (smooth consistency)									
Paté (corny consistency)									
Chopped food									
Regular food									
Thin liquid									
Thickened liquid									
Carbonated liquid (Samarin)									
Water-soluble contrast material									
Bread									
Other									

Therapeutic strategies

Sensory stimulation

   Thermal–tactile stimulation

   Push down with a spoon against the tongue

   Larger bolus volume

   Cold sour bolus—sorbet

   Chewing

Postural techniques

   Chin tuck

   Head back

   Head rotated to damaged side

   Head rotated

   Head tilt to stronger side

Swallowing techniques

   Supraglottic swallow

   Super supraglottic swallow

   Effortful swallow

   Mendelsohn manoeuvre

Recommended treatment:
Diet modification:

Table 3 Protocol for therapeutic videoradiographic swallowing examination. Radiology Department, University Hospital MAS, Malmö

Examination number: .... Date of examination: ....

Name: .... Person no ....

Medical diagnosis: ....

Remitter: ....

Examination performed by: ....

		Consistencies				
		Thin liquid	Thick liquid	Pudding	Puree	Solid bolus
Lateral view						
Oral preparation	Normal	0	0	0	0	0
	Incomplete lip closure	1	1	1	1	1
	Delayed bolus preparation	2	2	2	2	2
	Diffuse spreading of bolus in oral cavity	2	2	2	2	2
Oral phase	Normal	0	0	0	0	0
Leakage	Anterior	1	1	1	1	1
		2	2	2	2	2
	Posterior	1	1	1	1	1
		2	2	2	2	2
Tongue movements	Normal coordination	0	0	0	0	0
	Inefficient	1	1	1	1	1
Mastication	Normal	0	0	0	0	0
	Inefficient	1	1	1	1	1
Delayed bolus transport	Mild	1	1	1	1	1
	Moderate	2	2	2	2	2
Regurgitation into nasal cavity		1	1	1	1	1
Dissociation	<0.5 s	0	0	0	0	0
	0.5–2 s	1	1	1	1	1
	3–5 s	2	2	2	2	2
	>5 s	3	3	3	3	3

(continued)

Table 3 (continued)

Pharyngeal phase

Laryngeal elevation	Normal	0	0	0	0	0
Movements of hyoid bone	Reduced	1	1	1	1	1
	Anterior movement incomplete	2	2	2	2	2
	Elevation absent	3	3	3	3	3
Epiglottic movement	Normal	0	0	0	0	0
	Incomplete	1	1	1	1	1
Vestibulum penetration/aspiration	No	0	0	0	0	0
	Subepiglottic penetration	1	1	1	1	1
	Supraglottic penetration	2	2	2	2	2
	Tracheal penetration	3	3	3	3	3
Constrictor muscles/retention	No	0	0	0	0	0
	Weak muscles, with or without mild retention	1	1	1	1	1
	Paresis one segment, with or without moderate retention	2	2	2	2	2
	Severe paresis, with or without severe retention	3	3	3	3	3
Pharyngo-oesophageal segment	Normal opening	0	0	0	0	0
	<25% impaired	1	1	1	1	1
	25–50% impaired	2	2	2	2	2
	>50% impaired	3	3	3	3	3

Frontal view

Unilateral paresis
Bilateral paresis
Vocal fold closure

Comments
Total points

In the treatment of the dysphagic patient, a team approach is often necessary and one of the most important partnerships is between speech/language pathologists and dieticians (Heiss et al. 2010). Another type of interdisciplinary management is described in a study from 2005 (Denk and Bigenzahn 2005).

A critical component in the treatment of dysphagic patients is providing accurate *information*. *To inform and explain current problems in an understandable way* is essential for the patient, family members and nursing staff in terms of heightening awareness and understanding of the dysfunction, and highlighting the necessity for swallowing precautions and treatment. The successful rehabilitation of a dysphagic patient will, to a large extent, depend on the implementation of a team approach, with the patient and family as key components of the team.

Education of the medical and nursing staff regarding how to observe potential swallowing problems and hosting routine patient care rounds facilitates appropriate patient referrals and expedites the care of dysphagic patients.

7.1   The Postural Techniques

Change of head or body posture is relatively easy for most dysphagic patients to perform and can successfully eliminate misdirected swallows (penetration/aspiration) of liquids 75–80% of the time and is widely known and used among several speech/language pathologists (Logemann 1998; Okada et al. 2007; McCulloch 2010). *Head down* (*chin tuck*) widens the valleculae, pushes the tongue base backwards towards the pharyngeal wall, places the epiglottis in a more posterior position and narrows the entrance to the larynx. This position is used in cases where there is a reduction in posterior tongue base motion, unilateral laryngeal dysfunction, delayed initiation of pharyngeal swallow and reduced laryngeal closure. For patients with weak pharyngeal constrictor muscles, a chin tuck position makes the difficulties worse, especially when swallowing a masticated bolus, which could lead to increased retention in the pharyngeal recess and postswallow aspiration (Shanahan et al. 1993; Welch et al. 1993; Bülow et al. 1999; Baylow et al. 2009). But chin tuck can reduce the depth of misdirected swallows (penetration/aspiration) (Bülow et al. 2001).

If the *head back* posture is used, gravity can facilitate more efficient clearance of the oral cavity when oral transit is disturbed; however, good airway protection and pharyngeal swallowing mechanics must be present for safe implementation of this posture. When the *head is rotated to the damaged side*, the passage through the damaged or weakened side is reduced, permitting primary bolus passage through the stronger side. The *head rotation posture also pulls* the cricoid cartilage away from the posterior pharyngeal wall and facilitates passage into the cervical oesophagus as in the case of decreased pharyngo-oesophageal segment opening (Logemann et al. 1989). *Head tilt to the stronger side results in* bolus passage down on the stronger side in the case of unilateral oral and pharyngeal weakness. *Lying down on one side* will take advantage of the gravity effect on pharyngeal retention, and reduce the likelihood of aspiration of residue after the swallow in cases of reduced pharyngeal contraction.

7.2   Sensory Improvement Techniques

Techniques such as thermal–tactile stimulation and bolus manipulation are designed to improve oral sensory awareness and improve the timing of swallow initiation (Lazzara et al. 1986; Rosenbek et al. 1996; Lim et al. 2009; Teismann et al. 2009). Furthermore, bolus can be manipulated in different ways, such as giving a sour bolus, a cold bolus, a larger-volume bolus and a bolus that requires chewing. Pressure applied to the tongue during spoon administrations of food may also facilitate productive tongue movement towards a functional swallow.

7.3   Swallowing Manoeuvres

The four different techniques that are designed to change a selected aspect of the physiological process of pharyngeal swallow include supraglottic swallow, super supraglottic swallow, effortful swallow and the Mendelsohn manoeuvre (Logemann 1998; Logemann and Kahrilas 1990; Kahrilas et al. 1992). Swallowing manoeuvres showed during videofluoroscopy a greater range of hyoid bone displacement (van der Kruis et al. 2010) Despite their proven effectiveness in some patients, the complexity of the manoeuvres often precludes their usage with a patient experiencing language-cognitive impairment, pulmonary disease, deconditioning and fatigue.

7.4 Supraglottic Swallow and Super Supraglottic Swallow

The primary purpose of these techniques is to ensure airway protection prior to and throughout the swallow. The techniques include instructing patients to (1) take a breath, hold it and, in the super supraglottic swallow, bear down, (2) swallow, (3) clear their throat without inhaling, and (4) dry swallow. It has been shown that instructing patients to hold their breath "hard" and "bear down" results in optimal glottic and supraglottic closure (Martin et al. 1993; Logemann 1998).

The purpose by bearing down in the super supraglottic swallow technique is to assist the closure of the posterior glottis and the false vocal folds.

7.5 Effortful Swallow

The purpose of this technique is to increase posterior motion of the tongue base during pharyngeal swallow. The increase in tongue base retraction associated with the manoeuvre should facilitate improved bolus clearance from the valleculae (Logemann 1998). This technique can also reduce the depth and severity of misdirected swallows (penetration/aspiration) (Bülow et al. 2001). In later studies, effortful swallow was studied from different perspectives by using electromyography and pharyngeal manometry (Huckabee 2006; Witte et al. 2008).

For effortful swallow, patients should be instructed to squeeze hard with all of their tongue muscles when they swallow.

7.6 Mendelsohn Manoeuvre

The purpose of this manoeuvre is to increase the duration and extent of laryngeal elevation and thereby increase the width and duration of (pharyngo-oesophageal) cricopharyngeal opening (Logemann 1998). Following early relaxation of the cricopharyngeal muscle, the pharyngo-oesophageal segment is pulled open as the cricoid cartilage is moved away from the posterior pharyngeal wall during upward and forward movement of the hyoid bone and larynx. The functional result of this technique is to facilitate bolus passage through the pharyngo-oesophageal segment and decrease the degree of piriform residue (Lazarus et al. 1993; Wheeler-Hegland et al. 2008).

For the Mendelsohn manoeuvre, the patient should be instructed as follows:
- Pay attention to your neck by swallowing your saliva several times.
- Try to feel how your Adam's apple lifts and lowers as you swallow.
- Swallow again, and when you feel the Adam's apple lift, keep it in its highest position by squeezing the muscles of your tongue and neck for several seconds.

7.7 Oral Motor Exercises

From the performance of specialized exercises of the striated musculature of the tongue, pharynx and cervical oesophagus region, there is some evidence to suggest that it is possible to improve muscle strength and range of motion (Logemann 1983, 1995; Sonies 1993). The exercise programme must be individually adapted depending on the specific type(s) of swallowing impairment, and clearly documented and explained to ensure independent patient implementation whenever possible. Some exercises have prescribed intensities and frequencies, such as the Shaker exercise (Shaker et al. 1997). Other isometric strengthening exercises are usually introduced in a hierarchy of difficulty, with a gradual increase in intensity and frequency. From what is known about skeletal muscle physiological function in other parts of the body, it is likely that the patient will need to continue an exercise maintenance programme even after functional swallowing skills have been acquired.

7.8 Diet Modification

Food and liquid texture modifications are often found to be necessary from results of the therapeutic swallowing study, and to enable the patient to maintain adequate oral nutrition. We have found that it is often a problem to communicate the different textures between health care professionals. The terminology and the different textures may be very different from one health care setting to another. In a study from 2010, Wendin et al. (2010) tried to develop a system of objective, quantitative and well-defined food texture categories by using a combination of sensory and rheological measurements.

Table 4 Disorders documented on videofluoroscopy and their management. (Modified from Martin 1994)

Radiographic presentation	Cognitive and sensory stimulation, oral motor exercises, diet modification, alternative nutrition	Head positioning	Manoeuvres
Oral phase Anterior leakage due to incomplete lip closure Oral residue Posterior leakage due to spill over tongue base Delayed bolus preparation Diffuse spreading of bolus in oral cavity Inefficient tongue movements and mastication Delayed bolus transport Aspiration before pharyngeal swallow Regurgitation into nasal cavity	Optimize liquid/food texture Sufficient bolus volumes Intraoral placement to unimpaired side Labial resistive exercises Buccal range of motion exercises and resistive exercises Lingual range of motion exercises and resistive exercises Bolus control exercises Thickened liquids, cold liquids, semisolids, soft solids Controlled bolus volume Thickened liquids and semisolids Bolus hold exercises	Head tilt to unimpaired side	Lip pursing Double swallow Supraglottic swallow
Dissociation Delayed initiation of pharyngeal swallow	Thermal–tactile stimulation Thickened liquids Cold stimulus Controlled bolus volume Bolus hold exercises	Chin tuck	Supraglottic swallow
Pharyngeal phase Laryngeal elevation reduced Movements of hyoid bone Elevation incomplete, anterior movement incomplete Incomplete closure of epiglottis Misdirected swallows Vestibulum laryngis Subepiglottic penetration Supraglottic penetration Tracheal penetration/aspiration Weakness of constrictor muscles: Mild, moderate or severe retention Unilateral, pocketing in valleculae or/and piriform sinus Bilateral, pocketing in valleculae or/and piriform sinuses	Controlled bolus volume Slightly thickened liquids Thinned semisolids Cold stimulus Thickened liquids Thermal–tactile stimulation Bolus hold exercises Controlled bolus volume Liquids, semisolids and soft solids Hard swallow Controlled bolus volume Liquids and thinned semisolids	Chin tuck Head rotation towards impaired side Head tilt towards unimpaired side Head rotation	Mendelsohn manoeuvre Mendelsohn manoeuvre Supraglottic swallow Supraglottic swallow Double swallow Modified supraglottic swallow Double swallow Modified supraglottic swallow
Pharyngo-oesophageal segment Impaired opening Regurgitation from oesophagus to piriform sinuses	Liquids, semisolids and soft solids Controlled bolus volumes		Mendelsohn manoeuvre Double swallow Modified supraglottic swallow
Absent pharyngeal swallow	Thermal–tactile stimulation Tube feeding.		

Examples include changes from thin to thickened liquids, or vice versa, and from soft solids to pureed foods. Even though these texture modifications appear to be simply strategies to improve swallow safety and efficiency, several factors must be considered when making these recommendations: (1) patient tolerance and preference; (2) adequate nutrition and hydration; (3) cultural considerations regarding food items and textures. (Garcia et al. 2005). We have also found that carbonated liquids (Bülow et al. 2003) can be a good option for many patients, and may be better accepted than thickened liquids.

7.9   Oral Versus Non-oral Feeding

A tube feeding method, such as nasogastric tube, percutaneous endoscopic gastrostomy (PEG) or jejunostomy, is sometimes the only safe and efficient avenue for feeding in severely dysphagic patients. It is a common occurrence for a patient to have tube feedings as the primary source of nutrition and hydration, with safe supplementation of small amounts of modified food and liquid textures for pleasure and optimizing quality of life.

It has been found that dysphagic stroke patients who were recommended a thickened-fluid dysphagia diet failed to meet their fluid requirements, but this was not the case in patients with an enteral feeding and intravenous fluid regime (Finestone et al. 2001).

Dziewas et al. (2008) analysed if a nasogastric tube worsens dysphagia in patients with an acute stroke. Their results showed that a correctly placed nasogastric tube did not cause a worsening of stroke-related dysphagia.

Logemann et al. (2008) analysed what information clinicians use when recommending oral versus non-oral feeding in oropharyngeal dysphagic patients.

8   Therapeutic Strategies

Therapeutic strategies are given in Table 4.

9   Conclusion

In the therapeutic swallowing study a trained speech/language pathologist and a radiologist collaborate in performing the examination. The competence of the two specialists provides an opportunity for a complete visualization and analysis of the entire swallowing sequence. Testing swallowing function with various bolus volumes and textures, and the implementation of trial therapeutic strategies are integral components of the examination. Despite the strengths and clinical utility of the therapeutic swallowing study, there are several limitations with interpretation of test results across swallowing centres. There is lack of standardization regarding the textures of contrast materials, differing terminology and methods of analysis, and generally suboptimal intersubject reliability regarding the rating of swallowing function. Clearly there is a need for multicentre collaboration to determine salient features that warrant analysis on the therapeutic swallowing study, standardization of rating scales and the association of these ratings with patient functional outcomes and quality of life. The evaluation of oropharyngeal swallowing function is in its infancy, and we expect that the number of evidenced-based studies will increase across centres in Europe and the USA to assist us in further determining the optimal test protocols, item analysis and treatment strategies for improved swallowing function in our dysphagic patients.

References

Adnerhill I, Ekberg O, Groher ME (1989) Determining normal bolus size for thin liquids. Dysphagia 4:1

Ashford J, McCabe D, Wheeler-Hegland K, Frymark T, Mullen R, Musson N, Schooling T, Hammond CS (2009) Evidence-based systematic review: oropharyngeal dysphagia behavioral treatments: part III—impact of dysphagia treatments on populations with neurological disorders. J Rehabil Res Dev 46(2):195–204

Baylow HE, Goldfarb R, Taveira CH, Steinberg RS (2009) Accuracy of clinical judgment of the chin-down posture for dysphagia during the clinical/bedside assessment as corroborated by videofluoroscopy in adults with acute stroke. Dysphagia 24(4):423–433

Bingjie L, Tong Z, Xinting S, Jianmin X, Guijun J (2010) Quantitative videofluoroscopic analysis of penetration-aspiration in post-stroke patients. Neurol India 58(1):42–47

Bodén K, Hallgren A, Witt Hedström H (2006) Effects of three swallow maneuvers analyzed by videomanometry. Acta Radiol 47(7):628–633

Bülow M, Olsson R, Ekberg O (1999) Videomanometric analysis of supraglottic swallow, effortful swallow and chin tuck in healthy volunteers. Dysphagia 14:67–72

Bülow M, Olsson R, Ekberg O (2001) Videomanometric analysis of supraglottic swallow, effortful swallow and chin tuck in patients with pharyngeal dysfunction. Dysphagia 16:190–195

Bülow M, Olsson R, Ekberg O (2003) Videoradiographic analysis of how carbonated thin thickened liquids affect the physiology of swallowing in subjects with aspiration on thin liquids. Acta Radiol 44:366–372

Carnaby G, Hankey GJ, Pizzi J (2006) Behavioural intervention for dysphagia in acute stroke: a randomised controlled trial. Lancet Neurol 5:31–37

De Pippo KL, Holas MA, Reding MJ (1992) Validation of the 3-ounce water swallow test for aspiration following stroke. Arch Neurol 49:1259–1261

Denk DM, Bigenzahn W (2005) Management of oropharyngeal dysphagia. Current status. HNO 53(7):661–672

Dodds WJ, Logemann JA, Stewart ET (1990a) Radiological assessment of abnormal oral and pharyngeal phases of swallow. AJR Am J Roentgenol 154:965–974

Dodds WJ, Stewart ET, Logemann J (1990b) Physiology and radiology of the normal oral and pharyngeal phases of swallowing. AJR Am J Roentgenol 154:993–1963

Donner M (1988) The evaluation of dysphagia by radiography and other methods of imaging. Dysphagia 1:49–50

Dziewas R, Warnecke T, Hamacher C, Oelenberg S, Teismann I, Kraemer C, Ritter M, Ringelstein EB, Schaebitz WR (2008) Do nasogastric tubes worsen dysphagia in patients with acute stroke? BMC Neurol 23 8:28

Ekberg O (1986) Posture of the head and pharyngeal swallow. Acta Radiol Diagn 27:691–696

Ekberg O (1990) The role of radiology in evaluation and treatment of neurologically-impaired patients with dysphagia. J Neurol Rehabil 4:65–73

Ekberg O (1992) Radiologic evaluation of swallowing. In: Groher ME (ed) Dysphagia. Diagnosis and management, 2nd edn. Butterworth-Heineman, Boston, pp 163–195

Ekberg O, Bülow M, Ekman S, Hall G, Stading M, Wendin K (2009) Effect of barium sulphate contrast medium on rheology and sensory texture attributes in a model food. Acta Radiol 50(2):131–138

Finestone HM, Foley NC, Woodbury MG, Greene-Finestone L (2001) Quantifying fluid intake in dysphagic stroke patients: a preliminary comparison of oral and nonoral strategies. Arch Phys Med Rehabil 82(12):1744–1746

Garcia JM, Chambers E, Molander M (2005) Thickened liquids: practice patterns of speech language pathologists. Am J Speech Lang Pathol 14(1):4–13

Gates J, Hartnell GG, Graminga GD (2006) Videofluoroscopy and swallowing studies for neurologic disease: a primer. Radiographics 26(1):e22

Groher ME, Crary MA, Carnaby Mann G, Vickers Z, Aguilar C (2006) The impact of rheologically controlled materials on the identifications of airway compromise on the clinical and videofluoroscopic swallowing examinations. Dysphagia 21(4):218–225

Heiss CJ, Goldberg L, Dzarnoski M (2010) Registered dieticians and speech-language pathologists: an important partnership in dysphagia management. J Am Diet Assoc 110(9):1290, 1292–1293

Huckabee ML, Steele CM (2006) An analysis of lingual contribution to submental surface electromyographic measures and pharyngeal pressure during effortful swallow. Arch Phys Med Rehabil 87(8):1067–1072

Jones B, Donner MW (1989) How I do it: examination of the patient with dysphagia. Dysphagia 4:162–172

Kahrilas PJ, Logemann JA, Gibbons P (1992) Food intake by maneuver: an extreme compensation for impaired swallowing. Dysphagia 7:155–159

Lazarus CL, Logemann JA, Gibbons P (1993) Effects of manoeuvres on swallowing function in a dysphagic oral cancer patient. Head Neck 15:419–424

Lazzara G, Lazarus C, Logemann J (1986) Impact of thermal stimulation on the triggering of the swallow reflex. Dysphagia 1:73–77

Lim KB, Lee HJ, Lim SS, Choi YI (2009) Neuromuscular electrical and thermal-tactile stimulation for dysphagia caused by stroke: a randomized controlled trial. J Rehabil Med 41(3):174–178

Linden P, Sibens A (1983) Dysphagia: predicting laryngeal penetration. Arch Phys Med Rehabil 64:281–283

Logemann JA (1983) Evaluation and treatment of swallowing disorders. Pro-Ed, Austin

Logemann JA (1986) A manual for the videofluoroscopic evaluation of swallowing. College-Hill Press, Boston

Logemann JA (1995) Dysphagia: evaluation and treatment. Folia Phoniatr Logop 47(3):140–164

Logemann J (1998) Evaluation and treatment of swallowing disorders. Pro-Ed, Austin

Logemann JA (2008) Treatment of oral and pharyngeal dysphagia. Phys Med Rehabil Clin N Am 19(4):803–816, ix

Logemann JA, Kahrilas PJ (1990) Relearning to swallow post CVA: application of maneuvers and indirect biofeedback: a case study. Neurology 40:1136–1138

Logemann JA, Kahrilas PJ, Kobara M, Vakil NB (1989) The benefit of head rotation on pharyngoesophageal dysphagia. Arch Phys Med Rehabil 70:767–771

Logemann JA, Lazarus CL, Phillips Keely S, Sanches A, Rademaker AW (2000) Effectiveness of four hours of education in interpretation of radiographic studies. Dysphagia 15:180–183

Logemann JA, Rademaker A, Pauloski BR, Antinoja J, Bacon M, Bernstein M, Gaziano J, Grande B, Kelchner L, Kelly A, Klaben B, Lundy D, Newman L, Santa D, Stachowiak L et al (2008) What information do clinicians use in recommending oral versus nonoral feeding in oropharyngeal dysphagia patients? Dysphagia 23(4):378–384

Martin BJW (1994) Treatment of dysphagia in adults. In: Reiff Cherney L (ed) Clinical managements of dysphagia in adults and children. Aspen, Gaithersburg, pp 153–183

Martin BJW, Logemann JA, Shaker R, Dodds WJ (1993) Normal laryngeal valving patterns during three breath-hold manoeuvres: a pilot investigation. Dysphagia 8:11–20

Martin-Harris B, Jones B (2008) The videofluorographic swallowing study. Phys Med Rehabil Clin N Am 19: 769–785

Martin-Harris B, Logemann JA, McMahon S, Schleicher MA, Sandidge J (2000) Clinical utility of the modified barium swallow. Dysphagia 15:136–141

Martin-Harris B, Brodsky MB, Michel Y, Castell DO, Schleicher M, Sandidge J, Maxwell R, Blair J (2008) MBS measurement tool for swallow impairment—MBSImp: establishing a standard. Dysphagia 23:392–405

McCabe D, Ashford J, Wheeler-Hegland K, Frymark T, Mullen R, Musson N, Hammond CS, Schooling T (2009) Evidence-based systemtic review: Oropharyngeal dysphagia behavioural treatments. Part IV—impact of dysphagia treatment on individuals' postcancer treatments. J Rehabil Res Dev 46(2):205–214

McCulloch TM, Hoffman MR, Ciucci MR (2010) High-resolution manometry of pharyngeal swallow pressure events associated with head turn and chin tuck. Ann Otol Rhinol Laryngol 119(6):369–376

Murray J (1999) Videofluoroscopic examination. In: Manual of dysphagia assessment in adults. Singular, San Diego, pp 113–151

Nathadwarawala KM, Nicklin J, Wiles CM (1992) A timed test of swallowing capacity for neurological patients. J Neurol Neurosurg Psych 55:822–825

Nathadwarawala KM, Mc Groary A, Wiles CM (1994) Swallowing in neurological outpatients: use of a timed test. Dysphagia 9:120–129

Okada S, Saitoh E, Palmer JB, Matsuo K, Yokoyama M, Shigeta R, Baba M (2007) What is the chin-down posture? A questionnaire survey of speech language pathologists in Japan and in the United States. Dysphagia 22(3):204–209

Pauloski BR (2008) rehabilitation of dysphagia following head and neck cancer. Phys Med Rehabil Clin N Am 19(4):889–928, x

Rosenbek JC, Roecker EB, Wood JL, Robbins J (1996) Thermal application reduces the duration of stage transition in dysphagia after stroke. Dysphagia 11:225–233

Shaker R, Kern M, Bardan E, Taylor A, Stewart ET, Hoffamnn RG et al (1997) Augmentation of deglutitive upper esophageal sphincter opening in the elderly by exercise. Am J Physiol 272:G1518–G1522

Shanahan TK, Logemann JA, Rademaker AW, Pauloski BR, Kahrilas PJ (1993) Chin-down posture effect on aspiration in dysphagic patients. Arch Phys Med Rehabil 74:736–739

Sonies BC (1993) Remediation challenges in treating dysphagia post head/neck cancer. A problem-oriented approach. Clin Commun Disord 3(4):21–26

Speyer R, Baijens L, Heijnen M, Zwijnenberg I (2010) Effects of therapy in oropharyngeal dysphagia by speech and language therapists: a systematic review. Dysphagia 25(1):40-65.

Splaingard ML, Hutchins B, Sulton LD, Chauhuri G (1988) Aspiration in rehabilitation patients: videofluoroscopy vs bedside clinical assessment. Arch Phys Med Rehabil 69:637–640

Teismann IK, Steinsträter O, Warnecke T, Suntrup S, Ringelstein EB, Pantev C, Dziewas R (2009) Tactile thermal oral stimulation increases the cortical representation of swallowing. BMC Neurosci 10:71

Van der Kruis JG, Baijens LW, Speyer R, Zwijnenberg I (2010) Biomechanical analysis of hyoid bone displacement in videofluoroscopy: a systematic review of intervention effects. Dysphagia 26(2):171–182 . doi:10.1007/s00455-010-9318-9

Welch MV, Logemann JA, Rademaker AW, Kahrilas PJ (1993) Changes in pharyngeal dimensions effected by chin tuck. Arch Phys Med Rehabil 74:178–181

Wendin K, Ekman S, Bülow M, Ekberg O, Johansson D, Rothenberg E, Stading M (2010) Objective and quantitative definitions of modified food textures based on sensory and rheological methodology. Food Nutr Res 54:5134. doi:10.3402/fnr.v54i0.5134

Wheeler-Hegland KM, Rosenbeck JC, Sapienza CM (2008) Submental sEMG and hyoid movement during Mendelsohn maneuver, effortful swallow, and expiratory muscle strength training. J Speech Lang Hear Res 51(5):1072–1087

Witte U, Huckabee ML, Doeltgen SH, Gumbley F, Robb M (2008) The effect of effortful swallow on pharyngeal manometric measurements during saliva and water swallowing in healthy participants. Arch Phys Med Rehabil 89(5):822–828

Zammit-Maempel I, Chapple C-L, Leslie P (2007) Radiation dose in videofluoroscopic swallow studies. Dysphagia 22(1):13–15

Zenner PM, Losinski DS, Mills RH (1995) Using cervical auscultation in the clinical dysphagia examination in long-term care. Dysphagia 10(1):27–31

Surgical Aspects of Pharyngeal Dysfunction, Dysphagia, and Aspiration

Hans F. Mahieu and Martijn P. Kos

Contents

H. F. Mahieu (✉)
ENT Department, Meander Medical Center,
Amersfoort, The Netherlands
e-mail: hf.mahieu@meandermc.nl

M. P. Kos
ENT Department, Waterland Hospital,
Purmerend, The Netherlands
e-mail: martijn.kos@gmail.com

Abstract

Surgical treatment of oropharyngeal dysphagia and aspiration resulting from different disorders is a difficult issue. Sometimes the aim of the surgery is complete correction of the disorder (e.g., extraluminal obstruction), but more often no more than a reduction of the symptoms can be achieved (e.g., laryngeal suspension). The most frequent disorders eligible for surgical treatment are described and some others are described as examples of possible surgical approaches. The surgical techniques described are aimed at preservation or restoration of the function of the larynx and pharynx.

1 Introduction

Surgical treatment is presently only feasible for some disorders in the pharyngeal or esophageal phase of swallowing and is hardly an option in the oral phase. This is because the oral phase primarily consists of transportation of the bolus into the pharynx by shaping, lifting, and compression of the tongue. Surgical reconstruction of the tongue as a reconstructive part of extensive head and neck surgery can at best create a mass in the mouth to facilitate compensatory techniques of rehabilitation of swallowing. It is an illusion to try to restore the versatile and complex movements of the mobile tongue by surgical means.

Even in disorders in the pharyngeal or esophageal phase, where surgical therapy can theoretically or technically be applied, a large proportion of patients will not be eligible for surgical treatment because either they are not fit to undergo surgery or their

O. Ekberg (ed.), *Dysphagia*, Medical Radiology. Diagnostic Imaging, DOI: 10.1007/174_2011_357,
© Springer-Verlag Berlin Heidelberg 2012

underlying disorder is too rapidly progressive for them to benefit from a surgical procedure with a considerable recovery period.

The options for surgical treatment of swallowing disorders are dependent on the specific localization and type of the dysfunction. In the case of anatomical disorders, such as Zenker's diverticulum (ZD), surgery can be indicated.

In severe cases of dysphagia caused by retropharyngeal masses (e.g., osteophytes of cervical spine, benign tumors, and meningoceles) surgery is also often the treatment of choice. It is important to realize that bolus obstruction because of external compression usually occurs in the area of the pharynx and upper esophageal sphincter (UES) (C4–C7) and not lower in the esophagus. This is because of the rather strict midline location of the upper alimentary tract in this area as a consequence of the attachments of the pharynx and esophageal inlet posteriorly to the relatively rigid structures of the cricoid and thyroid, located in the midline of the neck. Because of this fixation to the laryngeal cartilages, the otherwise flexible and pliable structures of the pharynx and esophagus cannot divert from the midline. Thus, even relatively small anterior bony fragments of the cervical spine at this level cannot be easily circumnavigated by the bolus, which can result in obstruction. Below the UES, the esophagus has much more flexibility and freedom to deviate laterally, so even much larger osteophytes or large tumors lower in the neck or mediastinum rarely cause an obstruction of the bolus.

If the propulsive forces of the pharynx are inadequate to propel the bolus in the esophagus because of weakness of the constrictor pharyngeal musculature or in the case of dysfunction of the UES because of late or insufficient opening of this sphincter, a myotomy of the UES can be considered. If the propulsive forces of the pharynx are insufficient and severe aspiration occurs as a consequence of concomitant insufficient laryngeal elevation, a laryngeal suspension procedure can be considered.

Cancer treatment is, understandably, directed at survival, so a dysfunctional larynx and a dysfunctional pharynx are often considered as "collateral damage." Such a problem is then often addressed by bypassing the dysfunctional larynx and pharynx with a percutaneous gastrostomy. It would, however, be beneficial for some of these dysphagic patients if more functionally oriented surgical approaches were

considered, some examples of which are described in the following paragraphs. The more extensive procedures are described in another chapter.

In the case of aspiration in laryngeal paralysis, frequently seen after vagal nerve injury in surgery of the brainstem or neck, some authors also state that medialization thyroplasty should be performed as therapy additional to, for instance, UES myotomy (Flint et al. 1997). However, medialization thyroplasty only addresses anterior glottic insufficiency, whereas aspiration in glottic insufficiency mainly occurs posteriorly. If glottic insufficiency is to be addressed in addition to UES myotomy to reduce aspiration, it seems more logical to perform an arytenoid adduction, which is mainly directed at closure in the posterior part of the glottis. Both arytenoid adduction and medialization thyroplasty are procedures mainly for voice augmentation and will not be described here.

It is impossible within the scope of this chapter to describe all the surgical procedures which have been used for treatment of dysphagia resulting from pharyngeal or laryngeal dysfunction; therefore, we will restrict our descriptions to more often used techniques and some examples of other surgical approaches.

The goal of surgery for oropharyngeal dysphagia is usually not to normalize the swallowing act, but to improve bolus passage and/or prevent or minimize aspiration with preservation of a functional larynx. It is, of course, essential to extensively counsel the patient before the surgery and give extensive information concerning the expected outcome as well as the risks of the procedure.

2   Specific Pathology and Surgical Procedures

2.1   Zenker's Diverticulum

ZD, or hypopharyngeal diverticulum, is a relatively common problem encountered by head and neck surgeons. It consists of an acquired pouch in the dorsal wall of the hypopharynx, located at the level of the transition from the relatively wide hypopharynx to the narrow esophageal inlet. It is formed by herniation of mucosa and submucosa, protruding between the fibers of the cricopharyngeal muscle (below) and the inferior constrictor muscles (above).

It is important to realize that many conditions which on their own account can cause dysphagia are often present in patients who also have ZD. Sometimes the initial treatment should first be targeted at these other causes instead of performing a diverticulotomy. There is evidence from a postmortem study (Van Overbeek 1997) that ZD can occur without causing symptoms. If ZD is symptomatic, the prevailing complaints of ZD are dysphagia, regurgitation of undigested food, gurgling noises in the neck, a neck mass, fetor ex ore, coughing and aspiration especially in the supine position, weight loss, and, in extreme cases, an absolute food passage block. These complaints are predominantly caused by retention of food and fluid in the diverticulum, which, when sufficiently large and filled, can compress the esophagus.

Many different treatment strategies have been proposed for ZD. Traditionally, external treatment modalities were used, by some still today, most often consisting of diverticulectomy combined with cricopharyngeal myotomy.

Endoscopic surgical treatments are less extensive than the external surgical approach. All are directed toward transecting the diverticuloesophageal wall or "spur," so that an ample passage and overflow from the diverticulum into the esophagus is achieved. Since the diverticuloesophageal wall contains the cricopharyngeal and part of the upper esophageal musculature, division of this wall automatically results in a transmucosal myotomy of these muscles. The only difference in the endoscopic treatments is the technique used to divide the diverticuloesophageal wall. The endoscopic treatment was first described in 1917 by Mosher (1917), who endoscopically incised the diverticuloesophageal wall.

Dohlman and Mattson (1960) developed an endoscope with a slit in the distal end, so that the diverticuloesophageal wall could be fixed between the two lips of the endoscope. They then coagulated the wall and divided it with a diathermic knife. This method was refined by Van Overbeek et al. (1984), who modified the endoscope and started using the operating microscope coupled to a CO_2 laser, which enabled better control and more precise division of the diverticuloesophageal wall (Mahieu et al. 1996). Further development of laser techniques, with the introduction of the Acuspot in the early 1990s, facilitated precision and control of the surgical endoscopic technique. In the same period, endoscopic

diverticulotomy with a stapler technique was introduced (Collard et al. 1993).

In a study (Kos et al. 2009) describing our experiences with different endoscopic treatment modalities over the years, we found that in the modern microendoscopic CO_2 laser diverticulotomy 86.7% of 61 patients were free of dysphagic complaints as evaluated 1 year after treatment and repetitive surgery was required in only 13% of the patients. Mediastinitis, the most feared complication, was not encountered in this treatment modality. The results and complication ratio of the microendoscopic CO_2 laser diverticulotomy are comparable to the reported results of the recently introduced endoscopic stapler diverticulotomy, and indicate that CO_2 laser treatment is an excellent treatment modality. In approximately 10% of patients, emphysema of the neck is found, and is not necessary related to the presence of mediastinitis.

The principle of endoscopic treatment is the transection of the diverticuloesophageal wall, which contains the cricopharyngeal muscle, thereby achieving an ample overflow from the diverticulum to the esophagus. It is not necessary to completely divide the wall down to the floor of the large diverticulum; this would only increase the possibility of a perforation in the diverticulum to the mediastinum. If symptoms persist in patients with larger diverticula, repetition of the endoscopic procedure is usually possible. Our results show that a large ZD is not a contraindication for endoscopic treatment, and that there is no higher complication rate in these patients. Almost 70% of these patients experienced total relief of symptoms, and no higher recurrence rate was found.

Nowadays, endoscopic stapler diverticulotomy is used by many surgeons as the treatment of choice. This technique uses a telescope instead of a microscope to visualize the diverticulum. Besides the sharp incision of the diverticuloesophageal wall by the blade of the instrument, this procedure involves sealing the wound edges with multiple rows of staples. This sealing is said to prevent mediastinitis and perioperative bleeding, and should immediately allow oral intake and thus shorter hospitalization. The outcome results are comparable to those of laser endoscopic diverticulotomy. Cook et al. (2000) reported complete relief in 71% of patients ($n = 74$). Saetti et al. (2006) reported complete relief or a significant reduction of symptoms in all patients ($n = 106$), 19.8% of them requiring repeat surgery after a median of 15 months. Although not reported by Cook et al. and Saetti et al., fatal outcome after mediastinitis has also been reported (Mirza et al. 2003).

An obvious disadvantage of the stapler technique is that smaller diverticula (less than 2 cm) cannot be easily treated because of the difficult introduction of the stapler and because exposure of the operating field can cause difficulties that can lead to a higher conversion rate to external procedures than that seen with laser endoscopic treatment. By use of the microscope in the microendoscopic laser technique, a superior view and superior control are obtained without the view being impaired by instruments. Our experience is that if the stapler is introduced, visualization of the tip of the instrument and visualization of the cutting of the wall are often not possible; thus, this method provides less control and accuracy in our hands. We will therefore describe the laser microendoscopic method in more detail.

Flexible endoscopic treatment of ZD is also performed by gastroenterologists, employing diathermy needle-knife techniques or laser techniques with fibers (Tang et al. 2008; Seaman et al. 2008; Christiaens et al. 2007). The reported series are small. Often multiple fiber-optic treatments are necessary, mainly owing to inferior visualization of the operating field, to obtain results similar to those obtained by to rigid endoscopic procedures. If general anesthesia is contraindicated, this can be considered as an alternative treatment.

Although the development of malignancies in a ZD has been described, the incidence is so low that it does not justify preventive surgical treatment of an asymptomatic ZD in our opinion. Furthermore, the efficacy of such preventive surgery is very questionable in the light of reported recurrence rates of ZD.

2.1.1   Surgical Technique

To facilitate the location of the esophageal inlet, patients are requested to swallow a thread with a small metal weight attached to one end and taped to the cheek with the other end the evening before surgery. In more than 80% of cases, the metal weight had passed into the esophagus, thus facilitating identification of the esophageal inlet for introduction of the bitipped endoscope (Dohlman and Mattson 1960; Van Overbeek et al. 1984) (Fig. 1). First, careful

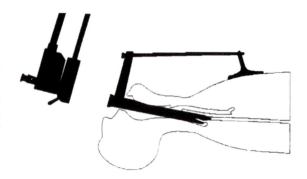

Fig. 1 Microendoscopic procedure with a CO_2 laser and a bitipped diverticulosope

Fig. 2 Zenker's diverticulum before (*left*) and after (*right*) endoscopic treatment. The cricopharyngeal muscle (*asterisk*) located in the esophagodiverticular wall is automatically sectioned during division of this wall

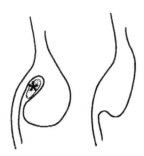

endoscopic examination is performed to exclude malignancy in the diverticulum.

Division of the diverticuloesophageal wall is than performed under microscopic control with the CO_2 laser until an ample communication between the diverticulum and the esophagus has been established. Usually, this means dividing the diverticuloesophageal wall over three quarters to four fifths of its height, sometimes less in extremely large diverticula (Fig. 2).

Postoperative management consists prophylactic antibiotics for 5 days, a feeding tube (often not used but placed at the time of surgery under direct vision, so that if necessary a way for nutritional intake can be guaranteed), and 24 h oral feeding. If no fever or emphysema is present the day following treatment, feeding is started on clear liquid and 12 h later on thick liquid. The feeding tube is removed if no fever or emphysema develops after 24 h oral feeding.

Contraindications for endoscopic treatment are as follows: malignancy in the diverticulum; extreme fixation of the cervical spine in an abnormal position, precluding safe endoscopy; suspicion of a large vessel in the diverticuloesophageal wall. In these cases external diverticulectomy with cricopharyngeal myotomy can be performed.

2.2 Neuromuscular Dysfunction of Pharyngeal Constrictors and the UES

Opening of the esophageal inlet to enable passage of the bolus from the pharynx into the esophagus is achieved by a combination of (1) elevation and anterior displacement of the larynx, which assists in the esophageal inlet being pulled open, (2) relaxation of the UES, and (3) passive dilatation of the esophageal inlet as a consequence of the propulsion of the bolus being pushed downward by contraction of the pharyngeal constrictor muscles. Failure of UES relaxation, or other forms of cricopharyngeal dysfunction, as well as diminished pharyngeal constrictor activity leads to an obstruction of bolus passage (Cook 1993) and can result in aspiration of food and saliva. Usually, deglutition of the solid bolus is more affected than deglutition of liquids because a large opening of the esophageal inlet is required to enable the passage of a solid bolus, whereas a minor opening of the esophageal inlet will allow passage of liquids. Various conditions affect the complex coordinated actions of neuromuscular structures in the pharyngeal, laryngeal, and UES regions. They can be divided in neurogenic, myogenic, idiopathic, and iatrogenic causes (Guily et al. 1994; Kelly 2000). Adaptation of food bolus consistency can be the first step in treating oropharyngeal dysphagia. In severe cases, replacement of oral alimentation by nutrition via a gastrostomy can be considered. However, this is not always a satisfactory alternative because swallowing of saliva persists and the patient is denied the quality-of-life aspects associated with the enjoyment and social aspects of eating.

The first UES myotomy was described by Kaplan (1951). The surgery was performed using an open transcervical approach in a patient following poliomyelitis. This was and continues to be the technique of choice for many head and neck surgeons, although since 1994 endoscopic laser-assisted transmucosal myotomy has been used increasingly.

The surgical intervention of UES myotomy consists of sectioning of all the muscles that constitute the functional UES unit, the last centimeters of the inferior constrictor muscles, the cricopharyngeal muscle, and the first few centimeters of the cervical esophagus, resulting in an incision of approximately 6 cm in an adult. Although myotomy is an action directed at the functional UES unit, oropharyngeal dysphagia is commonly associated with impairment of the pharyngeal musculature as the major pathophysiological factor and is less frequently caused by true cricopharyngeal dysfunction. Because correction of the weak or absent pharyngeal musculature is not possible presently, reduction of the resistance of the UES by means of a myotomy is the most logical approach to facilitate bolus propulsion. The reduced resistance of the UES will then allow opening of the esophageal inlet.

Recently, we analyzed our patients with longstanding dysphagia and/or aspiration problems of different causes who underwent UES myotomy as single surgical treatment (Kos et al. 2010). Preoperative and postoperative manometry and videofluoroscopy were used to assess swallowing and aspiration. Initial and long-term results after more than 1 year demonstrated success in 75% of the patients. The best outcomes were observed in patients with dysphagia of unknown origin, non-cancer-related iatrogenic cause, and neuromuscular disease. All successful patients had full oral intake with a normal bolus consistency without clinically significant aspiration. It was concluded that in select cases of oropharyngeal dysphagia success may be achieved by UES myotomy with restoration of oral intake of normal bolus consistency. Our long-term success rate of more than 75% is in line with that of other studies (Guily et al. 1994; Coiffier et al. 2006). Often it is said (Cook and Kahrilas 1999) that absence of pharyngeal constrictor activity is a contraindication for UES myotomy. In contrast to these statements, our results demonstrate that even in cases with absent or almost absent pharyngeal constrictor activity, UES myotomy can be successful.

Patient selection is essential and requires a complete medical history and clinical examination including functional endoscopic examination of swallowing (Leder et al. 2005), videofluoroscopy, and manometry. Esophagogastroscopy and 24-h pH-metry are usually only performed if they are indicated. We consider only severe gastroesophageal reflux to be a contraindication for UES myotomy.

We feel that it is important to perform videofluoroscopy and manometry postoperatively to evaluate the dysphagia status and determine whether myotomy has been complete. If the result of UES myotomy is not successful owing to insufficient pharyngeal propelling combined with insufficient laryngeal elevation, additional laryngeal suspension can be considered (Kos et al. 2008).

It is important to realize that in cases of slow progressive neuromuscular disease, alleviation of dysphagia by UES myotomy can be no more than temporary and can extend to many years of relief of dysphagic problems. However, in rapidly progressive neuromuscular disease, for example, amyotrophic lateral sclerosis, UES myotomy is not indicated.

Chemical UES myotomy by use of botulinum toxins can be helpful as a diagnostic treatment and can be indicated in patients with a high comorbidity. It is, however, often performed under general anesthesia, and repetitive treatments are needed (Moerman 2006). Dilatation usually gives temporary relief and is only indicated in cases where fibrosis of the UES unit is expected (Hatlebakk et al. 1998). Endoscopic myotomy, an adaptation of the endoscopic laser Zenker diverticulotomy, has increased in popularity in the last decade (Takes et al. 2005). It requires less surgical time and a shorter postoperative hospital stay than external myotomy. Institutions that perform endoscopic Zenker diverticulotomy can easily adjust their technique and perform endoscopic UES myotomy. In the absence of the diverticular wall between the diverticulum and the UES as is present in ZD, the diverticuloscope can now be used to "catch" the cricopharyngeal muscle between both blades of the endoscope and sever the muscle fibers and overlying mucosa with the CO_2 laser. Since in this case the mucosal barrier is breached, antibiotic prophylaxis is advised.

Having extensive experience in both techniques, we prefer the external UES myotomy approach as the treatment of choice for oropharyngeal dysphagia. It is our considered opinion that the accuracy of sectioning of the muscles over the entire length of the functional UES unit is better and the risk of local stenosis is less with an external approach. We use endoscopic UES myotomy in cases of recurrent dysphagia after previous external UES myotomy and in cases with poor quality of the skin of the neck or a poor exposure of the neck. Known potential risks of external myotomy are wound infection, pharyngocutaneous fistula, and paralysis of the recurrent laryngeal nerve (Brigand

et al. 2007). In our study of 28 cases we observed none of these complications.

2.2.1 Surgical Technique

The external UES myotomy starts with an endoscopy to assess the larynx, the pharynx, and the esophagus. A tube with an inflatable balloon or cuff (e.g., Sengstaken tube no. 16; Rusch, Kernen, Germany) is then introduced into the esophageal entrance to facilitate the UES myotomy. A left-sided approach of the UES is preferred because the esophagus is usually located slightly left of the trachea and the midline and this enables a better exposure of the UES. The most important complication of an external UES myotomy is a recurrent nerve palsy. The risk of the patient developing a recurrent nerve palsy later as a consequence of other disease is much higher on the left side than on right side. If paralysis of the recurrent laryngeal nerve is already present, then the myotomy should consequently be performed on that side.

A J-shaped incision is made along the anterior border of the sternocleidomastoid muscle curving toward the midline 1–2 cm above the sternum. The omohyoid muscle and if necessary the superior thyroid artery are transected for a good exposure. The head is tilted to the contralateral side and the UES myotomy is performed extending from the lower thyropharyngeal musculature, through the cricopharyngeal muscle, and down to the longitudinal fibers of the upper esophageal musculature (usually resulting in a total myotomy length of 5–6 cm, Fig. 3). This procedure is facilitated by the inflated balloon in the UES which stretches the muscle fibers and thus allows very precise sectioning of the UES musculature (Fig. 4a). After myotomy, the balloon is deflated (Fig. 4b), and while it is being retracted from the mouth, air is blown through the tube and with saline placed in the external wound this enables an additional check of the integrity of the UES mucosa. A minor perforation can be found by the escape of air bubbles. Before closure of the neck, a nasogastric feeding tube is placed, and this is carefully guided through the pharynx and UES by external palpation and gentle pressure of the surgeon's finger in the opened neck. A strict nonoral intake policy is valid for all patients in the first two postoperative days. If the integrity of the mucosa has not been breached, there is no indication for prophylactic antibiotics.

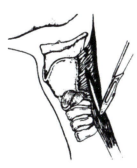

Fig. 3 Upper esophageal sphincter (UES) myotomy is performed extending from the lower constrictor pharyngeal musculature, through the cricopharyngeal muscle, and down to the longitudinal fibers of the upper esophageal musculature

Swallowing rehabilitation starts on the third post-operative day if there have been no signs of perforation or local infection. In the first few days of the rehabilitation, edema can interfere with the swallowing act, but prolonged delay of swallow training is not considered favorable because of the possible development of local fibrosis and consequently stenosis of the UES. Patients leave the hospital after a safe and adequate oral intake has been achieved. If they fail to accomplish a sufficiently safe oral intake despite extensive postoperative swallowing rehabilitation, percutaneous endoscopic gastrostomy (PEG) feeding or adequate dietary adjustments might be necessary so that the patient can safely manage at home.

2.3 Severe Aspiration in Oropharyngeal Dysphagia

In patients with chronic aspiration and recurrent pneumonia, often a strict PEG feeding policy is applied or a total laryngectomy or some other type of permanent anatomic or functional separation of the airway and digestive tract is performed. However, in selected cases it is possible to preserve or restore oral intake with a functional larynx by a laryngeal suspension procedure in combination with myotomy of the UES. This procedure should be considered if aspiration is caused by a combination of deficient deglutitive laryngeal elevation, lack of pharyngeal constrictor activity, and insufficient opening of the esophageal inlet.

UES myotomy is the most frequently used surgical technique for treating dysphagia and aspiration. Often, however, it proves to be insufficient to prevent aspiration. If we take into consideration the normal physiological processes of deglutition, there is evidence (Kahrilas et al. 1988) that the most important

factor responsible for opening of the esophageal inlet is not relaxation of the UES, nor passive opening as a consequence of the propulsion of the bolus being pushed downward by the peristaltic contraction of the pharyngeal constrictor muscles, but deglutitive laryngeal elevation (Fig. 5). Because the UES is attached to the larynx, anterior and cranial displacement of the larynx during the pharyngeal phase of the swallowing act results in opening of the esophageal inlet. Simultaneous relaxation of the UES facilitates the opening of the esophageal inlet, and propulsive activity of the pharyngeal musculature improves the passage of the food bolus.

In addition to being the most important factor in opening of the esophageal inlet, the anterior and cranial displacement of the larynx also results in other mechanisms that help to protect the airway from aspiration. The larynx is pulled out of the way of the food bolus's path, the epiglottis is lowered over the laryngeal entrance as a roof protecting the airway, and the larynx is pulled under the base of the tongue, thus providing a partial cover of the laryngeal inlet. Such a situation can be obtained surgically by means of a laryngeal suspension procedure, during which the larynx is permanently fixed in the position that it would normally acquire during the swallowing act.

Since Edgerton and Duncan (1959) and Desprez and Kiehn (1959) first described laryngeal suspension as a technique for improving function after surgical resection of the anterior floor of the mouth, this technique has been used by many surgeons (Calcatarra 1971; Goode 1976; Tiwari et al. 1993; Fujimoto et al. 2007) as an integral part of major ablative surgery entailing loss of the mandibular–hyoid integrity or extended partial laryngectomy. The intent in these cases is to restore the continuity between the laryngeal–hyoid complex and the mandible and/or floor of the mouth musculature. This is of major importance for restoration of deglutitional function and prevention of aspiration in such cases.

Most alternative surgical procedures used for treatment of severe aspiration are associated with a permanent tracheostoma and loss of normal phonation. The procedures proposed include total laryngectomy, laryngeal closure, epiglottopexy, and laryngeal diversion (Lindeman 1975; Laurian et al. 1986; Kitahara et al. 1993; Habal and Murray 1972; Mongomery 1975; Sasaki et al. 1980; Hawthorne et al. 1987). It is our considered opinion that for some

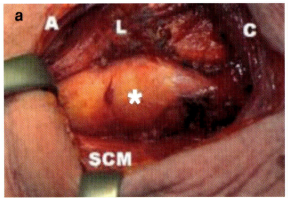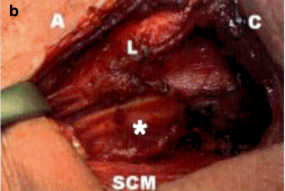

Fig. 4 a Image after the sectioning of the UES muscles with an inflated balloon (*asterisk*) endoluminally positioned in the esophageal entrance. **b** Image after the sectioning of the UES muscles with the balloon (*asterisk*) endoluminally positioned in the esophageal entrance but deflated. *A* anterior sternocleidomastoid muscle, *C* cranial, *L* larynx, *SCM* sternocleidomastoid muscle

of these patients with severe aspiration, surgical laryngeal suspension in combination with UES myotomy provides a less mutilating alternative, with preservation of normal phonation and respiration without permanent tracheostomy.

Our results (Kos et al. 2008) demonstrated that in nine of 17 patients (59%) long-term full oral intake without aspiration was achieved. In three patients (18%) partial improvement of deglutition was achieved, but these patients remained partly dependent on gastrostomy feeding for adequate nutrition. In two patients (12%) aspiration (of saliva) was reduced and no more aspiration pneumonias occurred, but these patients were unable to achieve even modified oral intake. In three patients (18%) a total laryngectomy could not be avoided, in two after initial success and as a result of progression of neuromuscular disease. None of the patients succumbed to aspiration pneumonia. In more than half of our patients (59%) life-threatening aspiration was successfully treated by UES myotomy and laryngeal suspension with full restoration of oral intake.

The goal of the laryngeal suspension and UES myotomy procedure is not to normalize the swallowing act, but to prevent life-threatening aspiration with preservation of a functional larynx. Even patients who were not able to achieve sufficient oral intake after the procedure had fewer problems with aspiration. The voice quality does not seem to change after elevation of the larynx. Because of potential postoperative airway compromise and anticipated difficulties with intubation as a result of the displaced larynx,

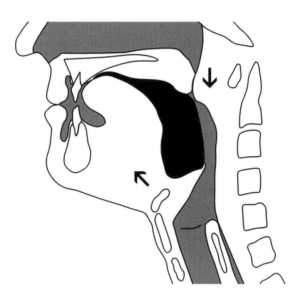

Fig. 5 Early pharyngeal phase of deglutition. Note the anterior and superior displacement of the hyoid and descending propulsive activity of constrictor pharyngeal muscles

elective temporary tracheotomy is routinely performed in all patients.

It seems advisable to include lower esophageal sphincter (LES) manometry in the preoperative diagnostic workup to rule out the possibility of an insufficient LES, since severe reflux is considered a contraindication to laryngeal suspension. After laryngeal suspension and UES myotomy, preexisting reflux can become worse, because this procedure abolishes the protective function of the UES against reflux. This situation can lead to severe aspiration of

Fig. 6 The UES myotomy and laryngeal suspension procedure. **a** UES myotomy; thyrohyoid approximation by an Ethibond 0 (Ethicon, Somerville, NJ, USA) suture tied as a mattress suture over polytetrafluoroethylene (GORE-TEX) bolsters on the thyroid cartilage and around the body of the hyoid bone. **b** Thyrohyoid complex suspended from the mandible by Ethibond 0 sutures, which have been passed around body of the hyoid bone and through holes drilled in the mandible

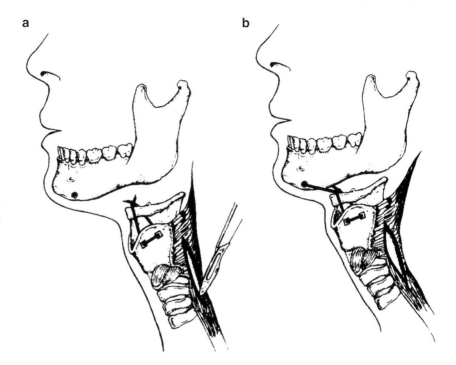

gastric refluxate, even in those cases in which the laryngeal suspension and UES myotomy allows relatively safe oral intake.

All patients who are eligible for this type of surgery have severe dysphagia and intractable aspiration despite intensive previous nonsurgical, and sometimes also surgical, treatment. Laryngeal suspension should be considered a procedure that can only partly compensate for the functional deglutitive deficiency and thus hopefully prevent aspiration. Patients who are unable or unwilling to accept these uncertainties in the outcome are not good candidates for the procedure. To avoid unrealistic expectations, patients should be made to understand that the goal of the surgical procedure is to prevent aspiration, and not to improve the swallowing act itself. Normal deglutition will never be achieved.

In patients who, because of a loss of sensation, did not notice their aspiration (silent aspiration) before the operation, the postoperative situation can be disappointing, because propulsion of the food bolus is not normalized and these patients fail to notice the improvement with respect to the aspiration. It is, of course, essential to extensively inform the patient before the operation of the expected outcome of the procedure. For these patients with a loss of sensibility, perhaps the option of additional restoration of

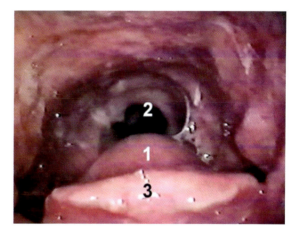

Fig. 7 View of the larynx and the esophageal inlet following laryngeal suspension, obtained with a 90° telescope during spontaneous respiration. *1* posterior surface of cricoid plate, *2* wide-open esophageal inlet, *3* epiglottis

sensibility by neural anastomosis may be helpful (Aviv et al. 1997).

2.3.1 Surgical Procedure

The surgical procedure (Fig. 6) starts with a UES myotomy as described already. All infrahyoid prelaryngeal muscles are severed to prevent traction of the laryngeal–hyoid complex in the caudal direction after surgery. A laryngeal suspension is performed by

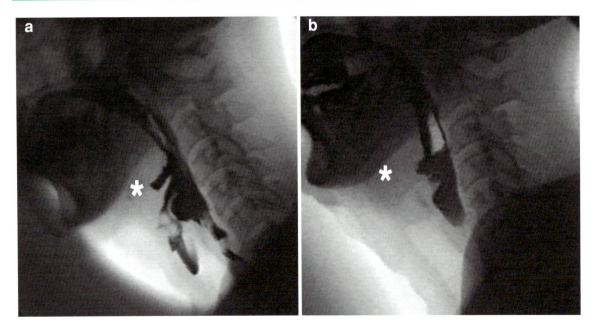

Fig. 8 Preoperative and postoperative videofluoroscopy. **a** Videofluoroscopic frame showing severe aspiration in the late pharyngeal phase before laryngeal suspension and UES myotomy. Note the absent pharyngeal constrictor activity and absent laryngeal elevation. **b** Videofluoroscopic frame in the late pharyngeal phase after laryngeal suspension and UES myotomy showing no aspiration. Note the position of the suspended larynx and epiglottis. *Asterisks* body of hyoid bone

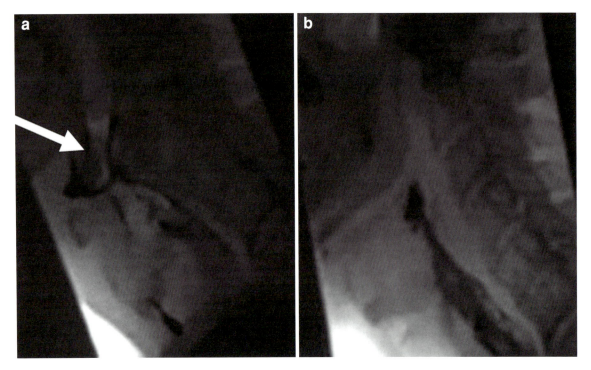

Fig. 9 Videofluoroscopic images of a 70-year-old patient with severe dysphagia and aspiration. **a** Preoperative image showing osteophytes at C3–C4 causing primary aspiration due to mechanical obstruction of the hypopharynx and esophageal inlet, and impairment of the epiglottis in its attempt to close the laryngeal inlet during the pharyngeal phase. **b** Image after removal of osteophytes showing normal bolus passage without obstruction

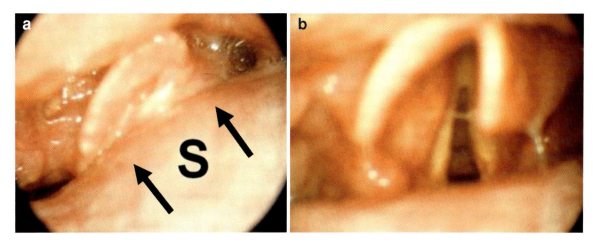

Fig. 10 Preoperative (**a**) and postoperative (**b**) endoscopic views of the larynx and pharynx. The retropharyngeal swelling (*S*) was caused by the meningoceles compressing and obstructing the laryngeal inlet as well as the esophageal inlet.

Postoperatively, free laryngeal inlet and normalized pharyngeal dimensions. Remaining asymmetric fold in the epiglottis due to prior prolonged compression by the meningoceles

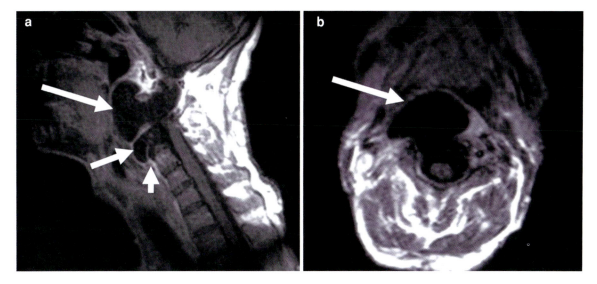

Fig. 11 Preoperative sagittal and axial T1-weighted magnetic resonance image revealing three meningoceles at the level of C3–C6. The two cranial and largest meningoceles protruding anterior to the cervical spine, the smallest remained intervertebral

approximating the thyroid cartilage and the hyoid bone with polytetrafluoroethylene (GORE-TEX; permanent) sutures and Vicryl 0 (Ethicon, Somerville, NJ, USA; resorbable but strong enough to overcome initial traction) tied over a polytetrafluoroethylene sheet to prevent rupturing of the thyroid cartilage and by pulling this laryngeal-hyoid complex toward the chin by two Ethibond (Ethicon) sutures, as well as the

polytetrafluoroethylene sutures, which are passed through drill holes in the mandible just posterior to the angle of the chin and anterior to the foramen of the mental nerve and are then tied. To prevent over-correction and consequent airway compromise, laryngoscopy is performed just before tying the sutures to ensure that the epiglottis and the base of the tongue do not completely obstruct the larynx. This is not

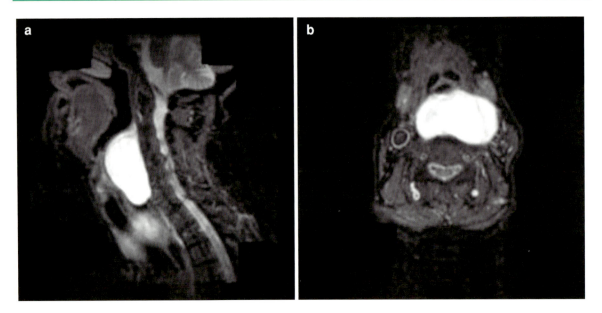

Fig. 12 T1 preoperative saggital and axial magnetic resonance images demonstrating the large retropharygeal tumor

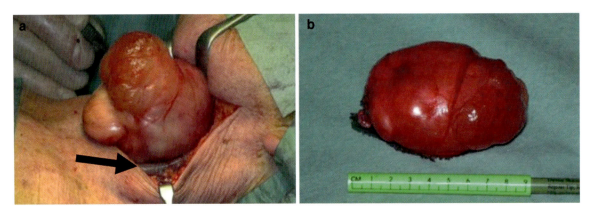

Fig. 13 a Removal of the tumor by an anterolateral approach. The longitudinal axis of the tumor was approximately 9 cm. **b** Tumor protruding through neck incision. *Arrow* jugular vein

always easy to estimate, because at this moment the intratracheal tube is still in place, preventing complete obstruction of the laryngeal inlet.

If the patients did not already have a PEG tube, they are given a transnasal feeding tube for the initial postoperative period. It is advisable to perform a temporary tracheotomy to guarantee a patent airway in the postoperative period, because as a consequence of the laryngeal suspension, the laryngeal entrance is displaced anteriorly and cranially (Fig. 5), interfering with intubation in the case of airway compromise. This tracheotomy should be performed at the end of

the procedure, after the actual laryngeal suspension procedure, so as not to limit the extent of the laryngeal suspension (Figs. 7, 8).

2.4 Dysphagia Caused by Extraluminal Compression

2.4.1 Anterior Cervical Osteophytes

Anterior cervical osteophytes are a common but rarely symptomatic finding mostly seen in the geriatric population. They can occur in cases of

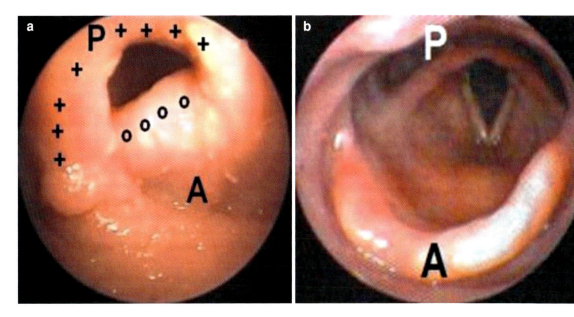

Fig. 14 a Endoscopic view of the semicircular oropharyngeal stenosis fixed to the epiglottis in a patient following radiotherapy for T1 oropharyngeal carcinoma. **b** Five-year postoperative endoscopic view of the larynx demonstrating only minor remains of the stenosis at the oropharyngeal level and an unobstructed view of the glottis. *Circles* the free edge of the epiglottis, *crosses* semicircular strictures attached to the epiglottis, *A* anterior, *P* posterior

degenerative disk disease, as part of the physiological or accelerated ageing process, but are most marked in diffuse idiopathic skeletal hyperostosis, also known as Forestier's disease (Resnick et al. 1975; Matan et al. 2002). If symptomatic, dysphagia appears to be the most common presentation, caused by mechanical obstruction of the pharyngoesophageal segment by anterior cervical hyperostosis. Exclusion of other causes of dysphagia is mandatory before blaming cervical osteophytes for dysphagic complaints. The surgical procedure is performed in collaboration with an orthopedic surgeon (Fig. 9).

Dysphagia is mostly seen in cases of cervical anterior osteophytes, mainly because C4–C7 are most often affected and compression at this level causes obstruction of the esophagus. Secondary aspiration can occur in patients with severe obstruction of the esophagus due to stasis. Primary aspiration can be caused by large osteophytes at C3–C4 directly interfering with laryngeal elevation and closure in the swallowing act. Primary aspiration can also occur as a consequence of vocal fold immobility due to damage of neural structures by the osteophytes (Giger et al. 2006). Dyspnea as a result of compression of the

pharynx and larynx is extremely rare (Matan et al. 2002). More common head and neck symptoms are pain and problems with sensation (as a consequence of compression of the cervical spine or vertebral artery), Horner's syndrome (Brandenberg and Leibrock 1986), and obstructive sleep apnea (Girgis et al. 1982). Dysphagia is often more severe with extension than with flexion of the neck. Complaints are more pronounced for solid boluses than for liquid boluses.

Diagnostic investigation should include laryngoscopic ENT examination. A lateral plain radiograph can be helpful in evaluation of the cervical spine for congenital or degenerative changes. Computed tomography or magnetic resonance imaging with sagittal reconstruction is advised to enable location of anterior bony lesions in relation to the surrounding soft tissues, large vessels, and nerve sheets. Dynamic videofluoroscopy is an important diagnostic tool, in which the patient swallows a liquid and solid bolus so that the dynamic process of deglutition can be evaluated. The level and cause of obstruction can be determined if dynamic videofluoroscopy is combined with conventional imaging of the spine. Manometry can be helpful to exclude coordination disorders of UES function.

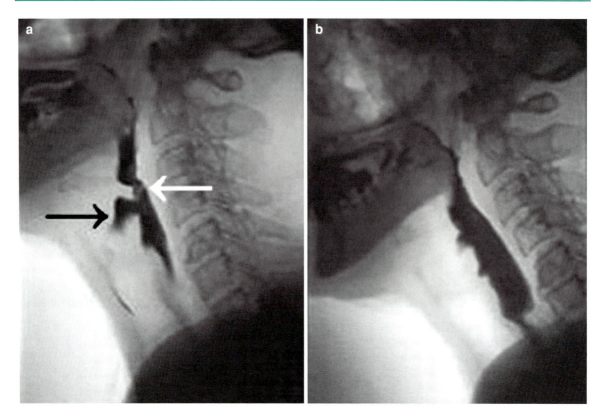

Fig. 15 Same case as in Fig. 14. **a** Preoperative videofluoroscopy demonstrating the oropharyngeal stenosis (*white arrow*), penetration of contrast material in the larynx (*black arrow*), primary aspiration into the trachea, and an almost absent pharyngeal constrictor muscle activity. **b** Postoperative videofluoroscopy in the pharyngeal phase revealing complete reduction of oropharyngeal stenosis, an increased bolus passage, and no penetration or aspiration. Of course, the pharyngeal constrictor activity is still insufficient

The treatment of patients with diffuse idiopathic skeletal hyperostosis depends on the degree of the symptoms. Initial therapy involves adaptation of food consistency. Conservative treatment with nonsteroidal anti-inflammatory drugs and antibiotics can be successful in cases with an inflammatory component (Oga et al. 1993). The symptoms will often have a more acute or subacute character in these cases.

When dysphagia is directly caused by obstruction of bony protrusions, the symptoms will be more chronic and slowly progressive. In these cases, or when there are more severe symptoms such as chronic aspiration and weight loss, surgical intervention should be considered (Richter 1995). Especially in older patients, who have a diminished cough reflex and thus an elevated risk of developing aspiration pneumonia, surgical treatment may be indicated.

Surgical approaches include anterolateral, posterolateral, and transoral approaches. Our preferred approach is anterolateral, because it provides optimal exposure of the large cervical vessels and vagal nerve and a good exposure of the prevertebral space, but it does place the recurrent laryngeal nerve at greater risk than the other approaches (Akhtar et al. 2000). The posterolateral approach offers wide exposure of the prevertebral space but requires more retraction of the carotid sheath (Carrau et al. 1990). The transoral approach has the advantage of cosmetic appeal as well as limited risk to the aforementioned structures compared with the anterolateral and posterolateral approaches. However, the disadvantages include limited exposure as well as the potential risk of fascial infection or osteomyelitis due to a contaminated surgical field.

Spondylodesis is only indicated in the case of instability after removal of cervical hyperostosis (Richter 1995; Krause and Castro 1994). If sufficient anterior ossification remains between the vertebrae, there is a low risk of postoperative cervical instability.

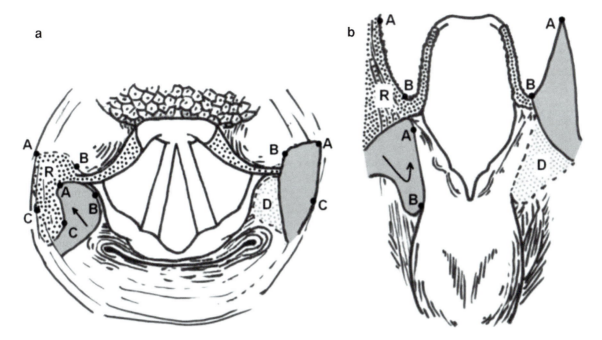

Fig. 16 **a** Craniocaudal and **b** posteroanterior views of the larynx and hypopharynx: the pharyngoplasty procedure. In each case the *left side* shows the situation after dissection and resecting the strictures, and before transpositioning of the mucosal flap from the piriform sinus, and the *right side* shows the situation after transpositioning of the mucosal flap and suturing. The raw surface of the epiglottis edges remained uncovered. The raw surface of the lateral free edge of the epiglottis and pharyngeal wall is marked with *R*. The donor site of the transposition flap is marked with *D* and its corresponding end position points are marked with *A*, *B*, and *C*

2.4.2 Dysphagia and Dyspnea Caused by Multiple Cervical Anterior Meningoceles

Type 1 neurofibromatosis may present with a wide spectrum of pathological anomalies. Very rarely it may present as a spinal meningocele, a protrusion of spinal meninges through a defect in the vertebral column or foramina. The pathogenesis of the lesion remains unclear, but several theories have been proposed, such as trauma (Freund and Timon 1992), dural (Bensaid et al. 1992), and/or regional bony dysplasia (Erkulurawatra et al. 1979). Magnetic resonance imaging is the preferred diagnostic tool for most spinal abnormalities. This modality accurately demonstrates the morphologic properties of a lesion, and changes in the longitudinal contour of the spinal cord can easily be detected. Computed tomography can be helpful in showing a relation of nervous structures to complex bony anatomy or in patients unable to undergo magnetic resonance imaging.

Meningoceles may be asymptomatic, and do not necessarily require treatment. The probability of the gradual enlargement of the meningocele with time and the possibility that it may cause pain, dysphagia, and dyspnea should be weighed against the risks of surgical resection of the meningocele. The goal of surgical treatment of a basal meningocele is ligation of its neck at the intervertebral foramina and resection of the sac. Figures 10 and 11 demonstrate a patient with type 1 neurofibromatosis who harbored a large retropharyngeal mass, consisting of two cervical meningoceles, causing dysphagia and dyspnea, and requiring surgical removal. The procedure is performed in collaboration with a neurosurgeon.

An anterior–lateral surgical extrapharyngeal approach is used for optimal exposure of the anterior cervical spine. A transoral approach is advised against because of contamination of the surgical field and the risk of postoperative meningitis. Surgery may be difficult because of dural defects and fragility

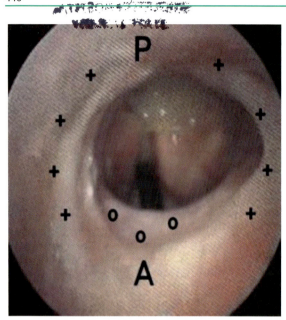

Fig. 17 Endoscopic view of the larynx of another patient demonstrating a similar, but less severe stricture (*crosses*) of the free edge of the epiglottis (*circles*) and the lateral pharyngeal walls and the arytenoids with the posterior part of the vocal folds below. In this case the esophageal stenosis was complete in continuity with an obliteration of the piriform sinus bilaterally. *A* anterior, *P* posterior

of the meningocele. A postoperative lumbar drain to diminish cerebrospinal fluid pressure is advisable.

Following excision, respiration as well as deglution normalized.

2.4.3 Dysphagia and Dyspnea Caused by a Retropharyngeal Tumor Mass

Dysphagia and dyspnea can be caused by any retropharyngeal tumor of benign or malignant origin. Here we describe an example of a 87-year-old female patient with severe dysphagia and dyspnea caused by a large retropharyngeal myxofibrosarcoma.

Myxofibrosarcoma is one of the most common sarcomas in the field of orthopedic surgery. Typically, it grows in the subcutaneous tissue of the extremities in elderly persons. Myxofibrosarcomas in the head and neck region are rare, and only a few cases of the disease in this area have been reported. Following excision, respiration as well as deglution normalized (Figs. 12, 13).

2.5 Strictures and Fibrosis of the Pharynx and UES

Fibrosis and strictures of the pharynx and UES are usually the result of caustic ingestion or chemoradiation and occasionally external neck trauma. Even though the nutritional status of the patient can easily be restored by tube feeding, swallowing problems generally have a considerable impact on quality of life and might also lead to social isolation (de Boer et al. 1995). Strictures are usually found in the hypopharynx or cervical esophagus, but also at more cranial levels in the pharynx. Depending on the stricture site, dyspneic complaints can be induced besides dysphagia and life-threatening aspiration. Usually (repeated) endoscopic bougienage or balloon dilations can be a successful treatment strategy (Piotet et al. 2008). Other treatment options have to be considered if stricture formation has advanced to complete stenosis or if the stricture is at a more cranial pharyngeal level.

2.5.1 Mucosal Flap Pharynxplasty with the CO_2 Laser

Strictures of the oropharynx are rare and complex problems. Severe stricture formation can occur between the lateral edges of the epiglottis and the lateral and posterior pharyngeal walls. In one patient who underwent radiotherapy for a T1 oropharyngeal carcinoma of the soft palate (Figs. 14, 15) such a stricture left a lumen of no more than 3–4 mm. Dyspnea in exercise became apparent as well as obstruction for larger food fragments in this segment, each time also obstructing his airway. The microendoscopic use of the CO_2 laser provided an excellent approach to release these strictures from the epiglottis with excellent visualization and working space. Mucosal pharyngeal reconstruction flaps can be transpositioned to prevent recurrent contracture and stricture formation. A tracheotomy under local anesthesia was first performed to improve the working space and visualization and secure the airway. Despite the impaired pharyngeal and tongue-base muscle activity and loss of laryngeal elevation and closure, near normal oral intake was achieved in this case. However, even the possibility of restoring minimal oral intake can provide a great improvement in the quality of life and is therefore worthwhile to try to achieve (Figs. 16, 17).

Fig. 18 **a** Preoperative videofluoroscopy demonstrating stenosis in the postcricoid area (*white arrow*) and severe aspiration (*black arrow*). **b** Postoperative videofluoroscopy demonstrating bolus passage into the esophagus with moderate residual stenosis and absence of aspiration

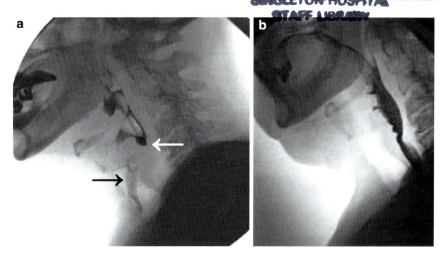

2.5.2 Anterograde–Retrograde Rendezvous Dilation for Complete Hypopharyngeal or UES Stenosis

Hypopharyngeal or UES strictures are commonly managed with bougie dilatation as long as there some lumen is still to be found. Laurell et al. (2003) reported a 78% success rate with dilatation of hypopharyngeal strictures secondary to radiotherapy for head and neck malignancies. Patients with moderate to severe strictures required one to eight dilations. The reported mortality rate was 5% secondary to esophageal perforation.

In the case of complete obstruction of the hypopharynx/cervical esophagus, an anterograde–retrograde dilatation technique can be considered. In this technique a guide wire retrogradely introduced through a (preexistent) percutaneous gastrostomy and the lumen of the esophagus can safely be detected from the hypopharyngeal side without creating a false route in the mediastinum, with the risk of mediastinitis. Often a rigid endoscope is required to enter the esophagus from below, because flexible endoscopes tend to curl up inside the stomach instead of passing through the LES into the esophagus. After the lumen has been resorted, intermittent anterograde bougie dilatation is often required.

The anterograde–retrograde rendezvous technique was first described by van Twisk et al. (1998), and several other small series were reported later (Petro et al. 2005; Maple et al. 2006). The advantage of this technique is that a stenosis can be punctured with a dilation guide wire away from the mediastinum,

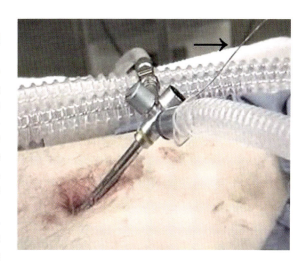

Fig. 19 Rigid endoscope introduced through the percutaneous endoscopic gastrostomy opening with a Savary dilation wire (*arrow*) introduced. The flexible tube attached to the endoscope is used for insufflation purposes

avoiding a false route in this direction and thus reducing the risk of mediastinitis. Sometimes transillumination is used from both sides to determine the direction of puncture. If the stenosis extends over a longer distance, anterograde dissection with a blunt instrument or the CO_2 laser can be performed toward an illuminated poststenotic lumen. Most patients treated this way have responded well to subsequent serial dilations and most have been able to discontinue gastrostomy tube use (van Twisk et al. 1998; Petro et al. 2005; Maple et al. 2006) (Figs. 18, 19).

3   Conclusion

As in all elective surgical procedures, the dysphagic patient has to be fit enough to overcome the stress related to general anesthesia, the surgical procedure, and the recovery period. However, the patent with a severe dysphagic problem is often not in a good condition and many patients have serious comorbidity. This restricts the use of a surgical treatment option in many cases. Furthermore, not all disorders resulting in oropharyngeal dysphagia can be successfully corrected surgically. Therefore, only a minority of dysphagic patients will be able to benefit from surgical treatment. However, the results presented in this chapter show that it is worthwhile to take into consideration the several procedures which have been described, in order to optimize the quality of life of the dysphagic patient. Since the focus of this chapter was on the surgical treatment of oropharyngeal dysphasia and no mention was made of swallowing rehabilitation, it should be stated that in almost all patients following surgical treatment, with the exception of patients with extraluminal compression and patients with ZD, an extensive postoperative swallowing rehabilitation program is an integral part of the treatment.

References

Akhtar S, O'Flynn PE, Kelly A, Valentine PM (2000) The management of dysphagia in skeletal hyperostosis. J Laryngol Otol 114:154–157

Aviv JE, Mohr JP, Blitzer A et al (1997) Restoration of laryngopharyngeal sensation by neural anastamosis. Arch Otolaryngol Head Neck Surg 123:154–160

Bensaid AH, Dietmann JL, Kastler B et al (1992) Neurofibromatosis with dural ectasia and bilateral symmetrical pedicular clefts: report of two cases. Neuroradiology 34:107–109

Brandenberg G, Leibrock LG (1986) Dysphagia and dysphonia secondary to anterior cervical osteophytes. Neurosurgery 18:90–93

Brigand C, Ferraro P, Martin J, Duranceau A (2007) Risk factors in patients undergoing cricopharyngeal myotomy. Br J Surg 94:978–983

Calcatarra T (1971) Laryngeal suspension after supraglottic laryngectomy. Arch Otol 94:306–309

Carrau RL, Cintron FR, Astor F (1990) Transcervical approaches to the prevertebral space. Arch Otolaryngol Head Neck Surg 116:1071–1073

Christiaens P, De Roock W, Van Olmen A, Moons V, D'Haens G (2007) Treatment of ZD through a flexible endoscope with a transparent oblique-end hood attached to the tip and a monopolar forceps. Endoscopy 39(2):137–140

Coiffier L, Périé S, Laforêt P, Eymard B, St Guily JL (2006) Long-term results of cricopharyngeal myotomy in oculopharyngeal muscular dystrophy. Otolaryngol Head Neck Surg 135:218–222

Collard JM, Otte JB, Kestens PJ (1993) Endoscopic stapling technique of esophagodiverticulostomy for ZD. Ann Thorac Surg 56:573–576

Cook IJ (1993) Cricopharyngeal function and dysfunction. Dysphagia 8:244–251

Cook IJ, Kahrilas PJ (1999) AGA technical review on management of oropharyngeal dysphagia. Gatroenterology 116:455–478

Cook RD, Huang PC, Richtsmeier WJ, Scher RL (2000) Endoscopic staple-assisted esophagodiverticulostomy: an excellent treatment of choice for ZD. Laryngoscope 110:2020–2025

de Boer MF, Pruyn JF, van den Borne B, Knegt PP, Ryckman RM et al (1995) Rehabilitation outcomes of long-term survivors treated for head and neck cancer. Head Neck 17(6):503–515

Desprez JD, Kiehn CL (1959) Method of reconstruction following resection of the anterior oral cavity and mandible for malignancy. Plast Reconstr Surg 24:238–249

Dohlman G, Mattson O (1960) The endoscopic operation for hypopharyngeal diverticula. Arch Otolaryngol 71:744–752

Edgerton MT, Duncan MM (1959) Reconstruction with loss of the hyomandibular complex in excision of large cancers. Arch Surg 78:425–436

Erkulurawatra S, El Gammal T, Hawkins JB et al (1979) Intrathoracic meningoceles and neurfibromatosis. Arch Neurol 36:557–559

Flint PW, Purcell LL, Cummings CW (1997) Pathophysiology and indications for medialization thyroplasty in patients with dysphagia and aspiration. Otolaryngol Head Neck Surg 116:349–354

Freund B, Timon C (1992) Cervical meningocele presenting as a neck mass in a patient with neurofibromatosis 1. J Laryngol Otol 106:463–464

Fujimoto Y, Hasegawa Y, Yamada H et al (2007) Swallowing function following extensive resection of oral or oropharyngeal cancer with laryngeal suspension and cricopharyngeal myotomy. Laryngoscope 117:1343–1348

Giger R, Dulguerov P, Payer M (2006) Anterior cervical osteophytes causing dysphagia and dyspnea: an uncommon entity revisited. Dysphagia 21(4):259–263

Girgis JH, Guirguis NN, Mourice M (1982) Laryngeal and pharyngeal disorders in vertebral ankylosing hyperostosis. J Laryngol Otol 96:659–664

Goode RL (1976) Laryngeal suspension in head and neck surgery. Laryngoscope 86:349–355

Guily JL, Perie S, Willig TN, Chaussade S, Eymard B, Angelard B (1994) Swallowing disorders in muscular diseases: functional assessment and indications of cricopharyngeal myotomy. Ear Nose Throat J 73:34–40

Habal MB, Murray JE (1972) Surgical treatment of life-endangering chronic aspiration pneumonia: use of an epiglottic flap to the arytenoids. Plast Reconstr Surg 59:305–311

Hatlebakk JG, Castell JA, Spiegel J, Paoletti V, Katz PO, Castell DO (1998) Dilatation therapy for dysphagia in patients with UES dysfunction–manometric and symptomatic response. Dis Esophagus 11:254–259

Hawthorne M, Gray R, Cottam C (1987) Conservative laryngectomy (an effective treatment for severe aspiration in motor neurone disease). J Laryngol Otol 101:283–285

Kahrilas PJ, Dodds WJ, Dent J et al (1988) Upper esophageal sphincter function during deglutition. Gastroenterology 95:52–62

Kaplan S (1951) Paralysis of deglutition, a post-poliomyelitis complication treated by section of the cricopharyngeus muscle. Ann Surg 133:572–573

Kelly JH (2000) Management of UES disorders: indications and complications of myotomy. Am J Med 108:43S–46S

Kitahara S, Ikeda M, Ohmae Y et al (1993) Laryngeal closure at the level of the false vocal cord for the treatment of severe aspiration. J Laryngol Otol 107:826–828

Kos MP, David EF, Aalders IJ, Smit CF, Mahieu HF (2008) Long-term results of laryngeal suspension and UES myotomy as treatment of life-threatening aspiration. Ann Otol Rhinol Laryngol 117:574–580

Kos MP, David EF, Mahieu HF (2009) Endoscopic CO$_2$-laser Zenker's diverticulotomy revisited. Ann Otol Rhinol Laryngol 118(7):512–518

Kos MP, David EF, Klinkenberg-Knol EC, Mahieu HF (2010) Long-term results of external UES myotomy for oropharyngeal dysphagia. Dysphagia 25(3):169–176

Krause P, Castro WH (1994) Cervical hyperostosis: a rare cause of dysphagia. Case description and bibliographical survey. Eur Spine J 3:56–58

Laurell G, Kraepelien T, Mavroidis P, Lind BK, Fernberg JO et al (2003) Stricture of the proximal esophagus in head and neck carcinoma patients after radiotherapy. Cancer 97:1693–1700

Laurian N, Shvili Y, Zohar Y (1986) Epiglotto-aryepiglottopexy: a surgical procedure for severe aspiration. Laryngoscope 96:78–81

Leder SB, Acton LM, Lisitano HL, Murray JT (2005) Fiberoptic endoscopic evaluation of swallowing (FEES) with and without blue-dyed food. Dysphagia 20:157–162

Lindeman RC (1975) Diverting the paralysed larynx: a reversible procedure for intractable aspiration. Laryngoscope 85:157–180

Mahieu HF, de Bree R, Dagli SA, Snel AM (1996) The pharyngoesophageal segment: endoscopic treatment of ZD. Dis Esophagus 9:12–21

Maple JT, Petersen BT, Baron TH, Kasperbauer JL, Wong Kee Song LM, Larson MV (2006) Endoscopic management of radiation-induced complete upper esophageal obstruction with an antegrade-retrograde rendezvous technique. Gastrointest Endosc 64(5):822–828

Matan AJ, Hsu J, Fredrickson A (2002) Management of respiratory compromise caused by cervical osteophytes: a case report and a review of the literature. Spine J 2:456–459

Mirza S, Dutt SN, Irving RM (2003) Iatrogenic perforation in endoscopie stapling divetiiculotomy for pbaryngeal pouches. J Laryngol Otol 117:93–98

Moerman MB (2006) Cricopharyngeal Botox injection: indications and technique. Curr Opin Otolaryngol Head Neck Surg 14:431–436

Mongomery WW (1975) Surgery to prevent aspiration. Arch Otolaryngol 101:679–682

Mosher HP (1917) Webs and pouches of the oesophagus: their diagnosis and treatment. Surg Gyn Obstet 25:175–187

Oga M, Mashima T, Iwakuma T, Sugioka Y (1993) Dysphagia complications in ankylosing spinal hyperostosis and ossification of the posterior longitudinal ligament. Spine 18:391–394

Petro M, Wein RO, Minocha A (2005) Treatment of a radiation-induced esophageal web with retrograde esophagoscopy and puncture. Am J Otolaryngol 26(5):353–355

Piotet E, Escher A, Monnier P (2008) Esophageal and pharyngeal strictures: report on 1,862 endoscopic dilatations using the Savary-Gilliard technique. Eur Arch Otorhinolaryngol 265(3):357–364

Resnick D, Shaul SR, Robins JM (1975) Diffuse idiopathic skeletal hyperostosis (DISH): Forestier's disease with extraspinal manifestations. Radiology 115:513–524

Richter D (1995) Ventral hyperostosis of the cervical spine—a rare differential diagnosis of dysphagia. Chirurg 66:431–433

Saetti R, Silvestrini M, Peracchia A, Narne S (2006) Endoscopic stapler-assisted Zenker's diverticulotomy: which is the best operative facility? Head Neck 28(12):1084–1089

Sasaki CT, Milmoe G, Yanagisawa E (1980) Surgical closure of the larynx for intractable aspiration. Arch Otolaryngol 106:422–423

Seaman DL, de la Mora Levy J, Gostout CJ, Rajan E, Knipschield M (2008) A new device to simplify flexible endoscopic treatment of ZD. Gastrointest Endosc 67:112–115

Takes RP, van den Hoogen FJ, Marres HA (2005) Endoscopic myotomy of the cricopharyngeal muscle with CO$_2$ laser surgery. Head Neck 27:703–709

Tang SJ, Jazrawi SF, Chen E, Tang L, Myers LL (2008) Flexible endoscopic clip-assisted Zenker's diverticulotomy: the first case series (with videos). Laryngoscope 118(7):1199–1205

Tiwari R, Karim ABM, Greven AJ et al (1993) Total glossectomy with laryngeal preservation. Arch Otolaryngol Head and Neck Surg 119:945–949

Van Overbeek JJ (1997) The hypopharyngeal diverticulum. Endoscopic treatment and manometry (thesis). VanGorcum, Assen

Van Overbeek JJ, Hoeksema PE, Edens E (1984) Microendoscopic surgery of the hypopharyngeal diverticulum using electrocoagulation or carbon dioxide laser. Ann Otol Rhinol Laryngol 93:34–36

van Twisk JJ, Brummer RJ, Manni JJ (1998) Retrograde approach to pharyngo-esophageal obstruction. Gastrointest Endosc 48(3):296–299

The Post-Operative Pharynx and Larynx

Anita Wuttge-Hannig and Christian Hannig

Contents

A. Wuttge-Hannig (✉)
Gemeinschaftspraxis für Radiologie,
Strahlentherapie und Nuklearmedizin,
Dres. Wuttge-Hannig-Rosskopf-Schepp-Sindelar,
Karlsplatz 3–5, 80335 Munich, Germany
e-mail: Olle.Ekberg@med.lu.se

C. Hannig
Institut für Röntgendiagnostik des Klinikums rechts der
Isar, Technische Universität München, Ismaningerstrasse
22, 82756 Munich, Germany

Abstract

Dysphagia is often seen in patients following surgery to the pharynx and larynx. It may be due to altered anatomy, altered physiology or altered function. Dysfunction may be due to sensory disturbances or altered biomechanics due to resection of muscles or repositioning of muscles. Radiotherapy with or without chemotherapy often contributes substantially to dysfunction. Mucosal abnormalities are best evaluated during endoscopy while extraluminal abnormalities including tumour recurrence are evaluated with MR or CT.

1 Introduction

Considerable progress has been made in the past few years in the diagnosis and treatment of swallowing disorders of neurological, anatomic or vascular origin. The treatment has been expanded to include patients with cancer and others with a rather limited time prognosis (Cantarella 1998; Denk et al. 1997; Groher 1992; Hannig and Wuttge-Hannig 1987, 1999; Hannig et al. 1989; Wuttge-Hannig and Hannig 1999; Lazarus et al. 2000; Leonard et al. 2001; Logemann et al. 1994).

This chapter will deal with patients who have undergone ear, nose and throat (ENT) surgery, minor or extensive and/or radio-, chemo- and the more recent use of radioimmunotherapy and gamma-knife therapy etc., including the sequelae of therapy (Eisbruch et al. 2002; Furia et al. 2000).

O. Ekberg (ed.), *Dysphagia*, Medical Radiology. Diagnostic Imaging, DOI: 10.1007/174_2012_650,
© Springer-Verlag Berlin Heidelberg 2012

The development in recent years of newer diagnostic and therapeutic modalities, including combined surgical and chemotherapeutic and radiotherapeutic schemes resulting in cure or remission even in advanced tumour stages, prompted the urgency to be aware and recognise swallowing complications before sequelae such as aspiration pneumonia become apparent (Hannig et al. 1995a, 1991; Jung and Adams 1980; Walther et al. 1990).

The differentiation between anatomical causes and functional origins related to sensory disturbances which often occur a year or two following the original treatment requires precise analysis in order to initiate appropriate therapy (Hannig and Wuttge-Hannig 1999; Wuttge-Hannig and Hannig 1995). It is also important to exclude submucosal spread of tumour, which may escape endoscopic detection (Wuttge-Hannig et al. 2001). Late consequences of subcutaneous and muscular fibrosis may occur resulting in the restriction of the antero-superior movement of the larynx during swallowing (Hannig 1995).

1.1 Altered Anatomy

Dysphagia is often the result of the altered anatomy following surgery such as laryngectomy, whereby separation of the larynx from the anterior pharyngeal wall produces a so-called pharyngeal tube seen especially in wider resections of pharyngeal structures. The configuration and diameter of the pharyngeal tube can vary with different surgical and sewing methods producing wide morphological variations in the radiological appearance (Hannig et al. 1994, 1996; Hannig 1995; Jung and Adams 1980; Martin et al. 1993) (Fig. 1).

The medical literature reports 15–20 % of dysphagia in partial and total laryngectomized patients (Di Santis et al. 1983; Hannig 1995). In our own series of 312 patients treated for laryngeal cancer, 37 % complained of dysphagia and 19 % of an annoying globus sensation. The higher incidence in our patients is probably due to stricter pre-selection of our interdisciplinary group, a heightened awareness as well as better patient education and compliance.

Post-therapeutic dysphagia following laryngectomy may be caused by the following pathology:
- Tumour recurrence (Fig. 2).
- Scarring and benign stenosis (Fig. 3).

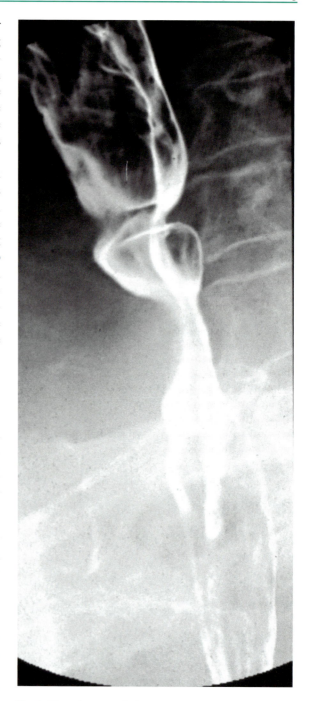

Fig. 1 Normal post-surgical anatomy of the pharyngeal tube after total laryngectomy. The pseudoglottis is seen as a circular narrowing

- Functional disorder of the "pharyngeal tube" and the pharyngo-esophageal transit zone (pseudoglottis) (Fig. 4).

Functional disorders are difficult to diagnose with video endoscopy or conventional radiological procedures but

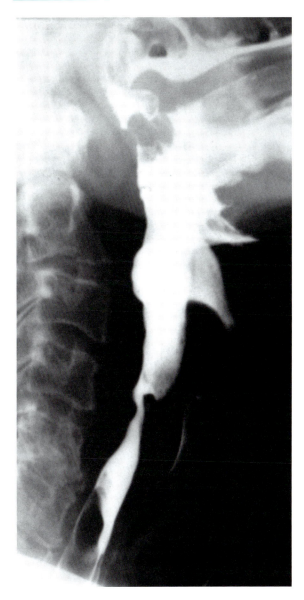

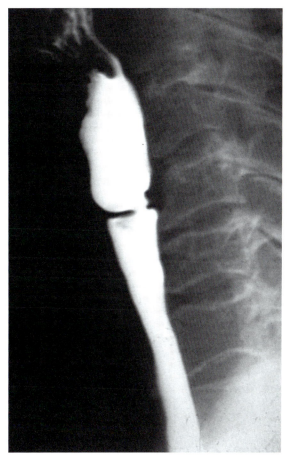

Fig. 3 Web due to scarring after radiation therapy

Fig. 2 Laryngectomy. Tumour recurrence with stenosis of the pharyngeal tube

require observation of the dynamics of swallowing and analysis of the altered motility of the post-surgical laryngo pharynx. This is the only way to differentiate among functional changes due to tumour recurrence or scarring.

1.2 Adapted Physiology of Swallowing

During the pharyngeal phase of swallowing, the force of the dorsal and lateral wave, the counterbalance of the larynx, the tongue base combined with the occlusion of the soft palate maintain the pressure needed to compress and move the bolus of food. The anatomic loss of soft tissue material causes important disturbances in the propulsion of the bolus (Dodds et al. 1975; Gates 1980; Gay et al. 1984; Hannig 1995). Surgical resection of part of the tongue base or floor of the mouth is a frequent cause of poor bolus preparation and compression in the oral cavity, thus hindering the trigger for an adequate swallowing reflex. The normal swallowing reflex is effected by an "input summation" needed to reach a critical limit (Kennedy and Kent 1988). This limit is rarely reached in patients treated for an oral-cavity carcinoma, therefore delaying the trigger in the secondary (valleculae) or tertiary area (piriform sinuses) or even quaternary area (laryngeal vestibule). Mucositis and mucosal atrophy due to radiation treatment can also cause trigger delay or absence. The restoration of the mucosal tissue integrity in the pharynx may restore

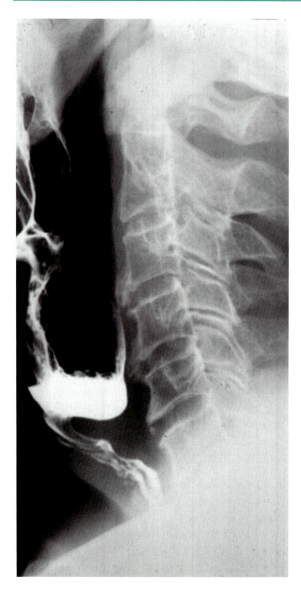

Fig. 4 Laryngectomy. Hypertrophic pseudoglottis with obstruction of the bolus transport

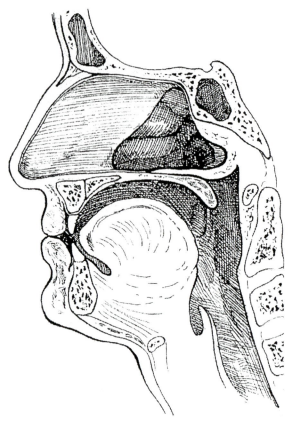

Fig. 5 Adult pharynx

the normal trigger but is frequently incomplete because of the rather permanent xerostomia. It may take 2–3 years of post-radiological treatment for restoration of the integrity of the mucosa. After combined radio-chemo treatment it may never be restored. In the latter patients, lesions in the trigger system occur in the receptors rather than the afferent limb of the loop (Fig. 5).

Children with a cleft palate present a special group of patients (Bosma et al. 1966; Isberg et al. 1990; Ren et al. 1993; Rubesin et al. 1987) (Fig. 6). The maturation of the swallowing reflex, which in nursing children occurs in the secondary area (the valleculae), cannot be brought up in time to the first area as is the case in adults, namely the arch of the fauces and dorsal pharyngeal wall, because the pressure generation in the oropharynx is inadequate. The lack of counter balance of the soft palate during swallowing may cause a compensatory downward movement by the tongue base in order to propagate the bolus into the pharynx.

A unilateral incision of the pharynx causes likewise lack of propagation and transport of the bolus retaining part of the bolus in the ipsilateral vallecula and piriform sinus. The most serious motility change occurs as a result of resection of the larynx and the resulting motility changes of the "neopharynx" referred to as the "pharyngeal tube" (Fig. 7). In such patients, even a hypertonic dorsal wave is incapable of producing a competent peristaltic wave. The pharyngeal pressure generation is not sufficient to passively open the upper oesophageal sphincter (UES).

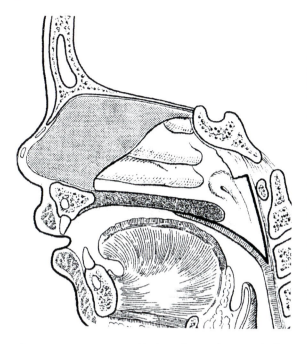

Fig. 6 Infantile pharynx with short distance between the base of the tongue and the laryngeal vestibule

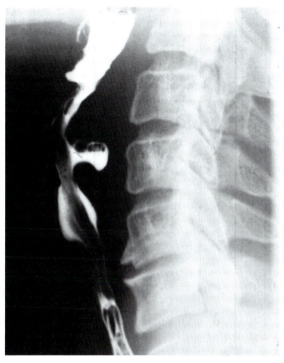

Fig. 7 Laryngectomy. Motor disturbance of the dorsal pharyngeal wall with diverticulum between the middle and inferior constrictors

We demonstrated that in patients with a hypotonic wave and a normal UES at least 40 mm Hg manometric pressure is needed for the passive opening of the dissected pharyngoesophageal segment.

1.3 Adaptation Methodology

In our swallowing-impaired patients we use an iso-osmolar iodine solution (Isovist®-Iotrolan) which causes no lung damage in case of aspiration. (The hyperosmolar preparations may cause pulmonary oedema) (Hannig et al. 1994; Hannig 1995). The contrast medium is mixed with the type of food that causes the swallowing difficulty. This can be solid, semi-solid, crumbly or liquid.

In patients after surgery for a cleft palate or following partial or complete laryngectomy we also have the patient perform different sounds and vocals, such as "coca-cola", "in the garden grows an apple tree", "kakadu". The elasticity of the pharynx and larynx is tested by the use of Valsalva (Fig. 8) and Mueller manoeuvres producing a maximal distension or collapse of the pharynx. This allows us to check for an occult neoplastic process of scarring.

1.4 Morphological and Functional Swallowing Abnormalities

A wide variety of morphological and functional swallowing abnormalities can be seen following ENT neoplasm surgery. The causes vary with the different types of surgery. Oral, pharyngeal, laryngeal and thyroid neoplasms are treated with a variety of procedures ranging from laser excision, wide resection, horizontal and transverse pharyngeal resection, partial or total laryngectomy or thyroidectomy, including combinations of therapy with or without hyperthermia present with different forms of dysphagia. Post-therapeutic changes related to vascular surgery of the neck, combinations of chemo- and radiation treatment may also result in dysphagia.

1.5 Laryngectomy

The incidence of dysphagia and globus pharyngis following total laryngectomy is around 50 % and rises with additional radiotherapy. Radiotherapy alone

Fig. 8 **a**, **b** Oro-hypopharyngeal neoplasm of the posterior wall best demonstrated by Valsalva manoeuvre

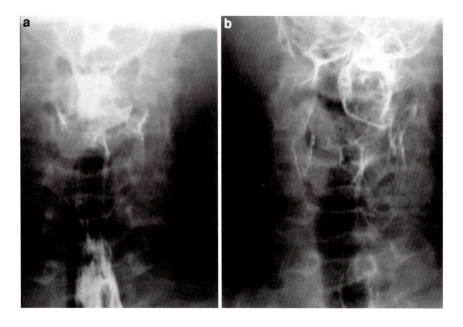

causes less of the latter but causes more frequently loss of sensation resulting in "trigger" delay. The displacement of the larynx results in loss of compression of the anterior pharyngeal wall, resulting in a hyper-competent dorsal wave of the reformed pharyngeal tube. Lateral compression during peristalsis is also deficient. The propulsion force is accomplished by the rotation of the tongue base which can result in hyper-excursion compensating for the dorsal pharyngeal wall (Hannig et al. 1994; Jung and Adams 1980; Mills 1973; Pauloski et al. 2002). A too large resection of the tongue base may cause severe dysphagia. A deficient opening of the reconstructed pharyngeal wall and the sphincter sleeve results in dysphagia. Hypotonicity of the pharyngeal tube may prevent the passive opening of the reconstructed sphincter. A hyperactive sphincter could also be responsible for solid-state dysphagia. Since voice prosthesis users form sounds with the reconstructed sphincter sling, a perfect voice quality correlates frequently with the degree of dysphagia. Our own patients favoured sacrificing the discomfort for a better voice quality (Hannig et al. 1994, 1993a).

Another cause of dysphagia is displacement of a voice prosthesis, particularly a too high implanted or a too steeply inclined prosthesis, causing food impaction and both solid and liquid dysphagia. Table 1 lists the changes in the area of the UES and pharynx in relation to the associated clinical symptoms. In one-third of patients the dysphagia could be related to functional disorders. Post-radiation and post-therapeutic scar stenosis or membranous stenosis is quite frequent but a recurrence is rare. In two-thirds of our patients with dysphagia, dysfunction of the motility of the pharynx or the UES could be identified. In asymptomatic patients slight dysmotility of the UES is still seen but is much less than in the symptomatic patients. The obstruction during a delayed opening of the UES was less than 20 % in those patients. UES function was assessed using planimetry and frame-by-frame analysis. The median delay caused by the dysmotility of the UES was 47.5 ms, considerably longer than the 24.5 ms in the asymptomatic patients. Two-thirds of our symptomatic patients had dysphagia and one-third only globus sensation. We were interested to see that there was a correlation between the extent of swallowing symptoms and the hypercontraction of the neopharynx. Table 2 shows the median values of time of peristalsis, the time of pharyngeal passage and the constrictor ratio (maximal protrusion of the dorsal pharyngeal wave in relation to the sagittal diameter of the C3 vertebral body). The median obstruction of the area of the pharyngo-esophageal segment due to a dysfunction of the sphincter was 35 % in the symptomatic group. It is remarkable how the time of peristalsis and time of pharyngeal passage was absolutely abnormal in the dysphagic patients. In Table 2,

Table 1 Dysphagia present in laryngectomie

	Causing dysphagia (%)	Not causing dysphagia (%)
Delayed opening of the UES	51	49
Premature closure of the UES	65	35
Incomplete opening of UES	70	30
Hypopharyngeal diverticula	52	48
Web	54	46
Reduced contractility/scarring of the pharyngeal tube	80	20
Tumor recurrence	31	69

n = 246, male: female = 77 %: 23 %, median age 61.5 aa

Table 2 Dysphagia present in laryngectomie alterations in pharyngeal timing in relation to dysphagia

	Causing dysphagia	Not causing dysphagia	Normal value
Dysphagia	Dysphagia	Value	
Time of pharyngeal peristalsis	1047 ms	763 ms	617 ms
Time of pharyngeal passage	868 ms	721 ms	615 ms
Depth of constriction wave (quotient)	0.60	0.69	0.47

n = 246, male: female = 77 %: 23 %, median age 61.5 aa

the motility disorders of the pharyngeal tube and the UES are presented in relation to the time measurements. As expected, due to the altered anatomy after laryngectomy, the constriction ratio was quite high in both the symptomatic and asymptomatic patients. Due to the loss of the laryngeal counter pressure, the dorsal peristaltic wave gets unusually prominent. In addition to the dysfunction of the neoglottis (formed by the UES) we see a second constricted area in the cervical oesophagus just below the UES. This "second sphincter" showed a functional pattern comparable to the UES. The exact pathomechanism of this second hyper-contractile zone is yet unknown. It might be the effect of regulation of the airflow during the oesophageal voice production.

In a large number of patients with a delayed emptying of the pharynx due to insufficient peristalsis we were able to observe a marked compensation by the tongue-base, a virtual "tongue pump" (Hannig 1995).

This tongue pump consists of an accentuated caudo-dorsal movement of the floor of the mouth together with the tongue base moving the bolus through the pharynx and the UES. In some patients, an additional hyper excursion of the Passavant cushion and the region of the superior constrictor pharyngis was noted

(a temporary long contact of the dorsal pharyngeal wall and tongue base). Quite often, scarring resulted in reduced contractility of the reconstructed pharynx or of a narrow pharyngeal canal. In Fig. 9 the scar was caused by radiotherapy. In other patients, it could be the result of chronic inflammation or in a poor healing of a post-operative fistula.

1.6 Hemi-pharyngectomy

There are two main types of partial pharyngeal resections. The horizontal resection (Fig. 9) is uncommon today, due to long-term complications from the interruption of the constrictor muscles resulting in deficient bolus propulsion. The more common longitudinal resection includes resection of the unilateral vallecula and piriform sinus and reconstruction of the pharyngeal tube by means of suturing the dorsal and anterior pharyngeal wall, often in combination with a myocutaneous flap. This reconstructed pharyngeal structure does not participate in the normal constriction due to relative weakness of the muscles. The bolus often remains on the resected side and can be cleared out of the pharynx

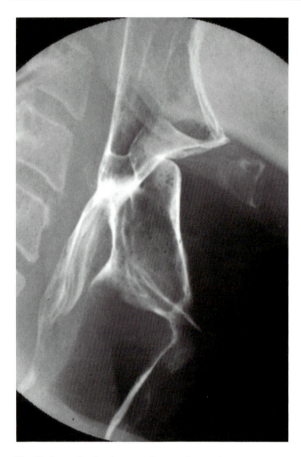

Fig. 9 Supraglottic pharyngo-laryngeal resection

only through the healthy hemi-pharynx (Hannig and Wuttge-Hannig 1999; Hannig 1995).

1.7   Post-Therapeutic Pharyngeal Cancer

In cancers of the oral cavity, the floor of the mouth, tongue, tonsils, pharynx and UES, the morphological and functional changes correspond to the type and extent of therapy (Hannig and Wuttge-Hannig 1999; Rosen et al. 2001; Zuydam et al. 2000). This may include simple resection, additional radio- or combined radio-chemotherapy. Less frequent forms of therapy such as combinations with hyperthermia are rare and will not be considered in our comparative studies (Fig. 10).

Table 3 summarises the functional disorders. Combined radiation and chemotherapy and surgery alone present similar problems, whereas radiation therapy alone presents the least. The most severe problems occur

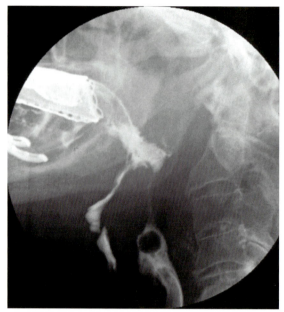

Fig. 10 Fistulation to the residual tongue base after partial tongue resection and radiochemotherapy

when surgery is followed by radiotherapy whereby in addition to the trigger problem related to the surgery, additional fibrosis related to the radiotherapy occurs. Differences in the severity and type of aspiration related to the different treatment modalities are illustrated in Table 4. Aspiration turns out to be most frequent in radiotherapy in combination with chemotherapy in which the negative effects of receptor destruction, hypostimulation and mucosal damage are added to the radiation and chemotherapy combination. Nevertheless, surgery alone causes the highest incidence of aspiration followed by radiotherapy alone and surgery plus radiotherapy. The high number of aspiration complications related to radiotherapy alone could be due to the fact that it usually involves older patients who could not tolerate a combined protocol. Table 5 lists the morphological alterations relative to the therapeutic protocol. As expected radiotherapy alone, surgery alone and radio-chemotherapy cause less problems.

1.8   Cleft Palate

A palatal cleft causes social stigma due to the external aesthetic image, the palato-rhinolalia and the nasal penetration of the bolus during swallowing (Engelke et al. 1991; Engelke 1994; Hannig et al. 1993b).

Table 3 Functional alterations due to ENT cancer-therapy

	Surg n = 37 (%)	Rth n = 47 (%)	Surg + Rth n = 92 (%)	Rth + Chemo n = 145 (%)
Bolus formation	46	11	87	25
Premature leaking out of the oral cavity	85	37	77	44
Delayed trigger of the swallowing reflex	49	78	88	81
Penetration in the laryngeal vestibule	40	19	76	72
Aspiration	75	71	79	75
Reduced coughing reflex	–	6	32	8
Laryngeal antero-cranial- movement	24	22	73	43
Dysfunction of the UES	65	9	86	56

n = 321, m: f = 67:33, mean age = 55.7 aa

Table 4 Type and severity of aspiration due to ENT cancer-therapy

	Surg 27/32 82 %	Rth 36/45 80 %	Surg + Rth 78/92 79 %	Rth + Chemo 112/145 77 %
Predeglutitive	16	24	36	47
Grade I	4	9	10	21
Grade II	4	6	9	9
Grade III	6	5	9	9
Grade IV	2	4	8	8
Intradeglutitive	3	0	13	21
Grade I	–	–	2	3
Grade II	2	–	4	7
Grade III	1	–	3	9
Grade IV	–	–	4	2
Postdeglutitive	8	12	29	44
Grade I	2	3	12	15
Grade II	2	2	9	13
Grade III	4	5	5	10
Grade IV	–	2	3	6
Combined forms	15	7	51	49

n = 321, m: f = 67:33, mean age = 55.7 aa

The anatomical shortening and the functional restriction of the soft palate include the post-therapeutic scar after closure of the defect. The above can lead to a velo-pharyngeal insufficiency.

An analysis of the velo-pharyngeal closing mechanism should be done before and after surgery (Thumfart et al. 1996; Bergeron et al. 1984; Croft et al. 1981; Dalston et al. 1985; Engelke et al. 1991; Engelke 1994; Hannig and Wuttge-Hannig 1992; Hannig et al. 1993b, 1995b; Hartmann et al. 1972; Hess et al. 1994, 1995a, b, 1996a, b; Herzog et al. 1993). The early use of surgical occlusion and/or prosthesis may help achieve proper maturation from the infantile to the adult swallowing reflex pattern. The nursing infant adapts safely to the anatomical changes. The first segment of the nearly horizontal aditus laryngis, which remains very narrow to the base of the tongue, together with the large valleculae and the long soft palate, permits a two-chamber separation of the pharynx. The infant is, thus, able to fill up the valleculae with usually three suctions during breathing. Only after three stimulations of the tongue base can the swallowing

Table 5 Morphologic Alterations due to ENT Cancer-Therapy

	Surg n = 20 (%)	Rth n = 47 (%)	Surg + Rth n = 92 (%)	Rth + Chemo n = 145 (%)
Fibrosis of the subepidermal tissue	11	62	72	48
Fibrosis of muscles	–	52	82	58
Adhesions skin-larynx	15	49	74	48
Adhesions larynx-prevertebral fascia	–	48	72	27
Stenosis by scarring	12	42	66	53
Oral defects	78	–	58	18
Pharyngeal defects	29	11	61	7
Laryngeal defects	32	–	48	–
Recurrence	–	07	11	21

n = 321, m: f = 67:33, mean age = 55.7 aa

reflex, located very deep in the pharynx, be triggered. Mastication assists in the development of the orally directed swallowing reflex. Tactile stimulations are also helpful in this process. According to Croft et al. (1981), four types of velo-pharyngeal occlusion mechanisms can be identified: sagittal, coronal, circular and circular with a Passavant cushion (Fig. 11).

The commonly used tools are: lateral radiography of the cranium, a pantogram of the dental arcade, video-fluoroscopy and the 16-slice helical CT already separated in spatial but not temporal resolution in the electron beam tomogram. In the future, MRI will be the imaging modality of choice especially in infants and young adults in whom the radiation dose is critical and where many radiograms in different planes have to be used. A very accurate appreciation of the velum motility and the swallowing competence allows one to decide which therapeutic approach would be most favourable: simple augmentation of the dorsal wall (Hynes) or the more complicated velo-pharyngoplasty (Sanvenero-Roselli) (Horch et al. 1993; Sader et al. 1994, 1995, 1997, 2001; Skolnick et al. 1989). Post-therapeutic evaluation of the velum performance assists in the decision whether a re-operation or a conservative programme is to be pursued.

2 Post-Traumatic, Post-Lesional and Post-Surgical Brain Lesions

A large spectrum of damage to the CNS and peripheral nervous system can result in dysphagia (Hannig 1995; Wuttge-Hannig and Hannig 1995). In neurologically impaired patients, conservative rehabilitative methods

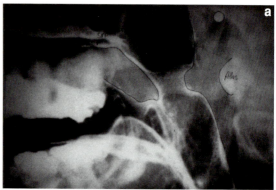
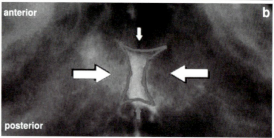

Fig. 11 Cleft. **a** Insufficient nasopharyngeal closure with attempt of a Passavant's compensation. **b** Circular compensation with major action of the lateral pharyngeal constrictors in hemiaxial projection

are the procedures of choice. Surgery might cause further damage to the trigger area. The Munich rehabilitative strategy is generally adopted for such patients. Therapy is planned based on dynamic swallowing analysis. A division and grading analysis into pre-, intra-, and post-deglutitive aspiration and its severity is done. The accurate study of the multiple patho-mechanisms allows us to design a programme individually tailored for each patient, which gives the best results and is most cost-effective (Hannig et al. 1995a; Hannig and Wuttge-Hannig 1999).

A unilateral functional defect or hypotonicity suggests a unilateral cerebral event, whereas a bilateral defect suggests a neuromuscular disorder (Wuttge-Hannig and Hannig 1995). Dilatation of the hypopharynx is common in trumpet players and singers and is bilateral. The study can identify neurogenic, myogenic and reflux induced disorders. The reflux episodes could be due to the 10th cranial nerve. The differentiation is important since in myogenic dysfunction simple drug use might solve the problem, which is not the case in vagal dysfunction where not only the UES but also the oesophageal clearing function is compromised. A myotomy of the UES should only be performed in rare cases. Oesophago-pharyngeal and tracheal aspiration would result from a surgical dilatation of the PE segment. The passive opening of the UES can be influenced by the Mendelsohn manoeuvre, but if there is a spasm of the UES conservative therapy is rarely adequate. Further reconstructive surgery should be undertaken only after a long-term rehabilitative trial. In the latter patient, the separation of the alimentary and respiratory canal should only be a last choice. If the patient possesses good cognitive capacity the use of alternative positional manoeuvres could be used. This is especially important in the planning of a laryngo-hyoido-mentopexy procedure planned via dynamic imaging. This surgical technique necessitates deglutition in the upright position (Hannig 1995). In 1996 Mahieu described a similar method as "laryngeal suspension", which was performed in a large number of aspirating patients but which excluded the tracheal stabilisation (Fig. 12). ENT and neurologists use botulism toxin injections. Newer applications of the latter may cure oesophageal motility disorders causing dysphagia. Within Thumfart's group in Innsbruck and at the ENT departments in Turin and Milan botox injections are frequently used (Cantarella 1998; Pastore et al. 1997; Thumfart et al. 1996).

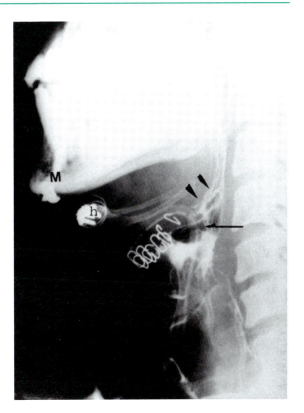

Fig. 12 Laryngo-hyoido-mentopexy in a patient with an intradeglutitive aspiration due to a resection of an ependymoma of the IVth ventricle

3   Scarring and Post-Surgical Instabilities of the Pharynx

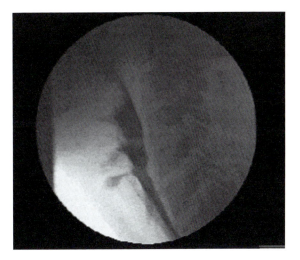

Fig. 13 Patient after surgery and radiotherapy for a thyroid cancer 25 years previously. Fistulation below the level of the arytenoid cartilages

Dysphagia is quite frequent as a result of muscular dissection in vascular (Fig. 13) and orthopaedic surgery of the cervical spine area (Hannig and Wuttge-Hannig 1999; Hannig 1995). In surgical unilateral procedures, an out-pouching of the weaker hemi-pharynx may occur due to a less effective lateral constrictor wave.

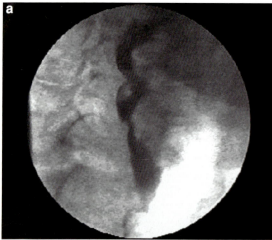

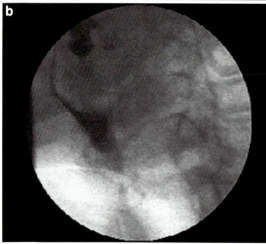

Fig. 14 Patient with dysphagia due to a patch insertion in the right carotid artery. **a** By turning the head to the left side the bolus passage is obstructed. **b** By turning the head to the right side a good clearance of the pharynx can be achieved

The therapeutic approach in such cases depends on the extent of weakness of the unilateral pharynx. If there is a relatively weak pharyngeal wall the bolus will end up in this weak hemi-pharynx and will not be cleared out of it. If there is a scar or hypertonicity of the surgical side, the contralateral side will transport the bolus well. A trial of the best manoeuvre by means of dynamic imaging will yield the best results. The raising or inclination of the head may result in a different pre-load to the external laryngeal musculature. The swallowing disorder may get even more complex by adhesions of the skin of the neck to the larynx frequently after surgery for thyroid tumours (Fig. 14).

4   Conclusion

Dynamic imaging in swallowing disorders defines the pathophysiology of the disorder and determines the method of rehabilitation of the post-therapeutically impaired deglutition. Myo- or neurogenic disorders can be identified. The oral and pharyngo-esophageal interaction can be studied. The advantage of this method of study lies in its ability to produce the high spatial and temporal resolution of the very fast motility between the oral cavity and entrance into the oesophagus. This procedure may also provide hints as to the localisation of the neurological focus, although the nature of the underlying disease is rarely identified by this technique alone. The studies permit individual tailoring of rehabilitation and the most cost-effective method.

References

Bergeron RT, Osborn AG, Sam PM (1984) Head and neck imaging. CV Mosby, St Louis

Bosma JF, Truby HM, Lind J (1966) Distortions of the upper respiratory and swallowing motions in infant having anomalies of the upper pharynx. Acta Paediatr Scand 163:111–128

Cantarella G (1998) Definizione ed epidemiologia dei disturbi della deglutizione. Centro Richerce e Sudi Amplifon, Raccolta bibliografica Seminario Turbe della deglutizione: attualità diagnostiche e terapeutiche, pp 12–17

Croft CB et al (1981) Patterns of velopharyngeal valving in normal and cleft palate subjects: a multi view videofluoroscopic and nasoendoscopic study. Laryngoscope 91:265–271

Dalston RM et al (1985) The diagnosis of velopharyngeal insufficiency. Clin Plastic Surg 12:685–695

Denk DM, Swoboda H, Schima W, Eibenberger K (1997) Prognostic factors for swallowing rehabilitation following head and neck cancer surgery. Acta Otolaryngol 117:769–774

Di Santis DJ, Balfe DM, Koehler RE, Lee KT (1983) Barium examination on the pharynx after vertical hemilaryngectomy. AJR 141:335–339

Dodds WJ, Hogan WJ, Lynden SB, Stewart ET, Stef JJ, Arndorfer RC (1975) Quantitation of pharyngeal motor function in normal human subjects. J Appl Physiol 39:692–696

Eisbruch A, Lyden T, Bradford CR, Dawson LA, Haxer MJ, Miller AE, Teknos TN, Chepeha DB, Hogikyan ND, Terrell JE, Wolf GT (2002) Objective assessment of swallowing dysfunction and aspiration after radiation concurrent with chemotherapy for head-and-neck cancer. Int J Radiat Oncol Biol Phys 53:23–28

Engelke W (1994) Videoendoskopische Untersuchungen des velopharyngealen Sphinkters bei Gesunden und bei Gaumenspaltpatienten. Dtsch Z Mund Kiefer Gesichtschir 18:190–195

Engelke W et al (1991) Elektromagnetische Artikulographie: Eine neue Methode zur Untersuchung von Bewegungsfunktionen des Gaumensegels. Folia Phoniatr 43:147–152

Furia CL, Carrara-de Angelis E, Martins NM, Barros AP, Carneiro B, Kowalski LP (2000) Videofluoroscopic evaluation after glossectomy. Arch Otolaryngol Head Neck Surg 126:378–383

Gates GA (1980) Upper esophageal sphincter: pre- and postlaryngectomy—a normative study. Laryngoscope 90:454–464

Gay I, Crisin R, Elidan J (1984) Myotomy of the cricopharyngeal muscle. A treatment for dysphagia and aspiration in neurological disorders. Rev Laryngol Otol Rhinol (Bord) 105:271–274

Groher M (1992) Dysphagia—diagnosis and management, 2nd edn. Butterworth-Heinemann, Boston

Hannig C (1995) Functional fluoroscopic diagnosis of pharynx and esophagus. Springer, Berlin

Hannig C, Wuttge-Hannig A (1987) Stellenwert der Hochfrequenzkinematographie in der Diagnostik des Pharynx und Ösophagus. Röntgenpraxis 40:358–377

Hannig C, Wuttge-Hannig A (1992) Cineradiography in pre- and postoperative evaluation of cleft patients. In: 6th Annual Meeting of the European Society of Head and Neck Radiology. Karlsruhe, Oct. 7–10

Hannig C, Wuttge-Hannig A (1999) Radiological functional diagnosis of swallowing disorders in neuological diseases and in posttherapeutic oncological ENT-diseases. In: Bartologme G, Buchholz DW, Feussner H, Hannig C, Neumann S, Prosiegel M, Schöter-Morasch H, Wuttge-Hannig A (eds) Schluckstörungen Diagnostik und Rehabilitation Hrsg, 2nd edn. Urban und Fischer Verlag, München, pp 65–110

Hannig C, Wuttge-Hannig A, Hörmann M, Herrmann IF (1989) Kinematographische Untersuchungen des Pathomechanismus der Aspirationspneumonie. ROFO Fortschr Geb Rontgenstr Nuklearmed 150:260–267

Hannig C, Wuttge-Hannig A, Clasen B, Kellermann S, Volkmer C (1991) Dysphagia of the treated laryngeal cancer—detection of functional and morphological changes by cineradiography. Bildgebung Imaging 58:141–145

Hannig C, Feussner H, Stein H (1993a) Cineradiography and radiomanometry in the pre- and postoperative evaluation of cricopharyngeal dysfunction. Scientific Programme and Abstracts, ECR 93. Springer International 1993:111

Hannig C, Wuttge-Hannig A, Daschner H, Sader R (1993b) Pre- and postoperative evaluation of cleft-patients by cineradiographic imaging. Scientific Programme and Abstracts, ECR 93. Springer International 273

Hannig C, Stein H, Wuttge-Hannig A, Hess U (1994) Diagnosis of cricopharyngeal dysfunction using simultaneous videomanometry and cinemanometry. In: 3rd Annual dysphagia research society meeting, Oct 14–16, 1994 McLean, Virginia, USA

Hannig C, Hess U, Sader R, Sinz J (1995a) Einfluss des velopharyngealen Abschlusses auf die OP-planung. In: Symposium "Moderne Chirurgi der Kieferfehlstellungen". Klinik und Poliklinik für Mund-Kiefer-Gesichtschirurgie, Technische Universität München, März 24–25

Hannig C, Wuttge-Hannig A, Hess U (1995b) Analyse und radiologisches Staging des Typs und Schweregrades einer Aspiration. Der Radiologe 35:741–746

Hannig C, Hess U, Wuttge-Hannig A, Volkmer C (1996) Dysphagie nach Laryngektomie—morphologische versus funktionelle Veränderungen. ROFO Fortschr Geb Rontgenstr Nuklearmed Suppl 164:95

Hartmann H et al (1972) Zur Frage der Intelligenz und sozialen Entwicklung von Kindern mit Lippen-, Kiefer-Gaumenspalten. Prax Kinderpsychol Kinderpsychiatr 21:1–10

Herzog M et al (1993) Röntgenbefunde nach sekundärer bzw tertiärer Osteoplastik bei Lippen-Kiefer-Gaumen-Spalten. Fortschr Kiefer Gesichtschir 38:64–66

Hess U, Hannig C, Sader R, Cavallaro A, Wuttge-Hannig A, Zeilhofer H (1994) Assessment of the velopharyngeal closure with high-frequence-cineradiography for preoperative planning of maxillary advancement, ICHNR, Washington, June 15–19.

Hess U, Hannig C, Weiss W, Sader R, Zeilhofer H, Wuttge-Hannig A, Merl T (1995a) Die Videokinematographie in der prä- und postoperativen Diagnostik der Lippen-Kiefer-Gaumen-Spalte. Radiologe 35:712–715

Hess U, Hannig C, Weiss W, Sader R, Zeilhofer HF, Wuttge-Hannig A, Merl T (1995b) Die Videokinematographie in der prä- und postoperativen Diagnostik der Lippen-Kiefer-Gaumenspalten. Radiologe 35:712–715

Hess U, Hannig C, Cavallaro A, Sader R (1996a) Die postoperative Kontrolle der seskundären Velopharyngoplastik mit Hilfe der Kinematographie. 77. Deutscher Röntgenkongress, Mai 15–18, 1996, Wiesbaden. ROFO Fortschr Geb Rontgenstr Nuklearmed 164:95

Hess U, Hannig C, Sader R, Cavallaro A, Wuttge-Hannig A, Zeilhofer H (1996b) Die Bewertung des velopharyngealen Verschlusses zur präoperativen Planung der Oberkiefervorverlagerung. Röntgenpraxis 49:25–26

Horch HH et al (1993) Klinische Ergebnisse nack sekundärer Kieferspaltosteoplastik im Wechselgebiss für Lippen-Kiefer-Gaumenspalten. Fortschr Kiefer Gesichtschir 38:61–64

Isberg A (1990) Radiographic examination of velopharyngeal function. In: Delbaso A (ed) Maxillofacial imaging. Saunders, Philadelphia

Jung TK, Adams GL (1980) Dysphagia in laryngectomised patients. Otolaryngol Head Neck Surg 88:25–33

Kennedy JG, Kent RD (1988) Physiological substrates of normal deglutition. Dysphagia 3:24–38

Lazarus CL, Logemann JA, Pauloski BR, Rademaker AW, Larson CR, Mittal BB, Pierce M (2000) Swallowing and tongue function treatment for oral and oropharyngeal cancer. J Speech Lang Hear Res 43:1011–1023

Leonard JR, Kendall KA, Johnson R, McKenzie S (2001) Swallowing in myotonic muscular dystrophy: a videofluoroscopic study. NY State Dent J 82:979–985

Logemann JA, Gibbons P, Rademaker AW, Pauloski BR, Kahrilas PJ, Bacon M, Bowman J, McCracken E (1994) Mechanism of recovery of swallow after supraglottic laryngectomy. J Speech Hear Res 37:965–974

Mahieu HF (1996) Aspiration in the late pharyngeal phase: UES dysfunction or defective laryngeal mobility? In: 2nd International symposium on laryngeal and tracheal reconstruction, Mai 22–26, 1996, Monte Carlo Proceedings, p 33

Martin BJ, Schleicher MA, O'Connor A (1993) Management of dysphagia following supraglottic laryngectomy. Clin Commun Disord 3:27–36

Mills CP (1973) Dysphagia in pharyngeal paralysis treated by cricopharyngeal sphincterotomy. Lancet 1:455–457

Pastore A, Marchese Ragona R, De Grandis D (1997) Il ruolo della tossina botulinica nelle turbe dello sfintere esofageo superiore. Corso intensivo teorico-pratico: Diagnostica e terapia die disturbi della deglutitzione. Milano 30–31.10.1997 (abstract book, pp 20–25)

Pauloski BR, Rademaker AW, Logemann JA, Lazarus CL, Newman L, Hamner A, MacCracken E, Gaziano J, Stachowiak L (2002) Swallow function and perception of dysphagia in patients with head and neck cancer. Head Neck 24:555–565

Ren YF, Isberg A, Henningsson G (1993) Interactive influence of a pharyngeal flap and adenoid on maxillofacial growth in cleft lip and palate patients. Cleft Palate Craniofac J 30:144–149

Rosen A, Rhee TH, Kaufman R (2001) Prediction of aspiration in patients with newly diagnosed untreated advanced head and neck cancer. Arch Otolaryngol Head Neck Surg 127:975–979

Rubesin SE, Jones B, Donner MW (1987) Radiology of the adult soft palate. Dysphagia 2:8–17

Sader R, Horch HH, Herzog M, Zeilhofer HF, Hannig C, Hess U, Bünte E, Böhme G (1994) Hochfrequenz-Videokinematographie zur objektiven Darstellung des velopharyngealen Verschlussmechanismus bei Gaumenspaltenpatienten. Fortschr Kieferorthop 55:169–175

Sader R, Horch HH, Zeilhofer HF, Deppe H, Hannig C, Hess U (1995) High-frequency cineradiography for objective three dimensional rendering of velopharyngeal closure in cleft patients. In: Kärcher H (ed) Functional surgery of the head and neck. RM-Druck u Verl, Graz, pp 31–36

Sader R, Zeilhofer HF, Horch HH (1997) Maxillary advancement and velopharyngeal closure in cleft patients. In: Lee ST, Huang M (eds) Transaction 8th International congress on cleft palate and related anomalies. Stamford Press Pte Ltd, Singapore, pp 651–654

Sader R, Zeilhofer HF, Dietz M, Bressmann T, Hannig C, Putz R, Horch HH (2001) Levatorplasty, a new technique to treat hypernasality: anatomical investigations and preliminary clinical results. J Craniomaxillofac Surg 29:143–149

Skolnick ML (1989) Videofluoroscopic studies of speech in patients with cleft palate. Springer, Berlin

Thumfarth WF, Potoschnig C, Dapunt U, Nekahm D (1996) Diagnostic and surgical systems for management of aspiration and swallowing disturbances. In: 2nd International symposium on laryngeal and tracheal reconstruction, Monte Carlo Proceedings, p 31

Walther EK, Rodel R, Deroover M (1990) Rehabilitation of deglutition in patients with pharyngeal carcinoma. Laryngorhinootologie 69:360–368

Wuttge-Hannig A, Hannig C (1995) Radiologische Differentialdiagnose neurologisch bedingter Schluckstörungen. Der Radiologe 35:733–740

Wuttge-Hannig A, Hannig C (1999) Anatomy of swallowing In: Bartologme G, Buchholz DW, Feussner H, Hannig C, Neumann S, Prosiegel M, Schöter-Morasch H, Wuttge-Hannig A (eds) Schluckstörungen Diagnostik und Rehabilitation Hrsg (2. Auflage). Urban und Fischer Verlag, München, pp 1–11

Wuttge-Hannig A, Beer A, Gebhardt A, Hellerhoff P, Wuttge R, Hannig C (2001) Alternative methods for the diagnostic of deglutition. In: Schindler O, Ruoppolo G, Schindler A (eds) Deglutologie. Omega Edizioni

Zuydam AC, Rogers SN, Brown JS, Vaughan ED, Magennis R (2000) Swallowing rehabilitation after oro-pharyngeal resection for squamous cell carcinoma. Br J Oral Maxillofac Surg 38:513–518

Dysphagia Evaluation and Treatment After Head and Neck Surgery and/or Chemo-radiotherapy for Head and Neck Malignancies

Antonio Schindler, Francesco Mozzanica, and Filippo Barbiera

Contents

A. Schindler (✉) · F. Mozzanica
Department of Biomedical and Clinical Sciences
"L. Sacco", University of Milan, Via GB Grassi,
74 20157 Milan, Italy
e-mail: antonio.schindler@unimi.it

F. Barbiera
Unità Operativa di Radiologia "Domenico Noto",
Azienda Ospedali Civili Riuniti "Giovanni Paolo II",
92019 Sciacca, Italy

Abstract

Tumors of the head and neck represent 3.2 % of newly diagnosed cancers; both surgery and chemo-radiotherapy are valid treatment options for head and neck cancer. In many head and neck cancer patients, dysphagia, malnutrition and aspiration pneumonia are found and significantly impact on quality of life. Dysphagia is related to the tumor itself, or consequences of its treatment. A large number of surgical procedures, according to tumor site and extension, patient age, and general conditions, have been developed and are reviewed in this chapter. Swallowing disorders are related to both the surgical approach (open or endoscopic) and the tissue removed; while surgery for oral and oro-pharyngeal cancers mainly impact on oral control, oral peristalsis and mastication, partial laryngeal surgery interferes with airway protection mechanisms, and complete laryngeal removal may be complicated with hypopharyngeal strictures. Different chemo-radiotherapy protocols are available nowadays and are reviewed here; dysphagia may arise in the first two years or even many years afterwards and is mainly related to increased oro-pharyngeal transit time, reduced tongue and pharyngeal strength, restricted laryngeal and hyoid elevation, poor vestibule and true vocal fold closure and possibly abnormal upper esophageal sphincter function. The primary treatment goal of dysphagia in head and neck cancer patients is maintaining functional oral feeding and preventing aspiration and thoracic complications. All patients treated for a head and neck cancers should have access to a dysphagia specialist and to an instrumental investigation in order to establish adequate treatment.

O. Ekberg (ed.), *Dysphagia*, Medical Radiology. Diagnostic Imaging, DOI: 10.1007/174_2012_606,
© Springer-Verlag Berlin Heidelberg 2012

1 Introduction

Tumors of the head and neck are not rare, representing 3.2 % of newly diagnosed cancer (Curado and Hashibe 2009). Incidence and prevalence may vary due to several factors: geographical area, area within the head and neck , age, and treatment. Both surgery and chemoradiotherapy are valid treatment options for head and neck cancers and the roles of these two approaches have changed considerably over time; in fact, the evolution of the treatment of head and neck cancers can be divided into three main periods. The first was focused on curing patients using radical surgical procedures; the second was developed to preserve speech, using sound oncological principles. The final and current period is of organ-sparing protocols utilizing a combination of radiation, chemotherapy and surgery (Genden et al. 2007; Haigentz et al. 2009; Genden et al. 2010).

In many of the patients with head and neck cancer, dysphagia as well as its complications (malnutrition and aspiration pneumonia), are commonly found and significantly impact on health and quality of life (QOL) (Gallo et al. 2009; Manikantan et al. 2009; Schindler et al. 2006). Different factors may contribute to the presence of dysphagia: the tumor itself, the treatment and, in a small percentage of patients, associated diseases, such as Parkinson's or stroke. Swallowing studies in patients with head and neck cancers revealed signs of dysphagia prior to treatment in up to 59 % of the population; pharyngeal tumors appeared to be more often associated with dysphagia compared to oropharyngeal or laryngeal tumors and swallowing function worsened significantly with increased tumor stage (Pauloski et al. 2000; Stenson et al. 2000; Van der Molen et al. 2009a). Appropriate management of dysphagia in this non-uniform population requires a team approach, with strict collaboration between various professions including surgeons, oncologists, radiotherapists, dentists, phoniatricians, speech and language pathologists, and dieticians; a precise understanding of the disease, the treatment protocols, and the patient's will are necessary before swallowing assessment and rehabilitation planning (SIGN 2006). In this chapter, only the main treatment options, for head and neck cancers, both surgical and non-surgical, are reviewed, with the aim of describing the impact on swallowing and the dysphagia management of these patients.

2 Surgical Options for Head and Neck Malignancies

A large number of surgical procedures, according to tumor site and extension as well as the patient's age and general condition, have been developed over time to treat head and neck malignancies. Head and neck cancers are often treated with curative intent despite frequent presentation with advanced-stage disease, an intent that must be balanced with the potential for long-term morbidity following aggressive local and regional therapies. Head and neck cancers are classified as either "resectable," or technically "unresectable," due to regional invasion of critical structures; while "unresectable" tumors are often best treated with chemoradiotherapy, several curative-intent treatment options currently exist for resectable tumors. The advantages of surgery as primary therapy include complete pathological staging for determination of patient prognosis as well as the potential for sparing some patients subsequent radiotherapy (RT), with or without chemotherapy with its attendant toxicity. However, possible disadvantages of primary surgery include morbidity of the procedure, postoperative functional impairment, or, when the patient is not able to avoid postoperative treatment, the toxicity of both surgical and subsequent adjuvant therapy.

In most surgical procedures of the oral cavity, pharynx and larynx a tracheotomy is performed in order to prevent respiratory failure in case of oedema, upper airway obstruction or peri-operative bleeding. Appropriate management of the tracheotomy and of the cannula are required in order to restore swallowing in the best possible way.

2.1 Surgery for the Oral Cavity Malignancies

The oral cavity extends from the lip to the junction of the hard and soft palate above and to the line of the circumvallate papillae below; therefore the regions of the oral cavity include buccal mucosa, upper and lower alveolar ridges, the retromolar trigone, the anterior two-thirds of the tongue, the floor of the mouth, and the hard palate. Surgical procedures for tumors of the oral cavity vary according to the site and the dimension of the tumor; while for tumors

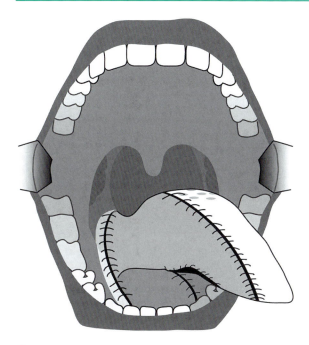

Fig. 1 Schematic drawing of split-thickness brachial flap after resection of half of the tongue and mouth floor

<4 cm surgery can be the only treatment option, for larger tumors chemo-radiotherapy is usually preferred. The challenge of surgery for malignancies of the oral cavity is to perform an adequate resection and then to provide the best functional reconstruction (de Bree et al. 2008). In fact, extensive surgical resections are often required, leading to major physical defects that can-not be repaired by primary mucosal closure or skin grafting. Surgical reconstruction aims to repair the physical deficit, while restoring functional deficits. Reconstruction techniques are diverse and vary by anatomical region. Split-thickness skin grafts are the mainstay for small, superficial defects of the oral cavity (Fig. 1); the pectoralis major myocutaneous flaps provide soft tissue for large floor-of-mouth and tongue resections, while myocutaneous or osteomyocutaneous free flaps are the reconstructive methods of choice for oral cavity defects. The radial fore-arm flap is the most widely used free flap, while if bone is required for mandibular reconstruction fibula, iliac crest or scapula, free flaps can be used.

2.1.1 Glossectomies

Tongue cancer surgery may vary depending on three main variables: extension of tongue resection, access

to the tumor, and reconstruction. Depending on the site and extension of the tumor, the possible tongue resections are: marginal glossectomy (resection of one-quarter of the tongue), hemiglossectomy (resection of half of the tongue along the midline), hemiglossomandibulectomy (resection of half of the tongue and a portion of the mandible), and near total glossectomy.

After marginal glossectomy or hemiglossectomy, swallowing disorders are usually temporary and are mainly related to clumsiness in tongue movement and difficulties in triggering the swallowing re-flex. Clumsiness in tongue movement may impact on both control of material in the mouth and lingual peristalsis. When lingual resection exceeds 50 % of the tongue, effects on swallowing are more severe. In particular, lingual peristalsis and oral control may be severely reduced (Fig. 2a, b); patients' diets may be restricted to liquids and thinned paste, and tilting of the head backward to allow gravity to carry material into the pharynx is often required.

2.1.2 Commando Procedures

The "commando procedure" (COMbined MANDibulectomy and Neck Dissection Operation) is a surgical procedure for malignant tumors of the floor of the oral cavity, involving resection of portions of the mandible in continuity with the oral lesion and radical neck dissection. Segmental mandibulectomy is considered only when there is gross invasion of the cancellous part of the bone by oral cancer, for primary bone tumors of the mandible, metastatic tumors of the mandible, invasion of inferior alveolar nerve or canal by tumor, and for massive soft-tissue disease around the mandible. In the other cases, since there are no lymphatic channels passing through the mandible, there is no need to perform an in-continuity composite resection of the uninvolved mandible; in order to gain access to the large primary oral cancer, a mandibulotomy can be performed without the need to sacrifice the normal intervening mandible (Shah 2009).

Reconstructive surgery following resection for oral cancer is considered when there is functional or esthetic loss of structures in the oral cavity. Superficial surgical defects of the mucosa and underlying soft tissues can be adequately reconstructed using a skin graft, while larger defects of the tongue exceeding one-half of the tongue or large surface areas of the floor of the mouth, gum and buccal

Fig. 2 Videofluoroscopic images of a patient after hemiglossectomy; poor oral control with stasis in the floor of the mouth and spillage in the hypopharynx (**a**) as well as aspiration (**b**) are visible

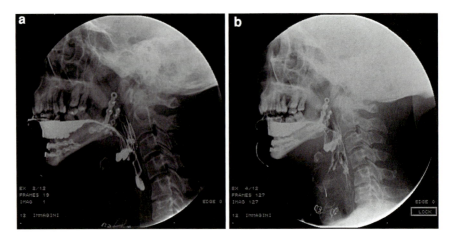

mucosa, require a free-tissue transfer. A radial forearm free flap provides excellent tissue for resurfacing mucosal defects and underlying soft tissue deficiencies. The radial forearm flap is also an excellent choice for reconstruction of any substantial resection of the tongue. Fibula free flap reconstruction is currently the choice of reconstruction for defects following segmental mandibulectomy in any part of the mandible. While other free flaps are available (from iliac crest, scapula and the radial forearm), the fibula provides the maximum length and bone stock to achieve a satisfactory reconstruction of the lower jaw.

After resection of the anterior floor of the mouth, swallowing is strictly related to surgical closure technique, but it is usually preserved. If the tongue is sutured into the surgical defect, however, impairment of control of the bolus and of lingual peristalsis and mastication will arise. After lateral mouth floor resection, severe swallowing impairment may arise if the base of the tongue is involved in the surgical procedure; lingual propulsion and oral transit time will be reduced and material will collect in the lateral sulcus and/or in the crevices.

2.2 Surgery for Oro-Pharyngeal Malignancies

The oropharynx consists of four sections: the soft palate, tonsil, base of the tongue, and pharyngeal wall. The survival outcomes of therapy for these tumors remain essentially the same, regardless of the treatment combination employed. The most important factor affecting long-term outcome following initial treatment of oro-pharyngeal cancer is the stage of disease at the time of presentation. In the past, surgery, followed by RT, was standard. However, at present, concurrent chemo-radiotherapy appears to be the preferred choice of therapy. Surgical intervention would be considered for tumors of minor salivary gland origin or squamous cell carcinoma that remains persistent after chemo-radiotherapy or recurs after chemo-radiotherapy. Surgical access to neoplasms of the oropharynx can be obtained via a mandibulotomy (Fig. 3), lateral pharyngotomy or transoral robotic surgery (TORS) (Weinstein et al. 2007). Early-stage tumors offer excellent cure rates; however, once regional lymph node metastases have taken place, a significant drop in the cure rate is to be expected. Early diagnosis and implementation of appropriate surgical treatment based on tumor and patient factors, selective management of regional lymph node metastases at risk, and involvement of multidisciplinary teams for implementation of adjuvant RT or chemo-radiotherapy, have all contributed to improvements in survival of patients with oral cancers in the last few decades. Contemporary surgical techniques of tumor resection and reconstruction are essential to improve the quality of life of patients following surgical resection due to oro-pharyngeal cancer.

Surgery for oro-pharyngeal tumors impact on both oral and pharyngeal stages of swallowing. Tongue propulsion will be reduced, and there may be nasal regurgitation as well as delayed or reduced triggering of the swallowing reflex and pharyngeal peristalsis, that lead to oral and pharyngeal residue. Occasionally, cricopharyngeal sphincter difficulties may also arise.

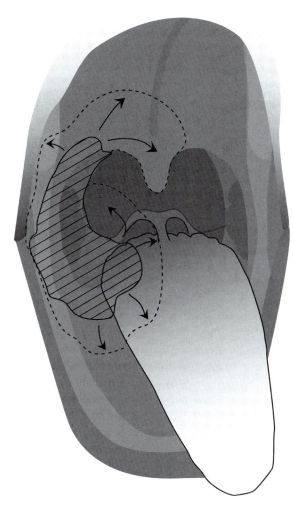

Fig. 3 Schematic drawing of transmaxillar-oropharyngectomy; the *arrows* indicate possible diffusione of the tumor

2.2.1 Mandibulotomy Access

Surgical access to the posterior oral cavity and oropharynx can be accomplished via a multitude of approaches, including pull-through glossotomy and pharyngotomy. In the pull-through technique, once the hypoglossal and lingual nerves are identified, the floor of the mouth mucosa and extrinsic tongue muscles are divided and the tongue is dropped into the neck (Fig. 4); when pharyngotomy is performed, neck dissection is associated and resection of the upper portion of the thyroid cartilage is necessary, before incision into the pharyngeal wall. The most widely used access is the mandibulomy, in particular the lip-splitting mandibulotomy approach. This involves a lower lip-splitting incision, followed by a mandibular

osteotomy, which is fixated at the end of the surgery. It provides the widest and most reliable access to the deep anatomy of the posterior oral cavity and oropharynx and lends exposure to virtually any site in the upper aerodigestive tract, including the nasopharynx, hypopharynx, parapharyngeal spaces, and clivus.

2.2.2 Lateral Pharyngotomy Access

Lateral pharyngotomy access is useful for small tumors of the base of the tongue and pharyngeal walls. The pharynx is entered posterior to the thyroid ala on the least diseased side. Once in the pharynx, the larynx is retracted to the opposite side. This allows a good view of the posterior pharyngeal wall, opposite lateral wall, and base of tongue. If more superior exposure is needed, the pharyngotomy can be extended across the vallecula or this approach can be combined with a lateral mandibulotomy.

2.2.3 Transoral Robotic Surgery

Robotic surgery is performed utilizing the da Vinci surgical system. The surgeon sits at the console and controls micromanipulators, which in turn are connected to a robotic cart at the patient's bedside. In TORS, three arms are routinely utilized (Genden et al. 2009).

2.3 Surgery for Laryngeal Malignancies

The era of surgical treatment began in 1873 when Billroth first described the surgical procedure of total laryngectomy (TL), the "gold standard" for advanced-stage laryngeal carcinoma. Despite its efficacy as an oncologic procedure, complete loss of the larynx is a devastating experience that results in significant diminution of QOL for many individuals. The consequences of TL include loss of nasal function, poor cough, swallowing difficulties, lung function changes and, above all, loss of the normal voice. Therefore, the challenge for the head and neck surgeon has not been significantly improving the cure rate for laryngeal cancers because the survival data for the radical laryngectomy have remained quite constant when adjusted for tumor site and stage, but reducing the morbidity associated with the treatment (Dworkin et al. 2003; Levine et al. 1997). Not surprisingly, the evolution in the management of laryngeal cancer has been to establish surgical as well as non-surgical protocols with overall survival equivalent to TL but better QOL (Genden et al. 2007).

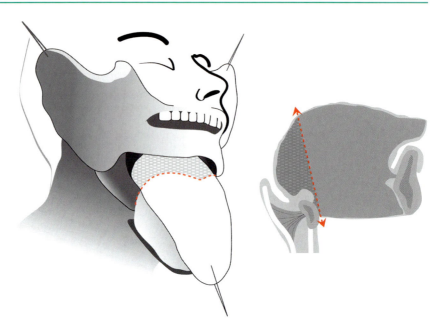

Fig. 4 Schematic drawing of pull-through glossotomy

2.3.1 Partial Laryngectomies

There are several surgical options for treating laryngeal carcinoma, that allow resection of the tumor with oncologically safe margin and preserve laryngeal function. While fronto-lateral partial resections have been used in the past, horizontal partial laryngectomies are currently more popular; horizontal partial laryngectomies include supraglottic partial laryngectomy (SGL) and supracricoid laryngectomies (SCL).

Frontolateral vertical laryngectomy consists of a vertical laryngectomy with removal of the anterior commissure; a lateral thyrotomy is performed on both sides, the vocal fold with the anterior commissure is removed and the remaining vocal fold is sutured to the thyroid cartilage. SGL consists of resecting the whole supraglottic portion of the larynx, including both ventricular folds and the epiglottis (Fig. 5). Depending on the size and site of the tumor, SGL may be extended into the base of the tongue or may include one arytenoid (Marandas et al. 1987). SCLs are conservative surgical techniques for the treatment of selected laryngeal carcinomas; two reconstruction techniques, cricohyoidoepiglottopexy (CHEP) and cricohyoidopexy (CHP) are used, depending on whether the epiglottis is preserved or not (Adamopoulos et al. 2000; Brasnu 2003; Labayle and Bismuth 1971; Laccourreye et al. 1987, 1990, 1995, 1996; Levine et al. 1997; Piquet et al., 1974; Piquet and Chevalier 1991). In SCL, both ventricular and vocal folds as well

as the entire thyroid cartilage are resected, while at least one arytenoid cartilage is spared; in SCL with CHP (Fig. 6) the epiglottis and pre-epiglottic space are also resected, while in SCL with CHEP they are spared (Fig. 7). In the past few years, in addition to open SCL, endoscopic CO_2 laser SCLs have been developed; this surgical approach reduces anterior neck muscles and nerve involvement (Weinstein et al. 2007; Jong-Lyel et al. 2008). Volitional sphincteric approximation of the mobile arytenoids cartilage and base of tongue, in the case of CHP, or epiglottis, in the case if CHEP, allow neoglottal closure and airway protection (Fig. 8), (de Vincentiis et al. 1996, 1998; Luna-Ortiz et al. 2004; Naudo et al. 1997, 1998).

The advantage of partial laryngectomies over TL is that a permanent tracheostomy is not required since the main laryngeal functions (respiration, phonation and swallowing) are preserved, when at least one functioning cricoarytenoid joint is maintained, facilitating neoglottal competency (Bron et al. 2000). Compensatory mechanisms with reorganization of the stepwise sequence of neuromuscular events, lasting several months, are necessary to restore swallowing (Woisard et al. 1996; Yuceturk et al. 2005). Satisfactory functional results of both voice and swallowing after partial laryngectomies have been reported by various authors (Crevier-Buchman et al. 1995, 1998; Zacharek et al. 2001); however, significant alterations have become inevitable and long-term outcome

Fig. 5 Schematic drawing of horizontal sovraglottic laryngectomy

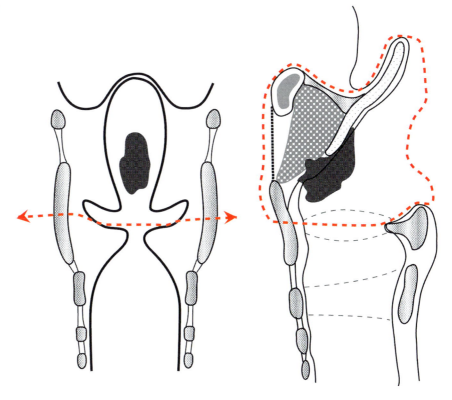

showed mild to moderate dysphagia in the majority of patients (Schindler et al. 2006, 2009).

While vertical partial laryngectomy usually does not impact on swallowing, horizontal partial laryngectomies are associated with dysphagia mainly due to airway protection impairment, and they require appropriate management by a swallowing therapist; in all the reported case series, a small but significant percentage of patients developed aspiration pneumonia and a few did not achieve the ability to eat by mouth. Severity of dysphagia and recovery time are mainly related to amplitude of resection: after SGL swallowing recovers sooner than after SCL with CHP, but SGL extended to the base of the tongue is associated with more severe dysphagia compared to SGL. Insufficient laryngeal vestibule and/or glottis closure during the pharyngeal phase of swallowing is seen in all these patients, and appropriate laryngeal closure needs to be acquired after surgery (Rademaker et al. 1993). While upper airway protection deficit is the main cause of dysphagia, other factors should be considered: superior laryngeal nerve function is often impaired, leading to a reduced laryngeal sensation; laryngeal elevation can also be damaged and upper

esophageal sphincter opening reduced. Finally, a delayed swallowing reflex is found in a significant percentage of patients (Fig. 9).

In the long term aspiration is found in about 40 % of patients who underwent SCL and who are by mouth feeded (Fig. 10); nonetheless, pulmonary CT scans fail to find significant differences compared to COPD patients, suggesting that in this population, a mild chronic aspiration is well tolerated (Simonelli et al. 2010).

2.3.2 TL and Laryngopharyngectomy

TL is the widely accepted standard for surgical treatment of advanced laryngeal and hypopharyngeal tumors. TL includes removal of all laryngeal and associated structures, from the hyoid bone and the epiglottis superiorly to the tracheal rings inferiorly, with varying amounts of the hypopharynx and thyroid gland. It can be extended to the base of the tongue, pharynx and trachea as well as prelaryngeal soft tissues including the skin (Fig. 11). When the tumor originates in the hypopharynx or there is a hypopharyngeal extension of laryngeal carcinoma, a partial or total laryngopharyngectomy may be needed. If the extension is limited, partial pharyngectomy is performed, while

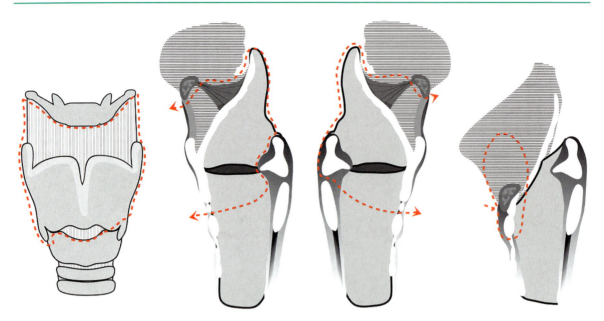

Fig. 6 Schematic drawing of surpacricoid laryngectomy with crico-hyodo-pexy (CHP); only one arytenoid is spared

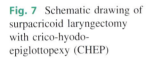

Fig. 7 Schematic drawing of surpacricoid laryngectomy with crico-hyodo-epiglottopexy (CHEP)

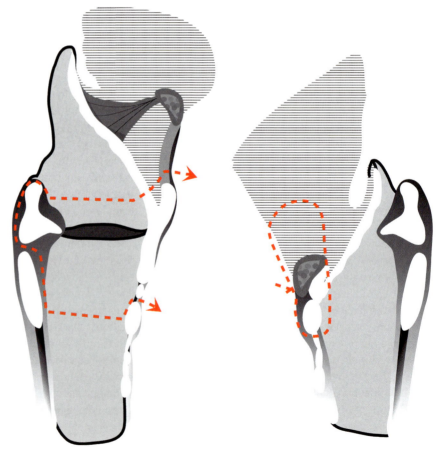

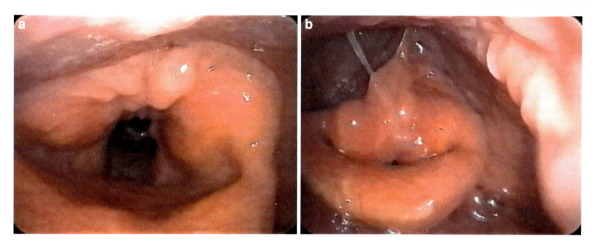

Fig. 8 Videoendoscopic laryngeal images of a patient who underwent supracricoid laryngectomy with crico-hyodo-epiglotto-pexy (CHEP); larynx during respiration (**a**) and phonation (**b**)

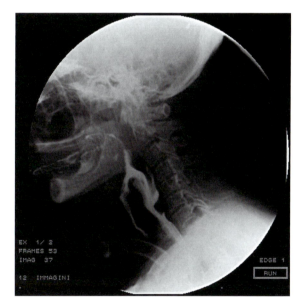

Fig. 9 Videofluoroscopic image of aspiration after surpacricoid laryngectomy with crico-hyodo-pexy (CHP); an incomplete opening of the upper esophageal sphincter is also visible

Fig. 10 Videofluoroscopic image of aspiration after surpacricoid laryngectomy with crico-hyodo-pexy (CHP) several years after the surgical procedure

with extensions of more than 50 % of the hypopharynx it is advisable to perform a total pharyngectomy. In case of extension to the esophagus, total laryngopharyngectomy with esophagectomy can be performed; the most frequently used reconstruction techniques are a tubed jejunum free flap, tubed pectoralis major flap and gastric pull-up (Remacle and Eckel 2010). After TL there is a significant modification of the aerodigestive tract, and the respiratory and digestive tracts are entirely separated: the mouth, pharynx and esophagus

act as the digestive system, while the trachea, directly attached to the skin of the neck, is the first section of the respiratory system.

Even if swallowing is usually well preserved and aspiration is not possible after TL, two-complications may lead to dysphagia: pharyngeoesophageal stenosis/stricture and esophageal motility disorders. Pharyngoesophageal stenosis/stricture may occur after large resections or as a consequence of adjuvant RT (Fig. 12). Outpatient dilatation is usually effective in restoring

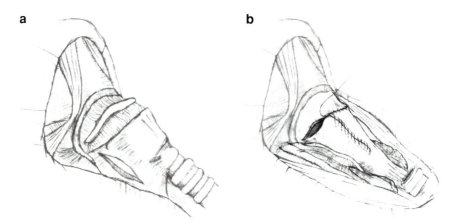

Fig. 11 Schematic drawing of total laryngectomy; incision of the muscle (**a**); suture of the pharynx (**b**). Taken from Remacle and Eckel 2010

swallowing, even if the dilatation procedure has to be repeated over time. In the unlikely situation that dilatation is unsuccessful, flap augmentation (e.g., pectoral major or jejunal free flap) may be necessary. Esophageal motility impairment has been found in patients after TL (Fig. 13): the amplitude of contractions is lower, and the number of nonperistaltic contractions is higher; besides, the duration of lower esophageal sphincter relaxation is shorter and the upper esophageal sphincter pressure is lower in laryngectomized patients than in control subjects (Dantas et al. 2002; Dantas et al. 2005).

2.4 Surgery for Neck Metastasis

Metastasis of head and neck malignancies to the neck lymph nodes are common and appropriate management of neck metastasis is as important as tumor treatment. Both surgical and non-surgical options are available; only surgical options will be considered in this paragraph. Several cervical lymph node dissections are currently used for the surgical treatment in patients with head and neck cancer. Neck dissections are classified, taking into account the lymph node groups (submental, submandibular, jugular, supraclavicular, paratracheal nodes) that are removed and the anatomic structures that may be preserved (spinal accessory nerve, sterno-cleidomastoid muscle). Based on this assumption, there are three anatomic types of neck dissections: radical, selective and extended. In radical neck dissection, *en bloc* removal of the lymph node bearing tissue of one side of the neck, from the inferior border of the mandible to the clavicle, and from the lateral border sterno-hyoid muscles to the anterior border of the trapezius, is performed. Included in the resection are the spinal

accessory nerve, the intrajugular vein and the sterno-cleidomastoid muscle. In selective neck dissection, only the lymph node groups at highest risk of containing metastases are removed. Extended neck dissections may include lymph nodes that are not routinely removed (retropharyngeal, upper mediastinal), or other structures that are not routinely removed (skin of the neck, carotid artery, vagus or hypoglossal nerve).

Even if neck dissection is considered not to impair swallowing, several important muscular and nerve structures for swallowing may be damaged during neck dissection, and there is evidence that swallowing modifications may arise (Hirai et al. 2010). In particular, a lower rest position of the hyoid bone and a decreased hyoid bone elevation have been described, together with penetration in a percentage of patients; no residue or pharyngeal transit time modifications were found. Recurrent laryngeal nerve injury and suprahyoid muscle resection are the most likely elements involved in the pathogenesis of swallowing impairment. Even if dysphagia is unlikely to develop following neck dissection, there is evidence that using a feeding tube is prolonged in patients with head and neck cancers who underwent neck dissections in addition to tumor treatment (Lango et al. 2010).

3 Chemo-radiotherapy for Head and Neck Malignancies

Chemo-radiotherapy can be delivered with curative intent (radical chemo-radiotherapy), in order to improve local control following surgery (adjuvant chemo-radiotherapy), or to provide symptomatic relief only (palliative chemo-radiotherapy). Chemotherapy is administered in

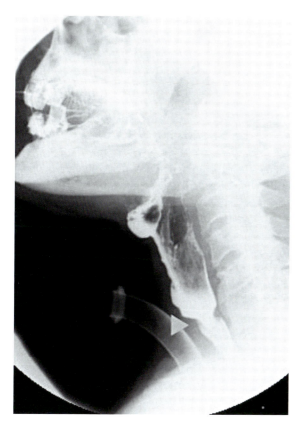

Fig. 12 Videofluoroscopic image of a mild stenosis (*arrow*) after total laryngectomy

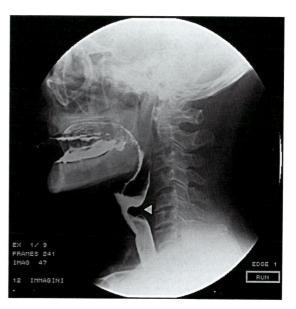

Fig. 13 Videofluoroscopic image of an hypertone of the upper esophageal sphincter (*arrow*) after total laryngectomy

combination with locoregional therapy to improve survival. The chemotherapic agents most widely used are cysplatinum (100 mg/m^2 on days 1, 22 and 43) and 5-Fluoro-Uracil, 5-FU (1 g/m^2 on days 1 and 4). RT uses ionizing radiation to treat malignancies. Ionizing radiation may be delivered as an external radiation beam targeting the tumor (external beam RT), or by directly implanting radioactive sources within the tumor (brachytherapy). External beam RT is usually fractionated, which means that the total dose is delivered over time in smaller doses or fractions. The dose of radiation that can be delivered to a tumor is limited by the tolerance of the surrounding normal tissues, which are also unavoidably irradiated during treatment. Generally, the dose of radiation per day is 1.8–2 Gy for 5 days a week for 6–7 weeks for a total of 70 Gy. Altered radiation fractionation regimens that incorporate acceleration and/or hyperfractionation have also been proposed; acceleration involves a reduction in overall treatment time, while hyperfractionation involves the use of multiple smaller dose fractions delivered at an increased frequency. The

latter improves locoregional control, but also increases acute toxicities for head and neck cancer patients (Harari 2005). The role of chemo-radiotherapy in Head and Neck cancer treatment increased significantly after the introduction of intensity-modulated RT (IMRT) (Liu et al. 2010). IMRT is an advanced mode of high-precision RT that utilizes computer-controlled linear accelerators to deliver precise radiation doses to a malignant tumor or specific areas within the tumor. IMRT allows for the radiation dose to conform more precisely to the three-dimensional shape of the tumor by modulating the intensity of the radiation beam in multiple small volumes. IMRT also allows higher radiation doses to be focused on regions within the tumor while minimizing the dose to surrounding normal critical structures. Typically, combinations of multiple intensity-modulated fields coming from different beam directions produce a custom tailored radiation dose that maximizes the tumor dose while also minimizing the dose to adjacent normal tissues.

3.1 Effects of Chemo-radiotherapy on Mucosa, Cartilage and Muscles

Concomitant chemo-radiotherapy protocols for locally advanced oropharynx carcinoma increases the overall survival rate but can cause significant and severe swallowing problems secondary to anatomic and functional

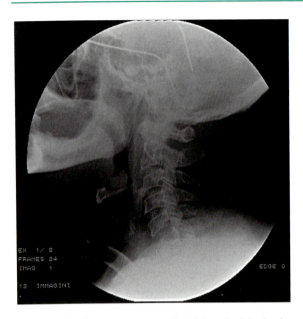

Fig. 14 Videofluoroscopic image of a thickened epiglottis after radiotherapy

changes occurring in the mucosa, cartilages and muscles that are involved in swallowing. In particular RT may induce edema, erythema, decreased acuity of taste buds, decreased production of the salivary glands, and desquamation of the skin that may eventually lead to atrophy and fibrosis of the connective tissues (Fig. 14). Xerostomia dryness of the mouth may impair normal oral functions (speech, chewing, and swallowing) because of insufficient wetting and decreased lubrication of the mucosal surfaces and of ingested food. Furthermore, the oral mucosa can become dry and atrophic, leading to frequent ulceration and injury. Finally, the shift in oral microflora towards cariogenic bacteria, the reduced salivary flow (oral clearance), and changes in saliva composition (decreased buffer capacity, pH, immunoprotein concentrations), may result in rapidly progressing radiation caries. In addition, concomitant chemo-radiotherapy affects the neuromuscular mechanism of swallowing resulting in multiple swallowing measure abnormalities, including increased oro-pharyngeal transit time, uncoordination of bolus movement through the oropharynx, reduced tongue-base contact with the posterior pharyngeal wall, restricted laryngeal and hyoid elevation and movement, poor vestibule and true vocal fold closure, possibly abnormal upper esophageal sphincter function and persistent pharyngeal residue and aspiration. These disorders are most likely the result of neuromuscular fibrosis and of increased apoptosis (Smith et al. 2000) and play the most important role in the genesis of dysphagia.

3.2 Effects of Chemo-radiotherapy on Swallowing

Chemo-radiotherapy plays a critical role in producing swallowing disorders in head and neck cancer patients (Eisbruch et al. 2002). A number of variables determines the incidence of late complications: total radiation dose, fraction size, radiated volume, interfraction interval, treatment techniques, use of IMRT and tissue-dose compensation, and location and size of the primary tumor (Dornfeld et al. 2007). Even if most of the widely described impairments occur in the first two years after chemo-radiotherapy, a number of oro-pharyngeal motility disorders can also be found many years after treatment (Jensen et al. 2007).

During RT, and in the first weeks afterwards, patients experience oral mucositis which severely impacts on oral intake. When oral and pharyngeal mucositis heals, a significant improvement in oral diet is seen and a correlation between healing from oral mucositis and oral intake is visible (Pauloski et al. 2011); nonetheless, oro-pharyngeal deficits are still visible. Oral phase impairment includes reduced mouth opening, reduced range of lingual motion, reduced lingual strength, impaired bolus formation, impaired bolus transport through the oral cavity, prolonged oral transit times and increased oral residue. As for the pharyngeal phase, several defects are found: reduced tongue base posterior movement, defective velopharyngeal closure, delayed triggering of the swallowing reflex, reduced pharyngeal contraction, reduced laryngeal elevation, reduced glottis and laryngeal vestibule closure, and reduced opening of the upper esophageal sphincter. Impairment is limited not only to motor function but to sensibility as well; several authors found reduced laryngeal sensibility, defective or absent laryngeal adductor reflex and silent aspiration in patients who underwent RT. Motor and sensibility impairment lead to reduced bolus clearance, residue and silent aspiration (Lazarus 2009); it is not surprising, therefore, that weight loss and malnutrition are commonly found in patients after RT for head and neck cancers.

Dysphagia may occur even many years after RT (Smith et al. 2000); even if the precise cause is not known, most authors agree that tissue fibrosis, peripheral neuropathy and sensibility impairment are responsible for late-onset dysphagia development. Xerostomia is usually found even years after chemoradiotherapy and significantly impacts on patients' perception of dysphagia and diet choices; however, there is no correlation between saliva weight and swallow function (Logemann et al. 2003).

4 Evaluation of Swallowing and Swallowing Disorder Complications after Surgery and/or Chemo-radiotherapy of Head and Neck Malignancies

Swallowing evaluation in patients after head and neck cancer treatment relies on the same principles of dysphagia of other origins: bedside clinical assessment and subsequent instrumental examination, either videofluoroscopy or fiberoptic endoscopic evaluation of swallowing (FEES). Before patient assessment, it is critical to have detailed information on the surgical procedure and the chemo-radiotherapy protocol; in fact, it is crucial to know which structures have been sacrificed or involved in an RT protocol. Clinical and instrumental examinations aim to understand the functions of the spared structures; in particular, motion range, strength, and timing of the remaining structures in swallowing and non-swallowing tasks are critical for understanding bolus transit.

Clinical examination is important for the understanding of tongue and mouth structures and functions; in particular, in patients with oral cancer, surgical and non-surgical treatment protocols may have seriously modified the anatomy and physiology of oral structures. FEES is recommended for a better definition of mucosal status, velopharyngeal and laryngeal motility as well as saliva and food residue. In particular, in the early phases after treatment, when tracheotomy is still in place, laryngeal assessment in retrograde vision through stoma access (Fig. 15) gives important information on laryngeal sensibility and aspiration mechanisms; besides, FEES may be repeated several times in order to establish when oral feeding may be initiated, avoiding exposure to X-rays. FEES with

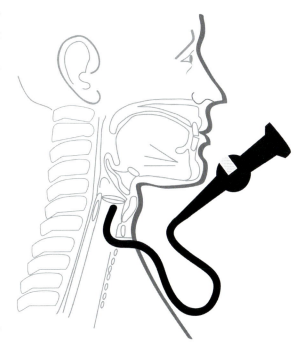

Fig. 15 Laryngeal assessment in retrograde vision through a stoma access

sensory testing is recommended if available, since laryngeal sensibility deficits are found in many patients (Schindler et al. 2010). Videofluoroscopy plays a critical role in establishing oral phase modification, severity of pharyngeal motion defects and mechanisms of pharyngo-esophageal segment dysfunctions.

The application of functional rating scales and dysphagia-specific quality of life measures, such as the M.D. Anderson Dysphagia Inventory or the SWAL-QOL, provide important information on the patient's perception of swallowing (Chen et al. 2001; McHorney and Robbins 2005). Use of these tools helps recognize patients' concerns, and helps define therapy goals (Speyer et al. 2011).

Assessment of dysphagia complications (malnutrition and pulmonary complication) in head and neck cancer patients does not differ from those of patients with dysphagia of other origins. Since the risk of malnutrition is very high, all head and neck cancer patients should be screened for nutritional status using a validated screening tool, appropriate to the patient population, such as the malnutrition universal screening tool.

5 Treatment of Swallowing Disorders after Surgery and/or Chemo-radiotherapy for Head and Neck Malignancies

All patients treated for head and neck cancers should have access to a dysphagia team and to an instrumental investigation, if needed, in order to establish adequate treatment. The primary treatment goal is to maintain functional oral feeding and prevent aspiration and thoracic complications (SIGN 2006); QOL improvement should be considered as a secondary, but not less important goal (Gillespie et al. 2004; Kulbersh et al. 2006).

Treatment mainly relies on swallowing rehabilitation, an emerging subspecialty of rehabilitation (Gamble et al. 2011). Swallowing rehabilitation can be divided into three main areas: preventative, compensatory and therapeutic exercises. While preventative rehabilitation after head and neck cancer surgery has been little explored but seems to reduce recovery time (Cavalot et al. 2009), there is a growing interest in prophylactic swallowing exercises prior to commencing RT (Mittal et al. 2003; Rosenthal et al. 2006; van der Molen et al. 2009b). These exercises focus on maintaining tongue, jaw, pharyngeal constrictor movement, hyo-laryngeal elevation, airway closure and upper esophageal sphincter opening; typically prescribed exercise are tongue range of motion, tongue strengthening, tongue base motion (effortful swallow, tongue-hold maneuver, gargle), jaw range of motion, Mendelsohn maneuver, Shaker exercise and super-supraglottic swallow. Efficacy and compliance data are emerging, but are not yet definitive. Compensatory strategies include postural changes (chin-tuck, head back, head tilt, head rotation, lying down), swallowing maneuvers (super-supraglottic swallow, Mendelsohn maneuver), and change in food consistency, temperature and taste; compensatory strategies are well developed in the field of swallowing rehabilitation and their rationale and application do not differ in head and neck cancer patients from patients with other dysphagia related diseases. Therapeutic exercises include a variety of exercises designed to increase motion range and/or muscle strength of specific muscle groups such as jaws, lips, tongue, closure of the airways and laryngeal elevation; these exercises include effortful swallow, Shaker exercise,

Mendelsohn maneuver, and tongue-hold maneuver, and they may be applied according to the residual swallowing deficit after cancer treatment. Efficacy of both compensatory strategies and therapeutic exercise have been the object of investigation, showing preliminary positive effects (Nguyen et al. 2007; McCabe et al. 2009).

Other treatment options for selected patients include application of prosthetic devices, surgery and enteral feeding. Prosthetic devices should be designed to provide maximum functional rehabilitation, as in the case of palatal obturators to prevent velo-pharyngeal insufficiency after oro-pharyngeal tumor resections. Surgical options include pharyngeal or cervical esophageal dilatation for hypopharyngeal or esophageal strictures, crycopharyngeal muscle myotomy for upper esophageal sphincter spasm, and application of fillers to reduce glottal insufficiency or tongue base deficits (Bergamini et al. 2010). Tube feeding is frequently adopted in the early phase after head and neck cancer treatment and a percentage of these patients remain on enteral feeding, even if there is not enough evidence to decide on the optimal feeding method (PEG or nasogastric tube); criteria to stop enteral feeding are mainly related to the severity of aspiration, even though there are differences in different centers (Logemann et al. 2008; Nugent et al. 2010).

Tracheostomy is frequently performed in head and neck cancer patients for prevention of complications due to post-operative edema or hemorrage, or where supraglottic and glottic edema may occur during chemoradiation. Management of the tracheostomy tube and removal timing differ in different centers and there is no consensus at the moment. However, the effect of tracheotomy and the tracheotomy tube have been the object of several investigations. It is reported that the presence of an inflated cuff may impact on the range of laryngeal motion and, as a result, airway protection and crico-pharyngeal opening (Ding and Logemann 2005). The possible causes of aspiration after tracheostomy may be divided into mechanical and neurophysiological factors. The mechanical factors are decreased laryngeal elevation and stasis of secretions in the upper airway and cervical esophagus due to local compressive forces exerted by the inflated cuff. The neurophysiological factors were desensitization of the protective cough reflex and a loss of co-ordination of laryngeal closure. Nonetheless, in most cases, swallowing deficit in tracheostomized patients is not related to the tracheotomy itself, but to the underlying disease that necessitated it (Leder et al. 2005; Leder and Ross 2010). Therefore, increased aspiration risk or improvement in swallowing function after decannulation seems a clinical impressions rather than a scientific evidence. Besides, it has to be emphasized that an inflated cuff is not protection against aspiration in tracheostomized patients. It is important that prior to decannulation, the supraglottic airway be evaluated to ensure successful removal of the tube; patients should undergo instrumental evaluation of swallowing in both a cuff-inflated and -deflated condition, thus returning those with adequate swallow function to oral intake.

References

Adamopoulos G, Yiotakis J, Stavroulaki P, Manolopoulos L (2000) Modified supracricoid laryngectomy with cricohyoidopexy series report and analysis results. Otolaryngol Head Neck Surg 123:288–293

Bergamini G, Presutti L, Alicandri Ciufelli M, Masoni F (2010) Surgical rehabilitation. Acta Otorhinolaryngol Ital 30:248–253

Brasnu DF (2003) Supracricoid partial laryngectomy with cricohyoidopexy in the management of laryngeal carcinoma. World J Surg 27:817–823

Bron L, Brossard E, Monnier P, Pasche P (2000) Supracricoid partial laryngectomy with cricohyoidoepiglottopexy and cricohyoidopexy for glottic and supraglottic carcinomas. Laryngoscope 110:627–634

Cavalot AL, Ricci E, Schindler A, Roggero N, Albera R, Utari C, Cortesina G (2009) The importance of preoperative swallowing therapy in subtotal laryngectomies. Otolaryngol Head Neck Surg 140:822–825

Chen AY, Frankowski R, Bishop-Leone J, Hebert T, Leyk S, Lewin J, Goepfert H (2001) The development and falidation of a dysphagia-specific quality-of-life questionnaire for patients with head and neck cancer. Arch Otolaryngol Head Neck Surg 127:870–876

Crevier-Buchman L, Laccourreye O, Weinstein G, Garcia D, Jouffre V, Brasnu D (1995) Evolution of speech and voice following supracricoid partial laryngectomy. J Laryngol Otol 109:410–413

Crevier-Buchman L, Laccourreye O, Wuyts FL, Monfrais-Pfauwadel MC, Pillot C, Brasnu D (1998) Comparison and evolution of perceptual and acoustic characteristics of voice after surpacricoid partial laryngectomy with cricohyoidoepiglottopexy. Acta Otolaryngol 118:594–599

Curado MP, Hashibe M (2009) Recent changes in the epidemiology of head and neck cancer. Curr Opin Oncol 21:194–200

Dantas RO, Aguiar-Ricz LN, Oliveira EC, Mello-Filho FV, Mamede RC (2002) Influence of esophageal motility on esophageal speech of laryngectomized patients. Dysphagia 17:121–125

Dantas RO, Aguiar-Ricz LN, Gielow I, Filho FV, Mamede RC (2005) Proximal esophageal contractions in laryngectomized patients. Dysphagia 20:101–104

de Bree R, Rinaldo A, Genden EM, Suárez C, Rodrigo JP, Fagan JJ, Kowalski LP, Ferlito A, Leemans CR (2008) Modern reconstruction techniques for oral and pharyngeal defects after tumor resection. Eur Arch Otorhinolaryngol 265:1–9

de Vincentiis M, Minni A, Gallo A (1996) Supracricoid laryngectomy with cricohyoidopexy (CHP) in the treatment of laryngeal cancer: a functional and oncologic experience. Laryngoscope 106:495–498

de Vincentiis M, Minni A, Gallo A, Nardo AD (1998) Supracricoid partial laryngectomies: oncologic and functional results. Head Neck 20:504–509

Ding R, Logemann JA (2005) Swallow physiology in patients with trach cuff inflated or deflated: a retrospective study. Head Neck 27:809–813

Dornfeld K, Simmons JR, Karnell L, Karnell M, Funk G, Yao M, Wacha J, Zimmerman B, Buatti JM (2007) Radiation dose to structures within and adjacent to the larynx are correlated with long-term diet - and speech - related quality of life. Int J Radiat Oncology Biol Phys 68:750–757

Dworkin JP, Meleca RJ, Zacharek MA, Stachler RJ, Pasha R, Abkarian GG, Culatta RA, Jacobs JR (2003) Voice and deglutition functions after the supracricoid and total laryngectomy procedures for advanced stage laryngeal carcinoma. Otolaryngol Head Neck Surg 129:311–320

Eisbruch A, Lyden T, Bradford CR, dawson LA, Haxer MJ, Miller AE, Teknos TN, Chepeha DB, Hogikyan ND, Terrel JE, Wolf GT (2002) Objective assessment of swallowing dysfunction and aspiration after radiation concurrent with chemotherapy for head- and- neck cancer. Int J Radiat Oncology Biol Phys 53:23–28

Gallo O, Deganllo A, Gitti G, Santoro L, Senesi M, Scala J, Boddi V, De Campora E (2009) Prognostic role of pneumonia in supracricoid and supraglottic laryngectomies. Oral Oncol 45:30–38

Gamble GL, Gerber LH, Spill GR, Paul KL (2011) The future of cancer rehabilitation: emerging subspecialty. Am J Phys Med Rehabil 90:S76–S87

Genden EM, Ferlito A, Silver CE, Jacobson AS, Werner JA, Suárez C, Leemans CR, Bradley PJ, Rinaldo A (2007) Evolution of the management of laryngeal cancer. Oral Oncol 43:431–439

Genden EM, Desai S, Sung CK (2009) Transoral robotic surgery for the management of head and neck cancer: a preliminary experience. Head Neck 31:283–289

Genden EM, Ferlito A, Silver CE, Takes RP, Suárez C, Owen RP, Haigentz M Jr, Stocckli SJ, Shaha AR, Rapidis AD, Rodrigo JP, Rinaldo A (2010) Contemporary management of cancer of the oral cavity. Eur Arch Otorhinolaryngol 267:1001–1017

Gillespie MB, Brodsky MB, Day TA, Lee FS, Martin-Harris B (2004) Swallowing-related quality of life after head and neck cancer treatment. Laryngoscope 114:1362–1367

Harari PM (2005) Promising new advances in head and neck radiotherapy. Annals of Oncology 16:vi13–vi19

Hirai H, Omura K, Harada H, Tohara H (2010) Sequential evaluation of swallowing function in patients with unilateral neck dissection. Head Neck 32:896–904

Haigentz M Jr, Silver CE, Corry J, Genden EM, Takes RP, Rinaldo A, Ferlito A (2009) Current trends in initial management of oropharyngeal cancer: the declining use of open surgery. Eur Arch Otorhinolaryngol 266:1845–1855

Jensen K, Lambertsen K, Grau C (2007) Late swallowing dysfunction and dysphagia after radiotherapy for pharynx cancer: frequency, intensity and correlation with dose and volume parameters. Radiother Oncol 85:74–82

Jong-Lyel R, Dong-Hyun K, Chan IP (2008) Voice, swallowing and quality of life in patients after transoral laser surgery for supraglottic carcinoma. J Surg Oncol 98:184–189

Kulbersh BD, Rosenthal EL, McGrew BM, Duncan RD, McColloch NL, Carrol WR, Magnuson JS (2006) Pretreatment, preoperative swallowing exercises may improve dysphagia quality of life. Laryngoscope 116:883–886

Labayle J, Bismuth R (1971) La laryngectomie totale avec reconstruction du larynx. Ann Otolaryngol Chir Cervicofac 219–228

Laccourreye H, Brasnu D, StGuily JL, Fabre A, Menard M (1987) Supracricoid hemilaryngopharyngectomy. Ann Otol Rhinol Laryngol 96:217–221

Laccourreye H, Laccourreye O, Weinstein G, Menard M, Brasnu D (1990) Supracricoid laryngectomy with cricohyoidopexy: a partial laryngeal procedure for selected supraglottic and transglottic carcinoma. Laryngoscope 100:735–741

Laccourreye O, Crevier-Buchmann L, Weinstein G, Biacabe B, Laccourreye H, Brasnu D (1995) Duration and frequency characteristics of speech and swallowing following supracricoid partial laryngectomy. Ann Otol Rhino Laryngol 104:516–521

Laccourreye O, Weinstein G, Naudo P, Cauchois R, Laccourreye H, Brasnu D (1996) Supracricoid partial laryngectomy after failed laryngeal radiation therapy. Laryngoscope 106:495–498

Lango MN, Egleston B, Ende K, Feignferd S, D'Ambrosio DJ, Cohen RB, Ahmad S, Nicolaou N, Ridge JA (2010) Impact of neck dissection on long-term feeding tube dependence in patients with head and neck cancer treated with primary radiation or chemoradiation. Head Neck 32:341–347

Lazarus CL (2009) Effects of chemoradiotherapy on voice and swallowing. Curr Opin Otolaryngol Head Neck Surg 17:172–178

Leder SB, Joe JK, Ross DA, Coelho DH, Mendes J (2005) Presence of a tracheotomy tube and aspiration status in early, postsurgical head and neck cancer patients. Head Neck 27:757–761

Leder SB, Ross DA (2010) Confirmation of no causal relationship between tracheotomy and aspiration status: a direct replication study. Dysphagia 25:35–39

Levine PA, Brasnu DF, Ruparelia A, Laccoureye O (1997) Management of advanced-stage laryngeal cancer. Otolaryngol Clin North Am 30:101–112

Liu WS, Hsin CH, Chou YS, Liu JT, Wu MF, Tseng SW, Lee JK, Tseng HC, Wang TH, Su MC, Lee H (2010) Long-term results of intensity-modulated radiotherapy concomitant with chemotherapy for hypopharyngeal carcinoma aimed at laryngeal preservation. BMC Cancer 10:102

Logemann JA, Pauloski BR, Rademaker AW, Lazarus CL, Mittal B, Gaziano J, Stachowiak L, MacCracken E, Newman LA (2003) Xerostomia: 12-month changes in saliva production and its relationship to perception and performance of swallow function, oral intake, and diet after chemoradiation. Head Neck 25:432–437

Logemann JA, Rademaker A, Pauloski BR, Antinoja J, Bacon M, Bernstein M, Gaziano J, Grande B, Kelchner L, Kelly A, Klaben B, Lundy D, Newman L, Santa D, Stachowiak L, Stangl-McBreen C, Atkinson C, Bassani H, Czapla M, Farquharson J, Larsen K, Lewis V, Logan H, Nitschke T, Veis S (2008) What information do clinicians use in recommending oral versus nonoral feeding in oropharyngeal dysphagic patients? Dysphagia 23:378–384

Luna-Ortiz K, Nunez-Valencia ER, Tamez-Velarde M, Granados-arcia M (2004) Quality of life and functional evaluation after supracricoid partial laryngectomy with cricohyoioepiglottopexy in Mexican patients. J Laryngol Otol 118:284–288

Manikantan K, Khode S, Sayed SI, Roe J, Nutting CM, Rhys-Evans P, Harrington KJ, Kazi R (2009) Dysphagia in head and neck cancer. Cancer Treat Rev 35:724–732

Marandas P, Luboinski B, Leridant AM, Lambert J, Schwaab G, Richrd JM (1987) La chirurgie fonctionelle dans les cancers du vestibule larynge. 149 cas traits a l'institut Gustave-Roussy. Ann Otolaryngol Chir Cervicofac 104:259–265

McCabe D, Ashford J, Wheeler-Hegland K, Frymark T, Mullen R, Musson N, Hammond CS, Schooling T (2009) Evidence-based systematic review: oropharyngeal dysphagia behavioural treatments. Part IV-impact of dysphagia treatment on individuals' postcancer treatments. J Rehab Res Devel 46:205–214

McHorney CA, Robbins J (2005) The SWAL-QOL and SWAL-CARE outcome tools for dysphagia. ASHA, Rockville, MD

Mittal BB, Pauloski BR, Haraf DJ, Pelzer HJ, Argiris A, Vokes EE, Rademaker A, Logemann JA (2003) Swallowing dysfunction-preventative and rehabilitation strategies in patients with head and neck cancers treated with surgery, radiotherapy and chemotherapy: a critical review. Int J Radiation Oncology Biol Phys 57:1219–1230

Naudo P, Laccourreye O, Weinstein G, Hans S, Laccourreye H, Brasnu D (1997) Functional outcome and prognosis factors after supracricoid partial laryngectomy with cricohyoidopexy. Ann Otol Rhinol Laryngol 106:291–296

Naudo P, Laccourreye O, Weinstein G, Jouffre V, Laccourreye H, Brasnu D (1998) Complications and functional outcome after supracricoid partial laryngectomy with cricohyoidoepiglottopexy. Otolaryngol Head Neck Surg 118:124–129

Nguyen NP, Moltz CC, Frank C, Vos P, Smith HJ, Nguyen PD, Nguyen LM, Dutta S, Lemanski C, Sallah S (2007) Impact of swallowing therapy on aspiration rate following treatment for locally advanced head and neck cancer. Oral Oncol 43:352–357

Nugent B, Lewis S, O'Sullivan JM (2010) Enteral feeding methods for nutritional management in patients with head and neck cancers being treated with radiotherapy and/or chemotherapy. The Cochrane library 3

Pauloski BR, Rademaker AW, Logemann JA, Stein D, Beery Q, Newman L, Hanchett C, Tusant S, MacCracken E (2000) Pretreatment swallowing function in patients with head and neck cancer. Head Neck 22:474–482

Pauloski BR, Rademaker AW, Logemann JA, Lundy D, Bernstein M, McBreen C, Santa D, Campanelli A, Kelchner L, Klaben B, Discekici-Harris M (2011) Relation of mucous membrane alterations to oral intake during the first year after treatment for head and neck cancer. Head Neck 33:774–779

Piquet JJ, Chevalier D (1991) Subtotal laryngectomy with crycohyoidoepilottopexy for the treatment of extended glottic carcinomas. Am J Surg 162:357–361

Piquet JJ, Desaulty A, Decroix G (1974) La crico-hyoido-epiglottopexie. Technique operatoire et resultats fonctionells. Ann Otolaryngol Chir Cervicofac 91:681–686

Rademaker AW, Logemann JA, Pauloski BR, Bowman JB, Lazarus CL, Sisson GA, Milianti FJ, Graner D, Cook BS, Collins SL, Stein DW, Beery QC, Johnson JT, Baker TM (1993) Recovery of postoperative swallowing in patients undergoing partial laryngectomy. Head Neck 15:325–334

Remacle M, Eckel HE (2010) Surgery of larynx and trachea. Springer, Berlin

Rosenthal DI, Lewin JS, Eisbruch A (2006) Prevention and treatment of dysphagia and aspiration after chemoradiation for head and neck cancer. C Clin Oncol 24:2636–2643

Schindler A, Favero E, Nudo S, Albera R, Schindler O, Cavalot AL (2006) Long-term voice and swallowing modifications after supracricoid laryngectomy: objective, subjective, and self-assessment data. Am J Otolaryngol 27:378–383

Schindler A, Favero E, Capaccio P, Albera R, Cavalot AL, Ottaviani F (2009) Supracricoid laryngectomy: age influence on long-term functional results. Laryngoscope 119:1218–1225

Schindler A, Ginocchio D, Peri A, Felisati G, Ottaviani F (2010) FEESST in the rehabilitation of dysphagia after partial laryngectomy. Ann Otol Rhinol Laryngol 119:71–76

Shah JP, Gil Z (2009) Current concepts in management of oral cancer–surgery. Oral Oncol 45:394–340

SIGN (Scottish Intercollegiate Guideline Network) (2006) Diagnosis and management of head and neck cancer. A national clinical guideline. 90

Simonelli M, Ruoppolo G, De Vincentiis M, Di Mario M, Calcagno P, Vitiello C, Manciocco V, Pagliuca G, Gallo A (2010) Swallowing ability and chronic aspiration after supracricoid partial laryngectomy. Otolaryngol Head Neck Surg 142:873–878

Smith RV, Kotz T, Beitler JJ, Wadler S (2000) Long-term swallowing problems after organ preservation therapy with concomitant radiation therapy and intravenous hydroxyurea. Arch Otolaryngol Head Neck Surg 6:384–389

Speyer R, Heijnen BJ, Baijens LW, Vrijenhoef FH, Otters EF, Roodenburg N, Bogaardt HC (2011) Quality of life in oncological patients with oropharyngeal dysphagia: validity and reliability of the Dutch version of the MD Anderson Dysphagia Inventory and the Deglutition Handicap Index. Dysphagia 26:407–414

Stenson KM, MacCracken E, List M, Haraf DJ, Brockstein B, Weichselbaum R, Vokes EE (2000) Swallowing function in patients with head and neck cancer prior to treatment. Arch Otolaryngol Head Neck Surg 126:371–377

Van der Molen L, Van Rossum MA, Ackerstaff AH, Smeele LE, Rasch CRN, Hilgers FJM (2009) Pretreatment organ function in patients with advanced head and neck cancer: clinical outcome measures and patients views. BMC Ear, Nose and Throat Disorders 9:10

Van der Molen L, van Rossum MA, Burkhead LM, Smeele LE, Hilgers FJ (2009b) Functional outcomes and rehabilitation strategies in patients treated with chemoradiotherapy for advanced head and neck cancer: a systematic review. Eur Arch Otorhinolaryngol 266:889–900

Weinstein GS, O'Malley BW Jr, Snyder W, Hockstein NG (2007) Transoral robotic surgery: supraglottic partial laryngectomy. Ann Otol Rhinol Laryngol 116:19–23

Woisard V, Puech M, Yardeni E, Serrano E, Pessey JJ (1996) Deglutition after supracricoid laryngectomy: compensatory mechanism and sequelae. Dysphagia 11:265–269

Yuceturk AV, Tarhan S, Gunhan K, Pabusu Y (2005) Videofluoroscopic evaluation of the swallowing function after supracricoid laryngectomy. Eur Arch Otorhinolaryngol 262:198–203

Zacharek MA, Pasha R, Meleca RJ, Dworkin JP, Stachler RJ, Jacobs JR, Marks SC, Garfield I (2001) Functional outcomes after supracricoid laryngectomy. Laryngoscope 111:1558–1564

Behavioural Treatment of Oropharyngeal Dysphagia: Bolus Modification and Management, Sensory and Motor Behavioural Techniques, Postural Adjustments, and Swallow Manoeuvres

Renée Speyer

Contents

Abstract

This chapter gives an overview of the most common behavioural techniques for treating oropharyngeal dysphagia, namely bolus modification and management, sensory and motor behavioural techniques, postural adjustments, and swallow manoeuvres. Each intervention is described along with its rationale. Furthermore, in light of the literature, the effects of dysphagia treatment are discussed as are some methodological issues that emerged from a review of outcome studies

1 Introduction

Evolution has endowed humans with an aerodigestive tract that facilitates the combined functions of breathing, vocalizing, and swallowing. The system poses a risk of aspiration and choking, however, as a result of the large supralaryngeal space created by the rather low position of the larynx in adults. Any dysfunction in this system may lead to swallowing problems, a condition known as dysphagia.

The effect on a person's health may be severe, as dysphagia can lead to dehydration, malnutrition, and aspiration pneumonia. It also affects people on a social and psychological level, making mealtimes stressful and taking the pleasure out of going to a restaurant. The possibility of suffocation, severe coughing, and vomiting may also heighten one's anxiety and lower self-esteem. All these consequences have a strong impact on quality of life as experienced by dysphagic patients (McHorney et al. 2002). Yet

R. Speyer (✉)
Mozartstraat 47, 6521 GB, Nijmegen,
The Netherlands
e-mail: r.speyer@online.nl

O. Ekberg (ed.), *Dysphagia*, Medical Radiology. Diagnostic Imaging, DOI: 10.1007/174_2011_350,
© Springer-Verlag Berlin Heidelberg 2012

studies on the effects of therapy in oropharyngeal dysphagia give little attention to the effects on quality of life (Speyer et al. 2010). In contrast, the literature on the effects of dysphonia or voice problems suggests that quality-of-life questionnaires are essential to multidimensional voice assessment (Speyer 2008).

Dysphagia can be caused by a variety of diseases (e.g. neurological causes such as cerebrovascular accidents or degenerative diseases). But it can also manifest itself as a side effect of treatment, for example, by radiation or surgical intervention in patients with head and neck cancer. Usually, a team of specialists will be involved in the diagnosis and treatment. Within a multidisciplinary context or interdisciplinary setting, each caregiver will focus on a particular aspect of the swallowing problems. In general, after the initial assessment and treatment by medical specialists, nurses may be the first to perform any bedside screening focused on dysphagia (Bours et al. 2009). Subsequently, speech therapists may take charge of any further assessment of the swallow mechanism, the choice of behavioural intervention, and the follow-up evaluation. In the event of malnutrition or dehydration, or if there is a severe nutritional risk, dieticians are involved to ensure the patient has a sufficient caloric intake and provide the patient with nutritional supplements if necessary. Additionally, occupational therapists, physiotherapists, social workers, or psychologists may be involved in the multidisciplinary management of dysphagia.

Depending on the dysphagic findings, swallowing treatment may include medical, surgical, and/or behavioural options (Crary and Groher 2003). The medical option could entail dietary modifications to address underlying disease (e.g. diabetes or hypertension) or pharmacological treatment (e.g. antireflux medication or mucolytics). The surgical option covers a range of interventions: to improve glottal closure by medialization thyroplasty or injection of biomaterials; to enhance airway protection (e.g. total laryngectomy); or to optimize the pharyngo-oesophageal segment opening by stretching the lumen of the segment by dilation, surgical myotomy of the cricopharyngeal muscle, or chemodenervation using botulinum toxin injection. This chapter focuses on the third option: treatment by speech therapists using behavioural techniques.

Langmore (2001) described three patterns of dysphagia: the ineffective swallow or incomplete bolus clearance; the misdirected swallow or impaired airway protection due to incomplete valving; and the delayed or mistimed swallow. Regarding the motor control of swallowing, the physiological parameters are intact sensation, briskness of initiation of movement, speed of movement, force or strength of movement, and amplitude of movement, as well as precision, timing, and coordination of movement. Therapeutic strategies used in swallowing therapy can be classified as rehabilitative and/or compensatory (Huckabee and Pelletier 1999). Interventions that are mainly intended to restore or improve the actual swallowing function are referred to as rehabilitative techniques. Compensatory techniques, in contrast, are intended to improve the ability to adapt and cope with the problem. Laryngeal adductor exercises to improve laryngeal valving are among the rehabilitative interventions, whereas strategies—such as the chin tuck posture—to improve laryngeal protection or the use of bolus modification are considered compensatory techniques.

Behavioural treatment of oropharyngeal dysphagia as performed by speech therapists may include a range of interventions: (1) bolus modification and management; (2) sensory and motor behavioural techniques; (3) postural adjustments; and (4) swallow manoeuvres—or any combination of these (Speyer et al. 2010). Bolus modification refers to adjusting the viscosity, volume, temperature, and/or acidity of the bolus. The second category includes oral motor exercises but also facilitation techniques that cover a variety of interventions, ranging from surface electrical stimulation to thermal application at the anterior faucial pillars. Behavioural techniques commonly used to modify the swallow mechanism are postural adjustments and swallow manoeuvres. Postural adjustments involve whole-body and head-position strategies. Swallow manoeuvres include the (super) supraglottic swallow, the Mendelsohn manoeuvre, the effortful swallow, the Masako manoeuvre, and the Shaker exercise, among others. Adjunctive biofeedback may be used to facilitate processes of complex motor learning. In the following sections, these techniques will be described in detail.

It is now widely accepted that medical treatments should be scrutinized by scientific methods. This implies that paramedical therapies should also be evaluated according to current standards of evidence-based medicine. An evaluation of therapy in oropharyngeal dysphagia thus falls squarely into this area of growing interest (Speyer et al. 2010). Besides describing the behavioural techniques commonly used in dysphagia therapy, studies should provide information on the effects of therapy in oropharyngeal dysphagia and the methodological issues that arise in the literature. Moreover, outcome studies are essential in order for caregivers to adjust and improve therapy for patients with oropharyngeal dysphagia.

2 Choice of Intervention Techniques

After medical and swallowing assessment, there may be a need for further intervention by speech therapists. However, many considerations may influence which intervention techniques are indicated for a particular patient.

First of all, many strategies require a patient's full cooperation as well as the capacity to follow complex instructions under the supervision of a therapist. It may be almost impossible to explain and teach certain strategies to patients with severe cognitive limitations. Furthermore, a patient has to be internally motivated or else have support from close relatives in order to keep trying. Having family support or motivated caregivers is essential, especially for the implementation of newly learned swallowing behaviours or compensation strategies in daily life.

When making decisions about oral feeding, one has to take the patient's general health into account. The estimated safety of oral intake must be set off against the risk of aspiration pneumonia. Concerns about malnutrition or frailty, particularly among the elderly (Rofes et al. 2011), may call for additional tube feeding combined with nutritional supplements. Oral feeding may be fatiguing and thus place a burden on the patient. But the taste and smell of food or drink may also be rewarding and motivating, allowing the patient to enjoy family meals. In fact, participating in daily dining routines might have a huge impact on the patient's quality of life. It is important to take a patient's food preferences and cultural background into account when advising on the possibilities of oral intake and on the use of food or liquid boluses in therapeutic settings. It should be realized that even when physicians and therapists consider oral intake to

be no longer safe, a patient may still refuse tube feeding because of the reduced quality of life associated with such an intervention.

Obviously, the choice of interventions is also determined by the medical diagnosis and corresponding prognosis for a disease. For example, for someone diagnosed with neuromuscular disease, rehabilitative techniques may result in fatigue and exhaustion instead of increased muscle strength. Also, if spontaneous recovery of the swallowing functions can be expected during the acute period after a recent cerebrovascular accident, compensatory techniques may suffice to achieve sufficient oral intake. On the other hand, in palliative care, intervention will be restricted to minimize the effects of the dysphagia and optimize a patient's quality of life during the dying phase (Veerbeek 2008).

Finally, cultural aspects may influence the way swallowing disorders are treated. Basically, care for dysphagia may be organized differently in different countries. National health systems may differ in the ratio of therapists to patients being hospitalized and treated. Or the training provided for therapists may differ with respect to the material being taught or the level of education required for certification. Besides national differences, the preferences or expertise of individual therapists will also influence the treatment. Decisions on therapy frequency, length of therapy sessions, and treatment period, as well as the behavioural techniques applied, all play a role in the outcome of swallowing therapy.

3 Behavioural Treatment of Dysphagia

Regarding the range of behavioural interventions used in oropharyngeal dysphagia, various strategies may be found in the literature. The most common techniques and therapeutic approaches that can be applied by speech and language therapists are covered in the following five subsections.

Bolus modification and management will be considered first, followed by sensory and motor behavioural techniques. Next, postural adjustments to facilitate swallowing will be presented. This third category includes general body positions such as lying down or side-lying. It also includes head positions, particularly adjustments such as head extension, flexion, rotation, or tilt. The fourth category consists of a variety of swallow manoeuvres: the supraglottic and super supraglottic swallow; the Mendelsohn manoeuvre; the effortful swallow; the Masako manoeuvre; and the Shaker exercise. Finally, the application of biofeedback will be discussed in the fifth subsection.

3.1 Bolus Modification and Management

Bolus modification and management is an approach that amounts to adjusting parameters such as viscosity, volume, temperature, and/or acidity of the bolus (Speyer et al. 2010). Modifying the rheologic properties of food and liquids may be one of the most common strategies applied by therapists. Ways to modify a food's consistency may vary from the use of commercial agents for thickening liquids to the blending of solid foods. By thickening thin liquids, clinicians seek to decelerate the bolus transport into the pharynx. By giving the patient more time to handle the bolus, one reduces the risk of penetration or aspiration. Thicker liquids may be helpful in the case of a delayed or mistimed swallow (Langmore 2001). Solid foods can be modified with a blender or masher. This reduces the need for chewing by smoothing the particulate nature of certain boluses or by blending foods of a mixed consistency. Patients who fatigue easily and are at risk of malnutrition may benefit from such a modified diet because of the diminished amount of effort required for swallowing. Those patients who have difficulty clearing a bolus may also show improved swallow behaviour when managing boluses of smoothed consistencies compared with handling crumbly or noncohesive foods. In the latter case, when food consistencies do not allow easy bolus-forming or preparation for swallowing, adding liquids may be considered. Smoothened bolus consistencies reduce the amount of pharyngeal residue, thereby reducing the risk of delayed aspiration as well. There is great variety in the clinical terminology used for different bolus consistencies, and consensus is lacking. However, to determine the effectiveness of modifying food and liquids in patients with oropharyngeal dysphagia and to compare study outcomes, uniform definitions for the rheologic properties of foods and liquids should be used (Dealy 1995).

To determine the appropriate volume of food or liquid boluses, the caregiver must know the patient's capacity to control and secure a safe oropharyngeal bolus transit with minimal amount of postswallow residue. Larger quantities may require optimal alertness of the swallow mechanism, whereas boluses that are too small may provide insufficient sensory stimulus to initiate the swallowing act, as seen in patients with Parkinson's disease (Baijens and Speyer 2009). Swallowing may also be influenced by temperature; colder boluses are thought to trigger a quicker onset of the swallowing reflex. Improved timing has also been found when using acid boluses (Logemann et al. 1995). Naturally, when applying bolus modification, one should keep in mind that achieving an optimal taste and smell—that is, adjusted to an individual's preference—will provide rewarding and motivating factors, which can improve the oral intake and in turn the health status of a patient.

3.2 Sensory and Motor Behavioural Techniques

Swallowing is the result of combined forces producing bolus passage through the pharynx and avoiding the larynx or airway (Langmore 2001). A normal sensory awareness in the oral cavity and pharynx is crucial to secure bolus manipulation and transportation. Lips, tongue, palate, and mandible have to operate in a coordinated order. Recruitment of adequate muscle strength, accuracy, and coordination thus results in a safe swallow. Therapists often draw upon sensory stimulation and oral motor exercises as part of dysphagia treatment in an effort to modify the swallow mechanism.

3.2.1 Oral Motor Exercises

The purpose of using oral motor exercises is to increase awareness of the bolus, to control and direct its passage, and to maximize the driving and propulsive force of the bolus in transit to the oropharynx. The exercises can address the various features of motor function: muscle strength, range of movement, muscle tone, steadiness, and accuracy. But regaining muscle function in terms of strength, range, and tone will in itself not result in normal swallowing unless the coordination of the swallow mechanism has been optimized as well.

During the oral phase of swallowing, labial awareness and control are essential to achieve adequate lip closure and prevent drooling. There are exercises for the tongue to improve bolus propulsion, which is created by posterior tongue thrust, and to diminish bolus pocketing or the amount of residue, as well as to reduce the risk of preswallow aspiration because of failure of bolus control (Robbins et al. 2007). Stretching exercises may improve the range of mandible movement in patients with reduced flexibility. Nasal regurgitation might be diminished by stimulating the soft palatal closure using velopharyngeal closure exercises.

3.2.2 Sensory Stimulation

Sensory stimulation activities may involve changing the taste of boluses or their temperature, applying pressure, or using neuromuscular electrical stimulation. It has been theorized that providing a sensory stimulus before a swallow attempt may serve as an alert or trigger to the nervous system and thereby help prepare the swallow mechanism for the subsequent swallow.

Effects of the use of sour boluses have been described in the literature, suggesting that an alteration is induced in swallowing behaviour—for instance, improved timing of the onset of swallowing (Logemann et al. 1995). Usually, tactile–thermal application procedures consist of cold, tactile stimuli. These may be presented to the anterior faucial pillars by stroking the pillars with an ice stick (Rosenbek et al. 1998) or with a cold laryngeal mirror taken from a cup of ice. These procedures are thought to reduce the delay in the initiation of swallowing, primarily in the pharyngeal phase. Besides temperature stimulation, pressure may be used to improve sensory awareness. For example, a spoon can be used to apply light pressure to the blade of the tongue during swallowing exercises.

3.2.3 Electrical Stimulation

The use of electrical stimulation has been the subject of several recent studies (Blumenfeld et al. 2006; Bülow et al. 2008; Ludlow et al. 2007; Power et al. 2006; Shaw et al. 2007). Surface electrical stimulation (neuromuscular electrical stimulation) activates muscles by stimulating the intact peripheral motor nerves. The main treatment goals are to strengthen weak muscles and to help in the recovery of motor control

(Freed and Wijting 2003). Stimulation at the motor level can be distinguished from stimulation at the sensory level. As defined by Ludlow et al. (2007), motor stimulation is the maximum tolerated stimulation level resulting in maximum muscle contraction without spasm. The level of sensory stimulation is set by gradually raising the intensity of the current until the patient reports the first sensation of stimulation, usually a tingling of the skin. Depending on the exact placement of skin electrodes in the neck and face, different groups of muscles are stimulated.

3.3 Postural Adjustments

Postural adjustment may involve head positioning strategies such as head-turn or chin-tuck manoeuvres or whole-body positioning strategies. In the literature, it has been shown that adjusting the head and/or body position can reduce or eliminate the risk of aspiration (Lewin et al. 2001; Logemann et al. 1994a; Rasley et al. 1993; Shanahan et al. 1993). Postural variations redirect and facilitate the bolus flow; they may improve oral and pharyngeal transit times, and they decrease the amount of residue after swallowing (Bogaert et al. 2003). These techniques are intended to change the dimensions of the oropharynx in order to accomplish a safer swallow by compensating for anatomic deficiencies, sensory loss, or a reduced propulsion or clearance of the bolus. Postural adjustments can be introduced as temporary techniques during the process of recovery of the swallowing function. Alternatively, they may become a permanent compensatory technique after rehabilitation to facilitate the changed swallow motor pattern or mechanism.

3.3.1 General Postural Adjustments

General postural adjustments usually concern body postures such as lying down or side-lying. Both of these postures reduce the effects of gravity during swallowing and the amount of postswallow residue. Side-lying may be beneficial when there is a difference in pharyngeal function between the left and the right side. The patient must lie down on the stronger side, thereby using gravity to direct the bolus or residue towards the stronger and/or more sensitive hemipharynx (Drake et al. 1997). However, changing the posture may have a negative influence on the oesophageal motor functions. Patients with suspected gastro-oesophageal reflux disease or poor oesophageal motility may benefit from an upright position during and after feeding. In the case of nocturnal reflux, head-of-bed elevation may be recommended during the night, thus reducing or prohibiting acid reflux from the oesophagus.

3.3.2 Head Postural Adjustment

Head postural adjustment includes the following positions: head flexion, head extension, head rotation, and head tilt. Head flexion, also called chin tuck, narrows the oropharynx and shortens the distance between the hyoid and the larynx, thus narrowing the laryngeal entrance (Bülow et al. 2001). It facilitates airway protection and may be used in patients with difficulties in oral control or timing. However, head flexion may also result in a weaker pharyngeal contraction during swallowing, causing problems of bolus propulsion in patients with pharyngeal weakness.

Unlike flexion, the aim of head extension is to widen the oropharynx by raising the chin, resulting in a head-back position. An extended head adjustment uses gravity for bolus propulsion into the pharynx. It may be useful in patients showing deficiencies in oral control and bolus transport during the oral (preparatory) phase of swallowing. Head extension can only be used in patients with an intact pharyngeal phase. Head extension may also have a negative impact on the pharyngo-oesophageal segment, increasing the intraluminal pressure and decreasing the duration of relaxation of the segment (Crary and Groher 2003). Furthermore, head extension reduces laryngeal closure. Thus, the swallowing outcome may deteriorate in patients with diminished laryngeal airway protection or deficits in pharyngo-oesophageal segment functioning.

The head rotation or head-turn manoeuvre is mainly used in patients with unilateral deficits (unilateral pharyngeal or vocal fold paralysis or paresis). Rotating the head towards the weakened side before swallowing results in the swallowing tract or piriform sinus on this damaged side being narrowed or even closed off. This directs the bolus down the stronger side (Logemann et al. 1989). The cricoid cartilage is pulled away from the posterior pharyngeal wall, reducing the pressure in the cricopharyngeal sphincter and thereby increasing the size of sphincter opening.

This, in turn, will reduce amount of bolus residue after swallowing as well as the risk of aspiration.

If the patient has unilateral oral and pharyngeal weakness on the same side, the head-tilt adjustment can be applied. When the head is tilted to the stronger side prior to the swallow, the bolus is directed down to the stronger side by utilizing the effects of gravity, thus reducing the amount of bolus residue (Rasley et al. 1993).

3.4 Swallow Manoeuvres

Apart from sensory and motor behavioural techniques or postural adjustments, behavioural swallowing therapy may combine a variety of swallow manoeuvres. These allow the patients to gain improved and voluntary control of the swallowing process, including bolus propulsion and airway protection. Many of these manoeuvres require active patient participation and intensive practice to induce the necessary physiological modification of the swallow mechanism.

3.4.1 Supraglottic Swallow

The supraglottic swallow manoeuvre may be suitable and advisable under certain conditions: in the event of restricted airway protection or risk of aspiration as a result of a delayed pharyngeal swallow, a reduced or late vocal fold closure, or laryngeal sensory deficits. The manoeuvre consists of several steps. Patients are first asked to inhale and hold their breath. Next, they place a bolus in the mouth and swallow while still holding their breath. Then, after swallowing and before inhaling, patients cough voluntarily. Finally, they swallow again. The aim of this manoeuvre is to close the vocal folds by holding one's breath and to clear any possible residue from the laryngeal vestibule that may have entered while swallowing (Logemann 1998). However, vocal fold closure may not always be achieved in patients when holding their breath.

3.4.2 Super Supraglottic Swallow

Patients who do not succeed in bringing about the required airway protective closure during the supraglottic swallow manoeuvre need to perform a forceful breath-hold or super supraglottic swallow manoeuvre. Adding force to the swallow manoeuvre increases the chances of establishing a complete vocal fold closure and may promote shorter swallowing transit times (Logemann 1998). Patient instruction is similar to that given during the supraglottic swallow manoeuvre, except for the request to bear down hard instead of just performing a swallow act. The rationale for applying either the supraglottic manoeuvre or the super supraglottic manoeuvre is similar. The difference lies in the amount of effort required. Bearing down causes the arytenoid muscles to be tilted anteriorly, closing the false vocal folds as well as the entrance to the trachea.

3.4.3 Mendelsohn Manoeuvre

The aim of the Mendelsohn manoeuvre is to increase the extent and duration of laryngeal elevation and thereby enhance the duration and width of the cricopharyngeal opening (Logemann 1999). While the upper oesophageal sphincter is open, bolus transfer may be facilitated, leaving less oropharyngeal residue. It is hypothesized that prolonging the swallow at the peak of hyolaryngeal elevation and pharyngeal contraction causes the frequency and the amount of aspiration to decline owing to improved upper oesophageal sphincter opening. The manoeuvre is designed for patients with a reduced range of laryngeal movement or a discoordinated swallow. Patients are instructed to press lightly on the thyroid cartilage with their fingers, keeping it in a raised position for several seconds directly after swallowing. Because the instruction to patients could be confusing and difficult to translate into practice, it may be advisable to offer adjunctive biofeedback such as surface electromyography during training. With electromyographic biofeedback, patients will have immediate visualization of their muscle activity while learning the Mendelsohn manoeuvre.

3.4.4 Effortful Swallow

The effortful swallow is also known as the hard swallow manoeuvre. The technique increases the posterior motion of the tongue base during the pharyngeal swallow, thereby improving bolus clearance from the valleculae (Logemann 1999). Thus, the effortful swallow may be recommended in the case of reduced posterior movement of the tongue base or reduced oropharyngeal pressure. During training, the patient is instructed to squeeze with maximal effort while swallowing. This manoeuvre is considered to be easily taught and easily implemented. However,

because it may be difficult to determine which muscles are being activated or recruited and to what degree, instrumental measurements or biofeedback (e.g. surface electromyography) may be useful during rehabilitation.

3.4.5 Masako Manoeuvre

During swallowing, the pharyngeal wall tends to bulge forwards, contacting the tongue base. It is hypothesized that pushing the tongue out and holding the anterior tongue between the teeth while swallowing will increase tongue base pressure and duration of contact with the posterior pharyngeal wall. This technique is known as the Masako manoeuvre or tongue holding. In the case of lingual weakness, for example after oral surgery, it might be considered a rehabilitative technique (Lazarus et al. 2002). By practising the Masako manoeuvre, the patient may train the pharyngeal wall to compensate for the lack of posterior tongue movement. The presumed result will be improved contact between the tongue base and the pharyngeal wall, thus creating a pressure source for bolus propulsion through the oropharynx. It is not advisable to combine this manoeuvre with swallowing food boluses because of the reduced duration of airway closure, the increased amount of residue after swallowing, and the increased delay in pharyngeal swallow initiation (Crary and Groher 2003).

3.4.6 Shaker Exercise

The Shaker exercise, otherwise known as the isotonic/isometric exercise, serves as rehabilitative training of the suprahyoid muscles responsible for the opening of the upper oesophageal sphincter. This manoeuvre may solve the problem of a reduced cricopharyngeal opening, thus decreasing the amount of postswallow residue. Patients are instructed to lie supine and raise their head without raising their shoulders. This position is maintained for about 1 min, after which the patient will rest before repeating this head-raising manoeuvre. A suprahyoid muscle-strengthening exercise programme has been found to be effective in patients with deglutitive failure due to an abnormal upper oesophageal sphincter opening. The exercise stimulates the restoration of oral feeding, diminishes the amount of postdeglutitive residue, and resolves aspiration (Shaker et al. 2002).

3.5   Adjunctive Biofeedback

Most swallow manoeuvres require complex learning or relearning of motor patterns by patients. The application of biofeedback as an adjunct to swallowing therapy may facilitate the learning processes and be valuable in enhancing the rate of motor learning. Several techniques can be used to reveal some of the internal physiological events, normal and abnormal, using visual or auditory signals. Patients will be able to manipulate these otherwise involuntary or unfelt events (Basmajian and Deluca 1985).

The literature describes positive effects of surface electromyographic feedback in dysphagia treatment (Bogaardt et al. 2009; Crary et al. 2004). For example, when surface electrodes are placed under the chin, between the front of the mandible and the hyoid, muscle activity in the submental muscles can be recorded. During therapeutic sessions, patients are asked to perform repeatedly the Mendelsohn manoeuvre while being provided with visual feedback of the electromyographic recordings that present muscle activity as a function of a time frame. Patients are able to judge for themselves the amount of success in prolonging the laryngeal excursion as they watch the surface electromyographic signal on a computer monitor, thus receiving immediate feedback on their swallowing performance (Bogaardt et al. 2009). Surface electromyographic feedback may help teach the patient muscle relaxation, straining, and strengthening, and the feedback may stimulate muscle coordination.

Other biofeedback techniques may be helpful in functional rehabilitation as well. The use of flexible videoendoscopic biofeedback in swallowing therapy, serving as pharyngeal image biofeedback, has been studied. It shorted the period of functional rehabilitation (Denk and Kaider 1997). Endoscopic feedback may be helpful to teach patients breath-hold manoeuvres such as the super supraglottic swallow or the supraglottic swallow. It can help by visualizing the degree of vocal fold closure or residue at the laryngeal vestibule. Instead of endoscopic recordings, videoradiographic recordings of swallowing may be used. Another technique, cervical auscultation, might be used to listen to swallow sounds as an adjunct to clinical swallowing assessment (Leslie et al. 2004). It has been speculated that swallow sounds provide audible cues that permit a reliable dichotomized classification of normal swallowing versus dysphagic swallowing with signs of penetration and/or aspiration.

4   Effects of Behavioural Treatment

It is not only treatments by physicians that have to be evaluated according to current standards of evidence-based medicine; so do interventions by allied health professionals. By extension, the therapy outcome of behavioural treatment of oropharyngeal dysphagia needs objective evaluation as well (Speyer et al. 2010). According to Logemann (1999), therapy procedures should not be implemented until data on their efficacy and positive outcomes have been published in peer-reviewed journals. Indeed, clinicians must be acquainted with the relevant literature in order to justify their choice of therapy strategies during the clinical decision-making process. Therapists are responsible for collecting clinical efficacy and outcome data on each of their patients. Only then can they objectify whether the goals set at the start of therapy have been adequately met at the end. Evidence-based practice is thereby the result of combining current research, the clinician's expertise, and the patient's values and preferences (Wheeler-Hegland et al. 2009).

Several reviews have been published summarizing the literature on the behavioural treatment of oropharyngeal dysphagia. Some narrative reviews provide extensive information about treatment possibilities (Logemann 2006). Other studies describe the effects of swallowing therapy in general as applied by speech and language therapists. The latter reviews are based on a systematic literature search using diverse electronic databases (Speyer et al. 2010). Furthermore, a few systematic reviews have restricted the literature search to certain types of therapy. Some are focused on neuromuscular electrical stimulation (Carnaby-Mann and Crary 2007; Clark et al. 2009). Others are confined to well-defined patient populations: for example, patients suffering from neurological disorders (Ashford et al. 2009) or oncological problems in the head and neck area (McCabe et al. 2009).

Therapists can thus turn to the existing literature for short, systematic overviews that will help them select therapeutic interventions when treating patients with oropharyngeal dysphagia. However, as many questions remain unsolved, clinicians will have to rely on their professional and clinical insights as well. For example, the success of therapy in a given patient population cannot necessarily be generalized to another population. Furthermore, behavioural dysphagia treatment may combine many different interventions for the same patient. The question is then, will the final outcome of therapy be equal to the sum of each component? Or will redundancy or antagonistic factors complicate the task of determining the actual efficacy of an individual patient's treatment? The literature thus has its shortcomings. But it still provides grounds for discerning trends in therapy success, even though methodological issues in outcome studies on oropharyngeal dysphagia remain to be addressed.

4.1   Trends in Treatment Effects

An overview of the literature on the behavioural treatment of oropharyngeal dysphagia shows statistically significant positive effects of therapy (Speyer et al. 2010). However, considering the major impact of dysphagia on a patient's quality of life (McHorney et al. 2003), the number of evidence-based studies is rather small. Only effect studies that meet certain quality criteria—notably concerning study design, patient attrition, randomization plus allocation of subjects to intervention groups, and blinding of outcome assessors—may provide information that is sufficiently reliable for the study outcome to be translated into clinical practice (Frymark et al. 2009; Speyer et al. 2010). Besides these methodological issues, it should be noted that the behavioural treatment of dysphagia frequently combines different interventions (Speyer et al. 2010). Thus, even though a combination of techniques has proven to be effective in eliminating or diminishing the symptoms, it may be hazardous to make any firm statements about the effectiveness of each of the separate elements. Still, a number of well-designed effect studies have demonstrated a positive therapy outcome of behavioural approaches in swallowing therapy. Therefore, some general conclusions may be drawn and certain trends may be distinguished.

One very common therapy intervention is bolus modification. In a study of two groups of dysphagic patients who had experienced aspiration pneumonia prior to therapy, Groher (1987) demonstrated that viscosity modulation (soft mechanical diet with thickened liquids versus pureed diet with thin liquids) could reduce the number of episodes of aspiration pneumonia. In a later study by Groher and McKaig (1995), the changes in dietary level in a group of persons in residential care were described after a single evaluation by a speech and language pathologist. On the basis of their findings, the authors concluded that many nursing home residents may be inappropriately assigned or maintained on mechanically altered diets. Regular reevaluation of the residents' dietary level was strongly advised. Several other studies have demonstrated the positive effects of increasing bolus viscosity in dysphagic patients. Clavé et al. (2006) found that changing the viscosity from that of liquid to that of nectar and pudding significantly improved the efficacy and safety of swallowing by reducing aspiration and penetration in patients with dysphagia. However, the timing of the swallow response and bolus kinetic energy were not affected, whereas increasing the bolus volume significantly impaired the efficacy and safety of swallowing. Similar effects were found in patients with unilateral vocal fold paralysis with aspiration and/or penetration (Bhattacharyya et al. 2003). In particular, paste bolus consistencies were found to be safer than thin liquids, as the paste led to much less penetration or aspiration despite a higher prevalence of pharyngeal residue. Increasing the bolus volume and viscosity in acute stroke patients (Bisch et al. 1994) led to decreased pharyngeal delay times. However, the patients exhibited very few significant effects of temperature on swallowing disorders or swallow measures. Hamdy et al. (2003) concluded that combined thermal (cold) and chemical (citrus) modification of water consistently altered swallowing behaviour after cerebral injury, resulting in slowed swallowing and reduced swallow capacity. On the other hand, Logemann et al. (1995) found an improved onset of the oral swallow in response to sour boluses compared with nonsour boluses in neurological patients. Increasing the bolus volume increased the amount of oral residue and the number of swallows but decreased the swallow times (oral transit time, pharyngeal delay time, and pharyngeal transit time). In conclusion, although bolus modification seems effective in therapy, further research will be needed.

Rehabilitation of the swallowing process may include an exercise programme consisting of diverse oral motor exercises. Even though the rationale seems obvious, a few studies have objectified the effects of intensive oral motor training. For instance, by means of an isometric lingual exercise programme, Robbins et al. (2007) demonstrated that lingual exercises enable acute and chronic dysphagic stroke patients to increase lingual strength, with associated improvements in swallowing pressure, airway protection, and lingual volume. Oral motor exercises such as tongue pull-back, yawn, and gargle tasks have also been found helpful to improve the maximum range of posterior movement of the tongue base (Veis et al. 2000). In a study by Nagaya et al. (2000), the initiation time of the swallowing reflex in dysphagic patients with Parkinson's disease was reduced significantly after a single session of swallowing training. That training consisted of tongue motion and resistance exercises, exercises to increase the adduction of the vocal folds, the Mendelsohn manoeuvre, and motion exercises for the neck, shoulders, and trunk. The orofacial regulation therapy of Castillo Morales, combining motor and sensory stimulation, indicated long-lasting improvement in oropharyngeal dysphagia in stroke patients, as measured by quality-of-life questionnaires, videofluoroscopy, and clinical evaluation (Hägg and Larsson 2004). In fact, many effect studies use oral motor exercises in combination with a variety of other intervention techniques, such as bolus modification, postural adjustments, and swallow manoeuvres (Denk et al. 1997; Elmståhl et al. 1990; Huckabee and Cannito 1999; Kiger et al. 2006; Martens et al. 1990; Masiero et al. 2007; Neumann 1993). Overall, the effects of therapy are positive. But because techniques are used in combination, the outcome of swallowing therapy cannot be attributed to any single oral motor training (Speyer et al. 2010).

A heightened sensory input may be achieved in several ways: by changing the volume, taste, or temperature of the bolus; by applying pressure; or with neuromuscular electrical stimulation. Bolus modification and management have already been discussed. Although no effect studies have been conducted on pressure application, considerable attention has been given to thermal application at the anterior faucial pillars, as studied by Rosenbek et al. (1991, 1996, 1998) in stroke patients. They were given intensive daily training using a chilled laryngeal mirror for repeated strokes on the pillars. Nonetheless, after 2 weeks of thermal application alternating with 2 weeks without it, there was no strong evidence that their dysphagia had improved (Rosenbek et al. 1991). A later study by Rosenbek et al. (1996) used a cross-over design to study the short-term effects of thermal application, comparing stroke patients' swallowing during 10 min in a treated and untreated condition. Swallowing durations were highly variable within an individual and across the patient group. Still, compared with no treatment, thermal stimulation reduced the duration of staged transition and total swallow duration. A third study (Rosenbek et al. 1998) investigated the effects of four intensities of tactile–thermal application combined with the effortful swallowing manoeuvre in acute stroke patients. Patients were randomly assigned to receive 150, 300, 450, or 600 trials of tactile–thermal application per week over a period of 2 weeks. No single treatment intensity emerged as superior. Overall, positive changes on an aspiration-penetration scale and decreased duration of stage transition did not reach clinical or statistical significance. Possibly, the observed changes might have been due to physiological recovery.

The effect of neuromuscular electrical stimulation on swallowing has been summarized in two recent systematic reviews (Carnaby-Mann and Crary 2007; Clark et al. 2009). Both indicate some small but significantly positive treatment effects. At the same time, they point out the need for additional research in this area. A few publications on neuromuscular electrical stimulation have appeared since the cut-off point for those two reviews. Some of these new studies provide cumulative evidence of the effectiveness of this therapeutic intervention as an adjunctive modality for treatment of swallowing disorders (Carnaby-Mann and Crary 2008), whereas others remain conservative in their conclusions. Ludlow et al. (2007) suggested that low levels of sensory stimulation might be an additional tool for dysphagia therapy, although emphasizing the need for further systematic studies. Others found no significant differences between neuromuscular electrical stimulation and traditional swallowing therapy in a group of stroke patients (Bülow et al. 2008). Future research will provide more evidence on whether or not neuromuscular electrical stimulation would be useful for patients with swallowing problems.

Various outcome studies have described the effects of postural changes, mainly head postural adjustments, which may affect the direction and speed of the bolus transport through the oropharynx. Overall, evaluations of therapy outcome, mainly in single-session study designs, have noted significant improvement from postural changes. For example, the use of head flexion or chin tuck in a group of aspirating patients with oesophagectomy (Lewin et al. 2001) and in a patient population with diverse neurological diseases (Shanahan et al. 1993) significantly reduced the number of patients who were aspirating. In a group of patients with unilateral dysphagia, head rotation towards the paretic side increased the fraction of the bolus swallowed and the opening diameter of the upper oesophageal sphincter (Logemann et al. 1989). However, studies on head tilt or general postural adjustments are rare and may be limited to single-case studies (Drake et al. 1997).

Behavioural swallow therapy may include diverse manoeuvres, such as the supraglottic swallow and the super supraglottic swallow. However, to determine the isolated effect of a single manoeuvre, studies must restrict the intervention protocol to one specific swallow manoeuvre. This would entail providing outcome data before and after this intervention, without introducing other treatment techniques during the same therapy period. In general, the treatment outcomes reported in the literature have been positive.

Logemann et al. (1994b) described an improved oral intake in patients after supraglottic laryngectomy when using the supraglottic swallow. When the super supraglottic swallow was applied in a group of patients with head and neck cancer (Logemann et al. 1997), fewer motility disorders were observed. Furthermore, the manoeuvre eliminated or reduced aspiration in some of the patients. With use of electromyographic biofeedback (surface electromyography) during the Mendelsohn manoeuvre in stroke patients and patients with head and neck cancer, the oral intake was improved and reflected a trend towards statistical significance (Crary et al. 2004). Evidence for the benefit of the effortful swallow is limited. For example, in two case studies by Lazarus et al. (2002) describing two patients with dysphagia as a result of oncological problems, using the effortful swallow seemed to help them attain near-normal swallowing pressures and an improved oropharyngeal clearing efficiency. The literature also provides little evidence for the benefit of the Masako manoeuvre, although the rationale has been well described (Fujiu et al. 1995; Fujiu and Logemann 1996). The Shaker or head-raising exercise was studied in a randomized controlled trial by Shaker et al. (2002) in a group of patients with dysphagia from diverse causes and an abnormal upper oesophageal sphincter opening. After a head-raising exercise programme, significant therapy effects were found. These included an improvement in the anteroposterior diameter of the sphincter opening and the anterior laryngeal excursion, a decrease in the amount of postdeglutitive residue, and the resolution of aspiration.

Several studies have been published on adjunctive biofeedback in dysphagia treatment with promising results. Denk and Kaider (1997) studied the use of videoendoscopic biofeedback in conventional therapy for patients with dysphagia associated with oncological disorders. Their main conclusion was that the functional rehabilitation period was shorter than in conventional therapy without adjunct biofeedback. In a study of tube-dependent stroke patients who had previously been treated by speech therapists without success, Bogaardt et al. (2009) demonstrated that using surface electromyography as biofeedback to standard exercises could result in a significantly positive change in oral intake. Some of these patients could have the percutaneous enteral gastrostomy tubes removed after therapy. In a study by Crary et al. (2004), the positive effects of electromyographic biofeedback on the functional oral intake in stroke patients and patients following treatment for head and neck cancer also showed a trend towards statistical significance. The findings of both studies are in line with the study outcome reported by Huckabee and Cannito (1999). In a population of chronic dysphagic patients with brainstem injury, they studied the effects of electromyographic biofeedback and cervical auscultation biofeedback in combination with traditional swallowing therapy, including swallow manoeuvres, oral motor exercises, and compensatory mechanisms. After therapy, significant improvements were observed in swallowing function as measured by severity ratings of videofluoroscopic swallowing studies, diet level, and pulmonary status.

Many more evidence-based studies have been published on issues related to outcomes in swallowing therapy using a combination of diverse intervention techniques (see the review by Speyer et al. 2010).

Actually, in daily practice, most clinicians or speech therapists will use a variety of treatment strategies instead of restricting therapy to a single technique. However, as stated before, it is hard to distinguish the particular contribution of each intervention in a behavioural therapy approach that is based on a combination of different techniques. Still, most of these studies show statistically significant, positive therapy effects (Carnaby et al. 2006; Kasprisin et al. 1989; Lin et al. 2003; Prosiegel et al. 2005). But no blanket answer can be given when trying to determine whether swallowing therapy is effective or not. Many questions about the effects of therapy in oropharyngeal dysphagia as applied by speech and language therapists remain unanswered, and many methodological problems still need to be resolved.

4.2 Methodology in Outcome Studies

An overview of the literature on the effects of behavioural swallowing therapy in oropharyngeal dysphagia raises some questions about evidence-based practice in this field. The diverse methodological problems to which many of the outcome studies attest warrant further attention. First, it is striking that, despite the great impact on a patient's quality of life, relatively few studies have been published on this subject. Furthermore, among the research that has been done, there is great diversity in study design and treatment protocols.

To evaluate treatment outcome, most effect studies use a limited set of assessment instruments. They strongly favour videofluoroscopy, which seems to be the gold standard in effect studies, whereas very few studies use quality-of-life questionnaires (Speyer et al. 2010). Since correlations between therapy effects as measured by different assessment tools may differ greatly, it may be difficult to draw comparisons between therapy outcome from studies not using similar tools. But even if studies do use the same assessment instrument, for example videofluoroscopic swallowing recording, the choice of outcome parameters, rating procedures, or protocols may differ considerably. Outcome parameters may be restricted to a single dichotomized variable such as the presence or absence of aspiration. But they may also consist of multiple complex temporal and/or spatial variables measured in digitized videofluoroscopic recordings

using specialized software packages (Clavé et al. 2006). There may be differences in the number of swallow trials performed, in the bolus consistencies and bolus volumes, or in the clinical cut-off points (e.g. wet voice, coughing, aspiration, or unsafe swallow as judged by the clinician during the videofluoroscopy). Many studies do not explain how the recordings have been assessed. A single expert or clinician can make the assessment during a patient's visit to an outpatient clinic for dysphagia. But the assessment could also be performed afterwards by a panel of blinded expert raters. Using panel ratings, one can gather information about the intra- and inter-rater reliability of scoring visuoperceptual variables in videofluoroscopic or fibre-optic endoscopic recordings of swallowing. The limited comparability may reflect the diversity of assessment protocols, in the absence of universal standardization. Furthermore, the frequent use of unvalidated or unreliable instruments or questionnaires may generate data that can neither be interpreted adequately nor make any useful contribution to formal assessment. Another issue is the enormous variation in the duration of therapies as found in the literature. Quite a few studies claim significant, usually short-term improvement after a single treatment session, such as when using postural adjustments or bolus modification. In contrast, other studies describe long series of therapy sessions. Very few trials have described any long-term treatment effects. The generalizability or comparability of effect data may be another problem. Treatment techniques that have been found effective in a specified patient population may not have the same positive therapy outcome when applied in a different group of dysphagic subjects with other etiological problems or patient characteristics, such as differences in age, severity of the dysphagic symptoms or underlying diseases, or motivation for therapy. Some studies use very small patient populations or restrict the number of therapists involved in treatment, thus introducing bias when no therapy effects may be found. The absence of significant therapy effects may be the result of a noneffective swallowing intervention. But if too few subjects or therapists have been included, the absence of clear effects may also be due to an underpowered study design or a clinician lacking sufficient expertise. A further methodological issue concerns blinding of the assessors or raters to the pre- and post-treatment data; another concerns the random allocation of patients to different treatment groups. In the case of controlled trials, the intention-to-treat principle must be applied to all participating patients. Studies that present outcome data but lack baseline measurements cannot be considered useful for determining therapy effects. But also studies intervening during a period of spontaneous recovery need to compensate for this positive tendency, for example by introducing a control group receiving no treatment (in the absence of any ethical objections) to enable group comparisons afterwards. Finally, the data or statistical analyses have to be well organized and documented.

The strength of the evidence supporting the key clinical recommendations for treatment is referred to as the level of evidence of a study (Siwek et al. 2002). The highest level of evidence can be achieved in randomized controlled trials. In the area of speech and language, however, many case studies have been published which are considered to be at the lower level of evidence. The literature abounds with examples of hierarchic schemes arranging study designs according to their presumed level of evidence. However, the methodological quality of an article is highly dependent on the degree to which the above-mentioned quality indicators have been taken into account, indicators such as the random allocation of subjects to an intervention or control group, the blinding of the outcome assessors, or patient attrition (Jüni et al. 2006; Khan et al. 2003). In light of the diverse methodological problems and the heterogeneity of study designs and therapies, statistical pooling of outcome data remains a hazardous challenge.

5   Conclusion

This chapter has given an overview of the most common behavioural intervention techniques in oropharyngeal dysphagia, pointing out new developments in the field. However, it has also emphasized the need for more evidence-based research and clinical trials. Progress in that direction is needed to objectify the effects of the intervention techniques, giving due attention to the reliability and validity of the measurement tools used.

References

Ashford J, McCabe D, Wheeler-Hegland K, Frymark T, Mullen R, Musson N, Schooling T, Smith Hammond C (2009) Evidence-based systematic review: Oropharyngeal dysphagia behavioral treatments. Part III—impact of dysphagia treatments on populations with neurological disorders. J Rehabil Res Dev 46(2):195–204

Baijens LW, Speyer R (2009) Effects of therapy for dysphagia in Parkinson's disease. Syst Rev Dysphagia 24(1):91–102

Basmajian JV, Deluca CJ (1985) Muscles alive. Their functions revealed by electromyography. Wiliams and Wilkins, Baltimore

Bhattacharyya N, Kotz T, Shapiro J (2003) The effect of bolus consistency on dysphagia in unilateral vocal cord paralysis. Otolaryngol Head Neck Surg 129(6):632–636

Bisch EM, Logemann JA, Rademaker AW, Kahrilas PJ, Lazarus CL (1994) Pharyngeal effects of bolus volume, viscosity, and temperature in patients with dysphagia resulting from neurologic impairment and in normal subjects. J Speech Hear Res 37:1041

Blumenfeld L, Hahn Y, Lepage A, Leonard R, Belafsky PC (2006) Transcutaneous electrical stimulation versus traditional dysphagia therapy: a nonconcurrent cohort study. Otolaryngol Head Neck Surg 135(5):754–757

Bogaardt HCA, Grolman W, Fokkens WJ (2009) The use of biofeedback in the treatment of chronic dysphagia in stroke patients. Folia Phoniatr Logop 61:200–205

Bogaert E, Goeleven A, Dejaeger E (2003) Effectmeting van therapeutische interventies tijdens radiologisch slikonderzoek. Tijdschr Geneeskd 59(22):1410–1414

Bours GJ, Speyer R, Lemmens J, Limburg M, De Wit R (2009) Bedside screening tests vs. videofluoroscopy or fibreoptic endoscopic evaluation of swallowing to detect dysphagia in patients with neurological disorders: systematic review. J Adv Nurs 65(3):477–493

Bülow M, Olsson R, Ekberg O (2001) Videomanometric analysis of supraglottic swallow, effortful swallow, and chin tuck in patients with pharyngeal dysfunction. Dysphagia 16:190–195

Bülow M, Speyer R, Baijens L, Woisard V, Ekberg O (2008) Neuromuscular electrical stimulation (NMES) in stroke patients with oral and pharyngeal dysfunction. Dysphagia 23:302–309

Carnaby G, Hankey GJ, Pizzi J (2006) Behavioural intervention for dysphagia in acute stroke: a randomised controlled trail. Lancet Neurol 5:31–37

Carnaby-Mann GD, Crary MA (2007) Examining the evidence on neuromuscular electrical stimulation for swallowing: A meta-analysis. Arch Otolaryngol Head Neck Surg 133:564–571

Carnaby-Mann GD, Crary MA (2008) Adjunctive neuromuscular electrical stimulation for treatment-refractory dysphagia. Ann Otol Rhinol Laryngol 117(4):279–287

Clark H, Lazarus C, Arvedson J, Schooling T, Frymark T (2009) Evidence-based systematic review: Effects of neuromuscular electrical stimulation on swallowing and neural activation. Am J Speech Lang Pathol 18:361–375

Clavé P, De Kraa M, Arreola V, Girvent M, Palomera E, Serra-Prat M (2006) The effect of bolus viscosity on swallowing function in neurogenic dysphagia. Aliment Pharmacol Ther 24:1385–1394

Crary MA, Groher ME (2003) Adult swallowing disorders. Elsevier, New York

Crary MA, Carnaby GD, Groher ME, Helseth E (2004) Functional benefits of dysphagia therapy using adjunctive sEMG biofeedback. Dysphagia 19:160–164

Dealy JM (1995) Official nomenclature for material functions describing the response of a viscoelastic fluid to various shearing and extensional deformations. J Rheol 39(1):253–265

Denk DM, Kaider A (1997) Videoendoscopic biofeedback: a simple method to improve the efficacy of swallowing rehabilitation of patients after head and neck surgery. ORL J Otorhinolaryngol Relat Spec 59:100–105

Denk DM, Swoboda H, Schima W, Eibenberger K (1997) Prognostic factors for swallowing rehabilitation following head and neck cancer surgery. Acta Otolaryngol (Stockh) 117(5):769–774

Drake W, O'Donoghue S, Bartram C, Lindsay J, Greenwood R (1997) Eating in side-lying facilitates rehabilitation in neurogenic dysphagia. Brain Inj 11:137–142

Elmståhl S, Bülow M, Ekberg O, Petersson M, Tegner H (1990) Treatment of dysphagia improves nutritional conditions in stroke patients. Dysphagia 14:61–66

Freed M, Wijting Y (2003) VitalStim Certification Program. Training manual for patient assessment and treatment using VitalStim electrical stimulation. Chattanooga Group, Hixson

Frymark MA, Schooling T, Mullen R, Wheeler-Hegland K, Ashford J, McCabe D, Musson N, Smith Hammond C (2009) Evidence-based systematic review: oropharyngeal dysphagia behavioural treatments. Part II—background and methodology. J Rehabil Res Dev 46(2):175–184

Fujiu M, Logemann JA (1996) Effect of a tongue holding maneuver on posterior pharyngeal wall movement during deglutition. Am J Speech Lang Pathol 5:23–30

Fujiu M, Logemann JA, Pauloski BR (1995) Increased postoperative posterior pharyngeal wall movement in patients with anterior oral cancer: preliminary findings and possible implication for treatment. Am J Speech Lang Pathol 4:24–30

Groher ME (1987) Bolus management and aspiration pneumonia in patients with pseudobulbar dysphagia. Dysphagia 1:215–216

Groher ME, McKaig TN (1995) Dysphagia and dietary levels in skilled nursing facilities. J Am Geriatr Soc 43:528–532

Hägg M, Larsson B (2004) Effects of motor and sensory stimulation in stroke patients with long-lasting dysphagia. Dysphagia 19(4):219–230

Hamdy S, Jilani S, Price V, Parker C, Hall N, Power M (2003) Modulation of human swallowing behaviour by thermal and chemical stimulation in health and after brain injury. Neurogastroenterol Motil 15:69–77

Huckabee M, Cannito M (1999) Outcomes of swallowing rehabilitation in chronic brainstem dysphagia: a retrospective evaluation. Dysphagia 14:93–109

Huckabee M, Pelletier C (1999) Management of adult neurogenic dysphagia. Singular Publishing Group, San Diego

Jüni P, Altman DG, Egger M (2006) Assessing the quality of randomised controlled trials. In: Egger M, Smith GD, Altman DG (eds) Systematic reviews in health care: meta-analysis in context, 2nd edn. BMJ Publishing Group, London

Kasprisin AT, Clumeck Nino-MurciaM (1989) The efficacy of rehabilitative management of dysphagia. Dysphagia 4:48–52

Khan KS, Kunz R, Kleijnen J, Antes G (2003) Systematic reviews to support evidence-based medicine. How to review and apply findings of healthcare research. Royal Society of Medicine Press, Oxford

Kiger M, Brown CS, Watkins L (2006) Dysphagia management: an analysis of patient outcomes using VitalStim therapy compared to traditional swallow therapy. Dysphagia 21(4):243–253

Langmore SE (2001) Endoscopic evaluation and treatment of swallowing disorders. Thieme, New York

Lazarus C, Logemann JA, Song CW, Rademaker W, Kahrilas PJ (2002) Effects of voluntary maneuvers on tongue base function for swallowing. Folia Phoniatr Logoped 54(4):171–176

Leslie P, Drinnan MJ, Finn S, Ford GA, Wilson JA (2004) Reliability and validity of cervical auscultation: a controlled comparison using videofluoroscopy. Dysphagia 19:231–240

Lewin JS, Hebert TM, Putnam JB, DuBrow RA (2001) Experience with the chin tuck maneuver in postesophagectomy aspirators. Dysphagia 16:216–219

Lin L, Wang S, Chen S, Wang T, Chen M, Wu S (2003) Efficacy of swallowing training for residents following stroke. J Adv Nurs 44(5):469–478

Logemann JA (1998) Evaluation and treatment of swallowing disorders. PRO-ED, Austin

Logemann JA (1999) Behavioral management for oropharyngeal dysphagia. Folia Phoniatr Logop 51:199–212

Logemann JA (2006) Medical and rehabilitative therapy of oral, pharyngeal motor disorders. GI Motil Online. doi: 10.1038/gimo50

Logemann JA, Kahrilas PJ, Kobara M, Vakil NB (1989) The benefit of head rotation on pharyngoesophageal dysphagia. Arch Phys Med Rehabil 70:767–771

Logemann JA, Rademaker AW, Pauloski BR, Kahrilas PJ (1994a) Effects of postural change on aspiration in head and neck surgical patients. Otolaryngol Head Neck Surg 110(2):222–227

Logemann JA, Gibbons P, Rademaker AW, Pauloski BR, Kahrilas PJ, Bacon M, Bowman J, McCracken E (1994b) Mechanisms of recovery of swallow after supraglottic laryngectomy. J Speech Hear Res 37(5):965–974

Logemann JA, Pauloski BR, Colangelo L, Lazarus C, Fujiu M, Kahrilas PJ (1995) Effects of a sour bolus on oropharyngeal swallowing measures in patients with neurogenic dysphagia. J Speech Hear Res 38:556–563

Logemann JA, Roa Pauloski B, Rademaker AW, Colangelo LA (1997) Super supraglottic swallow in irradiated head and neck cancer patients. Head Neck 19:535–540

Ludlow CL, Humbert I, Saxon K, Poletto C, Sonies B, Crujido L (2007) Effects of surface electrical stimulation both at rest and during swallowing in chronic pharyngeal dysphagia. Dysphagia 22(1):1–10

Martens L, Cameron T, Simonsen M (1990) Effects of a multidisciplinairy management program on neurologically impaired patients with dysphagia. Dysphagia 5:147–151

Masiero S, Previato C, Addante S, Grego F, Armani M (2007) Dysphagia in post-carotid endarterectomy: a prospective study. Ann Vasc Surg 21(3):318–320

McCabe D, Ashford J, Wheeler-Hegland K, Frymark T, Mullen R, Musson N, Smith Hammond C, Schooling T (2009) Evidence-based systematic review: Oropharyngeal dysphagia behavioral treatments. Part IV—impact of dysphagia treatments on individuals' postcancer treatments. J Rehabil Res Dev 46(2):205–214

McHorney CA, Robbins J, Lomax K, Rosenbek JC, Chignell K, Kramer AE, Bricker DE (2002) The SWAL-QOL and SWAL-CARE outcomes tool for oropharyngeal dysphagia in adults: III. Documentation of reliability and validity. Dysphagia 17:97–114

McHorney CA, Bricker DE, Kramer AE, Rosenbek JC, Robbins JA, Chignell K, Logemann JA, Clarke C (2003) The SWAL-QOL and SWAL-CARE outcomes tool for oropharyngeal dysphagia in adults: I. Conceptual foundation and item development. Dysphagia 15(3):115–121

Nagaya M, Kachi T, Yamada T (2000) Effect of swallowing training on swallowing disorders in Parkinson's disease. Scand J Rehab Med 32:11–15

Neumann S (1993) Swallowing therapy with neurologic patients: results of direct and indirect therapy methods in 66 patients suffering from neurological disorders. Dysphagia 8:150–153

Power ML, Fraser CH, Hobson A, Singh S, Tyrrell P, Nicholson DA, Turnbull I, Thompson DG, Hamdy S (2006) Evaluating oral stimulation as a treatment for dysphagia after stroke. Dysphagia 21(1):49–55

Prosiegel M, Höling R, Heintze M, Wagner-Sonntag E, Wiseman K (2005) Swallowing therapy: a prospective study on patients with neurogenic dysphagia due to unilateral paresis of the vagal nerve, Avellis' syndrome, Wallenberg's syndrome, posterior fossa tumours and cerebellar hemorrhage. Acta Neurochirurg Suppl 93:35–37

Rasley A, Logemann JA, Kahrilas PJ, RAdemaker AW, Pauloski BR, Dodds WJ (1993) Prevention of barium aspiration during videofluoroscopic swallowing studies: value of change in posture. AJR Am J Roentgenol160:1005–1009

Robbins J, Kays SA, Gangnon RE, Hind JA, Hewitt AL, Gentry LR, Taylor AJ (2007) The effects of lingual exercise in stroke patients with dysphagia. Arch Phys Med Rehabil 88(2):150–158

Rofes L, Arreola V, Cabré M, Almirall J, Campins L, García-Peris P, Speyer R, Clavé P (2011) Diagnosis and management of oropharyngeal dysphagia and its nutritional and respiratory complications in the elderly. Gastroenterol Res Prac 2011:13. doi:10.1155/2011/818979

Rosenbek JC, Robbins J, Fishback B, Levine RL (1991) Effects of thermal application on dysphagia after stroke. J Speech Hear Res 34:1257–1268

Rosenbek JC, Roecker EB, Wood JL, Robbins J (1996) Thermal application reduces the duration of stage transition in dysphagia after stroke. Dysphagia 11:225–233

Rosenbek JC, Robbins J, Willford WO, Kirk G, Schiltz A, Sowell TW, Deutch SE, Milanti FJ, Ashford J, Gramigna GD, Fogarty A, Dong K, Rau MT, Prescott TE, Lloyd AM, Sterkel MT, Hansen JE (1998) Comparing treatment intensities of tactile-thermal application. Dysphagia 13:1–9

Shaker R, Easterling C, Kern M (2002) Rehabilitation of swallowing by exercise in tube-fed patients with pharyngeal dysphagia secondary to abnormal UES opening. Gastroenterology 122:1314–1321

Shanahan TK, Logemann JA, Rademaker AW, Pauloski BR, Kahrilas PJ (1993) Chin-down posture effect on aspiration in dysphagic patients. Arch Phys Med Rehabil 74:736–739

Shaw GY, Sechtem PR, Searl J, Keller K, Rawi TA, Dowdy E (2007) Transcutaneous neuromuscular electrical stimulation (VitalStim) curative therapy for severe dysphagia: myth or reality? Ann Otol Rhinol Laryngol 116(1):36–44

Siwek J, Gourlay ML, Slawson DC, Shaughnessy AF (2002) How to write an evidence-based clinical review article. Am Fam Physician 65(2):251–259

Speyer R (2008) Effects of voice therapy: a systematic review. J Voice 22(5):565–580

Speyer R, Baijens LWJ, Heijnen MAM, Zwijnenberg I (2010) Effects of therapy in patients with dysphagia by speech and language therapists: a systematic review. Dysphagia 25(1):40–65

Veerbeek L (2008) Care and quality of life in the dying phase: the contribution of the Liverpool care pathway for the dying patient. Dissertation, Erasmus University Rotterdam

Veis S, Logemann JA, Colangelo L (2000) Effects of three techniques on maximum posterior movement of the tongue base. Dysphagia 15:142–145

Wheeler-Hegland K, Frymark T, Schooling T, McCabe D, Ashford J, Mullen R, Smith Hammond C, Musson N (2009) Evidence-based systematic review: oropharyngeal dysphagia behavioral treatments. Part V—applications for clinicians and researchers. J Rehabil Res Dev 46(2):215–222

Rheological Aspects of Swallowing and Dysphagia

Edmundo Brito-de la Fuente, Olle Ekberg,
and Críspulo Gallegos

Contents

Abstract

Dysphagia is a combination of symptoms affecting a person's ability to swallow. On the other hand, swallowing is about transferring of liquids and boluses from the mouth into the stomach. Boluses may have several solid-like consistencies and drinks may have different viscosities. Because rheology is the study of the deformation and flow of matter; the connection between swallowing and rheology and thus dysphagia is clear. This rheology science helps to better understand how a bolus is deformed and thus flowing during the swallowing process. Knowledge of the deformability and flow of a bolus is important to better understand dysphagia, or swallowing impairment. This chapter is organized as follows. Section 2 gives a short description of the material functions or rheological properties. Rheological data of products used for dysphagia are used as examples. Section 3 focuses on the rheological aspects of oral processing and bolus transportation. This is followed by a practical example on how to design new products for the nutritional management of dysphagic patients. The chapter ends with some concluding remarks.

E. Brito-de la Fuente (✉)
Innovation and Development Centre Clinical Nutrition
and Pharmaceuticals, Science Production and Technology,
Fresenius Kabi Deutschland GmbH,
61440 Oberursel, Germany
e-mail: edmundo.brito@fresenius-kabi.com

O. Ekberg
Department of Clinical Sciences/Medical Radiology,
Shane University Hospital, Lund University,
205 02 Malmö, Sweden

C. Gallegos
Departamento de Ingeniería Química,
Universidad de Huelva,
21071 Huelva, Spain

1 Introduction

Eating and drinking are essential activities of humans. Swallowing is a complex mechanism involving many muscles and nerves aiming to transport a bolus into the stomach. Because boluses may have several solid-like consistencies and drinks may have different viscosities, rheology is involved. This science helps to better understand how a bolus is deformed or flows during the

O. Ekberg (ed.), *Dysphagia*, Medical Radiology. Diagnostic Imaging, DOI: 10.1007/174_2011_362,
© Springer-Verlag Berlin Heidelberg 2012

swallowing process. Knowledge of the deformability and flow of a bolus is important to better understand dysphagia, or swallowing impairment. This chapter is organized as follows. Section 2 gives a short description of the material functions or rheological properties. Rheological data of products used for dysphagia are used. Section 3 focuses on the rheological aspects of oral processing and bolus transportation. This is followed by a practical example on how to design new products for the nutritional management of dysphagic patients. The chapter ends with some concluding remarks.

2　Rheology Fundamentals

2.1　Basic Concepts of Rheology

"Rheology," a term invented by Prof. Eugene Bingham of Lafayette College in Easton (PA, USA), is defined as "the study of the deformation and flow of matter" (Walters 2010).

It is well accepted that a given material can behave as a solid or a liquid depending on the timescale of the deformation process (Gallegos and Walters 2010). In other words, the mechanical properties of all materials are time-dependent, i.e., they vary with time in response to an applied load or deformation. This phenomenon is simply a consequence of the second law of thermodynamics, according to which a portion of the imparted energy of deformation is always dissipated as heat by viscous forces even while the rest may be stored elastically. The dissipation is neither instantaneous nor infinitely slow and is therefore a rate process. It is this that renders the physical properties time-dependent (Emri 2010). THe rheological behavior of materials ranges from virtually purely elastic (no dissipation) to virtually purely viscous (instantaneous dissipation), showing both elastic and viscous properties in between. The behavior of many materials such as puddings for dysphagia nutritional support typically falls between the extremes and such materials are defined as viscoelastic. The behavior may be expressed suitably by the Deborah number, De, the ratio of the characteristic time of the material, λ, on which molecular rearrangements take place and the characteristic time of the deformation process, T (Reiner 1964):

$$De = \frac{\lambda}{T}. \qquad (1)$$

High Deborah numbers correspond to solid-like behavior and low Deborah numbers correspond to liquid-like behavior. A material can appear solid-like either because it has an infinite characteristic time or because the deformation process is very fast. One obvious consequence of this is that even mobile liquid systems with very low characteristic times can behave like elastic solids when exposed to a very fast deformation process (viscoelastic liquids). In contrast, solid-like materials will be able to flow for a time (viscoelastic solids).

2.2　Linear Viscoelastic Behaviour

Viscoelastic materials possess both viscous and elastic properties in differing degrees. For a viscoelastic material, internal stresses depend not only of the instantaneous deformation, but also on the whole past history of deformation. When a material is deformed, thermodynamic forces immediately begin to operate to restore the minimum-energy state. Movement from the rest state represents storage of energy. If a material is submitted to deformations or stresses small enough so that its rheological functions do not depend on the value of the deformation or stress, the material response is said to be in the linear viscoelasticity range (Gallegos and Martínez-Boza 2010).

Consider the function $\gamma(t)$ as representative of some cause (shear strain) acting on a given material, and the shear stress, $\sigma(t)$, the effect resulting from this cause (Dealy and Wissbrun 1995). A variation in shear strain occurring at time t_1 will produce a corresponding effect at some time later, t, which can be expressed as

$$\sigma(t) = G(t - t_1)\delta\gamma(t_1). \qquad (2)$$

$G(t-t_1)$ is known as the relaxation function, or the relaxation modulus, which is a property of the material and relates cause and effect. It is a function of the time delay between cause and effect.

A series of N changes in the shear strain, each occurring at a different time, will contribute cumulatively to the stress at some later time (Boltzmann superposition principle). Thus,

$$\sigma(t) = \sum_{i=1}^{N} G(t - t_i)\delta\gamma(t_i). \qquad (3)$$

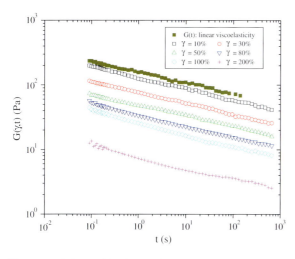

Fig. 1 Evolution with time of the linear and nonlinear relaxation modulus for a selected enteral pudding formulation

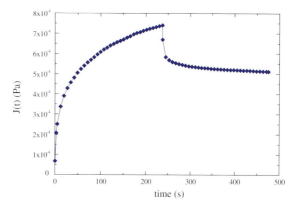

Fig. 2 Typical evolution of the creep compliance with the elapsed time, in the linear viscoelasticity region, for a selected pudding formulation

If the change in strain occurs continuously, the sum may be replaced by an integral:

$$\sigma(t) = \int_{-\infty}^{t} G(t - t')\mathrm{d}\gamma(t'). \qquad (4)$$

This linear constitutive equation is appropriate to describe the behavior of materials subjected to shear deformation, which is one of the most relevant types of deformation concerning the food swallowing process. However, this equation can be generalized for any type of deformation that can be applied to the material.

To gain information on the influencing function that relates cause and effect, a number of small strain experiments are used in rheology. Some of the more common techniques are stress relaxation, creep, and sinusoidal oscillations (Ferry 1980; Macosko 1994; Dealy and Wissbrun 1995; Barnes 2000). Different experimental methods are used because they may be more convenient for a particular material or because they provide data over a particular time range.

2.2.1 Stress Relaxation

Stress relaxation after a step strain is the fundamental way in which the relaxation modulus is defined. In this experiment, a sample is suddenly deformed at a given strain, γ_0, and the resulting stress is measured as a function of time. The relaxing stress data can be used to determine $G(t)$:

$$G(t) = \frac{\tau(t)}{\gamma_0}. \qquad (5)$$

The evolution of the linear relaxation modulus for a selected enteral pudding formulation is presented in Fig. 1.

Knowledge of the evolution of the linear relaxation modulus with time is essential to model the nonlinear viscoelastic behavior of complex fluids, as will be reviewed in Sect. 2.3.

2.2.2 Creep

Creep experiments are particularly useful for studying certain practical applications where long times are involved. In a creep experiment, a constant stress, σ_0, is instantaneously applied on a sample, and the resulting strain is recorded versus time. The strain values obtained as a function of time can be used to calculate the compliance, $J(t)$, as follows:

$$J(t) = \frac{\gamma(t)}{\tau_0}. \qquad (6)$$

A typical evolution of the creep compliance with time for a selected pudding formulation is shown in Fig. 2. This creep compliance function is independent of the shear stress applied in the linear viscoelasticity range.

2.2.3 Small Amplitude Oscillatory Shear

The most common type of test to characterize the linear viscoelastic behavior of complex fluids is the small amplitude oscillatory shear.

In a similar way to performing relaxation or creep tests over a range of time, oscillatory tests over a range of frequencies can be conducted. It is obvious that short times correspond to high frequencies, and long times correspond to low frequencies.

In this test, the material is subjected to a simple shearing deformation by applying a sine-wave-shaped input of stress or strain (Macosko 1994; Dealy and Wissbrun 1995; Barnes 2000). If a sinusoidal strain is applied, the shear strain as a function of time is given by

$$\gamma(t) = \gamma_0 \sin(\omega t), \tag{7}$$

where γ_0 is the strain amplitude and ω is the frequency.

By differentiating, one obtains the evolution of shear rate with time:

$$\dot{\gamma}(t) = \gamma_0 \omega \cos(\omega t) = \dot{\gamma}_0 \cos(wt), \tag{8}$$

where $\dot{\gamma}$ is the shear rate amplitude.

The resulting stress is measured as a function of time:

$$\sigma(t) = \sigma_0 \sin(\omega t + \delta), \tag{9}$$

where σ_0 is the stress amplitude and δ is a phase shift, also known as the loss angle.

The stress data can be analyzed by decomposing the stress wave into two waves of the same frequency, one in phase with the strain wave ($\sin \omega t$) and the other 90° out of phase with this wave ($\cos \omega t$):

$$\sigma = \sigma' + \sigma'' = \sigma' \sin \omega t + \sigma'' \cos \omega t. \tag{10}$$

Two dynamic moduli can be then defined:

$$G' = \frac{\sigma'_0}{\gamma_0}, \tag{11}$$

the elastic, storage, or in-phase modulus, and

$$G'' = \frac{\sigma''_0}{\gamma_0}, \tag{12}$$

the viscous, loss, or out-of-phase modulus.

The loss tangent is given by

$$\tan \delta = \frac{G''}{G'}, \tag{13}$$

In addition, a complex modulus, G^*, can be defined as

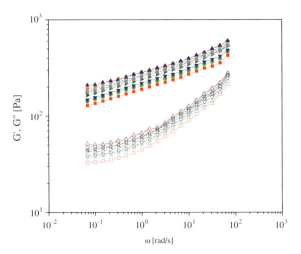

Fig. 3 Evolution of the storage and loss moduli with frequency for a selected enteral nutrition pudding as a function of ageing

$$\sigma_0 = |G^*|\gamma_0, \tag{14}$$

G' and G'' being its real and imaginary parts, respectively:

$$G^*(\omega) = G'(\omega) + iG''(\omega). \tag{15}$$

For a purely elastic material, there is no viscous dissipation, no phase shift, and the loss modulus is zero. In contrast, there is no energy storage for a purely viscous liquid, the storage modulus being zero and the loss angle being 90°.

Typical evolutions of the storage and loss moduli with frequency for a selected enteral nutrition pudding as a function of ageing are shown in Fig. 3.

Another way to interpret the results obtained from small amplitude oscillatory shear tests is in terms of a sinusoidal strain rate. Two new material functions are then defined:

$$\sigma(t) = \dot{\gamma}_0[\eta'(\omega) \cos(\omega t) + \eta''(\omega) \sin(\omega t)], \tag{16}$$

where

$$\eta' = \frac{\sigma''_0}{\dot{\gamma}_0} = \frac{\sigma_0}{\dot{\gamma}_0} \sin \delta = \frac{G''}{\omega}, \tag{17}$$

and

$$\eta'' = \frac{\sigma'_0}{\dot{\gamma}_0} = \frac{\sigma_0}{\dot{\gamma}_0} \cos \delta = \frac{G'}{\omega}. \tag{18}$$

The complex viscosity is

$$\eta^*(\omega) = \eta'(\omega) - i\eta''(\omega) \qquad (19)$$

and its magnitude is

$$|\eta*| = \frac{\sigma_0}{\dot{\gamma}_0} \sqrt{(\eta')^2 + (\eta'')^2}. \qquad (20)$$

The reciprocal of the complex modulus is also defined as an additional oscillatory material function, the complex compliance, J^*:

$$J^*(\omega) = \frac{1}{G*(\omega)} = J'(\omega) + iJ''(\omega), \qquad (21)$$

where the real and imaginary components of the complex compliance are related to those of the complex modulus by

$$J'(\omega) = \frac{G'(\omega)}{G'^2(\omega) + G''^2(\omega)}, \qquad (22)$$

and

$$J''(\omega) = -\frac{G''(\omega)}{G'^2(\omega) + G''^2(\omega)}. \qquad (23)$$

2.2.4 Linear Viscoelastic Behaviour Modeling

For dispersions with complex microstructure, their dynamic linear viscoelastic behavior can be described by a generalized Maxwell model (Mackley et al. 1994; Madiedo and Gallegos 1997a, b):

$$G' = G_e + \sum_{i=1}^{N} G_i \frac{(\omega\lambda_i)^2}{1 + (\omega\lambda_i)^2}, \qquad (24)$$

$$G'' = \sum_{i=1}^{N} G_i \frac{\omega\lambda_i}{1 + (\omega\lambda_i)^2}, \qquad (25)$$

where G_e is the elastic modulus. This model considers a superposition of a series of N independent relaxation processes, each process having a relaxation time, λ_i, and a relaxation strength, G_i. The resulting distribution or spectrum of relaxation times can be used to compare the mechanical behavior of complex fluids.

On the other hand, in the case of the linear relaxation modulus,

$$G(t) = \sum_{i=1}^{N} G_i[\exp(-t/\lambda_i)]. \qquad (26)$$

However, Madiedo and Gallegos (1997a, b) have also used a continuous relaxation, or retardation, spectrum, $H(\lambda)$, to represent the linear viscoelasticity data of food emulsions, which provides a continuous function of relaxation times, λ, rather than a discrete set. Thus, the linear relaxation modulus and the dynamic viscoelasticity functions are now defined as

$$G(t) = \int_{-\infty}^{\infty} H(\lambda)[\exp(-t/\lambda)]d(\ln\lambda), \qquad (27)$$

$$G'(\omega) = G_e + \int_{-\infty}^{\infty} H(\lambda)\frac{\omega^2\lambda^2}{1 + \omega^2\lambda^2}d(\ln\lambda), \qquad (28)$$

and

$$G''(\omega) = \int_{-\infty}^{\infty} H(\lambda)\frac{\omega\lambda}{1 + \omega^2\lambda^2}d(\ln\lambda). \qquad (29)$$

As the spectra cannot be directly obtained from experimentation, the problem that generally arises is the calculation of these spectra from experimental data for a given linear viscoelasticity function. This, of course, implies inverting the corresponding integral equation relating the spectrum with the selected material function. However, it is well known that the resolution of these equations is an ill-posed problem, as small changes in the rheological functions give rise to strong oscillations in the spectra. For that reason, many approximation methods have been developed to perform such calculations (Madiedo and Gallegos 1997a, b).

2.3 Nonlinear Viscoelastic Behaviour

At sufficiently large deformations, many products for dysphagia nutritional support show nonlinear viscoelastic characteristics. This behavior is clearly

observed, for instance, by applying increasing deformation during relaxation tests or by characterizing the
viscous flow behavior of these formulations in a wide
range of shear rates.

2.3.1 Viscous Flow Behaviour

Thus, as a consequence of their complex microstructure, complex fluids (e.g., puddings for dysphagia nutritional support) show linear viscoelastic
characteristics at a sufficiently small deformation, and
a non-Newtonian viscous response in a certain range
of shear rates. The flow curve of a non-Newtonian
fluid shows an apparent viscosity, the shear stress
divided by the shear rate, which depends on the flow
conditions, e.g., shear rate, and, sometimes, even on
the kinematic history of the fluid element under
consideration (see Sect. 2.3.2).

Complex materials may show different types of
non-Newtonian behavior. However, the most common one found in dysphagia nutritional support
products rheology is the shear-thinning behavior. This
viscous response is characterized by a continuous
decrease in the apparent viscosity as the shear rate
increases (Partal and Franco 2010).

However, most shear-thinning fluids with a complex microstructure also exhibit Newtonian regions at
low and high shear rates. The resulting constant viscosity values at very low and high shear rates are
known as the zero-shear-rate-limiting viscosity, η_0,
and the high-shear-rate-limiting viscosity, η_∞. Thus,
the apparent viscosity of a shear-thinning fluid
decreases from η_0 to η_∞ with increasing shear rate.
These fluids are known as "structured fluids" because
the shear rate affects the microstructure of the material and their viscous behavior changes according to
the evolution of the microstructure. Data in a sufficiently wide range of shear rates may illustrate this
complete viscous behavior (see Fig. 4).

Several equations have been proposed to model the
non-Newtonian flow behavior of food dispersions.
Some of them have a theoretical basis, whereas others
are curve fittings which provide empirical relationships for the shear stress (or apparent viscosity) versus
shear rate curves (Bird et al. 1987; Carreau et al.
1997; Chhabra and Richardson 1999). The more
widely used viscosity models that may represent the
"structured" fluid response of these binders are
described next.

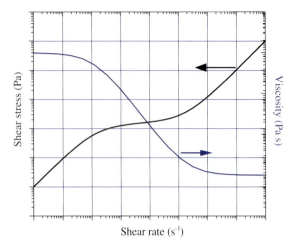

Fig. 4 Log–log plot of the viscous flow behavior of a standard
"structured" fluid

2.3.1.1 Ostwald–de Waele or Power-Law Model

The relationship between shear stress and shear rate
(plotted on a log–log scale) for a shear-thinning fluid
can often be approximated by a straight line over a
wide shear rate range (or stress):

$$\sigma = k\dot{\gamma}^n, \tag{30}$$

where k is the consistency index and n is the flow
index. Thus, the apparent viscosity for the so-called
power-law (or Ostwald–de Waele) fluid is given by

$$\eta = k\dot{\gamma}^{n-1}. \tag{31}$$

For $n = 1$, the fluid shows Newtonian behavior.
For a shear-thinning fluid, the index n ranges from 0
to 1, so the smaller the value of n, the greater is the
degree of shear thinning. The value of k can be
viewed as the value of the apparent viscosity at a
shear rate of unity.

2.3.1.2 Sisko's Model

This three-parameter model predicts a shear-thinning
region at intermediate shear rates and a Newtonian
viscosity, η_∞, at high shear rates:

$$\eta = \eta_\infty + k\dot{\gamma}^{n-1}, \tag{32}$$

where η_∞ is a high-shear-rate-limiting viscosity and
k and n are parameters related to the consistency and

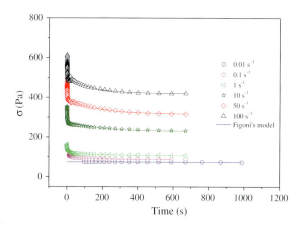

Fig. 5 Transient shear flow tests at different constant shear rates for a selected pudding formulation

flow indexes. With the use of the third parameter, this model provides a somewhat better fit to some experimental data, being particularly recommended to describe the material flow behavior in the high-shear-rate region.

2.3.1.3 Carreau's Model

On the basis of molecular network considerations, Carreau (1972) proposed the following viscosity model, which incorporates both low-shear-rate-limiting and high-shear-rate-limiting viscosities, η_o and η_∞:

$$\frac{\eta - \eta_\infty}{\eta_o - \eta_\infty} = \frac{1}{[1 + (\lambda\dot{\gamma})^2]^s}. \tag{33}$$

The parameter $\lambda = 1/\dot{\gamma}_c$, where $\dot{\gamma}_c$ is a critical shear rate for the onset of the shear-thinning region. On the other hand, s is a parameter related to the slope of the power-law region. This model can describe the so-called structural behavior over a very wide range of shear rate.

2.3.2 Transient Flow Behaviour

Shear viscosities of complex fluids for dysphagia nutritional support in many cases are not only a function of the applied shear stress or shear rate, but are also a function of the length of time for which the shear rate or stress is applied on the sample. A suitable way of measuring time-dependent effects during viscous flow is to follow the evolution of viscosity with time, after applying a constant shear rate (see Fig. 5). As can be deduced from this figure, the viscosity decreases with time to a steady-state value.

This behavior is known as thixotropy. All fluids that develop a certain level of complex microstructure can show this behavior. Thixotropy is a reversible phenomenon; that is, it reflects the finite time taken by the fluid to change its microstructure, which is fully recovered after cessation of the perturbation. The occurrence of thixotropy implies that the flow history of the fluid has to be taken into account when making predictions of its flow behavior.

Different models can be found in the literature that adequately describe the thixotropic response of complex fluids (Partal and Franco 2010). In this sense, Figoni's model has been successfully used to fit the transient flow behavior of enteral puddings for dysphagia nutritional support. Figoni's model is a stress-decay model with two kinetic functions:

$$\sigma - \sigma_e = (\sigma_{01} - \sigma_{e1})\exp(-k_1 t) + (\sigma_{02} - \sigma_{e2})\exp(-k_2 t), \tag{34}$$

where k_1 and k_2 are kinetic constants at short and long times, respectively. Subindexes 0 and e refer to initial and equilibrium stresses, respectively.

2.3.3 Nonlinear Viscoelasticity Modeling

One approach to describing nonlinear behavior (transient and steady state) of rheologically complex materials is based on continuum mechanics principles, aiming to establish a rheological constitutive equation to replace the Boltzmann principle (Eq. 4).

Wagner (1979) proposed the introduction of a nonlinear memory function in the constitutive equation for nonlinear viscoelasticity. Taking into account that the relaxation of stress following a large step strain (nonlinear relaxation modulus) can often be separated into time-dependent and strain-dependent factors (see Fig. 1, parallel lines in a log–log plot for different strains), Wagner proposed the use of a memory function, defined as the product of the linear memory function and the *damping function* (reflecting strain influence), an empirical function whose parameters are determined by fitting experimental data.

$m(t-t')$ is the memory function, related to the linear relaxation modulus by differentiation:

$$m(t - t') = \frac{dG(t - t')}{dt'}, \tag{35}$$

where t is the time at which the stress is evaluated and t' is a time prior to time t at which the stress is evaluated.

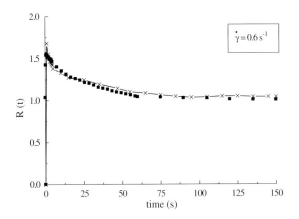

$\dot{\gamma} = 0.6\,\mathrm{s}^{-1}$

Fig. 6 Relationship between transient and steady-state stress values, and Wagner's model fitting, as a function of shear time for a selected pudding sample. *Squares* model predictions, *crosses* calculation from experimental values

If time–strain separability for the nonlinear relaxation modulus is possible, and considering only the simple shear component, one can express the Wagner model as

$$\sigma(t, \dot{\gamma}) = - \int_{-\infty}^{t} \frac{\mathrm{d}G(t - t')}{\mathrm{d}t'} h(\gamma)\gamma(t, t')\mathrm{d}t', \qquad (36)$$

where $\tau(t, \dot{\gamma})$ is the transient shear stress and $h(\gamma)$ is the damping function, which can be easily calculated from the ratio between the nonlinear relaxation modulus, $G(\gamma, t-t')$, and the linear relaxation modulus, $G(t-t')$ (Rolón-Garrido and Wagner 2009):

$$h(\gamma) = \frac{G(\gamma, t - t')}{G(t - t')}. \qquad (37)$$

Different types of damping functions have been proposed. For instance, according to Wagner,

$$h(\gamma) = \exp(-k\gamma), \qquad (38)$$

and assuming that the evolution of the linear relaxation modulus with time can be described by a generalized Maxwell model,

$$G(t) = \sum_{i=1}^{n} g_i \mathrm{e}^{\frac{-(t-t')}{\lambda_i}}. \qquad (39)$$

The steady-state viscosity is then

$$\eta(\dot{\gamma}) = \sum_{i=1}^{n} \frac{g_i \lambda_i}{(1 + k\lambda_i \dot{\gamma})^2}. \qquad (40)$$

Nevertheless, Quinchia et al. (2011) have also used a damping function described by the Soskey–Winter model, which fits fairly well the experimental results obtained with different types of emulsions, and more specifically, with puddings for dysphagia nutritional support:

$$h(\gamma) = \frac{1}{1 + a\gamma^b}. \qquad (41)$$

Figure 6 shows the experimental and calculated values of $R(t)$, the ratio between the shear stress after instantaneous imposition of a constant shear rate, $\sigma(t)$, and the steady-state stress, $\sigma(\infty)$, for a transient flow test conducted on a selected pudding. As can be observed, the Wagner model fits the experimental results obtained fairly well.

3 Rheology, Swallowing, and Dysphagia: State of the Art

3.1 Rheology and the Swallowing Process

There are several angles from which dysphagia may be analyzed. The medical side is perhaps the one has attracted most scientists and researchers in this field and this includes several medical disciplines such as neurology, radiology, and gastroenterology as well as speech and language pathologists and therapists. Nowadays, it is well accepted that the dysphagia management process begins with an interdisciplinary assessment from which a treatment plan is designed and developed with the goal of minimizing the risk of aspiration, pneumonia, malnutrition, and dehydration.

However, knowing that dysphagia is a combination of symptoms affecting a person's ability to swallow, one may analyze dysphagia from another angle, which is from a fluid kinematics/dynamics point of view. This may be considered as the "dysphagia engineering point of view." Fluid kinematics deals with describing the motion of fluids without necessarily considering the forces and moments that cause the motion. Fluid kinematics describes velocity, acceleration, and visualization of fluid motion. On the other hand, fluid dynamics deals with the analysis of the specific forces necessary to produce the motion.

A kinematic/dynamic analysis of dysphagia aims to gain insight into the mechanisms of bolus and liquid flow during swallowing. Because rheology is the study of the deformation and flow of matter, the connection between the dysphagia world and rheology is clear.

The velocity spectrum of bolus flow in the pharynx and esophagus has been determined using different techniques. The "gold standard" videofluoroscopy is the technique that has been most frequently used. Other nonradiological techniques such as high-resolution manometry (Takasaki et al. 2008; Bredenoord and Smout 2008; Bardan et al. 2006) and intraluminal impedance (Omari et al. 2006) have also been used to generate bolus transit velocity data, followed by a swallowing kinematic analysis but with lower frequency. An ultrasonic pulse Doppler imaging method has recently been added to list (Hasegawa et al. 2005).

Regardless of the technique used for kinematic analysis of dysphagia, it is clear that the bolus transit time and thus the velocity is highly dependent on the patient's medical conditions and the rheological properties of the bolus.

A nonexhaustive literature review of kinematic analysis of dysphagia is given in Table 1. The purpose is to show how the bolus transit velocity changes depending on the swallowing phase and the rheological properties of the bolus. The results in Table 1 clearly suggest that the bolus transit velocity is considerably higher for the pharyngeal phase than for the esophageal phase. On the other hand, as the bolus viscosity increases, the bolus transit velocity decreases, as expected.

With use of some of the information given in Table 1, and under the assumption that bolus deformation only occurs in shear, an estimation of the shear rates that may be associated with swallowing was performed, and the results are shown in Table 2. As the results clearly suggest, bolus deformation (i.e., shear rate) during the swallowing process is greater for the pharyngeal phase than for the esophageal phase. In general, one may see that the shear rate spectrum for the whole swallowing process goes from 1 to 1,000 l/s. This is in line with previous estimations (Steele et al. 2003). Experimental values in vivo are not available owing to the complex and irregular oral geometry and the lack of reliable techniques. However, several authors have tried to estimate shear rates associated with the swallowing process. Nicosia and Robbins (2001) using a rheological approach based upon parallel plates to simulate the squeezing effect of a

food bolus from the oral cavity into the pharynx predicted shear rates of 180,000 and 3,000 s^{-1} for bolus viscosities of 1×10^{-3} and 1 Pa s, respectively. These values are very unlikely in reality. On the other hand, Meng et al. (2005) estimated a shear rate around 400 s^{-1} for water; this value may be more reasonable than those shown in Table 2.

Regardless of the progress achieved from rheological sciences applied to bolus properties and experimental in vivo kinematic studies, health professionals in charge of the dietary management of dysphagia have hardly integrated this information in their guidelines for diet modification. As an example, the only association using a viscosity dimension is the USA is the American Dietetic Association (National Dysphagia Diet Task Force), which proposed different bolus viscosity categories on the basis of viscosity values estimated at only one shear rate of 50 s^{-1}. More details are given in the next section.

A kinematic systematic study with well-defined bolus rheological properties is still not available in the literature. The reader should note that also elongational flows are involved in the deformation of a food bolus, as clearly seen from videofluoroscopy and real-time magnetic resonance imaging (Imam et al. 2005; Buettner et al. 2001). The shape of the deformed bolus is typical of the shapes produced under elongational stretching. This is in line with the fact that many boluses exhibit extensional properties (Ekberg et al. 2009; Chen 2009). Unfortunately, little attention has been given to the role of elongational flows and dysphagia. So far, viscous properties are the only considered in the dysphagia world and with still too many limitations.

Rheology and swallowing are also connected at the diagnosis level. The "gold standard" technique is a videofluoroscopic swallowing study (VFSS). The swallowing process can be visualized using videoradiography, either by using a ready-to-use commercial contrast medium or by mixing food with barium sulfate ($BaSO_4$), making it radiopaque. Unfortunately, there is no standardization for how to perform a VFSS. For example, in USA, it is common to use commercial ready-to-use contrast media, but this is not the case in Europe. This lack of standardization leads to variability in practice and results and encourages individual speech pathologists, dieticians, and dysphagic food manufacturers to determine their own dietary consistencies.

However, what it is more important to mention here is the fact and recognition that the rheological

Table 1 Kinematic analysis of dysphagia

Reference	Bolus transit velocity (cm/s)	Comments
Pharyngeal phase		
Nguyen et al. (1997)	37.1 ± 1.1	Bolus head traversing the pharyngeal region. Data from multiple intraluminal impedance
	28.3 ± 2.1	Bolus head velocity decreases as viscosity increases
	9.6 ± 1.0	Mean pharyngeal propulsion velocity of bolus body
William et al. (2001)	42	Bolus head entering the UES. Data from high-resolution manometry
Omari et al. (2006)	8.13[a]	Bolus tail estimated from MII and videofluoroscopy
Hasegawa et al. (2005)	50	Transit time of 1 s
Bardan et al. (2006)	37.6 ± 8.1	Bolus head traversing the pharyngeal region. Data from videofluoroscopy
	10.3 ± 3.0	Bolus tail average velocity as the bolus traversed the pharynx and passed through the UES
Esophageal phase		
Li et al. (1994)	1–4	Peristaltic wave velocities from videofluoroscopy—Kahrilas et al. (1988)
Nguyen et al. (1997)	9.6 ± 1.4	Head liquid bolus (low viscosity); subjects in supine position. Data from MII
	14.2 ± 2.2	Head liquid bolus (low viscosity); subjects in upright position
	6.3 ± 0.8	Head high-viscosity bolus (yogurt); subjects in supine position
	5.0 ± 0.4	Body liquid bolus (low viscosity); subjects in supine position
	5.2 ± 0.8	Body liquid bolus (low viscosity); subjects in upright position
	4.0 ± 0.2	Body high-viscosity bolus (yogurt); subjects in supine position
	4.1 ± 0.1	Tail liquid bolus (low viscosity); subjects in supine position
	4.7 ± 0.2	Tail liquid bolus (low viscosity); subjects in upright position
	4.1 ± 0.2	Tail High viscosity bolus (yogurt); subjects in supine position
Srinivasan et al. (2001)	2.9[b]	Estimation from BTTs for applesauce. Data from MII
Mizunuma et al. (2009)	8[c]	Head liquid bolus—estimations based on bolus transfer time from CFD for a jelly

MII multiple intraluminal impedance, *UES* upper esophageal sphincter, *BTT* bolus transfer time, *CFD* computational fluid dynamics

[a] BTT(tail) = 0.664 s; h = 5.4 cm

[b] BTT(average) = 6.24 s; h = 18 cm; v = 1–4 ml applesauce

[c] BTT(head) = 0.5 s; h = 4 cm up to the epiglottis

properties of the radiopaque bolus prepared by mixing contrast medium (e.g., barium sulfate, $BaSO_4$) with normal food. In other words, means that barium sulfate is added to normal food usually liquids and/or purees and the final mixture is radiopaque, are quite different from those of the normal food used as a vehicle for the VFSS. If the results from the VFSS are extrapolated to dietary recommendations using foods without added barium, there may be a severe problem.

Ekberg et al. (2009) found significant differences in the rheological properties of a model food versus the same food but mixed with $BaSO_4$. In addition, the sensory texture dimensions of this model food were significantly affected by the added barium. Ould-Eleya and Gunasekaran (2007) reported significant differences in the rheological properties of both prethickened and videofluoroscopy fluids currently used for diagnosis and treatment of dysphagia. Sopade et al. (2007) studied the rheological properties of typical food powder thickeners and proposed equations to prepare matching VFSS fluids and obtain objective classification of the thickened fluids. More recently, our group (Brito-de la Fuente et al. 2010, 2011) proposed a rheological similarity approach by closing the gap with the rheological properties of VFFS fluids for the design of oral nutritional supplements having complex formulations.

3.2 Rheology in Nutritional-Support-Product Design

Malnutrition and dehydration are quite often a consequence of dysphagia. Neurogenic dysphagia impairs swallowing and thus reduces oral feeding, leading to malnutrition and/or dehydration (Ickenstein 2011; Cabre et al. 2010). However, dysphagia remains mainly a transport problem that has to be solved first, before thinking of nutrition, in particular if the swallowing function should be stimulated. Ideally, if the two problems can be solved at once by transferring under safer conditions high-quality nutrient boluses, then the quality of life of dysphagic patients may significantly increase (Brito-de la Fuente et al. 2010).

The nutritional management of dysphagic patients is fundamentally based upon the so-called diet modification of texture or consistency. However, in the frame of the concepts presented in this chapter, it is clear that modification of texture or consistency means, in general, changes in the rheological properties of the diet. Assessment of consistency, quite often called "viscosity," still remains quite subjective in the dysphagia world. The preparation, assessment of consistency/viscosity, and administration of thickened drinks to patients is universally subjective, and unfortunately, health care professionals responsible for prescribing the patient's modified diet have shown poor or little knowledge of this field and thus the wide range of viscous properties for the same dysphagia level or recommendation (Steele and Cichero 2008; Steele et al. 2003)

The rationale behind altering or modifying the consistency of foods and/or drinks is to change the rate at which food is transported through the pharynx and thus to reduce the risk of patients aspirating food because of their diminished swallowing reflex. Ideally, the most appropriate modification of food consistencies should follow from a clear assessment of the swallowing problem, as reviewed by Penman and Thomson (1998). However, this is not possible in all

Table 2 Estimated swallowing shear rates from bolus transit velocities

Swallowing phase	Liquid bolus kinematics velocity, V^c (cm/s)	Estimated shear rate, γ^d (l/s)
Pharyngeal		
Bolus head (maximum)[a]	35.5	931.7
Bolus tail (average)[a]	10	262
Esophageal		
From BTT (BTT = 6.12 s)[b]	2.94	4.7

[a] Anatomy—data from Battagel et al. (2002)
[b] Data based on MII from Srinivasan et al. (2001)
[c] Kinematics—data from Bardan et al. (2006)
[d] From capillary and peristaltic flow equations

cases and quite often health care professionals rely on national guidelines for the dietary management of dysphagia.

For example, the National Dysphagia Diet Task Force (2002) of the American Dietetic Association proposed terms for liquids and other viscoelastic fluids using viscosity measurements at 25°C and a single shear rate of 50 l/s. No scientific evidence or rationale has been given by the National Dysphagia Diet Task Force for the temperature and shear rate chosen for this scale. In fact, on the basis of sensorial analysis from lingual perception viscosity, a wide range of shear rates ranging from 5 to 1,000 s^{-1} have been proposed, and a value of 50 s^{-1} is the most frequently cited, perhaps because this value was adopted by the National Dysphagia Diet Task Force. These conditions have been challenged recently by our research group and others (Brito-de la Fuente et al. 2010; Quinchia et al. 2011; O'Leary et al. 2010; Steele et al. 2003). As shown in Sect. 3.1, from bolus transit velocities, shear rates may range from 1 to 1,000 l/s depending on the swallowing phase (see Table 2).

Moreover, in the UK, the British Dietetic Association (2009) recently reissued its *National Descriptors for Texture Modification in Adults* using again subjective descriptors from sensorial analysis. Quantitative measurement of viscosity is acknowledged to be presently impractical according to the British Dietetic Association and thus it is not performed by health care professional or others. This practice remains at all levels in hospitals and nursing home

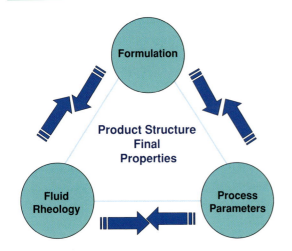

Fig. 7 Dynamic triad strategy for the design of oral nutritional supplements with rheological similarity to swallow barium test feeds

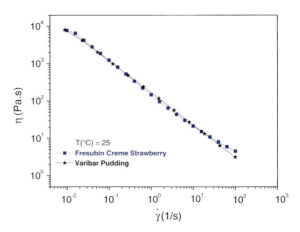

Fig. 8 Steady-shear viscosity curves for Varibar® pudding and Fresubin® crème

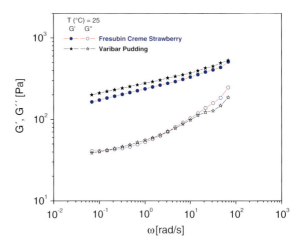

Fig. 9 Viscoelastic properties for Varibar® pudding and Fresubin® crème under dynamic linear oscillatory conditions

care settings, in spite of all the scientific evidence regarding the complex rheological properties (i.e., non-Newtonian behavior and thus shear-dependent viscosity) of different boluses found during swallowing (Quinchia et al. 2011; Ekberg et al. 2009; Steele and Cichero 2008; Germain et al. 2006; Clavé et al. 2006; Bülow et al. 2003) and the clinical evidence suggesting that the pharyngeal swallowing phase occurs at different bolus transit velocities and thus shear rates as shown in Sect. 3.1.

In summary, one of the major challenges confronting the dietary management of dysphagia is product consistency or more generally product rheological properties. This leads to the still fundamental question: is it possible to design better products for the dietary management of dysphagia under safety conditions? One answer to this question may be the design of nutritional products that are ready to swallow by following a rheological similarity approach; this means by matching the rheological properties of the fluids used for the diagnosis (e.g., swallow barium test feeds used in videofluoroscopy examination) with those of the bolus.

Brito-de la Fuente et al. (2010) have proposed a dynamic triad strategy for closing the gap between the rheological properties of the swallow barium test feeds and the ready-to-use product being designed (see Fig. 7). This strategy has been applied quite successfully in the design and commercial production of complex-structure oral nutritional supplements rich

in proteins with a pudding consistency (e.g., Fresubin® crème). The benchmark used for this design was the "gold standard" barium-based E-Z-EM product Varibar® pudding. The main rheological results of this exercise are described next.

Regarding viscous properties, Fresubin® crème showed shear-thinning behavior, i.e., a viscosity-decreasing function of the shear rate, matching the results for Varibar® pudding as seen in Fig. 8. Regarding viscoelastic properties, the G' values clearly confirm the gel-like behavior of both products, which means they are structured systems. For both products, the dynamic rheological properties can be considered to be essentially similar, as seen in Fig. 9.

These results suggest that it is possible to design oral nutritional supplements that exhibit rheological properties similar to those of $BaSO_4$ suspensions used for diagnosis of dysphagia. A complete rheological characterization of the final oral nutritional supplement was published elsewhere (Quinchia et al. 2011).

In a more recent publication, Brito-de la Fuente et al. (2011) describes an in-depth rheological characterization of prethickened foods and videofluoroscopy diagnostic fluids, showing the important role that rheology plays in the diagnosis and dietary management of dysphagia.

4 Conclusions

Dysphagia and rheology are closed interconnected. Regardless of the experimental technique used for the assessment of dysphagia, bolus flow properties play an important role to guarantee higher levels of safe swallowing.

Kinematic analysis of more dysphagic patients is needed to better understand how boluses with different rheological properties are transferred in different neurological or medical conditions. New techniques such as computational fluid dynamics applied to complex swallowing situations may be of high value for prediagnosis and diagnosis as well as an educational tool to increase the compliance patients under diet-modification programs.

The creation or design of novel foods for dietary management of dysphagia or the improvement of existing ones depends on a better understanding of the complex interrelationship between food structure and performance. More sophisticated experimental techniques coming from material sciences such as rheology play an important role in the design and development of new products for management of dysphagia. On the other hand, a better understanding of the flow properties of the fluids used for the videofluoroscopic assessment of dysphagia and later the recommendation of specific diets should be of high priority in the dysphagia world. Even though this knowledge is now being used to rationally design safer dysphagia products, this approach should be extended to different consistencies and nutritional profiles.

Finally, the incorporation of more knowledge on the role rheological properties play during swallowing is crucial for proper management of dysphagia.

References

Bardan E, Kern M, Arndorfer RC, Hofmann C, Shaker R (2006) Effect of aging on bolus kinematics during the pharyngeal phase of swallowing. Am J Physiol Gastrointest Liver Physiol 290:G458–G465

Barnes HA (2000) A handbook of elementary rheology. Institute of Non-Newtonian Fluid Mechanics, University of Wales, Aberystwyth

Battagel J, Johal A, Smith AM, Kotecha B (2002) Postural variations in oropharyngeal dimensions in subjects with sleep disordered breathing—a cephalometric study. Eur J Orthodont 24:263–276

Bird RB, Armstrong RC, Hassager O (1987) Dynamics of polymeric liquids: fluid dynamics, vol 1, 2nd edn. Wiley, New York

Bredenoord AJ, Smout AJPM (2008) High resolution manometry. Digest Liver Dis 40:174–181

British Dietetic Association (2009) National descriptors for texture modification in adults. British Dietetic Association, Birmingham

Brito-de la Fuente E, Quinchia L, Valencia C, Partal P, Franco JM, Gallegos C (2010) Rheology of a new spoon-thick consistency oral nutritional supplement (ONS) in comparison with a swallow barium test feed (SBTF). In: Proceedings Dysphagia Research Society 18th annual meeting, San Diego, CA, USA, 4–6 March 2010

Brito-de la Fuente E, Staudinger-Prevost N, Quinchia L, Valencia C, Partal P, Franco JM, Gallegos C (2011) Design of a new spoon-thick consistency oral nutrition supplement (ONS) using rheological similarity with a swallow barium test feed (SBTF) (Submitted to Dysphagia)

Buettner A, Beer A, Hannig C, Settles M (2001) Observation of the swallowing process by applications of videfluoroscopy and real time magnetic resonance imaging-consequences for retronasal aroma stimulation. Chem Sens 26:1211–1219

Bülow M, Olsson R, Ekberg O (2003) Videoradiographic analysis of how carbonated thin liquids and thickened liquids affect the physiology of swallowing in subject with aspiration on thin liquids. Acta Radiol 44:366–372

Cabre M, Serra-Prat M, Palomera E, Almirall J, Pallares R, Clavé P (2010) Prevalence and prognostic implications of dysphagia in elderly patients with pneumonia. Age Ageing 39(1):39–45

Carreau PJ (1972) Rheological equations from molecular network theories. Trans Soc Rheol 16:99–127

Carreau PJ, Dekee D, Chhabra RP (1997) Rheology of polymeric systems: principles and applications. Hanser, Munich

Chen J (2009) Food oral processing—a review. Food Hydrocolloids 23:1–25

Chhabra RP, Richardson JF (1999) Non-Newtonian flow in the process industries. Butterworth-Heinemann, Oxford

Clavé P, De Kraa M, Arreola V, Girvent M, Farré R, Palomera E, Serrat-Pratt M (2006) The effect of bolus viscosity on swallowing function in neurogénica dysphagia. Aliment Pharmacol Ther 24:1385–1394

Dealy JM, Wissbrun KF (1995) Melt rheology and its role in plastic processing. Chapman and Hall, London

Ekberg O, Bülow M, Ekman S, Hall G, Stading M, Wendin K (2009) Effect of barium sulfate contrast medium on rheology and sensory texture attributes in a model food. Acta Radiologica 2:131–138

Emri I (2010) Time-dependent behaviour of solid polymers. In: Gallegos C, Walters K (eds) Rheology: encyclopaedia of life support systems (EOLSS), UNESCO. Eolss, Oxford, pp 247–330

Ferry JD (1980) Viscoelastic properties of polymers. Wiley, New York

Gallegos C, Martínez-Boza FJ (2010) Linear viscoelasticity. In: Gallegos C, Walters K (eds) Rheology: encyclopaedia of life support systems (EOLSS), UNESCO. Eolss, Oxford, pp 120–143

Gallegos C, Walters K (2010) Rheology. In: Gallegos C, Walters K (eds) Rheology: encyclopaedia of life support systems (EOLSS), UNESCO. Eolss, Oxford, pp 1–14

Germain I, Dufresne T, Ramaswamy HS (2006) Rheological characterization of thickened beverages used in the treatment of dysphagia. J Food Eng 73:64–74

Hasegawa A, Otogure A, Kumagai H, Nakazawa F (2005) Velocity of swallowed gel food in the pharynx by ultrasonic method. J Jpn Soc Food Sci Technol 52:441–447

Ickenstein GW (2011) Diagnosis, treatment of neurogenic dysphagia. UNI-MED, Bremen

Imam H, Shay S, Ali A, Baker M (2005) Bolus transit patterns in healthy subjects: a study using simultaneous impedance monitoring, videoesophagram, and esophageal manometry. Am J Physiol Gastrointest Liver Physiol 288:G1000–G1006

Kahrilas PJ, Dodds WJ, Hogan WJ (1988) Effect of peristaltic dysfunction on esophageal volume clearance. Gastroenterology 94:73–80

Li M, Brasseur JG, Doods W (1994) Analyses of normal and abnormal esophageal transport using computer simulations. Am J Physiol Gastrointest Liver Physiol 266:G525–G543

Mackley MR, Marshall RTJ, Smeulders JB, Zhao FD (1994) The rheological characterization of polymeric and colloidal fluids. Chem Eng Sci 49:2551–2565

Macosko CW (1994) Rheology principles, measurements and applications. VCH, New York

Madiedo JM, Gallegos C (1997a) Rheological characterization of oil-in-water emulsions by means of relaxation and retardation spectra. Recent Res Devel Oil Chem 1:79–90

Madiedo JM, Gallegos C (1997b) Rheological characterization of oil-in-water food emulsions by means of relaxation and retardation spectra. Appl Rheol 7:161–167

Meng Y, Rao MA, Datta AK (2005) Computer simulation of the pharyngeal bolus transport of Newtonian and non-Newtonian fluids. Trans Inst Chem Eng Part C 83:297–305

Mizunuma H, Sonomura M, Shimokasa K, Ogoshp H, Nakamura S, Tayama N (2009) Numerical modelling and simulation on the swallowing of jelly. J Text Stud 40:406–426

National Dysphagia Diet Task Force (2002) National dysphagia diet: standardization for optimal care. American Dietetic Association, Chicago

Nguyen HN, Silny J, Albers D, Roeb E, Gartung C, Rau G, Metern S (1997) Dynamics of esophageal bolus transport in heathy subjects studied using multiple intraluminal impedancometry. Am J Physiol Gastrointest Liver Physiol 273:G958–G964

Nicosia MA, Robbins J (2001) The fluid mechanics of bolus ejection from the oral cavity. J Biomech 34:1537–1544

O'Leary M, Hanson B, Smith C (2010) Viscosity and non-Newtonian features of thickened fluids used for dysphagia therapy. J Food Sci 75(6):E330–E338

Omari TI, Rommel N, Szczesniak M, Fuentealba S, Dinning P, Davidson G, Cook I (2006) Assessment of intraluminal impedance for the detection of pharyngeal bolus flow during swallowing in healthy adults. Am J Physiol Gastrointest Liver Physiol 290:G183–G188

Ould-Eleya M, Gunasekaran S (2007) Rheology of barium sulfate suspensions and pre-thickened beverages used in diagnosis and treatment of dysphagia. Appl Rheol 17: 33137-1–33137-8

Partal P, Franco JM (2010) Non-Newtonian fluids. In: Gallegos C, Walters K (eds) Rheology: encyclopaedia of life support systems (EOLSS), UNESCO. Eolss, Oxford, pp 96–119

Penman JP, Thomson M (1998) A review of the textured diets developed for the management of dysphagia. J Hum Nutr Diet 11:51–60

Quinchia LA, Valencia C, Partal P, Franco JM, Brito-de la Fuente E, Gallegos C (2011) Linear and non-linear viscoelasticity of puddings for nutritional management of dysphagia. Food Hydrocolloids 25:586–593

Reiner M (1964) The Deborah number. Phys Today 17:62

Rolón-Garrido V, Wagner M (2009) The damping function in rheology. Rheol Acta 48:245–284

Sopade PA, Halley PJ, Cichero JAY, Ward LC (2007) Rheological characterisation of food thickeners marketed in Australia in various media for the management of dysphagia I: water and cordial. J Food Eng 79:69–82

Srinivasan R, Vela MF, Kartz PO, Tutuian R, Castell JA, Castell DO (2001) Esophageal function testing using multichannel intraluminal impedance. Am J Physiol Gastrointest Liver Physiol 280:G457–G462

Steele C, Cichero JA (2008) A question of rheological control. Dysphagia 23:199–201

Steele CM, Lieshout PHHM, Goff HD (2003) The rheology of liquids: a comparison of clinician's subjective impression and objective measurement. Dysphagia 18:182–195

Takasaki K, Umeki H, Enatsu K, Tanaka F, Sakihama N, Kumagami H, Takahashi H (2008) Investigation of pharyngeal swallowing function using high-resolution manometry. Laryngoscope 118(10):1729–1732

Wagner MH (1979) Zur Netzwerktheorie von Polymer-Schmelzen. Rheol Acta 18:33–50

Walters K (2010) History of rheology. In: Gallegos C, Walters K (eds) Rheology: encyclopaedia of life support systems (EOLSS), UNESCO. Eolss, Oxford, pp 15–30

Williams RB, Pal A, Brasseur G, Cook I (2001) Space-time pressure structure of pharyngo–esophageal segment during swallowing. Am J Physiol Gastrointest Liver Physiol 281:G1290–G1300

The Dietitian's Role in Diagnosis and Treatment of Dysphagia

S. Burton, A. Laverty, and M. Macleod

Contents

Abstract

This chapter aims to provide an overview of the registered dietitian's role and the commonplace feeding dilemmas presented at the practical level when applying the modified textured prescription for food and fluids in adults with dysphagia. The dietitian is one of a range of professionals involved in service provision, and there is an increased emphasis on an interdisciplinary and transdisciplinary team approach to care for people with dysphagia at both the acute and the community level. The role of the dietitian can be wide-ranging, from traditional nutritional management to a whole-systems approach encompassing screening, assessment, diagnosis and organisation of the modified textures within a dynamic nutritional framework. A person-centred approach is essential to provide nutrition in a mode which not only sustains nutrition and hydration integrity but also serves to enhance the individual's quality of life.

1 Introduction

The ideal approach to the management of dysphagia involves a multidisciplinary team (MDT) (Kemp 2001). The registered dietitian is an integral member of this team and fundamental to service provision in both the acute and the community setting (Heiss et al. 2010). The knowledge, skills and role of the registered dietitian within dysphagia include:

- Advising on nutritional requirements to minimise nutritional deterioration, including dehydration and

S. Burton · A. Laverty · M. Macleod (✉)
Abteilung Neurologie, m&i-Fachklinik Bad Heilbrunn,
Wörnerweg 30, 83670, Bad Heilbrunn, Germany
e-mail: marjorymacleod1950@yahoo.co.uk

O. Ekberg (ed.), *Dysphagia*, Medical Radiology. Diagnostic Imaging, DOI: 10.1007/174_2011_346,
© Springer-Verlag Berlin Heidelberg 2012

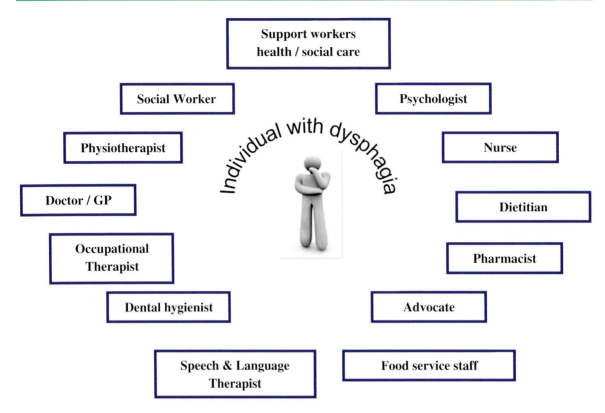

Fig. 1 Members of the multidisciplinary team (MDT) for dysphagia. (Adapted from Copeman and Hyland 2007)

different administration modalities such as oral, enteral and parenteral.

- Having the knowledge and experience to interpret height, weight and anthropometric measurements when assessing nutritional status.
- Using a holistic approach to assess, problem-solve and ensure that health and well-being needs are met.
- Using appropriate health facilitation skills within the therapeutic framework.
- Contributing to the application of a legal framework.
- Identifying, referring and working in partnership with health and social care colleagues, agencies and organisations.
- Addressing inequalities in health and social care.
- Advocating both formally and informally.
- Supporting individuals[1] and carers in decision-making.
- Educating the individual, carers and other members of the dysphagia team.

-----

[1]   As dysphagia is managed in both the acute and the community health (and social) care settings, the term 'individual' is used within the text to represent patient, client and service user.

- Using augmented/alternative communication for those with acquired and non-acquired cognitive impairments.
- Working in dynamic environments with individuals who may display unpredictable behaviours that present a challenge.
- Ensuring continuity of care across professional and organisational boundaries.

Membership of a typical MDT is shown in Fig. 1, with the individual with dysphagia being pivotal in assessment and all management decisions. A brief summary of roles is shown in Table 1.

Although the terms 'multidisciplinary' and 'interdisciplinary' are often used interchangeably, there is an important difference in function. The interdisciplinary team model expands the MDT process where collaboration (rather than just sharing information on uni-professional interventions) in setting team goals and team action plans results in more effective management (Dyer 2003). As so many disciplines are involved in the assessment and treatment of dysphagia, collaborative working within the MDT is essential to provide coordinated evidence-based and safe

Table 1 Roles of each member of the dysphagia multidisciplinary team (MDT). (Adapted from Copeman and Hyland 2007)

Member	Role
Individual with dysphagia and their carers	Participate in assessment, treatment and management decision-making where possible
	Inform MDT of any problems adhering to guidelines
	Inform MDT of any changes in clinical presentation
Advocate	Represents the individual's views, interests and rights
	Participates fully in decisions made about the individual's life
Clinical psychologist	Assessment, treatment and management of socio-emotional, behavioural and psychological aspects of dysphagia
Catering staff/carers in community settings	Adheres to eating and drinking guidelines
	Provision of attractive, nutritious and suitably fortified foods
	Provision of food and fluids of suitable consistency
	Provision of adequate amounts of food and fluid as required
Dietitian	Initial screening, assessment and diagnosis (*where trained*)
	Close liaison with speech and language therapist
	Assessment, treatment and management of nutrition and hydration
	Assessment of need for supplements and monitoring efficacy
	Assisted eating and drinking training
	Together with speech and language therapist supports decision-making in relation to artificial feeding
Physician/GP	Referral to relevant other professionals if dysphagia is suspected
	Medical investigation into the cause of dysphagia and treatments if required
	Prescribes medication in suitable presentations
Nurse	Initial screening (*where trained*)
	Implementation of dysphagia/feeding advice
	Monitors food and fluid intake as appropriate
	Liaison with dietitian and speech and language therapist
	Administers medication in the correct format
Occupational therapist	Assessment and management of the impact of physical and environmental factors
	Advice regarding adaptive equipment, technical skills and positioning at mealtimes
	Assisted eating and drinking training
Pharmacist	Advice on availability of medication in suitable presentations
	Checks side effects of medications in relation to dysphagic properties
	Advice on drug–nutrient interactions
Physiotherapist	Assessment, treatment and management of the respiratory system
	Advice on positioning when eating and drinking, including head control management
	Assisted eating and drinking training
Social worker	Assess, advise and coordinate a suitable care package for home in liaison with other professionals
Speech and language therapist	Assessment, diagnosis and monitoring of swallowing problems
	Advice on compensatory strategies
	Close liaison with dietitian
	Assisted eating and drinking training
	Together with dietitian supports decision-making in relation to artificial feeding

(continued)

Table 1 (continued)

Member	Role
Support workers in health/social care	Assistance with choosing appropriate foods and fluids
	Follows feeding guidelines in place such as correct environment, suitable posture, assisted eating

These roles are not exhaustive. All may be involved in risk assessment; MDT training, and best interests decision-making

person-centred care (National Patient Safety Agency 2007; Nazarko 2009).

In some areas, as a matter of necessity, such as a lack of skilled dysphagia therapists, pressure of response times within clinical pathways or professional development within extended roles of practice, the management of dysphagia is moving from the role-specific professions within an MDT framework to a transdisciplinary approach in practice where disciplines undertake similar and complementary roles (Butt and Lam 2005). Members of a team based on a transdisciplinary model share knowledge, skills and responsibilities, thus blurring traditional boundaries between the professions and enabling the delivery of effective and timely person-centred care (Dyer 2003).

2   Role in Diagnosis

2.1   Screening

The aim of screening is to inform and guide the safest management (Perry and Love 2001). During a routine nutritional assessment, the dietitian is in an ideal situation to observe potential signs and symptoms of dysphagia, especially in people who do not present with an overt neurological condition such as cerebrovascular accident, cerebral palsy, or motor neuron disease or a mechanical cause such as oesophageal stricture, injury or carcinoma. Insidious onset with symptoms such as unexpected weight loss, taking longer to eat and drink, and becoming increasingly selective with food choices can be missed or not seen as important by carers or indeed the person herself/ himself. Indices of malnutrition such as reduced serum levels of transferrin and albumin have been found to be present in people with severe dysphagia, although a statistically significant relationship has not been found (Brody et al. 2000). Biochemical and haematological data, however, could be additional

triggers for a detailed assessment to be undertaken following an initial screen. Thus, for individuals exhibiting signs of dysphagia, assessment and treatment can be conducted in a timely manner to avoid inappropriate feeding or long periods of starvation which could lead to malnutrition and/or refeeding syndrome (Davies 2002; Mehanna et al. 2009).

2.2   Assessment

Traditionally, it was the unique province of the speech and language therapist (SLT) to assess swallow and that of the dietitian to advise on how to meet nutritional needs within the textures allowed. Countries such as the USA and Canada have documented evidence which indicates that with appropriate training to enhance existing knowledge and skills, dietitians could be as proficient as SLTs at conducting swallowing assessments and making recommendations on suitable textures (Brody et al. 2000; Butt and Lam 2005). Within the UK, dietitians undertake dysphagia assessments in some stroke units, and according to the outcomes of the 2008 International Confederation of Dietetic Associations education and work survey (ICDA 2008), dietitians practising in other countries also fulfil this role, which includes the prescribing of modified foods and fluids. Close working with the SLT trained in dysphagia is essential, especially in more complex cases where instrumental assessment is required, such as the gold standard modified barium swallow or videofluoroscopy.

3   Role in Nutritional Management

This is the long-established role of the dietitian, who is lead professional in the assessment and treatment of malnutrition and dehydration (Crawford 2009). Individuals with dypshagia must be frequently monitored as their needs may constantly change. At all stages in the progression of dysphagia the dietitian should be consulted to ensure nutritional requirements are tailored to meet the individual's needs. Factors which need to be considered before making the initial and subsequent nutritional recommendations are highlighted as follows:

3.1 Nutrition

Hospitalised and institutionalised individuals on texture-modification regimens have suboptimal fluid, energy and protein intakes (Whelan 2001; Nowson et al. 2003; Wright et al. 2005). In addition, clinical practice reveals deficits in a range of macronutrients and micronutrients, requiring supplementation in both acute and community care. Nutritional intake has been shown to improve with targeted feeding assistance (Wright et al. 2008), although there are many other factors which have an effect on achieving adequate nutrition. These include the quality of food preparation and presentation and more person-specific influences such as the psychological burden of being unable to swallow without coughing, being unable to clear foods and fluids from the mouth and an inability to manage salivation. All these need to be taken into account when devising an individualised eating and drinking programme (Nazarko 2007).

In a qualitative study by Ekberg et al. (2002) less than half of the participants who experienced dysphagia-related symptoms found that eating was a pleasurable experience. Alarmingly, over 50% reported eating less, with 44% reporting weight loss and one third being still hungry and thirsty after their meals. Food that is not eaten is not nutritious whatever the merits of its nutritive constituents. Nutrition is much more than calculating an individual's requirements for nutrients and meeting recommendations. The art and skill of the dietitian lies in translating scientific evidence into practical solutions which must be fit for purpose, using a holistic and person-centred approach.

If consumption does not provide the nutrition required to match individual requirements, then either food enrichment which will increase nutrient density without increasing volume, or the prescription of oral nutritional supplements may be needed, and the adequacy of such measures will need close monitoring (Burton et al. 2009; Copeman and Hyland 2007;

National Institute for Health and Clinical Excellence 2006; Elia et al. 2005). The dietitian will recommend and monitor the usage of any specific oral nutritional supplements needed by the individual which will address their nutritional needs, taking into account taste and preparation preferences (Nazarko 2009). Nutritional management and treatment of dysphagia is further complicated by cognitive decline and the end-of-life pathway where any decision to commence enteral tube feeding should be carefully balanced against the individual's known wishes and impact on his/her quality of life (White et al. 2008).

It must be remembered that nasogastric or gastrostomy feeding does not significantly reduce aspiration risk even though such means of artificial nutrition can rectify any nutritional and hydration deficits. As Brotherton et al. (2006) demonstrated in their qualitative study of adults with a gastrostomy tube in situ, there are both positive and negative aspects to enteral tube feeding. Gastrostomy feeding may reduce the stress associated with mealtimes but results in a reduced quality of life by missed opportunities for social eating, disruptive sleep patterns and stoma site infections.

There is also a risk of rapid and undesired weight gain as standard energy predictive equations such as the Schofield and the Harris–Benedict equations overestimate energy requirements for some groups, such as people with profound and multiple physical and learning disabilities (Dickerson et al. 1999; Fairclough et al. 2008) and those with low resting energy expenditure due to hypothermia (Gervasio et al. 1997; Dickerson et al. 2003). The Parenteral and Enteral Nutrition Group recommends using the Schofield equation in the UK (Todorovic and Micklewright 2007). Whichever formula is used by clinicians, such equations and stress factors act primarily as an objective starting point for estimating energy and protein requirements.

Normal swallow requires well-coordinated timing of sensory and motor mechanisms to safely transport boluses of food. In individuals who have dysphagia, these processes may no longer work effectively and the need for texture modification is indicated to assist safety in moving foods (and liquids) from the oral cavity.

Currently there is no universal standard texture guidance to support the management of dysphagia. A recent review of the literature undertaken by the

Table 2 Texture descriptors of foods. (Reproduced with kind permission from Guntrum Ickenstein)

ASHA/ADA (2002) USA	SPA/DAA (2007) Australia	NPSA/RCSLT/BDA/NNG/HCA (2011) UK	IASLT/Irish Nutrition and Dietetic Institute (2009) Ireland
TMD level 3: advanced (soft foods that require more chewing ability)	Texture A: soft	Texture E: fork-mashable dysphagia diet; soft moist food needs some chewing	Texture A: soft
TMD level 2: mechanically altered (cohesive, moist, semisolid foods, requiring some chewing)	Texture B: minced and moist	Texture D: pre-mashed dysphagia diet food that is soft, tender and moist; needs very little chewing	Texture B: minced and moist
TMD level 1: pureed (homogenous, very cohesive, pudding-like, requiring very little chewing ability)	Texture C: smooth pureed	Texture C: thick puree dysphagia diet: smooth, uniform, does not require chewing	Texture C: smooth pureed
		Texture B: thin puree dysphagia diet; smooth, uniform, does not require chewing	Texture D: liquidised

ASHA American Speech Language Hearing Association, *ADA* American Dietetic Association, *SPA* Speech Pathology Australia, *DAA* Dietitians Association Australia, *NPSA* National Patient Safety Agency, *RCSLT* Royal College of Speech and Language Therapists, *BDA* British Dietetic Association, *NNG* National Nurses Nutrition Group, *HCA* Hospital Caterers Association, *IASLT* Irish Association of Speech and Language Therapists, *TMD* texture-modified diet

authors in preparation for this chapter revealed the availability of guidance documents produced by four countries (namely Australia, Ireland, the USA and the UK) (Table 2). All have the common aim of improving communication and enabling a more consistent approach to patient care (Atherton et al. 2007; Irish Nutrition and Dietetic Institute 2009; National Dysphagia Diet Task Force 2002; NPSA Dysphagia Expert Reference Group 2011). These documents were developed jointly by the SLTs and dietitians within these countries.

As shown in Fig. 2, the US and UK guidelines are similar in that they start with the least modified food texture and go through to the most modified, whereas the Australian and Irish guidelines are the reverse. Perhaps the first step in developing a universal system would be to have the trajectory of all descriptors, whether using a numerical or an alphabetical nomenclature, starting from the normal texture and running forward to the most modified.

In clinical practice, individuals who maintain the oral route seem to have fewer reflux problems than those who are nil by mouth. Nutrition and hydration therefore need to be supported for as long as possible by establishing a safe and effective eating environment, using texture modification and the judicious addition of supplements. In severe dysphagia and/or severe malnutrition, the dietitian and the SLT work together to support the individual and carers in the decision-making process, where the transition from an inadequate and unsafe oral route to the enteral feeding route is clinically recommended. Where the individual is unable to participate in the decision-making process and consent to treatment, best interests decisions should be made by the whole MDT.

3.2 Hydration

Healthy adults manage hydration through thirst. Individuals who have dysphagia may lack the ability to recognise thirst or may experience problems with swallowing normal fluids. Adequate hydration is essential for life and as there is no easy non-invasive method of monitoring hydration, the dietitian should consider fluid requirements when advising on dysphagia diets (Penman and Thomson 2008). Many of these individuals may have significant fluid loss due to poor oral control, ineffective management of salivation (drooling) or aspirating. It has been estimated that 1.5 l of parotid saliva is produced per day, with electrolyte losses of 169 mmol sodium and 28.5 mmol potassium (Lee 1974).

Country	Least modified foods	Most modified foods	Date of guidance doc.
USA	3	1	2002
UK	E	B	2011
Australia	A	C	2007
Ireland	A	D	2009

Fig. 2 Trajectory of food modification. (Reproduced with kind permission from Guntrum Ickenstein)

There is no scientific method to calculate fluid loss from drooling as each individual will produce different amounts of saliva and have different volumes of loss, depending on the ability to achieve mouth closure. One novel way of estimating these losses would be to weigh the towels or absorbent cloths (often used by individuals and carers to protect their clothing from getting wet), then reweigh them but keeping wet towels in a plastic bag to reduce evaporation. Fluid losses need to be replaced as part of day-to-day fluid requirements.

Traditionally, fluid requirements for adults are based on age and weight, so for an adult under 65 years the fluid requirement is 35 ml/kg; for adults over 65 years this is reduced to 30 ml/kg in a temperate climate (Todorovic and Micklewright 2007). Again, as there is no scientific method to calculate fluid loss from poor mouth seal, the 'towel method' as detailed above could be utilised. The individual could be given a known volume of fluid without food. On completion of the drink, the towel/cloth is reweighed, providing the practitioner with an estimate of fluid lost. This can be repeated on several occasions and at different times of the day. In clinical experience, the fluid lost could be as great as 50% of the fluid offered. This volume would also have some saliva present, but can give some observational information to inform judgement on fluid requirements or the ability to meet needs orally.

Modified or thickened fluids are often recommended as a management strategy by dietitians and SLTs (Butt and Lam 2005; Garcia et al. 2005). The effectiveness of using modified fluids has long been recognised (Khlemeier et al. 2001; Bhattacharyya et al. 2003; Clave et al. 2006; Logemann 2008; Robbins et al. 2008).

The dietitian and SLT will work closely with individuals who are at risk of ingesting thin fluids. They will advise the individual on all suitable drinks whilst taking into account personal preferences. A full dietary assessment will enable fluid from food sources to be calculated. The remainder of the fluid requirements would be only safely achievable with modified fluids or by parenteral or enteral feeding or with subcutaneous fluids . The dietitian will always work with the least restrictive option, as exclusions of food and drink would reduce the individual's quality of life (Ekberg et al. 2002).

The issue of thickened fluids in the management of dysphagia is complex. There is a need for universal standard thickness definitions. Typical descriptors are thin, nectar and honey (Table 3); however, these are subjective terms, which may lead to wide variations in the consistency of the modified fluid.

Evidence suggests that achieving appropriate consistency using subjective measures is not reliable, as commercial thickeners have different properties depending whether they are primarily starch-based or gum-based (Goulding and Bakheit 2000; Garcia and Chambers 2010; Garcia et al. 2010). In Queensland, a protocol has been produced with detailed information on methods of mixing and ways of assessing textures for the various commercial thickeners. This is an extremely useful resource and shows the different mixing preparatory processes needed for starch- and gum-based products (Queensland Health Dietitians 2007).

Table 3 Texture descriptors of fluids. (Reproduced with kind permission from Guntrum Ickenstein)

ASHA/ADA (2002) USA	SPA/DAA (2007) Australia	RCSLT/British Dietetic Association (2002) UK	IASLT/Irish Nutrition and Dietetic Institute (2009) Ireland
Nectar-like	Mildly thick	Naturally thick fluid	Grade 1: very mildly thick
Honey-like	Moderately thick	Stage 1: syrup	Grade 2: mildly thick
Spoon-thick	Extremely thick	Stage 2: custard	Grade 3: moderately thick
		Stage 3: pudding	Grade 4: extremely thick

Table 4 Properties of thickeners.

Starch-based thickeners	Gum-based thickeners
Particles expand like a balloon capturing the fluid, which means they often tend to keep on absorbing fluid and getting thicker. Affected by refrigeration. May continue to thicken over time	Interact with liquid by forming 'nets' that trap liquid. Require careful preparation and must be vigorously shaken or blended with base fluid, otherwise mixed consistency may result. If mixed correctly, they will maintain relatively stable viscosity over time
Can be added to hot or cold drinks	Hot liquids may need to be cooled then reheated
Less effective water binding than gum	Excellent water-binding properties
More prone to chemical reactions with base fluids, e.g. pulp, thickness, acid content	More stable, less likely to react to base fluid, although some drinks such as adult nutritional beverages contain ingredients that may interact and form clumps
Sensory perceptions: tendency to impart a starch grainy texture to fluids, enhanced flavour	Sensory perceptions: tendency to impart a slick flavour or texture, enhanced flavour
Metabolism and water absorption in the small intestine	Metabolism and water absorption in the large intestine

Amylase-resistant thickeners based on guar gum/guar gum starch combinations have been put forward as being beneficial for individuals who hypersalivate, although recent research questions this evidence (Hanson et al. 2011). From a pragmatic point of view, the best thickener to use will be that preferred by the person who has to ingest it day after day, as any scientific rationale proved or disputed should not override individual preference for taste, and achieving that elusive characteristic—consistent consistency. The dietitian will be able to advise a change in prescription as necessary, especially if an individual reports changes in gut function after the introduction of thickeners. Sensory characteristics of drinks (and foods) may be enhanced with thickeners (Longton et al. 2003; Matta et al. 2006; Pelletier 1997), which may contribute to non-compliance (Table 4).

Garcia et al. (2010) found that most health care providers were unable to consistently prepare modified liquids. Seventy-five percent could not prepare a honey texture and 31% could not replicate a syrup consistency despite following the manufacturers' instructions. In the UK, a small study has produced and tested a texture indicator model. This consists of four plastic tubes containing fluids of different viscosities aligned to the UK national descriptors. The tubes when inverted allow the fluid to flow from one compartment to the next, giving a visual indication of each texture (Anderson 2008).

The addition of thickener in fluids may lead to an increase in energy intake, resulting in weight gain, which may or may not be advantageous. The dietitian should consider the implications of the additional energy component, impact on weight and which thickener to use as the energy content of thickeners may differ. The dietitian should consider carefully the complex factors on a case-by-case basis to ensure that the individual receives hydration. It is essential that the dietitian calculates the volume of fluid and also the quantity of thickener required to inform and generate accurate medical prescriptions.

Just because thickened fluids reduce the risk of aspiration, this does not always result in adequate hydration (Finestone et al. 2001; Vivanti et al. 2009). A study by Whelan (2001) noted that individuals receiving prethickened drinks drank 100% more than those given drinks thickened with powdered thickeners. Variables such as temperature, rate of mixing, method of mixing and the base properties of the drink to be thickened all have an impact on the resultant texture. Timing is also a key consideration, especially for individuals who are slow to drink, with the product continuing to thicken in the cup (Garcia et al. 2008).

There is evidence to suggest that 'free' water may be an acceptable treatment option for individuals who have been assessed as requiring modified fluids (Panther 2005). The Frazier free water protocol has been developed by a unit in Canada, and allows individuals who have been identified at risk from thin liquids to drink plain water between meals. The authors theorise that if plain water is aspirated, then it is less likely to create pneumonia as the lungs have high moisture content and therefore have an ability to handle fluid. The safety of allowing patients to consume 'free' water is constantly an area of great debate. Where an individual has capacity and is unwilling to comply with thickened fluids, free water may be the safest acceptable oral option. Aspiration of saliva contaminated with pathogens can lead to pulmonary infection and so adherence to aggressive oral and dental care is essential especially where individuals are unable to clean their own teeth and gums (Panther 2005).

As far as possible, nutrition and hydration is provided orally. When careful feeding, hydration and adherence to recommendations do not result in a safe swallow and prevention of recurrent aspiration and malnutrition, then alternative and more aggressive routes of administration need to be explored with the individual and her/his carers (Stewart 2003). Even if the individual has been assessed as having an unsafe swallow, a risk management approach, especially if care is palliative, may offer the best quality of life for that person (Royal College of Physicians and British Society of Gastroenterology 2010).

3.3 Medication

Medications need to be administered in a format suited to the individual's safe swallowing capacity, especially if the route of administration is via an enteral feeding tube (White and Bradnam 2007). Prescribers are recommended to check not only the format of the preparation but also any contraindications which will apply for swallowing disorders. The knowledge and skills of the pharmacist within the MDT is crucial to safe medicines management. During assessment and treatment, medication reviews are essential to identify

any impact on the swallow as a result of medication (Nazarko 2007). The following examples are taken from the online resource DMR Health Standard 07-1 (2011).

- *Dysphagia as a side effect of medication*, e.g. medications that affect the smooth and striated muscles of the oesophagus involved in swallowing may cause dysphagia, such as preparations with anticholinergic and antimuscarinic effects.
- *Medications that cause xerostomia*, e.g. angiotensin-converting enzyme inhibitors, antihistamines and selective serotonin reuptake inhibitors, may interfere with swallowing by impairing the person's ability to move food.
- *Medications that cause movement disorders*, e.g. antipsychotic/neuroleptic medications which impact on the muscles of the face and tongue.
- *Dysphagia as a complication of the therapeutic action of the medication*, e.g. anti-epileptics, narcotics and other medications that depress the central nervous system can decrease awareness and voluntary muscle control that may affect swallowing.
- *Medications that can cause oesophageal injury and increase risk*, e.g. non-steroidal anti-inflammatory agents. These can cause dysphagia because of injury to the oesophagus as a consequence of local irritation.

Interactions between enteral tube feed formulations and medications can be clinically significant. As a general rule, if the absorption of a drug is affected by food or antacids, it is also likely to be affected by the feed, and a time lag between feeding and drug administration is necessary (British Association of Parenteral and Enteral Nutrition 2003). The dietitian will need to be aware of the prescribed medications and make the necessary adjustments to the timing of enteral tube feeding to minimise risk.

3.4 Quality of Life Issues

Any intervention should consider the four principles of medical ethics—respect for autonomy, beneficence, non-maleficence and justice (Beauchamp and Childress 2004) as well as the issue of consent, which always needs to be obtained for dietetic interventions. When dealing with the general population, one customarily obtains consent verbally. In clients with cognitive impairment, however, the issue about capacity to consent needs to be explored fully. When capacity to consent is being determined, it is essential to involve both the individual and the carers in the assessment and treatment process and to communicate openly (Burton et al. 2011).

Nutritional assessments can be conducted without considering whether the individual has ability to give consent to treatment, but in order to treat the individual, that individual's capacity must be determined. Determining capacity to consent must always be time- and decision-specific. It is important to remember that an individual should not be treated as unable to make a decision unless all practicable steps to help him/her have been taken without success. This includes the use of alternative forms of communication, for example:

- Short, concise, non-complex language.
- Body language.
- Eye pointing.
- Symbolised information.
- Photographs.
- Signing.
- Audio-visual.

In the UK, legislation exists to provide a legal framework for decision-making on behalf of adults who lack the capacity to make specific decisions for themselves. It also provides the means for adults, with the capacity to do so, to plan ahead in the event of future incapacity.

Readers are recommended to refer to the relevant legislation pertaining to their geographical work base as legislation may differ between countries. In the UK, for example, there are three different acts dealing with this issue, namely:

1. *In Scotland*, the Adults with Incapacity (Scotland) Act (Scottish Parliament 2000).
2. *In England and Wales*, the Mental Capacity Act 2005 (Department of Health 2005).
3. *In Northern Ireland*: Seeking Consent (Department of Health, Social Services and Public Safety 2003).

4 Education and Training Role

Carers and individuals with dysphagia may struggle with the day-to-day practical management of food and fluids (Ginocchio et al. 2009). Interactive and practical training sessions underpinned with theory and delivered in partnership with the SLT are an invaluable method of training, thus enabling people to experiment with using thickeners in a range of food and fluid preparations.

Key components of training for individuals with dysphagia and carers include:
Understanding the rationale for thickening and the risks of non-compliance.
Understanding the rationale for texture modification of foods and items which are prone to leaching.
Understanding the sensory properties of thickeners.
Understanding foods unsuitable for texture modification, e.g. pureed lettuce.
Menu planning to reduce repetition of using same foods, avoiding taste fatigue.
Correct preparation of textured foods to preserve nutritional content.
Correct preparation of thickened fluids depending on the type of thickener used.
Presentation to enhance compliance.
Food fortification using prescribed and non-prescribed products.
Correct usage of prescribed supplementary drinks and puddings.

Key components of training for health and social care professionals include:
Understanding the role and responsibilities of the dietitian.
Understanding the consequences of malnutrition in relation to dysphagia.
Understanding the rationale of nutritional consequences of texture modification.
Correct usage of any prescribed supplements, including type and amount of thickeners.

It has been shown that when implementing a diet for dysphagia, training enhances patient safety and increases energy intake (Dunne 2008; Garcia et al. 2010; Garcia and Chambers 2010). Dietitians along with the SLT are integral in training medical and nursing staff, health care assistants and carers at all levels on the recognition and consequences of dysphagia. Management options must also be included, so that all aspects of the swallowing mechanism and consequences of undernutrition can be highlighted and discussed.

5 Summary

The registered dietitian is one of a range of professionals involved in dysphagia management, and the role can be wide-ranging, from traditional nutritional management through to a whole-systems approach encompassing screening, assessment, diagnosis and organisation of the modified textures within a dynamic nutritional framework. A person-centred approach is essential to provide nutrition in a manner which not only sustains nutrition and hydration integrity but also serves to enhance the individual's quality of life. The dietitian's expertise lies in using the available clinical evidence, applying this to the individual's wider health and well-being needs, and devising and delivering targeted training to the individual, carers and other key health and social care professionals, so ensuring that the resultant recommendations are wholly person-centred.

References

Anderson D (2008) Training support staff to modify fluid consistancy for adults with learning disabilities and dysphagia: an efficacy study. Diet Today 44:14

Atherton M, Bellis-Smith N, Chichero JAY, Suter M (2007) Texture-modified foods and thickened fluids as used for individuals with dysphagia:Australian standardised labels and definitions. J Hum Nutr Diet 64S:523–576

British Association of Parenteral and Enteral Nutrition (2003) Drug administration via enteral feeding tubes: a guide for general practitioners and community pharmacists. http://www.bapen.org.uk/res_drugs.html Accessed 19 Feb 2011

Beauchamp TL, Childress JF (2004) Principles of biomedical ethics, 5th edn. Oxford University Press, Oxford

Bhattacharyya N, Kotz T, Shapiro J (2003) The effect of bolus consistency on dysphagia in unilateral vocal cord paralysis. J Otolaryngol Head Neck Surg 129:632–636

British Dietetic Association (2002) National descriptors for texture modification in adults. Joint working party of the British dietetic association and the royal college of speech and language therapists. British Dietetic Association, Birmingham

Brody RA, Touger-Decker R, VonHagen S, Maillet JO (2000) Role of registered dietitians in dysphagia screening. J Am Diet Assoc 101:179–180

Brotherton A, Abbott J, Aggett P (2006) Tne impact of percutaneous endoscopic gastrostomy feeding upon daily life in adults. J Hum Nutr Diet 19:355–367

Burton S, Cox S, Sandham SM (2009) Nutrtion, hydration and weight. In: Pawlyn J, Carnaby S (eds) Profound intellectual and multiple disabilities. Wiley-Blackwell, Oxford

Burton S, McIntosh P, Jurs A, Laverty A, Macleod M, Morrison L, Robinson N (2011) Weight management for adults with a learning disability living in the community. British Dietetic Association, Birmingham

Butt K, Lam P (2005) The role of the registered dietitian in dysphagia assessment and treatment. J Can Diet Pract Res 66:91–94

Clave P, De Kraa M, Arreola V, Girvent M, Farre R, Palomera E, Serra-Prat M (2006) The effect of bolus viscosity on swallowing function in neurogenic dysphagia. Aliment Pharmacol Ther 24:1385–1394

Copeman J, Hyland K (2007) Dysphagia. In: Thomas B, Bishop B (eds) Manual of dietetic practice, 4th edn. Blackwell, Oxford

Crawford C (2009) Dysphagia and people with profound intellectual and multiple disabilities. In: Pawlyn J, Carnaby S (eds) Profound intellectual and multiple disabilities. Wiley-Blackwell, Oxford

Davies S (2002) An interdisciplinary approach to the management of dysphagia. Prof Nurs 18:22–25

Department of Health (2005) Mental Capacity Act 2005: code of practice. Department of Constitutional Affairs. http://www.dca.gov.uk Accessed 7 Feb 2011

Department of Health, Social Services and Public Safety (2003) Seeking consent: working with people with learning disabilities. Department of Health, Social Services and Public Safety, Belfast

Dickerson RN, Brown RO, Gervasio JG, Hak EB, Hak LJ, Williams JE (1999) Measured energy expenditure of tube-fed patients with severe neurodevelopmental disabilities. J Am Coll Nutr 18:61–68

Dickerson RN, Brown RO, Hanna DL, Williams JE (2003) Energy requirements of non-ambulatory tube-fed adult patients with cerebral palsy and chronic hypothermia. Nutrition 19:741–746

DMR Health Standard 07-1 (2011) Guidelines for identification and management of dysphagia and swallowing risks attachment A. http://www.ct.gov/dds/lib/dds/health/attacha_med_dsyphagia_swallowing_risks.pdf Accessed 14 Feb 2011

Dunne P (2008) Balancing act. Nursing in the Community 9:19–20

Dyer JA (2003) Multidisciplinary, interdisciplinary and trans-disciplinary educational models and nursing education. Nurs Educ Perspect 24:186–188

Ekberg O, Hamdy S, Woisard V, Wuttge-Hannig A, Ortega P (2002) Social and psychological burden of dysphagia: its impact on diagnosis and treatment. Dysphagia 17:139–146

Elia M, Stratton R, Russell C, Green C (2005) The cost of disease related malnutrtion in the UK and economic considerations for the use of nutritional supplements (ONS) in adults. British Association of Parenteral and Enteral Nutrition, Worcester

Fairclough J, Burton S, Craven J, Ditchburn L, Laverty A, Macleod M (2008) Home enteral tube feeding for adults with a learning disability. British Dietetic Association, Birmingham

Finestone HM, Foley NC, Woodbury MG, Greene-Finestone L (2001) Quantifying fluid intake in dysphagic strok patients: a preliminary comparison of oral and nonoral strategies. Arch Phys Med Rehab 82:1744–1746

Garcia JM, Chambers E IV (2010) Managing dysphagia through diet modifications. Am J Nutr 110:26–33

Garcia JM, Chambers E IV, Matta Z, Clark M (2005) Viscosity measurement of nectar and honey thick liquids: product, liguid, and time comparisons. Dysphagia 20:325–335

Garcia JM, Chambers E IV, Matta Z, Clark M (2008) Serving temperature viscosity comparisons of nectar and honey-thick liquids: product, liquid and time comparisons. Dysphagia 23:65–75

Garcia JM, Chambers E IV, Clark M, Helverson J, Matta Z (2010) Quality of care issues for dysphagia: modifications involving oral fluids. J Clin Nurs 19:1618–1624

Gervasio JM, Dickerson RN, Brown RO, Matthews JB (1997) Chronic hypothermia and energy expenditure in a neurodevelopmentally disabled patient: a case study. Nutr Clin Pract 12:211–215

Ginocchio D, Borghi E, Schindler A (2009) Dysphagia assessment in the elderly. Nutr Ther Metabol 27:9–15

Goulding R, Bakheit AMO (2000) Evaluation of the benefits of monitoring fluid thickness in the dietary management of dysphagic stoke patients. Clin Rehabil 14:119–124

Hanson B, O'Leary M, Smith C (2011) The effect of saliva on the viscosity of thickened drinks. Dysphagia. doi:10.1007/s00455-011-9330-8

Heiss CJ, Goldberg L, Dzarnoshi M (2010) Registered dietitians and speech and language pathologists: an important partnership in dysphagia management. J Am Diet Assoc 110:1290–1293

ICDA (2008) Dietitians around the world: their education and their work. http://www.internationaldietetics.org/Downloads/2008-Report-on-Education-and-Work-of-Dietitians.aspx Accessed 22 Feb 2011

Ickenstein GW(2011) Diagnosis and treatment of neurogenic dysphagia. UNI-MED, Bremen

Irish Nutrition and Dietetic Institute (2009) Irish consiststency descriptors for modified fluids and foods. http://www.iaslt.ie/docs/public/information/Irish%20consistency%20descriptors%20for%20modified%20fluids%20and%20food.pdf Accessed 12 Feb 2011

Kemp S (2001) Restoring pleasure:nutritional management of dysphagia. Br J Community Nurs 6:284–289

Khlemeier KV, Palmer JB, Rosenberg D (2001) Effect of liquid bolus consistency and delivery method on aspiration and pharyngeal retention in dysphagia patients. Dysphagia 16:119–122

Lee HA (1974) Composition of some body external secretions. In: Lee HA (ed) Parenteral nutrition in acute metabolic illness. Academic, London

Logemann J (2008) A randomize study of three interventions for aspiration of thin liquids in patients with dementia or Parkinson's disease. J Speech Lang Hear R 51:173–183

Longton V, Chunn SS, Chambers E IV, Garcia JM (2003) Texture and flavor characteristics of beverages containing commercial thickening agents for dysphagia diets. J Food Sci 68:1537–1541

Matta Z, Chambers E IV, Garcia JM (2006) Sensory characteristics of beverages prepared with commercial thickeners used for dysphagia diets. J Am Diet Assoc 106:1049–1054

Mehanna H, Nankivell PC, Moledina J, Travis J (2009) Refeeding syndrome—awareness, prevention and management. http://www.headandneckoncology.org/content/1/1/4 Accessed 3 Feb 2011

National Dysphagia Diet Task Force (2002) National dysphagia diet. American Dietetic Association, Chicago

National Patient Safety Agency (2007) Ensuring safer practice for adults with learning disabilities who have dysphagia. http://www.nrls.npsa.nhs.uk/resources/?entryid45=59823 Accessed 24 Feb 2011

Nazarko E (2007) Nutrition part 5: dysphagia. Br J Healthcare Assistants 3:228–232

Nazarko E (2009) The clinical management of dysphagia in primary care. Br Community Nutr 13:258–264

National Institute for Health and Clinical Excellence (2006) Nutrition support in adults:oral nutrition support;enteral tube feeding and parenteral nutrition. http://www.nice.org.uk/nicemedia/pdf/cg032fullguideline.pdf Accessed 20 Feb 2011

Nowson CA, Sherwin AJ, McPhee JG, Wark JD, Flicker L (2003) Energy, protein, calcium, vitamin D and fibre intakes from meals in resedential care establishments in Australia. Asia Pac J Clin Nutr 12:172–177

NPSA Dysphagia expert reference group (2011) Dysphagia diet food texture descriptors. http://www.rcslt.org/members/publications/dysphagia_diet_texture_descriptions Accessed 1 Jun 2011

Panther K (2005) The Frazier free water protocol. Swallowing and swallowing disorders. Dysphagia 14:4–9

Pelletier CA (1997) A comparison of consistency and taste of five commercial thickeners. Dysphagia 12:74–78

Penman JP, Thomson M (2008) A review of the textured diets developed for the management of dysphagia. J Hum Nutr Diet 11:51–60

Perry L, Love CP (2001) Screeing for dysphagia and aspiration in acute stroke: a systematic review. Dysphagia 16:7–18

Queensland Health Dietitians (2007) Thickened fluids. http://www.health.qld.gov.au/nutrition/resources/txt_mod_tf.pdf Accessed 19 Feb 2011

Robbins J, Gensler G, Hind J, Logemann J, Lindblad A, Brandt D, Baum H, Lilienfeld D, Kosek S, Lundy D, Dikeman K, Kazandjian M, Gramigna G, McGarvey-Toler S, Gardner PJM (2008) Comparison of 2 interventions for liquid aspiration on pneumonia incidence. Ann Intern Med 148:509–519

Royal College of Physicians, British Society of Gastroenterology (2010) Oral feeding difficulties and dilemmas: a guide to practical care, particularly towards the end of life. Royal College of Physicians, Nottingham

Scottish Parliament (2000) Adults with Incapacity (Scotland) Act. The Stationery Office, Edinburgh

Stewart L (2003) Development of the nutrition and swallowing checklist, a screening tool for nutrition risk and swallowing risk in people with intellectual disability. J Int Dev Dis 28:171–187

Todorovic V, Micklewright A (2007) A pocket guide to clinical nutrition, 4th edn. Parenteral and Enteral Nutrition Group, Nottingham

Vivanti AP, Campbell KL, Suter MS, Hannan-Jones MT, Hulcombe JA (2009) Contribution of thickened drinks, food and enteral parenteral fluids to fluid intake in hospitalised patients with dysphagia. J Hum Nutr Diet 22:148–155

Whelan K (2001) Inadequate fluid intake in dysphagic stroke. Clin Nutr 20:423–428

White R, Bradnam V (2007) Handbook of drug administration via enteral feeding tubes. Pharmaceutical Press, London

White GN, O'Rourke F, Ong BS, Cordato DJ, Chan DKY (2008) Dysphagia:causes, assessment, treatment, and management. Geriatrics 63:15–20

Wright L, Cotter D, Hickson M (2005) The effectivensss of targetted feeding assistance to improve the nutritional intake of elderly dysphagic patients in hospital. J Hum Nutr Diet 21:555–562

Wright L, Cotter D, Hickson M, Frost G (2008) Comparison of energy and protein intakes of older people consuming a texture modified diet with a normal hospital diet. J Hum Nutr Diet 18:213–219

Direct and Indirect Therapy: Neurostimulation for the Treatment of Dysphagia After Stroke

Satish Mistry, Emilia Michou, Dipesh H. Vasant, and Shaheen Hamdy

Contents

Abstract

Swallowing problems (dysphagia) are common after brain injury, and can affect as many as 50% of patients in the period immediately after stroke. In some cases this can lead to serious morbidity, in particular malnutrition and pulmonary aspiration. Despite this, swallowing therapies remain controversial, with a limited evidence-base and little in the way of objective outcome measures providing scientific support for any observed changes. Moreover, swallowing can recover in some patients to a safe level within weeks, making it an interesting model for understanding brain recovery and compensation. A better understanding of these adaptive processes, seen during the spontaneous recovery phase, may help in developing therapeutic interventions capable of driving brain changes and encouraging the recovery process and is therefore a key goal for clinical neuroscience research which warrants systematic investigation. In this chapter, we review current knowledge and discuss some of the pioneering work conducted by researchers from both our laboratory and others in the field of human swallowing over the last decade. This chapter provides insights as to how the cerebral control of swallowing can be studied non-invasively in the human brain using neuroimaging tools and neurostimulation techniques. In addition, it also describes how using these neurostimulation techniques to manipulate the brain's natural capacity to reorganise (cortical plasticity) after injury or in response to new stimuli is helping in the process of developing novel therapies for the treatment of dysphagia and other motor disorders in humans.

S. Mistry · E. Michou · D. H. Vasant · S. Hamdy
Department of Inflammation Sciences,
Salford Royal NHS Foundation Trust,
University of Manchester, M6 8HD, Manchester, UK

S. Hamdy (✉)
Department of GI Sciences (Clinical Sciences Building),
Salford Royal NHS Foundation Trust,
Inflammation Sciences Research Group,
University of Manchester,
M6 8HD, Manchester, UK
e-mail: shaheen.hamdy@manchester.ac.uk

Abbreviations

DOSS	Dysphagia outcome and severity scale
fMRI	Functional magnetic resonance
PAS	Paired associative stimulation
PES	Pharyngeal electrical stimulation
PET	Positron emission tomography
rTMS	Repetitive transcranial magnetic stimulation
tDCS	Transcranial direct current stimulation
TMS	Transcranial magnetic stimulation

1   Introduction

For most of the world's population, swallowing, or deglutition, is a normal and effortless everyday task taken for granted. Despite this ease of performance, swallowing is now known to be a complex and dynamic sensorimotor activity involving 26 pairs of muscle, five cranial nerves and different levels of the central nervous system. This complexity emerges as a consequence of the common shared pathway between the respiratory and gastrointestinal tracts and is vital to ensuring the safe transport of ingested material from the mouth to the stomach for digestion without compromising the integrity of the airway. It is an integral component of feeding, learned during gestation, organized at birth (Hooker 1954) and essential for the continuation of life.

However, this complexity is also its "Achilles' heel", as any form of impairment (structural or neurogenic, see Table 1) in this co-ordination can become extremely debilitating. Unfortunately, this is often a reality for patients who suffer from swallowing difficulties or 'dysphagia' as a result of cerebral injuries such as Stroke (Singh and Hamdy 2006) or neurodegenerative diseases such as Parkinson's Disease (Michou and Hamdy 2010). Aspiration pneumonia is a common consequence of dysphagia (Johnson et al. 1993; Mann et al. 1999; DePippo et al. 1994; Kidd et al. 1995; Katzan et al. 2003; Cabre et al. 2010; Martino et al. 2005) and carries a significantly increased risk of morbidity and mortality (Katzan et al. 2003; Smithard et al. 1996). Moreover, neurogenic causes of dysphagia often lead to patients requiring enteral nutrition (Foley et al. 2009; Ha and

Hauge 2003) and increase the need for institutionalized care (Smithard et al. 2007).

Historically, the central neural control of swallowing was traditionally believed to be almost entirely dependent on brainstem reflexive mechanisms (Miller 2008; Jean 2001). However, in recent years, the role of the cerebral cortex in swallowing has received increased recognition and has been the subject of much research (Michou and Hamdy 2009). Its role in the control of human swallowing was first reported over a century ago by Bastian (1898), who described a patient suffering from dysphagia following a hemispheric stroke. Unsurprisingly, much of our understanding of the neural control of swallowing has come from invasive neurophysiological observations in animals, such as the seminal studies conducted by Miller and Sherrington (Miller 1920; Miller and Sherrington 1916). Replication studies by other authors (Jean 2001; Hamdy et al. 2001; Issa 1994; Weerasuriya et al. 1979; Goldberg et al. 1982; Huang et al. 1989; Yao et al. 2002; Sumi 1969; ten Hallers et al. 2004; Amarasena et al. 2003; Martin et al. 1997; Martin et al. 1999; Narita et al. 1999; McFarland and Lund 1993; Huang et al. 1988; Grelot et al. 1992) have shown that artificially stimulating cortical swallowing areas using invasive electrical microstimulation of either cortical hemisphere in anaesthetized animals, is capable of inducing full swallow responses visible to the investigator, providing evidence that swallowing musculature is bilaterally controlled. In humans, neural cartographer Wilder Penfield and colleagues (Penfield 1937), using the same technique of invasive electrical micro-stimulation in anaesthetized patients undergoing neurosurgery, demonstrated that stimulation of certain parts of the cerebral cortex could also induce swallowing. One of the first non-invasive studies of swallowing conducted in canines showed that with the use of transcranial magnetic stimulation (TMS) devices, stimulation of the cerebral cortex from the scalp surface could still elicit full swallowing responses (Valdez 1993). This may suggest that both hemispheres play an equal role in controlling swallowing (Martin and Sessle 1993); however, pathophysiological evidence resulting from cerebral injury such as stroke has begun to suggest that one hemisphere may show functional dominance over the other (Bastian 1898; Daniels and Foundas 1997; Robbins and Levin 1988; Meadows 1973) and that subsequent changes in

Table 1 Common causes of dysphagia

Structural causes of dysphagia	Causes of neurogenic dysphagia
• Amyloidosis	• Cerebral palsy
• Cervical spine osteophytes	• Guillan–Barre and other polyneuropathies
• Congenital anatomic abnormalities, e.g. cleft palate	• Head trauma[a]
	• Huntington's disease
• Iron and vitamin B12 deficiency	• Infectious disorders e.g. meningitis, syphilis, diphtheria, botulism, and encephalitis
• Oral malignancies of the tongue and palate	• Medication side effects
	• Motor neurone disease[a]
• Pharyngeal malignancy of the epiglottis, tongue base or larynx	• Multiple sclerosis[a]
	• Myasthenia gravis
• Salivary gland disease	• Myopathy, e.g. polymyositis, dermatomyositis, and sarcoidosis
• Skull base tumours	• Neoplasms, e.g. brain tumour
• Thyroid disease	• Parkinson's disease and other movement and neurodegenerative disorders
• Thyroid tumours	• Post-polio syndrome
• Zenkers diverticulum	• Progressive supranuclear palsy
	• Stroke[a, b]
	• Torticollis
	• Tardive dyskinesia
	• Wilsons disease

[a] Conditions which specifically cause pyramidal disease
[b] In the UK, stroke is the most common cause of neurogenic dysphagia

brain organization after lesion are crucial to recovery (Hamdy et al. 1996). Understanding how these changes in brain organization and activity correspond to normal and abnormal physiological function is, therefore, a key goal for clinical neuroscience research which warrants systematic investigation. Moreover, leaps in technological advancement and an increasing use of neurophysiological imaging and stimulation techniques have helped to improve our understanding of swallowing and its cortical control.

In addition to confirming the importance of multiple cortical sites in the control of swallowing, Positron Emission Tomography (PET) and Functional Magnetic Resonance (fMRI) studies have consistently shown bilateral activation in the Cerebellum during swallowing, with stronger activation reported in the left cerebellar hemisphere (Zald and Pardo 1999; Hamdy et al. 1999; Suzuki et al. 2003; Mosier and Bereznaya 2001; Mosier et al. 1999; Malandraki et al. 2009). Although current understanding of the contribution of the cerebellum in the control of swallowing is

extremely limited, there is some evidence from the animal literature which suggests that the cerebellum may be implicated in swallowing. For instance, in cats, throat contractions and overt swallowing are observed following cerebellar stimulation (Mussen 1927, 1930). High-intensity cerebellar stimulation using neurosurgically implanted cerebellar electrodes has also been shown to facilitate chewing, swallowing and predatory attack of prey in cats (Reis et al. 1973). A more recent study by Zhu et al. (2006) involving cerebellar stimulation in rats has also reported altered feeding regulation. In humans, further evidence for cerebellar involvement in swallowing comes from a recent neurophysiological study using non-invasive magnetic cerebellar stimulation. In this study, Jayasekeran et al. (2011) demonstrated that distinct motor responses can be induced in the pharyngeal musculature using single pulses of TMS. Together with findings from a paired-pulse experiment, they also indicate that cerebellar stimulation has the potential to excite the pharyngeal motor cortex (Jayasekeran et al. 2011). These results are encouraging; however, further research is required to see if this facilitation of the corticobulbar pathways can be exploited as a treatment option in dysphagia rehabilitation.

2   Current Management of Dysphagia

Current clinical guidelines for the treatment of dysphagic patients mainly constitutes helping patients to develop compensatory strategies to try and prevent complications whilst any natural recovery takes place (Speyer et al. 2009). Delivered by speech and language therapists in dysphagia rehabilitation, these strategies include a variety of head and neck exercises (chin tuck, head-turn or Mendelssohn manoeuvre) but with limited evidence to support their efficacy (Singh and Hamdy 2006). However methodological studies conducted with different modalities such as fMRI (Arima et al. 2011; Peck et al. 2010) are starting to appear in the literature. In addition, one behavioural exercise, described by Shaker et al. (2002), has been shown to reduce pharyngeal residue after swallowing by promoting opening of the upper oesophageal sphincter by reinforcing the actions of the suprahyoid muscles. Nonetheless, patients often become increasingly dependent during their lengthy hospital stays and are generally placed upon a modified-consistency diet or receive nothing orally if their symptoms are severe. Artificial feeding via either a nasogastric tube or percutaneous endoscopic gastrostomy is frequently resorted to, but has been shown to have no benefit in reducing the risk of pneumonia or aspiration or in improving patient outcomes (Norton et al. 1996; Dennis et al. 2005a, b). There is a role for enteral feeding in patients with restricted oral intake in order to maintain nutritional and hydration status, particularly if oral intake is restricted. This may keep alive patients who may have otherwise died but does not improve their quality of life or feeding independence.

3   Mechanisms of Recovery of Swallowing After Cerebral Cortex Damage

Given sufficient time, a large proportion of dysphagic stroke patients eventually recover the ability to swallow again (Mann et al. 1999; Barer 1989). The mechanism for this recovery, seen in many of the initially dysphagic stroke patients, has, however, remained controversial. As a first step towards understanding the mechanisms, midline structures involved in swallowing such as the pharyngeal, oesophageal, and mylohyoid musculature were mapped in healthy volunteers (Hamdy et al. 1996). The findings of this study demonstrated that in health, human swallowing musculature in the cerebral cortex was discretely and somatotopically represented in both hemispheres in the motor and premotor cortices. However, there were displays of interhemispheric asymmetry, independent of handedness, thereby implying the presence of dominant and non-dominant hemispheres. In a seminal study of swallowing in stroke using TMS, both dysphagic and non-dysphagic patients had the cortical topography of their pharyngeal musculature serially mapped over several months (Hamdy et al. 1996) (Fig. 1). The results from an earlier study by the same authors (Hamdy et al. 1996) taken together with the results of a follow-up study (Hamdy et al. 1998a) showed that the cortical map representation of the pharyngeal musculature in the undamaged hemisphere markedly increased in size in dysphagic patients who recovered swallowing, whereas there was no change in patients who had persistent dysphagia or in patients who were non-dysphagic throughout. Furthermore, the changes seen in the damaged hemisphere in any of the groups of patients were not significant. These observations imply that over a period of weeks or months, the recovery of swallowing after stroke may be reliant on compensatory strategies of cortical reorganization, through neuroplastic changes, mainly observed in the undamaged hemisphere.

More recently, the validity of early observations on the usefulness of TMS in the study of swallowing musculature organization and re-organization (Hamdy et al. 1996, 1998a) has been supported by evidence via TMS studies in oesophageal musculature by Khedr et al. (2008) and in mylohyoid musculature by Gallas et al. (2009), both of which illustrate the potential therapeutic role of neuroplastic changes in the unaffected hemisphere of dysphagic patients. This situation appears to differ from the recovery pattern observed for the limb muscles, where magnetic stimulation and fMRI studies, including the study by Hamdy et al. (1996) where limb function was used as a control for recovery pattern (Pascual-Leone et al. 2005;

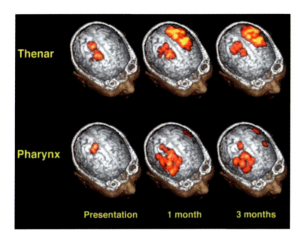

Fig. 1 Transcranial magnetic stimulation and magnetic resonance imaging co-registered representational map data from pharynx and thenar in a left hemisphere stroke patient. This patient, who was dysphagic at presentation, recovered swallowing function by 1 month, which was sustained at 3 months. Recovery of swallowing appears correlated to compensatory reorganization of the unaffected hemisphere, whereas hand recovery appears to occur in the damaged hemisphere [Reprinted from Hamdy et al. (1998a)]

Calautti et al. 2001; Marshall et al. 2000), have indicated that limb recovery after hemiparesis is more likely to result from an increase in the activity of the remaining viable cortex in the damaged hemisphere. In such cases, the scope for expansion of a normal connection from the undamaged part of the brain may be a limiting factor in recovery. However, cortical reorganization for limb function accompanied by functional changes has also been observed to occur within the contralesional hemisphere (Cramer et al. 1997; Ward et al. 2003). Thus it is well established that significant reorganizational change, observed as either beneficial or maladaptive, can occur in the adult cortex throughout life and after stroke lesions (Murphy and Corbett 2009). Furthermore, unmasking of existing connections, shifting of synaptic weighting and even sprouting of new dendritic connections and formation of new synapses are possible (Sanes and Donoghue 2000; Kaas 1997). Thus, neurorehabilitation strategies with neurostimulation interventions effectively applied to dysphagic stroke patients may deliver favourable outcomes by enhancing neuroplasticity in the uninjured hemisphere and accelerate the natural process of recovery.

4 Modulation of Brain Plasticity by Neurostimulation

There are a number of different neuroimaging and neurostimulation techniques that have been applied to the study of human cerebral control of swallowing and to experimentally manipulate cortical reorganizational mechanisms for therapeutic benefit. These studies show promising findings; however, clinical trials have proven challenging, with sample sizes being small and as a result none of these modalities are currently recommended for clinical use (Cheeran et al. 2009). In the following sections, we describe four such techniques used in several experimental trials in our laboratory.

4.1 Repetitive Transcranial Magnetic Stimulation

Repetitive TMS (rTMS) uses regularly repeated stimulation of a specific site over the cortex and is known as fast or high-frequency rTMS when used at rates above 1 Hz. In general, rates of stimulation of 1 Hz or below have inhibitory effects, whereas those above 1 Hz have excitatory effects on the cortex (Bailey et al. 2001; Ridding and Rothwell 2007). There are several potential applications of rTMS, including investigation and treatment of Parkinson's disease and other movement disorders (Muellbacher et al. 1999), epilepsy (Cantello 2002) and depression (Tassinari et al. 2003; Ziemann et al. 1998) as well as research into the neural mechanisms of vision (Gershon et al. 2003; Lisanby et al. 2002; Pascual-Leone et al. 1996) and language (Epstein 1998; Galletta et al. 2011; Tsujii et al. 2011). rTMS can also be used to investigate the functional relevance of cortical areas by creating 'virtual' lesions which interfere temporarily with neuronal function or it may be used to stimulate cortical reorganization, thereby altering function (Siebner et al. 2009). The direction of these changes of cortical excitability is dependent on the precise combination of several stimulation parameters used, such as the frequency and intensity of stimulation, and the intrinsic properties of the area being stimulated (Siebner et al. 2009).

The risks of the application of single-pulse TMS over the swallowing motor cortex are very low and no significant side effects have been shown to be produced in healthy individuals (Gow et al. 2004). However, much longer trains of stimulation are used in rTMS, and have the potential to induce seizures, especially when given at high intensities or frequencies and can also induce a spread of cortical excitation (Kandler 1990). Thus, guidelines based on the frequency and intensity of the stimulation applied (Wassermann 1998) were drawn up to limit rTMS applications in humans and have recently been updated by Rossi et al. (2009). There are a number of contraindications to the use of TMS because of the magnetic field produced; these include studying people with cardiac pacemakers, electronic implants and certain metal foreign bodies within the head as the coil may induce movement or heating. Patients with significant heart disease or raised intracranial pressure are at increased risk of complications following seizures and should be excluded, as should those on medications that are central nervous system active or lower the seizure threshold. Other contraindications include a history of epilepsy and pregnancy (Wassermann 1998; Rossi et al. 2009).

The pharyngeal motor cortex appears to be specifically responsive to stimulation at 5 Hz. When 100 pulses of rTMS are given over the cortex at 80% of pharyngeal threshold (capped at 120% of thenar threshold to comply with safety guidelines), there is increased excitability of the corticobulbar projection to the pharynx, which lasts for over 1 h (Gow et al. 2004). More recently, Jefferson et al. (2009a), applied differing trains of 5-Hz rTMS to pharyngeal motor cortex, ranging from 100 to 1,000 pulses. This work found that 250 pulses at low threshold intensities were as effective as longer or stronger 5-Hz rTMS trains at inducing plasticity in the swallowing motor system. Conversely, Mistry et al. (2007) have shown that by using an inhibitory 1-Hz rTMS paradigm for 10 min (600 magnetic stimulation pulses) at 120% of pharyngeal threshold, one can generate a unilateral virtual lesion in the pharyngeal motor cortex that affects swallowing neurophysiological function for up to 45 min and can also interfere with swallowing behaviour, as measured using reaction time swallowing tasks (Fig. 2).

This is of particular interest as translating neurostimulation therapies into patients with stroke is extremely challenging, because stroke is heterogeneous, often with intercurrent illness, and there are commonly problems with gaining consent. With the ability to generate virtual lesions in swallowing motor areas, we now have the opportunity to study function and recovery in a more controlled environment. Of importance, with the use of virtual lesions, we now have a potentially exciting model on which to test the efficacy of new neurostimulation techniques before progressing to trials in patient populations. Of relevance, (Jefferson et al. 2009a) were recently able to reverse the neurophysiological and behavioural effects of a virtual lesion to the inhibited pharyngeal motor cortex with contralateral 5-Hz rTMS, laying the foundation for the application of this technique in dysphagic stroke patients (Fig. 3).

In more recent literature, the use of rTMS has been explored in the treatment of dysphagia after stroke by several authors (Khedr et al. 2009; Verin and Leroi 2009). In the study by Khedr et al. (2009), excitatory 3-Hz rTMS (300 pulses at 120% of first dorsal interosseous motor threshold) was delivered for 10 min per day for five consecutive days to 26 unilateral hemispheric stroke patients with swallowing problems. Stimulation was delivered to the affected hemisphere, and according to the authors, resulted in a bilateral increase in brain excitability, 1 and 2 months after treatment, with an associated improvement in the symptoms and signs of dysphagia. However, the behavioural swallowing assessment was not standardized and contained little information regarding the patients' dysphagic problems. This is an important parameter, since the authors applied rTMS to the oesophageal cortical area without using other motor cortical areas as a control site. The second by Verin and Leroi (2009) attempted to decrease transcallosal inhibition between mylohyoid primary motor cortices by using an inhibitory 1-Hz rTMS paradigm. The authors applied 20 min of 1 Hz rTMS for five consecutive days to the healthy (unaffected) hemisphere of seven chronic dysphagic stroke patients (6 months after stroke) and assessed swallowing using videofluoroscopy. The study found a very modest decrease in the behavioural markers for swallowing impairment (aspiration–penetration scores) and in swallow reaction times. However, there was no control arm for the study against which comparisons could be made. Additionally, this model of rehabilitation has only been tested in healthy volunteers for changes in cortical excitability of hand musculature and hand function after stroke but has not

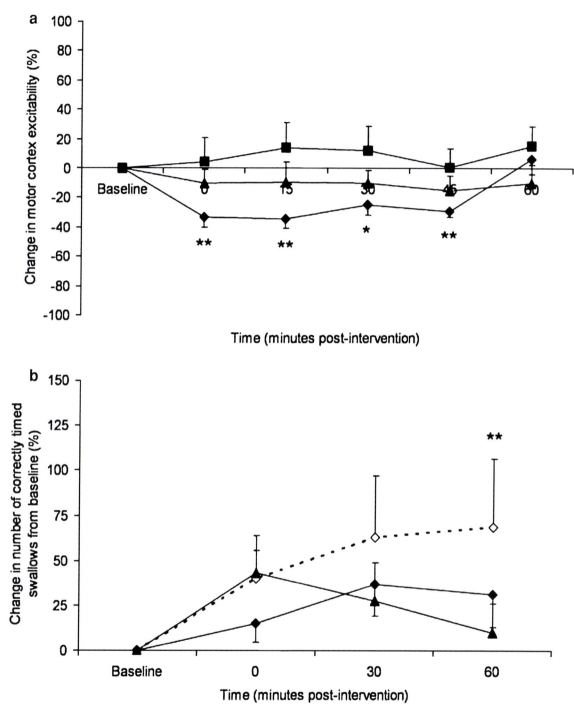

Fig. 2 Effects of inhibitory 1-Hz repetitive transcranial magnetic stimulation (rTMS) on swallowing neurophysiological function and behaviour. **a** Group mean change in pharyngeal and thenar motor evoked potential amplitudes (± standard error of the mean) from the baseline following (*diamonds*) 1 Hz rTMS over the dominant pharyngeal motor cortex. Inhibitory changes in responses evoked from the dominant pharyngeal motor cortex can be seen immediately and for up to 45 min after active rTMS (*single asterisk* $p < 0.004$, *double asterisk* $p < 0.001$, post hoc t tests) but are not consistently seen in hand motor cortex (*squares*). The non-dominant pharyngeal motor cortex (*triangles*) shows no change in excitability ($p = 0.7$). **b** Group mean change in successful challenge swallow trials from baseline following active 1-Hz rTMS applied to dominant (*Closed diamonds*) and non-dominant (*triangles*) pharyngeal motor cortices and after sham (*diamonds*). Successful swallow trials show a (anticipated) rise following sham 1 Hz rTMS but not after active stimulation of either hemisphere (*double asterisk* $p = 0.04$ post hoc t test) [Reprinted from Mistry et al. (2007)]

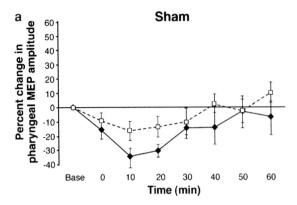

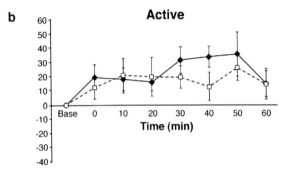

Fig. 3 Reversal of a virtual lesion in pharyngeal motor cortex using excitatory 5-Hz rTMS. Group mean change in pharyngeal motor evoked potential MEP amplitudes (± standard error of the mean) from the baseline over time following a virtual lesion. **a** Sham 5 Hz rTMS applied to the lesioned hemisphere has no effect on reversing excitability of both the lesioned (*diamonds*) and the non-lesioned (*squares*) hemispheres, which display decreased excitability for up to 50 min after lesion. **b** Active 5-Hz rTMS applied to the contralateral non-lesioned hemisphere completely reverses the effects of the virtual lesion on cortical excitability in both hemispheres [Reprinted from Jefferson et al. (2009a)]

been trialled for swallowing musculature; therefore, its feasibility is somewhat questionable. Nevertheless, application of the technique demonstrates the potential of neurostimulation in the modification of behaviour many months after cerebral injury.

4.2 Peripheral Stimulation

In contrast to direct (or transcranial) stimulation of the brain, it is also possible to modulate cortical plasticity by stimulation of peripheral nerves. There are a number of postulated mechanisms by which changes in swallowing occur following peripheral stimulation

(for a review, see Steele and Miller (2010); such as the notion that increasing the sensitivity of the mucosa may allow more effective triggering and modulation of the swallow in response to a bolus (de Lama Lazzara et al. 1986; Teismann et al. 2009) or retrograde activation of corticobulbar pathways may prime the brainstem swallowing centre and cortical neurones. Early work in anaesthetized animals (Doty 1951; Miller 1972) demonstrated that electrical stimulation of the superior laryngeal nerve branch of the vagus nerve can elicit swallowing motor activity, which is that of a 'stereotyped' nature (Jean 2001). In contrast, in humans, stimulation with the various techniques from the periphery has shown that there is a considerable variability in the elicitation of motor components of the swallowing motor action.

More recently published literature in humans demonstrates an increasing list of stimulation techniques capable of providing sensory information to sensory receptors and mechanoreceptors of the oral cavity, including thermal (de Lama Lazzara et al. 1986; Gisel 2008; Rosenbek et al. 1996, 1998), tactile (Rosenbek et al. 1996, 1998; Lamm et al. 2005; Ali et al. 1996), gustatory (Hamdy et al. 2003; Mistry et al. 2006), air pulse (Lowell et al. 2008; Soros et al. 2008; Theurer et al. 2005, 2009) and electrical stimulation of different oral regions, including the tongue (Lamm et al. 2005), palate (Park et al. 1997) and faucial pillars (Power et al. 2004, 2006). These paradigms provide an avenue for rehabilitation in dysphagia; however, careful characterization of the stimulation parameters must be conducted prior to any utilization in dysphagic patients. One example of the need for careful and methodological research into stimulation paradigms is that although it has been observed that stimulation of the faucial pillars increases cortical excitability (Power et al. 2004, 2006) and may reduce bolus transfer timings and increase swallowing safety immediately (Rosenbek et al. 1996, 1998), it does not appear to have any effect on other physiological abnormalities in dysphagia (Ali et al. 1996; Power et al. 2006). Stimulation of the tongue has not been shown to be of therapeutic benefit (Lamm et al. 2005) and palatal stimulation may be beneficial; however, the studies are limited by small sample sizes (Park et al. 1997). Studies using air pulse stimulation of the peritonsillar region have been more encouraging, with the results showing an associated urge to swallow after

Fig. 4 Effects of volitional water swallowing on (**a**) pharyngeal (*circles*) and oesophageal (*triangles*) motor cortical responses and (**b**) craniobulbar reflexes. Group mean responses were recorded for up to 60 min after 10 min of volitional water swallowing and compared to baseline [Reprinted from Fraser et al. (2003)]

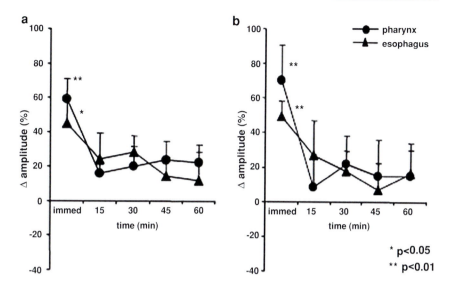

application and an increased rate of saliva swallowing as well as bilateral brain activations during fMRI in the regions known to be involved in swallowing (primary somatosensory cortex and thalamus, primary motor cortex, supplementary motor area, cingulate motor area and polymodal areas) (Lowell et al. 2008; Soros et al. 2008; Theurer et al. 2005, 2009).

A problem common to all the oral stimulation techniques is that if a therapeutic benefit is produced, the effects are only short-term, merely lasting for a few swallows (de Lama Lazzara et al. 1986; Rosenbek et al. 1996; Sciortino et al. 2003). Indeed, simply activating swallowing pathways by swallowing either water or flavoured solutions have been shown to significantly alter pharyngeal motor cortex excitability for up to 30 min (Mistry et al. 2006; Fraser et al. 2003) (Figs. 4, 5) and decrease swallow speed and volume per swallow (Hamdy et al. 2003; Chee et al. 2005).

Interestingly, the merits of neuromuscular electrical stimulation for the treatment of dysphagia (transcutaneous stimulation of the neck muscles) have been discussed at length both in clinical practice and in the literature (Carnaby-Mann and Crary 2007; Steele et al. 2007). However evidence of its efficacy, remains limited, with many of the published studies using a technique containing methodological flaws, the most important of which being the lack of a physiological and/or neurophysiological evidence base for its efficacy before progressing with its use in clinical trials on the dysphagic population.

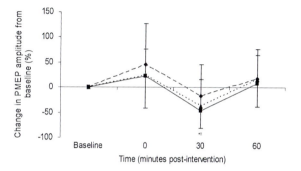

Fig. 5 Effects of swallowing neutral (water, *diamonds*), bitter (*squares*) and sweet (*triangles*) flavoured solutions on pharyngeal motor cortical responses. Group mean responses were recorded for up to 60 min after 10 min of volitional swallowing and compared to baseline ($p < 0.03$). *PMEP* pharyngeal motor evoked potential [Reprinted from Mistry et al. (2006)]

On the other hand, pharyngeal electrical stimulation (PES) has also been studied both in healthy volunteers and in the patient population. Short (5-Hz) trains of intraluminal PES delivered for 10 min have been shown to increase corticobulbar excitability, without affecting brainstem responses (Fraser et al. 2003; Hamdy et al. 1998b) (Fig. 6), increase blood-oxygenation level-dependent fMRI responses (Fraser et al. 2002) (Fig. 7) and are also able to improve levels of swallowing dysfunction assessed using videofluoroscopy following stroke (Fraser et al. 2002), for at least 30 min (Fig. 8).

On the basis of this early encouraging work (Fraser et al. 2002, 2003), Jayasekeran et al. (2010) sought to substantiate the mechanisms by which PES can help

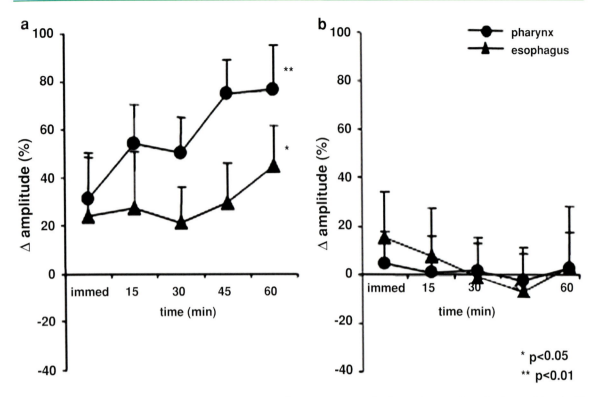

Fig. 6 Effects of pharyngeal electrical stimulation on corti-cobulbar and craniobulbar motor excitability. Group mean change in responses from the baseline **a** After stimulation, pharyngeal (*circles*) and oesophageal (*triangles*) cortical response amplitudes are increased at 45 min, reaching significance at 60 min. **b** Craniobulbar reflexes remain unaffected [Reprinted from Fraser et al. (2003)]

reverse both cortical and behavioural swallowing impairments in dysphagic stroke patients. Using the virtual lesion model of swallowing impairment developed by Mistry et al. (2007) described earlier, they studied the effects on both swallowing neurophysiological function and behaviour of active or sham PES after inducing a virtual lesion in healthy volunteers. Similarly to the reversal study of Jefferson et al. (2009a), they were able to show strong reversal of the neurophysiological and behavioural effects of a virtual lesion to the inhibited pharyngeal motor cortex with PES, laying the foundation for the application of this technique in dysphagic stroke patients (Fig. 9).

Moving forward, Jayasekeran et al. (2010) refined the treatment parameters in a dose–response study of PES in dysphagic stroke patients and assessed swallowing outcome using videofluoroscopy. They found that a stimulation regime of PES once a day for 3 days was the most practical and effective course of neurostimulation to reduce aspiration. In addition, the efficacy of PES was evaluated in a randomized clinical trial of 28 acute dysphagic stroke patients. The authors concluded that PES significantly improved swallowing performance and intriguingly reduced the length of hospital stay (Fig. 10), compared with the control group.

Therefore, although the evidence for some peripheral stimulation treatments and their use in clinical practice remains controversial (Speyer et al. 2009; Power et al. 2006; Foley et al. 2008), this pilot study by Jayasekeran et al. (2010) is the first randomized trial to show that bedside neurostimulation of the pharynx can be delivered in a safe and effective manner with encouraging results for reducing swallowing impairment and prolonged hospitalization. A larger, randomized controlled trial is now necessary and should clarify the therapeutic potential of PES in a wider clinical context.

4.3 Transcranial Direct Current Stimulation

Transcranial direct current stimulation (tDCS) is a novel technique in which a weak electric current (approximately 1–2 mA) is passed over the brain.

NO STIMULATION

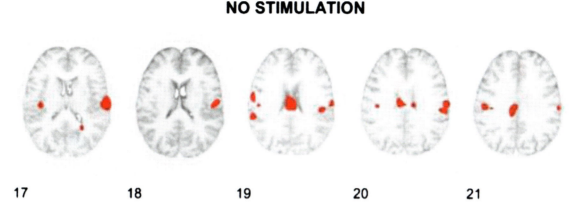

17   18   19   20   21

STIMULATION

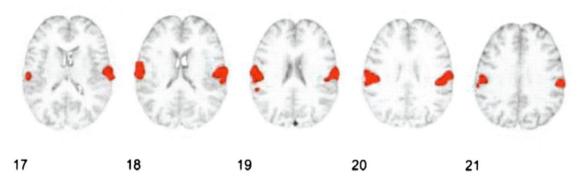

17   18   19   20   21

Fig. 7 Effects of pharyngeal electrical stimulation on cortical Blood-oxygenation-level-dependent functional magnetic resonance imaging signals in healthy subjects during volitional swallowing. Group mean activation data are shown as a series of normalized transverse brain slices, with no stimulation paradigm across the *top*, and the stimulation paradigm across the *bottom*. Activated pixels are shown in *red*, and brain slice numbers are indicated below the images. Greater bilateral functional activation occurs within sensorimotor cortex (Brodmann areas 3 and 4), and is most overt in slices 17–19, after pharyngeal stimulation compared to with stimulation ($p < 0.05$) [Reprinted from Fraser et al. (2002)]

It appears to be both safe and well tolerated (Nitsche and Paulus 2000) and has already been shown to alter the excitability and function of various parts of the nervous system depending on which site is stimulated (Gandiga et al. 2006; Maeda et al. 2000). In the clinical setting, tDCS also offers other advantages; the equipment needed is small and easily transportable, therefore, making it a more viable tool.

The direction of change of excitability is dependent on the position of the electrodes; excitability increases when the anode is placed over the motor cortex and the cathode is placed over the supraorbital ridge ('anodal' tDCS), whereas it decreases when the current flow is reversed ('cathodal' tDCS)

(Fregni et al. 2005; Takeuchi et al. 2005; Nitsche and Paulus 2001; Hummel et al. 2005). These effects are also dependent on the combination of parameters such as the current strength, duration of stimulation and electrode montage. The excitatory effects in the motor cortex produced with this technique are thought to be due to neuronal depolarization and possible hyperpolarization of inhibitory interneurones, whereas the inhibitory effects are thought to be caused by hyperpolarization of motor neurones.

It is a useful tool for sham-controlled studies as the current produces a mild tingling sensation on the scalp, lasting for approximately 20 s. Stimulation can therefore be given for 30 s, enough time to produce

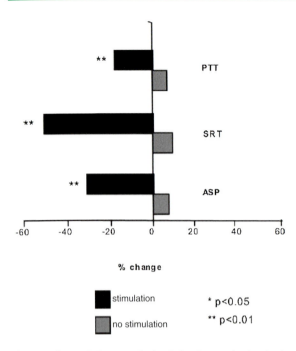

PTT

SRT

ASP

% change

■ stimulation   * p<0.05

□ no stimulation   ** p<0.01

Fig. 8 Effects of pharyngeal stimulation in acutely dysphagic stroke patients. Functionally beneficial reductions in pharyngeal transit time (*PTT*), swallowing response time (*SRT*), and aspiration (*ASP*) are seen after active stimulation (*black bars*) but not after no stimulation (*grey bars*) [Reprinted from Fraser et al. (2002)]

the initial sensation, but not long enough to induce any cortical changes (Nitsche and Paulus 2000).

In a recent study by Jefferson et al. (2009b), the parameters of tDCS that might be usefully applied to the swallowing regions of motor cortex were explored. The study found that the levels of stimulation applied to the hand motor cortex were not effective at changing excitability in the pharyngeal motor cortex. However, when higher or longer levels of current were applied, both excitatory (anodal) and inhibitory (cathodal) changes were induced (Fig. 11). It is therefore conceivable that anodal tDCS could be a new therapeutic avenue for dysphagic stroke patients.

Following on from this parameter-setting study, Kumar et al. (2011) very recently published data from a clinical trial of tDCS in 14 acute dysphagic stroke patients (seven real, seven sham). In this study, the authors applied a 5-day treatment of 2 mA of anodal tDCS for 30 min a day to the motor cortex of the unlesioned hemisphere (electrode placement was estimated using the international 10–20 system for -EEG for electrode placement and magnetic resonance image co-registration). Patients in both treatment arms were also given lemon-flavoured lollipops to suck, asked to perform effortful swallows and were given ice chips intermittently for dryness. Changes in the dysphagia outcome and severity scale (DOSS) score before stimulation compared with the DOSS score after the last session were used as the main outcome measure (O'Neil et al. 1999) with videofluoroscopy assessments made intermittently, unless DOSS scores could not be obtained. The authors reported that there was significant improvement in DOSS scores when comparing the actively treated group with the sham-treated group (p = 0.019). This would appear to be a potentially promising result; however, this study has several confounding limitations. The first is the amalgamation of several plasticity-inducing behavioural interventions (effortful swallows) and peripheral sensory interventions (lemon taste and cold tactile stimulation) which may have influenced the overall effects of the tDCS. Secondly, the use of the DOSS scale is not sufficient to give information about the improvement in swallowing behaviour and as such this information is lacking in this study. The authors, however, have acknowledged that they did not trial the optimal parameters of stimulation as identified by Jefferson et al. (2009b) as their protocol predated its publication.

4.4 Paired Associative Stimulation

Plastic changes of the motor and somatosensory cortical areas have also been investigated using TMS in the form of paired associative stimulation (PAS). This neurostimulation technique is capable of provoking long-lasting heterosynaptic plasticity in neuronal pathways through the near-synchronous combination of peripheral stimuli in the targeted muscle with cortical stimuli over the targeted muscle representational area in the motor cortex. PAS has been studied in many cerebral regions (Cruikshank and Weinberger 1996; Kelso and Brown 1986; Bindman et al. 1988; Iriki et al. 1991) both invivo (Baranyi and Feher 1981) and invitro (Hess and Donoghue 1994). The concept of this technique derives from evidence that peripheral input plays an important role in plastic reorganization of motor areas and can lead to long-lasting changes in cortical excitability of the targeted area, as already seen with the application of PES on swallowing musculature. Research in animal

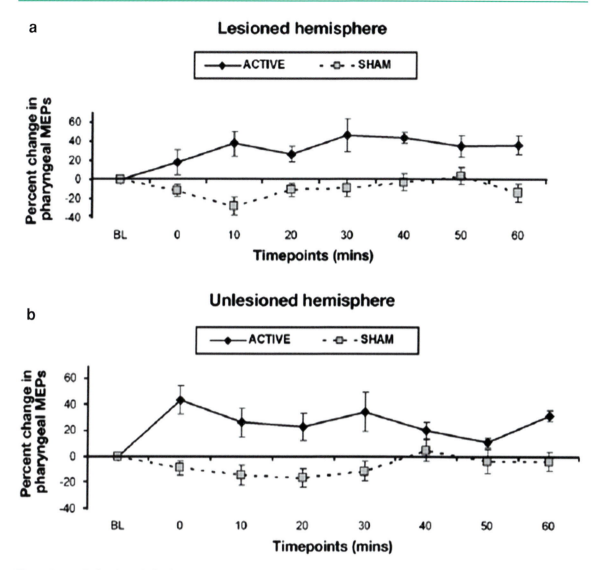

Fig. 9 Reversal of a virtual lesion in pharyngeal motor cortex using pharyngeal electrical stimulation (PES). Group mean change in pharyngeal motor evoked potential (*MEP*) amplitudes (± standard error of the mean) from the baseline over time following a virtual lesion. Sham PES (*squares*) had no effect on reversing excitability of both the lesioned (**a**) and the non-lesioned (**b**) hemisphere, which displayed decreased excitability for up to 40 min after lesion. Active PES (*diamonds*) however, completely reverses the effects of the virtual lesion on cortical excitability in both hemispheres [Reprinted from Jayasekeran et al. (2010)]

neocortical slices has shown that when a weak excitatory synaptic input repeatedly arrives at a neurone shortly before the neurone has fired an action potential, then the strength and efficacy of that connection is increased, whereas if the input arrives after the neural discharge, the strength of the connection is reduced (Dan and Poo 2006; Kirkwood and Bear 1994). Bi-directional modulation of synaptic efficacy in this manner is termed 'Hebbian plasticity' (Donoghue 1995).

Modulation of cortical networks in healthy volunteers using PAS was first described by Stefan et al. (2000), who paired low-frequency (peripheral) electrical median nerve stimulation with (central) TMS of the abductor pollicis brevis motor cortical representation. These findings for the limb muscles have since been replicated by several authors (Ridding and Taylor 2001; Stefan et al. 2002; McKay et al. 2002; Pyndt and Ridding 2004). The exact mechanism(s) underlying the induced changes

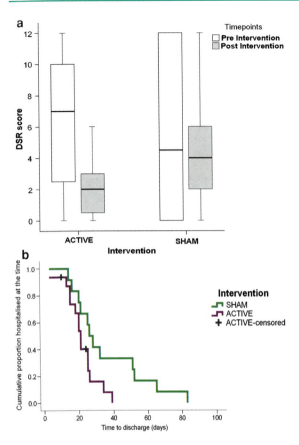

Fig. 10 Results of a randomized clinical trial of (PES) in dysphagic stroke patients. **a** Comparison of Dysphagia Severity Rating Scale (DSR) scores between active and sham treatment groups (U = 58.0, p = 0.04), indicates an improved feeding status in the active group after PES. **b** Kaplan–Meier plot showing the period of hospitalisation following either active or sham treatment. The active treatment group have a significantly shorter period of hospitalization compared with the sham treatment group when time-to-event analysis was used (log rank test p = 0.038). The censored data take into account two patients who died during hospitalization [Reprinted from Jayasekeran et al. (2010)]

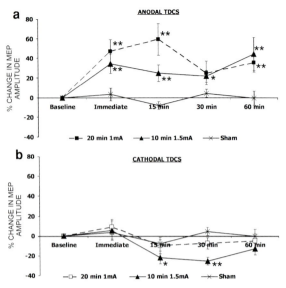

Fig. 11 Effects of transcranial direct current stimulation (tDCS) on pharyngeal motor cortex. Group mean change in pharyngeal motor evoked potential (MEP) amplitudes (± standard error of the mean) of the stimulated hemisphere from baseline over time after (**a**) anodal or (**b**) cathodal tDCS for 20 min at 1 mA (*squares*) or 10 min at 1.5 mA (*triangles*) or sham stimulation (*crosses*). Significant changes in excitability are seen following 10 min of 1.5 mA and 20 min of 1 mA anodal stimulation and 10 min of 1.5 mA cathodal stimulation with repeated-measures analysis of variance; *single asterisk t* test $p < 0.05$ compared with the baseline, *double asterisk t*-test $p < 0.05$ compared with both the baseline and sham treatment [Reprinted from Jefferson et al. (2009)]

is (are) yet to be fully elucidated; however, consensus amongst researchers is currently focusing towards the existence of no single mechanism. NMDA-dependent mechanisms, such as long-term potentiation and depression, are currently the putative candidates responsible for the induction of plastic changes in sensorimotor areas through activity-dependent modification of the existing cortical synapses (Stefan et al. 2000; Wolters et al. 2003). However, recent studies in the swallowing motor system have contributed additional information on the origin of, and the potential mechanisms involved in the induction of cortical changes.

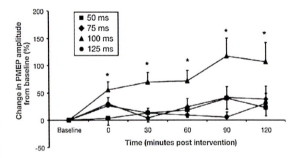

Fig. 12 Effects of paired associative stimulation (PAS) on pharyngeal motor cortex excitability. Group mean change (± standard error of the mean) in pharyngeal response amplitudes from the baseline are shown for PAS using inter-stimulus-intervals of 50 ms (*squares*), 75 ms (*diamonds*), 100 ms (*triangles*), and 125 ms (*circles*). PAS using an inter stimulus interval of 100 ms produced significant increases in excitability for up to 2 h (*single asterisk p < 0.002*, post hoc t tests). No significant changes were evident with the other interstimulus intervals. *PMEP* pharyngeal motor evoked potential

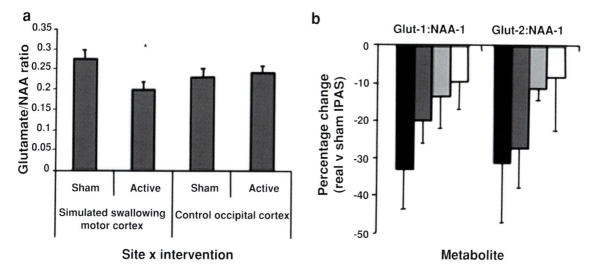

Fig. 13 Glutamate ratio changes after PAS measured by magnetic resonance spectroscopy. **a** Glut-1/NAA-1 ratio (group mean across all time points ± standard error of the mean) at the ipsilateral pharyngeal motor cortex and occipital cortex after real or sham PAS with an inter stimulus interval of 100 ms. An average reduction of approximately 25% is seen in cortical Glut-1/NAA-1 ratio levels at the stimulated site after real PAS compared with sham PAS *(asterisk p < 0.02)*. No significant change was seen at the occipital control site. **b** Percentage difference (group mean at each time point ± standard error of the mean) in both glutamate ratios at the ipsilateral pharyngeal motor cortex at four time points *(from dark to light columns* immediate, 30, 60, and 90 min respectively). All four measures show their greatest changes in the early period after intervention with a gradual return towards sham PAS. This contrasts with the changes in cortical excitability after PAS with an interstimulus intervals of 100 ms, where the effect builds up over 2 h. Glut glutamate, NAA N-acetylaspartate) [Reprinted from Singh et al. (2009)]

In 2009, Singh et. al. (2009) (Fig. 12) described a PAS protocol for inducing changes in pharyngeal motor cortical excitability. Using PES–(peripheral stimulation) and TMS (cortical stimulation) separated by a 100-ms inter-stimulus interval, Singh et al. (2009) were able to produce changes in cortical excitability that lasted for up to 2 h after stimulation, and for up to 8 h in a separate study in two subjects. Using magnetic resonance spectroscopy, they also demonstrated that the mechanism involved changes in intracortical glutamate levels within the cortex (Fig. 13).

Investigations into refinement of the PAS parameters described by Singh et al. (2009) have continued in our laboratory and have shown that PAS applied for just 10 min can induce changes in pharyngeal motor cortical excitability to the same magnitude as a 30-min protocol (Michou et al. 2009). Moreover, similarly to 5-Hz rTMS and PES, it is also capable of reversing the effects of a virtual lesion in both hemispheres when applied to the non-lesioned hemisphere. These data support the notion that interventions targeting the undamaged hemisphere may produce more favourable effects in terms of brain excitability than those targeting

the damaged hemisphere, with PAS being a strong potential candidate therapeutic intervention in stroke patients with dysphagia.

5   Conclusion

Direct and indirect forms of experimental neurostimulation therapies are developing rapidly and now provide new avenues for successful neurorehabilitation, founded on an understanding of how the brain reorganizes and compensates following injury. These approaches should lay the foundation for the design of future large-scale randomized controlled trials of non-invasive cortical and peripheral stimulation in dysphagic stroke patients and provide useful correlates for its potential application in other types of brain injury. It is hoped that such studies will provide more information as to whether neurostimulation can be a useful therapeutic tool or an adjunct to current clinical practice in the care of patients with dysphagia, so reducing the suffering and mortality associated with this distressing condition.

References

Ali GN, Laundl TM, Wallace KL, deCarle DJ, Cook IJ (1996) Influence of cold stimulation on the normal pharyngeal swallow response. Dysphagia 11(1):2–8

Amarasena J, Ootaki S, Yamamura K, Yamada Y (2003) Effect of cortical masticatory area stimulation on swallowing in anesthetized rabbits. Brain Res 965(1–2):222–238

Arima T, Yanagi Y, Niddam DM, Ohata N, Arendt-Nielsen L, Minagi S, Sessle BJ, Svensson P (2011) Corticomotor plasticity induced by tongue-task training in humans: a longitudinal fMRI study. Exp Brain Res 212(2):199–212

Bailey CJ, Karhu J, Ilmoniemi RJ (2001) Transcranial magnetic stimulation as a tool for cognitive studies. Scand J Psychol 42(3):297–305

Baranyi A, Feher O (1981) Synaptic facilitation requires paired activation of convergent pathways in the neocortex. Nature 290(5805):413–415

Barer DH (1989) The natural history and functional consequences of dysphagia after hemispheric stroke. J Neurol Neurosurg Psychiatry 52(2):236–241

Bastian HC (1898) A treatise on aphasia and other speech defects. Lewis, London

Bindman LJ, Murphy KP, Pockett S (1988) Postsynaptic control of the induction of long-term changes in efficacy of transmission at neocortical synapses in slices of rat brain. J Neurophysiol 60(3):1053–1065

Cabre M, Serra-Prat M, Palomera E, Almirall J, Pallares R, Clave P (2010) Prevalence and prognostic implications of dysphagia in elderly patients with pneumonia. Age Ageing 39(1):39–45

Calautti C, Leroy F, Guincestre JY, Baron JC (2001) Dynamics of motor network overactivation after striatocapsular stroke: a longitudinal PET study using a fixed-performance paradigm. Stroke 32(11):2534–2542

Cantello R (2002) Applications of transcranial magnetic stimulation in movement disorders. J Clin Neurophysiol 19(4):272–293

Carnaby-Mann GD, Crary MA (2007) Examining the evidence on neuromuscular electrical stimulation for swallowing: a meta-analysis. Arch Otolaryngol Head Neck Surg 133(6):564–571

Chee C, Arshad S, Singh S, Mistry S, Hamdy S (2005) The influence of chemical gustatory stimuli and oral anaesthesia on healthy human pharyngeal swallowing. Chem Senses 30(5):393–400

Cheeran B, Cohen L, Dobkin B, Ford G, Greenwood R, Howard D, Husain M, Macleod M, Nudo R, Rothwell J, Rudd A, Teo J, Ward N, Wolf S (2009) The future of restorative neurosciences in stroke: driving the translational research pipeline from basic science to rehabilitation of people after stroke. Neurorehabil Neural Repair 23(2):97–107

Cramer SC, Nelles G, Benson RR, Kaplan JD, Parker RA, Kwong KK, Kennedy DN, Finklestein SP, Rosen BR (1997) A functional MRI study of subjects recovered from hemiparetic stroke. Stroke 28(12):2518–2527

Cruikshank SJ, Weinberger NM (1996) Receptive-field plasticity in the adult auditory cortex induced by Hebbian covariance. J Neurosci 16(2):861–875

Dan Y, Poo MM (2006) Spike timing-dependent plasticity: from synapse to perception. Physiol Rev 86(3):1033–1048

Daniels SK, Foundas AL (1997) The role of the insular cortex in dysphagia. Dysphagia 12(3):146–156

de Lama Lazzara G, Lazarus C, Logemann J (1986) Impact of thermal stimulation on the triggering of the swallowing reflex. Dysphagia 1(2):73–77

Dennis MS, Lewis SC, Warlow C (2005a) Effect of timing and method of enteral tube feeding for dysphagic stroke patients (FOOD): a multicentre randomised controlled trial. Lancet 365(9461): 764–772

Dennis MS, Lewis SC, Warlow C (2005b) Routine oral nutritional supplementation for stroke patients in hospital (FOOD): a multicentre randomised controlled trial. Lancet 365(9461): 755–763

DePippo KL, Holas MA, Reding MJ, Mandel FS, Lesser ML (1994) Dysphagia therapy following stroke: a controlled trial. Neurology 44(9):1655–1660

Donoghue JP (1995) Plasticity of adult sensorimotor representations. Curr Opin Neurobiol 5(6):749–754

Doty RW (1951) Influence of stimulus pattern on reflex deglutition. Am J Physiol 166(1):142–158

Epstein CM (1998) Transcranial magnetic stimulation: language function. J Clin Neurophysiol 15(4):325–332

Foley N, Teasell R, Salter K, Kruger E, Martino R (2008) Dysphagia treatment post stroke: a systematic review of randomised controlled trials. Age Ageing 37(3):258–264

Foley NC, Martin RE, Salter KL, Teasell RW (2009) A review of the relationship between dysphagia and malnutrition following stroke. J Rehabil Med 41(9):707–713

Fraser C, Power M, Hamdy S, Rothwell J, Hobday D, Hollander I, Tyrell P, Hobson A, Williams S, Thompson D (2002) Driving plasticity in human adult motor cortex is associated with improved motor function after brain injury. Neuron 34(5):831–840

Fraser C, Rothwell J, Power M, Hobson A, Thompson D, Hamdy S (2003) Differential changes in human pharyngo-esophageal motor excitability induced by swallowing, pharyngeal stimulation, and anesthesia. Am J Physiol Gastrointest Liver Physiol 285(1):G137–G144

Fregni F, Boggio PS, Mansur CG, Wagner T, Ferreira MJL, Lima MC, Rigonatti SP, Marcolin MA, Freedman SD, Nitsche MA, Pascual-Leone A (2005) Transcranial direct current stimulation of the unaffected hemisphere in stroke patients. Neuroreport 16(14):1551–1555

Gallas S, Marie JP, Leroi AM, Verin E (2009) Sensory transcutaneous electrical stimulation improves post-stroke dysphagic patients. Dysphagia 25(4):291–297

Galletta EE, Rao PR, Barrett AM (2011) Transcranial magnetic stimulation (TMS): potential progress for language improvement in aphasia. Top Stroke Rehabil 18(2):87–91

Gandiga PC, Hummel FC, Cohen LG (2006) Transcranial DC stimulation (tDCS): a tool for double-blind sham-controlled clinical studies in brain stimulation. Clin Neurophysiol 117(4):845–850

Gershon AA, Dannon PN, Grunhaus L (2003) Transcranial magnetic stimulation in the treatment of depression. Am J Psychiatry 160(5):835–845

Gisel E (2008) Interventions and outcomes for children with dysphagia. Dev Disabil Res Rev 14(2):165–173

Goldberg LJ, Chandler SH, Tal M (1982) Relationship between jaw movements and trigeminal motoneuron membrane-potential fluctuations during cortically induced rhythmical jaw movements in the guinea pig. J Neurophysiol 48(1):110–138

Gow D, Rothwell J, Hobson A, Thompson D, Hamdy S (2004) Induction of long-term plasticity in human swallowing motor cortex following repetitive cortical stimulation. Clin Neurophysiol 115(5):1044–1051

Grelot L, Milano S, Portillo F, Miller AD, Bianchi AL (1992) Membrane potential changes of phrenic motoneurons during fictive vomiting, coughing, and swallowing in the decerebrate cat. J Neurophysiol 68(6):2110–2119

Ha L, Hauge T (2003) Percutaneous endoscopic gastrostomy (PEG) for enteral nutrition in patients with stroke. Scand J Gastroenterol 38(9):962–966

Hamdy S, Aziz Q, Rothwell JC, Singh KD, Barlow J, Hughes DG, Tallis RC, Thompson DG (1996) The cortical topography of human swallowing musculature in health and disease. Nat Med 2(11):1217–1224

Hamdy S, Aziz Q, Rothwell JC, Power M, Singh KD, Nicholson DA, Tallis RC, Thompson DG (1998a) Recovery of swallowing after dysphagic stroke relates to functional reorganization in the intact motor cortex. Gastroenterology 115(5):1104–1112

Hamdy S, Rothwell JC, Aziz Q, Singh KD, Thompson DG (1998b) Long-term reorganization of human motor cortex driven by short-term sensory stimulation. Nat Neurosci 1(1):64–68

Hamdy S, Rothwell JC, Brooks DJ, Bailey D, Aziz Q, Thompson DG (1999) Identification of the cerebral loci processing human swallowing with H2(15)O PET activation. J Neurophysiol 81(4):1917–1926

Hamdy S, Xue S, Valdez D, Diamant NE (2001) Induction of cortical swallowing activity by transcranial magnetic stimulation in the anaesthetized cat. Neurogastroenterol Motil 13(1):65–72

Hamdy S, Jilani S, Price V, Parker C, Hall N, Power M (2003) Modulation of human swallowing behaviour by thermal and chemical stimulation in health and after brain injury. Neurogastroenterol Motil 15(1):69–77

Hess G, Donoghue JP (1994) Long-term potentiation of horizontal connections provides a mechanism to reorganize cortical motor maps. J Neurophysiol 71(6):2543–2547

Hooker D (1954) Early human fetal behavior, with a preliminary note on double simultaneous fetal stimulation. Res Publ Assoc Res Nerv Ment Dis 33:98–113

Huang CS, Sirisko MA, Hiraba H, Murray GM, Sessle BJ (1988) Organization of the primate face motor cortex as revealed by intracortical microstimulation and electrophysiological identification of afferent inputs and corticobulbar projections. J Neurophysiol 59(3):796–818

Huang CS, Hiraba H, Murray GM, Sessle BJ (1989) Topographical distribution and functional properties of cortically induced rhythmical jaw movements in the monkey (Macaca fascicularis). J Neurophysiol 61(3):635–650

Hummel F, Celnik P, Giraux P, Floel A, Wu W-H, Gerloff C, Cohen LG (2005) Effects of non-invasive cortical stimulation on skilled motor function in chronic stroke. Brain 128(3):490–499

Iriki A, Pavlides C, Keller A, Asanuma H (1991) Long-term potentiation of thalamic input to the motor cortex induced by coactivation of thalamocortical and corticocortical afferents. J Neurophysiol 65(6):1435–1441

Issa FG (1994) Gustatory stimulation of the oropharynx fails to induce swallowing in the sleeping dog. Gastroenterology 107(3):650–656

Jayasekeran V, Singh S, Tyrrell P, Michou E, Jefferson S, Mistry S, Gamble E, Rothwell J, Thompson D, Hamdy S (2010) Adjunctive functional pharyngeal electrical stimulation reverses swallowing disability following brain lesions. Gastroenterology 138(5):1737–1746

Jayasekeran V, Rothwell J, Hamdy S (2011) Non-invasive magnetic stimulation of the human cerebellum facilitates cortico-bulbar projections in the swallowing motor system. Neurogastroenterol Motil 23(9):831–841

Jean A (2001) Brain stem control of swallowing: neuronal network and cellular mechanisms. Physiol Rev 81(2):929–969

Jefferson S, Mistry S, Michou E, Singh S, Rothwell JC, Hamdy S (2009a) Reversal of a virtual lesion in human pharyngeal motor cortex by high frequency contralesional brain stimulation. Gastroenterology 137(3):841–849 849 e1

Jefferson S, Mistry S, Singh S, Rothwell J, Hamdy S (2009b) Characterizing the application of transcranial direct current stimulation in human pharyngeal motor cortex. Am J Physiol Gastrointest Liver Physiol 297(6):G1035–G1040

Johnson ER, McKenzie SW, Sievers A (1993) Aspiration pneumonia in stroke. Arch Phys Med Rehabil 74(9):973–976

Kaas J (1997) Functional plasticity in adult cortex, in seminars in neuroscience. Academic Press: Orlando

Kandler R (1990) Safety of transcranial magnetic stimulation. Lancet 335(8687):469–470

Katzan IL, Cebul RD, Husak SH, Dawson NV, Baker DW (2003) The effect of pneumonia on mortality among patients hospitalized for acute stroke. Neurology 60(4):620–625

Kelso SR, Brown TH (1986) Differential conditioning of associative synaptic enhancement in hippocampal brain slices. Science 232(4746):85–87

Khedr EM, Abo-Elfetoh N, Ahmed MA, Kamel NF, Farook M, El Karn MF (2008) Dysphagia and hemispheric stroke: a transcranial magnetic study. Neurophysiol Clin 38(4):235–242

Khedr EM, Abo-Elfetoh N, Rothwell JC (2009) Treatment of post-stroke dysphagia with repetitive transcranial magnetic stimulation. Acta Neurol Scand 119(3):155–161

Kidd D, Lawson J, Nesbitt R, MacMahon J (1995) The natural history and clinical consequences of aspiration in acute stroke. QJM 88(6):409–413

Kirkwood A, Bear MF (1994) Hebbian synapses in visual cortex. J Neurosci 14(3 Pt 2):1634–1645

Kumar S, Wagner CW, Frayne C, Zhu L, Selim M, Feng W, Schlaug G (2011) Noninvasive brain stimulation may improve stroke-related dysphagia: a pilot study. Stroke 42(4):1035–1040

Lamm NC, De Felice A, Cargan A (2005) Effect of tactile stimulation on lingual motor function in pediatric lingual dysphagia. Dysphagia 20(4):311–324

Lisanby SH, Kinnunen LH, Crupain MJ (2002) Applications of TMS to therapy in psychiatry. J Clin Neurophysiol 19(4):344–360

Lowell SY, Poletto CJ, Knorr-Chung BR, Reynolds RC, Simonyan K, Ludlow CL (2008) Sensory stimulation activates both motor and sensory components of the swallowing system. Neuroimage 42(1):285–295

Maeda F, Keenan JP, Tormos JM, Topka H, Pascual-Leone A (2000) Interindividual variability of the modulatory effects of repetitive transcranial magnetic stimulation on cortical excitability. Exp Brain Res 133(4):425–430

Malandraki GA, Sutton BP, Perlman AL, Karampinos DC, Conway C (2009) Neural activation of swallowing and swallowing-related tasks in healthy young adults: an attempt to separate the components of deglutition. Hum Brain Mapp 30(10):3209–3226

Mann G, Hankey GJ, Cameron D (1999) Swallowing function after stroke: prognosis and prognostic factors at 6 months. Stroke 30(4):744–748

Marshall RS, Perera GM, Lazar RM, Krakauer JW, Constantine RC, DeLaPaz RL (2000) Evolution of cortical activation during recovery from corticospinal tract infarction. Stroke 31(3):656–661

Martin RE, Sessle BJ (1993) The role of the cerebral cortex in swallowing. Dysphagia 8(3):195–202

Martin RE, Murray GM, Kemppainen P, Masuda Y, Sessle BJ (1997) Functional properties of neurons in the primate tongue primary motor cortex during swallowing. J Neurophysiol 78(3):1516–1530

Martin RE, Kemppainen P, Masuda Y, Yao D, Murray GM, Sessle BJ (1999) Features of cortically evoked swallowing in the awake primate (Macaca fascicularis). J Neurophysiol 82(3):1529–1541

Martino R, Foley N, Bhogal S, Diamant N, Speechley M, Teasell R (2005) Dysphagia after stroke: incidence, diagnosis, and pulmonary complications. Stroke 36(12):2756–2763

McFarland DH, Lund JP (1993) An investigation of the coupling between respiration, mastication, and swallowing in the awake rabbit. J Neurophysiol 69(1):95–108

McKay DR, Ridding MC, Thompson PD, Miles TS (2002) Induction of persistent changes in the organisation of the human motor cortex. Exp Brain Res 143(3):342–349

Meadows JC (1973) Dysphagia in unilateral cerebral lesions. J Neurol Neurosurg Psychiatry 36(5):853–860

Michou E, Hamdy S (2009) Cortical input in control of swallowing. Curr Opin Otolaryngol Head Neck Surg 17(3):166–171

Michou E, Hamdy S (2010) Dysphagia in Parkinson's disease: a therapeutic challenge? Expert Rev Neurother 10(6):875–878

Michou E, Mistry S, Jefferson S, Hamdy S (2009) Reversibility in human swallowing motor cortex by paired cortical and peripheral stimulation to a unilateral virtual lesion: evidence for targetting the contralesional cortex. Gastroenterology 136(5):A-17–A-18

Miller FR (1920) The cortical paths for mastication and deglutition. J Physiol 53(6):473–478

Miller AJ (1972) Significance of sensory inflow to the swallowing reflex. Brain Res 43(1):147–159

Miller AJ (2008) The neurobiology of swallowing and dysphagia. Dev Disabil Res Rev 14(2):77–86

Miller FR, Sherrington CS (1916) Some observations on the buccopharyngeal stage of reflex deglutition in the cat. Q- J Exp Physiol 9:147–186

Mistry S, Rothwell JC, Thompson DG, Hamdy S (2006) Modulation of human cortical swallowing motor pathways after pleasant and aversive taste stimuli. Am J Physiol Gastrointest Liver Physiol 291(4):G666–G671

Mistry S, Verin E, Singh S, Jefferson S, Rothwell JC, Thompson DG, Hamdy S (2007) Unilateral suppression of pharyngeal motor cortex to repetitive transcranial magnetic stimulation reveals functional asymmetry in the hemispheric projections to human swallowing. J Physiol 585(Pt 2):525–538

Mosier K, Bereznaya I (2001) Parallel cortical networks for volitional control of swallowing in humans. Exp Brain Res 140(3):280–289

Mosier KM, Liu WC, Maldjian JA, Shah R, Modi B (1999) Lateralization of cortical function in swallowing: a functional MR imaging study. AJNR Am J Neuroradiol 20(8):1520–1526

Muellbacher W, Artner C, Mamoli B (1999) The role of the intact hemisphere in recovery of midline muscles after recent monohemispheric stroke. J Neurol 246(4):250–256

Murphy TH, Corbett D (2009) Plasticity during stroke recovery: from synapse to behaviour. Nat Rev Neurosci 10(12):861–872

Mussen AT (1927) Symposium on the cerebellum: (4) experimental investigations on the cerebellum. Brain 50(3–4):313–349

Mussen AT (1930) The cerebellum: the influence of the cortical reactions on the classification and the homology of the lobes and fissures in the cat, monkey and man. Arch Neurol Psychiatry 24(5):913–920

Narita N, Yamamura K, Yao D, Martin RE, Sessle BJ (1999) Effects of functional disruption of lateral pericentral cerebral cortex on primate swallowing. Brain Res 824(1):140–145

Nitsche MA, Paulus W (2000) Excitability changes induced in the human motor cortex by weak transcranial direct current stimulation. J Physiol 527(Pt 3):633–639

Nitsche MAMD, Paulus WMD (2001) Sustained excitability elevations induced by transcranial DC motor cortex stimulation in humans. Neurology 57:1899–1901

Norton B, Homer-Ward M, Donnelly MT, Long RG, Holmes GK (1996) A randomised prospective comparison of percutaneous endoscopic gastrostomy and nasogastric tube feeding after acute dysphagic stroke. BMJ 312(7022):13–16

O'Neil KH, Purdy M, Falk J, Gallo L (1999) The Dysphagia Outcome and Severity Scale. Dysphagia 14(3):139–145

Park CL, O'Neill PA, Martin DF (1997) A pilot exploratory study of oral electrical stimulation on swallow function following stroke: an innovative technique. Dysphagia 12(3):161–166

Pascual-Leone A, Rubio B, Pallardo F, Catala MD (1996) Rapid-rate transcranial magnetic stimulation of left dorsolateral prefrontal cortex in drug-resistant depression. Lancet 348(9022):233–237

Pascual-Leone A, Amedi A, Fregni F, Merabet LB (2005) The plastic human brain cortex. Annu Rev Neurosci 28:377–401

Peck KK, Branski RC, Lazarus C, Cody V, Kraus D, Haupage S, Ganz C, Holodny AI, Kraus DH (2010) Cortical activation during swallowing rehabilitation maneuvers: a functional MRI study of healthy controls. Laryngoscope 120(11):2153–2159

Penfield W, Boldrey E (1937) Somatic motor and sensory representation in the cerebral cortex of man as studied by electrical stimulation. Brain 60:389–443

Power M, Fraser C, Hobson A, Rothwell JC, Mistry S, Nicholson DA, Thompson DG, Hamdy S (2004) Changes in pharyngeal corticobulbar excitability and swallowing behavior after oral stimulation. Am J Physiol Gastrointest Liver Physiol 286(1):G45–G50

Power ML, Fraser CH, Hobson A, Singh S, Tyrrell P, Nicholson DA, Turnbull I, Thompson DG, Hamdy S (2006) Evaluating oral stimulation as a treatment for dysphagia after stroke. Dysphagia 21(1):49–55

Pyndt HS, Ridding MC (2004) Modification of the human motor cortex by associative stimulation. Exp Brain Res 159(1):123–128

Reis DJ, Doba N, Nathan MA (1973) Predatory attack, grooming, and consummatory behaviors evoked by electrical stimulation of cat cerebellar nuclei. Science 182(114):845–847

Ridding MC, Rothwell JC (2007) Is there a future for therapeutic use of transcranial magnetic stimulation? Nat Rev Neurosci 8(7):559–567

Ridding MC, Taylor JL (2001) Mechanisms of motor-evoked potential facilitation following prolonged dual peripheral and central stimulation in humans. J Physiol 537(2):623–631

Robbins J, Levin RL (1988) Swallowing after unilateral stroke of the cerebral cortex: preliminary experience. Dysphagia 3(1):11–17

Rosenbek JC, Roecker EB, Wood JL, Robbins J (1996) Thermal application reduces the duration of stage transition in dysphagia after stroke. Dysphagia 11(4):225–233

Rosenbek JC, Robbins J, Willford WO, Kirk G, Schiltz A, Sowell TW, Deutsch SE, Milanti FJ, Ashford J, Gramigna GD, Fogarty A, Dong K, Rau MT, Prescott TE, Lloyd AM, Sterkel MT, Hansen JE (1998) Comparing treatment intensities of tactile-thermal application. Dysphagia 13(1):1–9

Rossi S, Hallett M, Rossini PM, Pascual-Leone A (2009) Safety ethical considerations, and application guidelines for the use of transcranial magnetic stimulation in clinical practice and research. Clin Neurophysiol 120(12):2008–2039

Sanes JN, Donoghue JP (2000) Plasticity and primary motor cortex. Annu Rev Neurosci 23:393–415

Sciortino K, Liss JM, Case JL, Gerritsen KG, Katz RC (2003) Effects of mechanical, cold, gustatory, and combined stimulation to the human anterior faucial pillars. Dysphagia 18(1):16–26

Shaker R, Easterling C, Kern M, Nitschke T, Massey B, Daniels S, Grande B, Kazandjian M, Dikeman K (2002) Rehabilitation of swallowing by exercise in tube-fed patients with pharyngeal dysphagia secondary to abnormal UES opening. Gastroenterology 122(5):1314–1321

Siebner HR, Hartwigsen G, Kassuba T, Rothwell JC (2009) How does transcranial magnetic stimulation modify neuronal activity in the brain? Implications for studies of cognition. Cortex 45(9):1035–1042

Singh S, Hamdy S (2006) Dysphagia in stroke patients. Postgrad Med J 82(968):383–391

Singh S, Mistry S, Jefferson S, Davies K, Rothwell J, Williams S, Hamdy S (2009) A magnetic resonance spectroscopy study of brain glutamate in a model of plasticity in human pharyngeal motor cortex. Gastroenterology 136(2):417–424

Smithard DG, O'Neill PA, Parks C, Morris J (1996) Complications and outcome after acute stroke. Does dysphagia matter? Stroke 27(7):1200–1204

Smithard DG, Smeeton NC, Wolfe CD (2007) Long-term outcome after stroke: does dysphagia matter? Age Ageing 36(1):90–94

Soros P, Lalone E, Smith R, Stevens T, Theurer J, Menon RS, Martin RE (2008) Functional MRI of oropharyngeal air-pulse stimulation. Neuroscience 153(4):1300–1308

Speyer R, Baijens L, Heijnen M, Zwijnenberg I (2009) Effects of therapy in oropharyngeal dysphagia by speech and language therapists: a systematic review. Dysphagia 24(1):91–102

Steele CM, Miller AJ (2010) Sensory input pathways and mechanisms in swallowing: a review. Dysphagia 25(4):323–333

Steele CM, Thrasher AT, Popovic MR (2007) Electric stimulation approaches to the restoration and rehabilitation of swallowing: a review. Neurol Res 29(1):9–15

Stefan K, Kunesch E, Cohen LG, Benecke R, Classen J (2000) Induction of plasticity in the human motor cortex by paired associative stimulation. Brain 123(Pt 3):572–584

Stefan K, Kunesch E, Benecke R, Cohen LG, Classen J (2002) Mechanisms of enhancement of human motor cortex excitability induced by interventional paired associative stimulation. J Physiol 543(Pt 2):699–708

Sumi T (1969) Some properties of cortically-evoked swallowing and chewing in rabbits. Brain Res 15(1):107–120

Suzuki M, Asada Y, Ito J, Hayashi K, Inoue H, Kitano H (2003) Activation of cerebellum and basal ganglia on volitional swallowing detected by functional magnetic resonance imaging. Dysphagia 18(2):71–77

Takeuchi NMD, Chuma TMD, Matsuo YMD, Watanabe IMDP, Ikoma KMDP (2005) Repetitive transcranial magnetic stimulation of contralesional primary motor cortex improves hand function after stroke. Stroke 36(12):2681–2686

Tassinari CA, Cincotta M, Zaccara G, Michelucci R (2003) Transcranial magnetic stimulation and epilepsy. Clin Neurophysiol 114(5):777–798

Teismann IK, Steinstrater O, Warnecke T, Suntrup S, Ringelstein EB, Pantev C, Dziewas R (2009) Tactile thermal oral stimulation increases the cortical representation of swallowing. BMC Neurosci 10:71

ten Hallers EJ, Rakhorst G, Marres HA, Jansen JA, van Kooten TG, Schutte HK, van Loon JP, van der Houwen EB, van Loon JP, Verkerke GJ (2004) Animal models for tracheal research. Biomaterials 25(9):1533–1543

Theurer JA, Bihari F, Barr AM, Martin RE (2005) Oropharyngeal stimulation with air-pulse trains increases swallowing frequency in healthy adults. Dysphagia 20(4):254–260

Theurer JA, Czachorowski KA, Martin LP, Martin RE (2009) Effects of oropharyngeal air-pulse stimulation on swallowing in healthy older adults. Dysphagia 24(3):302–313

Tsujii T, Sakatani K, Masuda S, Akiyama T, Watanabe S (2011) Evaluating the roles of the inferior frontal gyrus and superior parietal lobule in deductive reasoning: a rTMS study. Neuroimage 58(2):640–646

Valdez DT, Salapatek A, Niznik G, Linden RD, Diamant NE (1993) Swallowing and upper esophageal sphincter contraction with transcranial magnetic-induced electrical stimulation. Am J Physiol, 264(2 Pt 1): G213–G219

Verin E, Leroi AM (2009) Poststroke dysphagia rehabilitation by repetitive transcranial magnetic stimulation: a noncontrolled pilot study. Dysphagia 24(2):204–210

Ward NS, Brown MM, Thompson AJ, Frackowiak RS (2003) Neural correlates of outcome after stroke: a cross-sectional fMRI study. Brain 126(Pt 6):1430–1448

Wassermann EM (1998) Risk and safety of repetitive transcranial magnetic stimulation: report and suggested guidelines from the international workshop on the safety of repetitive transcranial magnetic stimulation, June 5–7, 1996. Electroencephalogr Clin Neurophysiol 108(1): 1–16

Weerasuriya A, Bieger D, Hockman CH (1979) Basal forebrain facilitation of reflex swallowing in the cat. Brain Res 174(1):119–133

Wolters A, Sandbrink F, Schlottmann A, Kunesch E, Stefan K, Cohen LG, Benecke R, Classen J (2003) A temporally asymmetric Hebbian rule governing plasticity in the human motor cortex. J Neurophysiol 89(5):2339–2345

Yao D, Yamamura K, Narita N, Martin RE, Murray GM, Sessle BJ (2002) Neuronal activity patterns in primate primary motor cortex related to trained or semiautomatic jaw and tongue movements. J Neurophysiol 87(5):2531–2541

Zald DH, Pardo JV (1999) The functional neuroanatomy of voluntary swallowing. Ann Neurol 46(3):281–286

Zhu JN, Li HZ, Ding Y, Wang JJ (2006) Cerebellar modulation of feeding-related neurons in rat dorsomedial hypothalamic nucleus. J Neurosci Res 84(7):1597–1609

Ziemann U, Steinhoff BJ, Tergau F, Paulus W (1998) Transcranial magnetic stimulation: its current role in epilepsy research. Epilepsy Res 30(1):11–30

Intervention on the Esophagus

Jason D. Conway, David J. Ott, and Michael Y. Chen

Contents

Abstract

Currently, most interventions on the esophagus are performed by endoscopists. However, diagnostic imaging is often necessary prior to or after these interventions. This chapter reviews the roles of diagnostic radiological imaging as well as diagnostic and therapeutic endoscopy in the management of common esophageal diseases including hemorrhage, Barrett's esophagus and esophageal cancer, esophageal foreign bodies, achalasia, and peptic strictures.

1 Introduction

In the past, the evaluation of esophageal disease consisted mainly of diagnosis and possibly the use of surgical or radiation treatment. Major advancements in esophageal intervention have occurred in recent decades (Wallace 2004), especially with innovations with endoscopic techniques. The endoscopist will typically perform these interventional procedures, but imaging may be required during or after the procedure. Thus, the radiologist needs a thorough understanding of these newer techniques and knowledge of their radiographic appearances and potential complications. Interventional techniques in the esophagus center largely on the management of specific disorders or their complications. Important clinical conditions that may require evaluation and endoscopic management include treatment of esophageal hemorrhage, endoscopic mucosal ablation, removal of esophageal foreign bodies, pneumatic dilatation for treating achalasia, peptic stricture dilatation, and therapeutic or

J. D. Conway (✉)
Department of Gastroenterology,
Medical Center Boulevard,
Wake Forest University School of Medicine,
Winston Salem, NC 27157, USA
e-mail: jconway@wakehealth.edu

D. J. Ott · M. Y. Chen
Department of Radiology,
Medical Center Boulevard,
Wake Forest University School of Medicine,
Winston-Salem, NC 27157, USA

O. Ekberg (ed.), *Dysphagia*, Medical Radiology. Diagnostic Imaging, DOI: 10.1007/174_2012_607,
© Springer-Verlag Berlin Heidelberg 2012

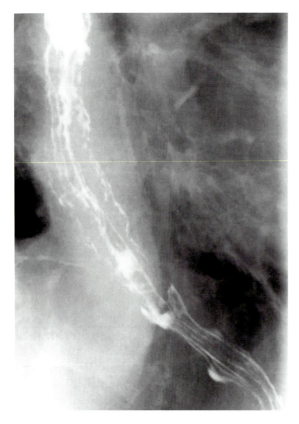

Fig. 1 Multiple linear varices in the lower esophagus

palliative management of esophageal malignancy, which often involves placement of metallic stents.

In this chapter, the evaluation and management of the following clinical conditions and procedures are discussed: (1) esophageal hemorrhage, (2) endoscopic mucosal ablation, (3) esophageal foreign bodies, (4) achalasia, especially the use of pneumatic dilatation, (5) peptic strictures, and (6) esophageal malignancy. The endoscopic procedures are reviewed and the role of imaging in assisting in the management of these disorders is discussed and illustrated. The newer metallic endoprostheses are emphasized because imaging is pivotal in their deployment, assessment, and subsequent evaluation.

2   Esophageal Hemorrhage

Endoscopy has become the primary method used for the diagnosis and potential treatment of upper gastrointestinal bleeding (Shah and Kamath 2010). Esophageal sources of hemorrhage are numerous but usually occur secondary to esophagitis, Mallory-Weiss tears, varices, or malignancies. Mallory-Weiss tears and varices are the most common causes of esophageal bleeding. The Mallory-Weiss tear is a longitudinal mucosal injury located at the esophagogastric junction that may follow an episode of vomiting with hematemesis. Esophageal varices are most often caused by portal hypertension related to cirrhosis in Western societies (Fig. 1). Thus, treatment of bleeding esophageal varices may be directed at the varices, alleviation of portal hypertension, or both.

Endoscopic techniques for control of esophageal bleeding include injection, thermal, and mechanical therapies (Wallace 2004). Injection of submucosal or intramural epinephrine or sclerosants can be effective in controlling hemorrhage from a number of esophageal lesions, or may be combined with other therapies to improve hemostasis. Thermal therapies and coaptive technology with the heater probe or BICAP (bipolar electrocoagulation) device are other options. The heater probe and BICAP device allow for effective and safe treatment of bleeding sites in the esophagus. This technology converts electrical energy to heat and causes a coaptive coagulation of the bleeding site when the device is applied with pressure. Hemoclips and variceal ligators are examples of mechanical therapies that may be used for nonvariceal or variceal hemorrhage.

Endoscopy plays a pivotal role in the diagnosis and management of esophageal variceal bleeding (Shah and Kamath 2010). Sclerotherapy involves injection of a sclerosant into or near the varix. Mechanical therapies can also be used to treat bleeding varices. Variceal ligation has emerged as the preferred method in the management of variceal hemorrhage; with the development of multiple banders, the need for an overtube or re-endoscopy has been eliminated. Balloon tamponade has been used for many years as an alternate method to temporarily control variceal bleeding by compression of the varices. Various balloon devices have been used, but the four-lumen Minnesota tube is considered to be the safest because secretions above the esophageal balloon can be aspirated continuously.

Complications from these therapeutic modalities are variable and include ulceration with recurrent hemorrhage, stricture formation, perforation, mediastinitis, and pleural effusions (Albillos et al. 2010; Kochhar et al. 1992; Sharara and Rockey 2001). Radiologic imaging has a limited role in the diagnosis of many of

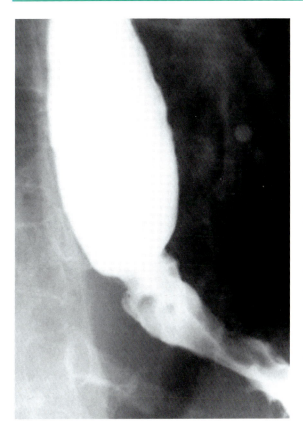

Fig. 2 Irregular, nodular narrowing at the lower end of the esophagus following endoscopic sclerotherapy. Repeat endoscopic examination showed a stricture and varices

the esophageal causes of upper gastrointestinal bleeding, although esophagitis, varices, and malignancies are often detected. Imaging may be more important in the evaluation of potential complications following these procedures (Fig. 2). In particular, a contrast esophagram can assess for perforation and stricture formation, although the latter complication has diminished with the newer therapies.

3 Mucosal Ablation

Endoscopic mucosal resection (EMR) and mucosal ablation of esophageal lesions are emerging techniques directed at the destruction or removal of superficial lesions involving the mucosal and submucosal layers of the organ. Endoscopic ultrasound is usually used to confirm that a lesion is limited to these layers of the esophageal wall prior to therapy (Larghi

et al. 2005). EMR often entails removal of the lesion after submucosal saline injection to elevate a lesion from the muscularis propria. The lesion is then removed with an electrocautery snare and retrieved for pathologic examination. Band-assisted mucosectomy utilizes a clear plastic cap with rubber bands similar to a variceal band ligator placed on the tip of the endoscope. The lesion can be sucked into the cap and a band placed to create a "pseudopolyp" that can then be removed with snare cautery (Seewald et al. 2006). Mucosal ablation may be performed using chemical, thermal, or mechanical methods. Modalities employed to ablate superficial lesions include multipolar electrocoagulation, argon plasma coagulation, photodynamic therapy, radiofrequency ablation, and cryotherapy (Garman et al. 2011). The depth of injury must be limited to the inner layers of the esophageal wall to avoid perforation, which is the major complication.

Barrett's esophagus is a complication of gastroesophageal reflux disease where the normal squamous mucosa of the distal esophagus is replaced with intestinal metaplasia. Rarely, Barrett's esophagus may lead to dysplasia and even progress to adenocarcinoma (Wiseman et al. 2011) (Fig. 3). Endoscopic ablation of dysplastic Barrett's esophagus has emerged as a popular alternative to both the passive "wait-and-watch" endoscopic surveillance strategy and the highly invasive esophagectomy strategy, with its substantial morbidity and mortality. The goal of endoscopic ablation is to remove the Barrett's epithelium, and allow regeneration of squamous mucosa in an alkaline milieu (usually with patients on high-dose proton pump inhibitor medications). Radiofrequency ablation (RFA) is the most common method of ablation and uses endoscopically placed electrodes on catheters to ablate the Barrett's mucosa. Over 80 % of patients can achieve complete eradication of their Barrett's with RFA (Shaheen et al. 2009). Cryotherapy using an endoscopically guided catheter to spray liquid nitrogen on the Barrett's is another method of ablation (Shaheen et al. 2010).

Complications related to mucosal ablation techniques will depend on the methods used, the types of lesions treated, and the experiences of the operators, and are similar to those discussed in the section on esophageal hemorrhage. Complications are rare but include stricture, pain, hemorrhage, perforation and

Fig. 3 a Tapered stricture (*arrows*) in the mid-esophagus with lower normal-appearing segment consistent with Barrett's esophagus, which was confirmed at endoscopic examination. **b** Irregular nodularity and stricture in lower esophagus in a patient with Barrett's esophagus. Endoscopy with multiple biopsies showed complicating adenocarcinoma

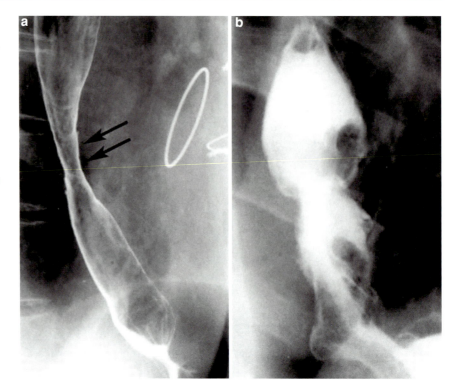

Fig. 4 a Frontal radiograph of chest shows "en-face" coin swallowed by a child with the appearance of the coin suggesting an esophageal location. **b** Lateral radiograph on the chest in the same patient shows the opposite orientation of the coin which is posterior to the trachea (T) and thus located in the esophagus

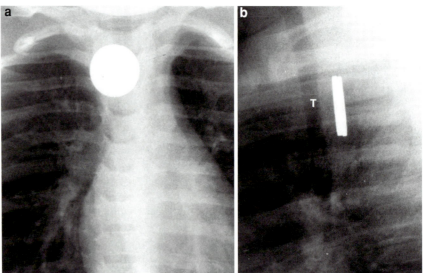

mediastinal processes (e.g., abscess). Radiologic imaging may be useful in pre-endoscopic evaluation of these patients, assessment of immediate complications (e.g., esophageal perforation or mediastinal abscess), or post-procedural evaluation of patients with potential symptomatic complications (e.g., dysphagia and stricture formation) (Levine 2005; Yamamoto et al. 2001).

4   Esophageal Foreign Bodies

Foreign body ingestion remains a common problem and although the actual incidence is difficult to estimate, reports indicate that between 1,500 and 2,750 deaths occur annually in the United States as a result of this problem (Ginsberg and Pfau 2010). Up to 90 % of

Fig. 5 **a** Food (*F*) impaction in the lower esophagus with small amount of contrast material progressing below the impaction. **b** Post-endoscopic removal of the food impaction, which was a meat bolus. Repeat contrast examination shows a stricture (*arrows*) and hiatal hernia

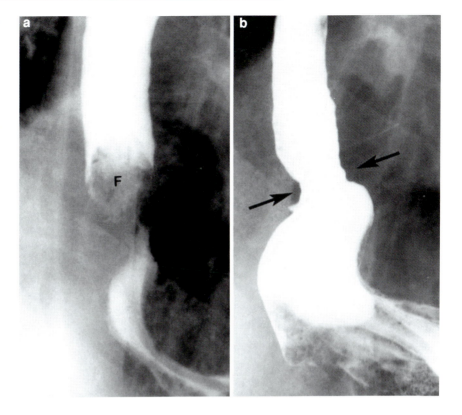

Fig. 6 **a** Food impacted in the lower end of the esophagus. Radiographic attempts at dis-impaction of the food using gas crystals were unsuccessful. **b** Food impaction was removed using several endoscopic accessories. Repeat contrast examination shows a mild stricture (*arrows*) and hiatal hernia

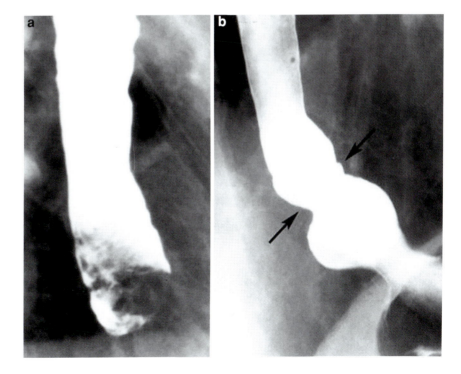

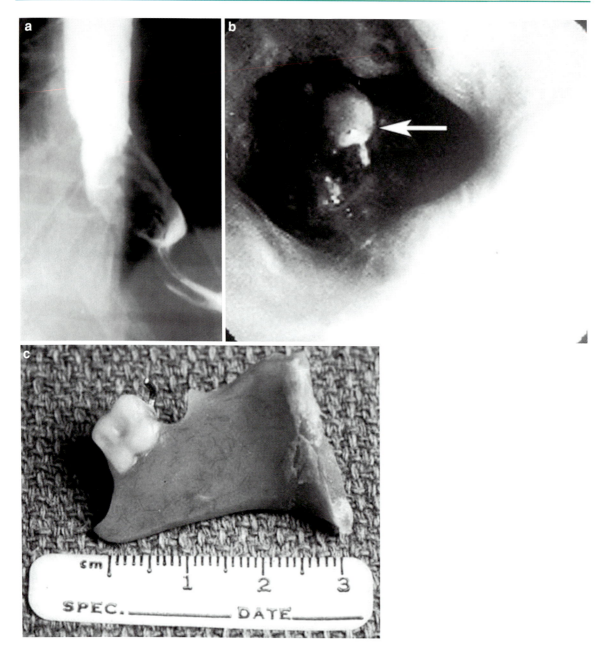

Fig. 7 a Patient swallowed a portion of a dental plate. Contrast esophagram shows a rectangular filling defect in the lower esophagus. **b** Endoscopic image shows a tooth (*arrow*) attached to the dental plate. **c** Photograph of the dental plate after endoscopic retrieval; no complications occurred during the procedure

swallowed objects that reach the stomach will pass uneventfully through the gastrointestinal tract, but the remaining 10 % may become lodged in the esophagus with subsequent risk to the patient. Potential complications from impacted esophageal foreign bodies include mucosal damage with bleeding, respiratory difficulty, luminal obstruction, perforation, and sinus tract and fistula formation to adjacent structures, which may lead to abscess, sepsis, and death. The goals of managing patients with potential esophageal foreign bodies include proper diagnosis, relief of symptoms, and prevention of complications.

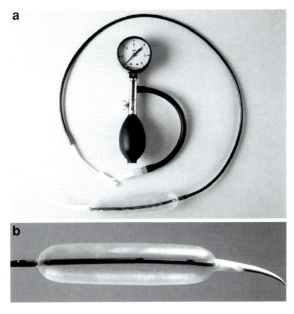

Fig. 8 a Microvasive pneumatic dilator (Boston Scientific, Watertown, MA), which is a popular instrument used to treat achalasia. b Inflated balloon end of the same dilator; balloons are available in various sizes, ranging from 3.0 to 4.0 cm

Foreign bodies in the esophagus typically impact at physiologic or pathologic areas of narrowing, with the most common site being the cervical inlet followed by the middle esophagus, and, least likely, the lower esophagus. In children, the foreign bodies seen most often include accidental ingestion of objects such as toys, coins, pins, batteries, and bones (Garza and Kaul 2010) (Fig. 4). Food impaction is more likely in adults, although other objects, such as dentures or partial dental plates, can be swallowed (Ayantunde and Oke 2006). The type and nature of the object ingested, the duration of impaction, the location of the ingested material, as well as other factors will determine the approach in treating the patient. The diagnosis and treatment of esophageal foreign bodies is usually performed with endoscopic techniques depending on these various considerations (Ginsberg and Pfau 2010); surgical exploration is rarely needed unless perforation or subsequent extra-luminal complications occur.

Radiologic imaging can be used for the initial evaluation of the patient with suspected esophageal foreign body impaction. Non-opaque foreign bodies in the esophagus can be evaluated with contrast examinations using water-soluble agents or barium suspensions; typically, only several swallows of the contrast

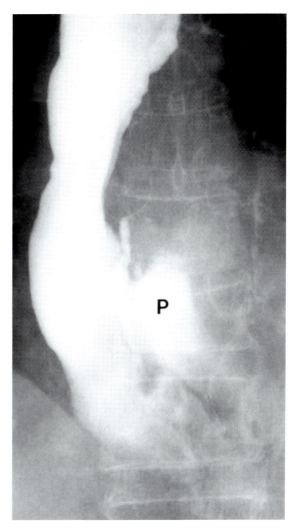

Fig. 9 Following pneumatic dilatation of the esophagus for achalasia, an intubated water-soluble contrast examination was performed which showed a large perforation (P) arising from the left lateral wall of the lower esophagus

material are needed to indicate the presence, size, and location of a non-opaque foreign body. The choice between the use of a water-soluble or a barium agent may depend on the suspected location of the foreign body (e.g., barium is safer if aspiration risk is high in a cervical impaction), on the preference of the clinician or radiologist, or on the possible presence of complications, such as perforation. If endoscopy may be needed to remove the foreign body after its diagnosis by radiologic examination, a water-soluble contrast is preferable since an opaque barium suspension prevents adequate visualization of the impacted material,

Fig. 10 Focal narrowing of the lower esophagus (*arrows*) due to peptic stricture

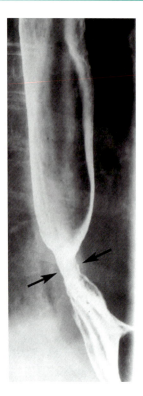

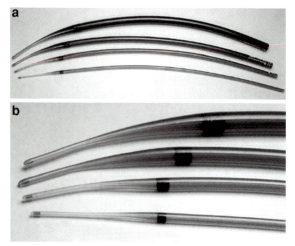

Fig. 11 a Savary-Gilliard esophageal dilators (Wilson-Cook Medical, Winston-Salem, NC) of various sizes. **b** Tapered tips of the same dilators. Sizes at the level of the dark rings are 20 mm (60F), 15 mm (45F), 11 mm (33F), and 8 mm (24F) from the top to bottom, respectively

making performance of the endoscopic procedure more difficult.

Depending on their structural nature (e.g., round and potentially mobile foreign bodies), radiologic removal of foreign bodies may be attempted (Fig. 5). For an acute distal food impaction, such as a piece of meat impacted in the lower esophagus, a radiologic approach using gas-crystals with water or a contrast material can be attempted (Kaszar-Seibert et al. 1990). The diagnosis of lower esophageal food impaction is first confirmed by radiological examination; the patient is then placed in the upright position and residual contrast material usually remains to outline the impacted material. The patient then ingests gas-producing crystals, followed immediately by water or dilute contrast material; the generation of gas above the food often propels it into the stomach, and the procedure can be repeated several times, as needed. The intravenous administration of glucagon (0.5–1.0 mg) may facilitate the passage of impacted food into the stomach using this technique (Colon et al. 1999). This method is successful and can be performed safely in most patients with lower esophageal food impactions.

Endoscopy can also be used for the diagnosis and, more importantly, the treatment of esophageal foreign bodies of various sizes and shapes, including sharp objects such as pins (Ginsberg and Pfau 2010). The endoscopic techniques employed to treat patients with foreign bodies in the esophagus will depend on several considerations, including the type of material impacted, but the therapeutic modality of choice is often endoscopic extraction (Narra and Al-Kawas 2010; Wu et al. 2011). Endoscopic accessories available for foreign body extraction include retrieval baskets, polyp grabbers, biopsy forceps, foreign body forceps, polypectomy snares, and overtubes (Fig. 6). Flexible (vs. rigid) endoscopic removal of a meat bolus is the preferred method of choice and can be performed much like standard endoscopic examinations. Coins, batteries, dental objects, and sharp and pointed objects require different and often more specific approaches (Fig. 7). The major risks of endoscopic removal include esophageal perforation, aspiration, and airway occlusion. Finally, following removal of a foreign body in the esophagus, regardless of the method used, a thorough radiographic or endoscopic examination should be performed to determine a potential underlying cause of the obstruction, such as a lower esophageal mucosal ring.

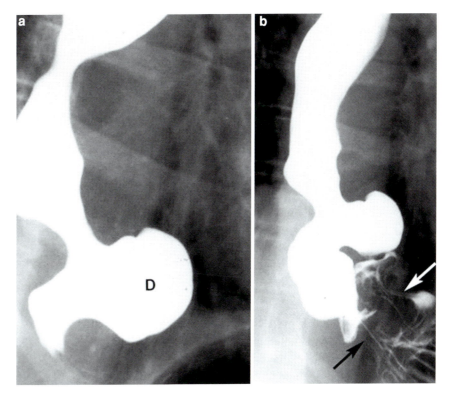

Fig. 12 **a** Pre-operative appearance of the lower esophagus in a patient with gastro-esophageal reflux disease showing a large epiphrenic diverticulum (*D*). **b** Following laparoscopic fundoplication, herniation of the operative site (*arrows*) has occurred. Patient developed recurrent symptoms of reflux disease several months after the procedure

5   Achalasia

Achalasia is characterized by aperistalsis of the esophagus and lower esophageal sphincter dysfunction (Francis and Katzka 2010). Treatment of achalasia involves reducing the functional obstruction of the sphincter to improve esophageal emptying and to relieve symptoms, such as dysphagia and regurgitation. Pneumatic dilatation of the esophagus (Fig. 8) and the modified Heller myotomy, which is now performed laparoscopically, are the most effective forms of therapy to treat achalasia (Francis and Katzka 2010; Imperiale et al. 2000). Local injection of botulinum toxin is performed under endoscopic guidance and may offer temporary relief by reducing the lower esophageal sphincter tone (Richter 2008).

The "open" Heller myotomy was the major alternative to pneumatic dilatation for the treatment of achalasia for many years, but is now done using laparoscopic techniques (Ackroyd et al. 2001; Katilius and Velanovich 2001; Patti and Herbella 2010). Similar to the open surgical methods, incision of the muscular layers of the esophagogastric junction over a short segment is performed laparoscopically. The addition

of an anti-reflux wrap (partial or total) following cardiomyotomy has been controversial, but a small percentage of patients will develop gastro-esophageal reflux, which may be alleviated by use of an anti-reflux procedure. Complications of this procedure may be immediate or delayed and include perforation at the operated site, gastro-esophageal reflux, and stricture; many of these potential complications can be evaluated with radiographic contrast examinations.

Pneumatic dilatation of the lower esophagus for the treatment of achalasia involves placement of an inflatable balloon across the esophagogastric junction using fluoroscopic guidance (Katz et al. 1998; Richter and Boeckxstaens 2011; Emami et al. 2008; Vaezi et al. 2002; Ott et al. 1991). Larger pneumatic dilators, which measure 3.0–4.0 cm in diameter, are available for this procedure, although a wide variety of different types of dilators were used in the past. The Rigiflex pneumatic dilator (Microvasive, Milford, MA) in the 30 or 35 mm sizes is commonly employed; a guidewire is placed into the stomach through an endoscope and its location verified fluoroscopically. The dilator is advanced over the guidewire and the balloon positioned at the esophagogastric junction. One or more inflations of the balloon can be

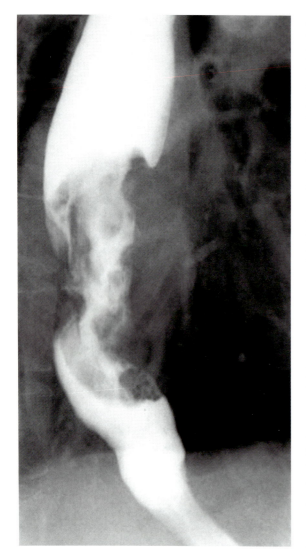

Fig. 13 Advanced, annular squamous cell carcinoma of the lower esophagus

studies, especially if esophageal intubation is used, there are conflicting reports on the value of the radiologic examination in predicting the clinical response of the patient. Parameters that have been studied include changes in the radiographic appearance of the esophagogastric region, rate of esophageal emptying using various contrast materials or radionuclide agents, type and size of the dilators and techniques used, inflation pressures generated and their duration, presence or absence of blood on the dilator, severity of chest pain during the procedure, and changes in manometric measurements, such as the lower esophageal sphincter pressure. Most investigations have shown that these parameters fail to predict the long-term results after pneumatic dilatation.

Regarding radiographic changes following pneumatic dilatation, an increase in the caliber of the esophagogastric junction commonly occurs following this procedure. In a compilation of six reports using various types of dilators and techniques, the mean caliber of the esophagogastric junction increased from pre-dilation widths of 2.3–4.7 mm to post-dilation calibers of 4.8–10.0 mm (Ott and Chen 1998). Clinical improvement in these investigations was seen in 59 to 88 % of the patients treated, but no significant correlation was found between the symptomatic response of the patient and the change in caliber of the esophagogastric region. In addition, the contour of the post-dilated esophagus (i.e., smooth vs. irregular) and the status of esophageal emptying (i.e., immediate vs. delayed) do not correlate well in predicting the long-term relief of patient symptoms (Ott et al. 1991). Thus, the main role of the radiographic examination used immediately following pneumatic dilatation for achalasia is to assess for serious complications, such as perforation, which may necessitate emergency surgery. Smaller intramural or confined perforations of the esophagus may also be seen in patients undergoing pneumatic dilatation and are often amenable to more conservative management.

performed; the impression from the lower esophageal sphincter is evident transiently by a constriction at the waist of the balloon, but disappears quickly. Potential complications include malplacement of the dilator, mucosal injury with bleeding, intramural hemorrhage, and perforation.

Radiographic evaluation of the esophagus following pneumatic dilation is useful to detect serious complications, such as perforation (Fig. 9), which occurs in about 5 % or less of patients using modern dilators (Ott et al. 1991; Vaezi et al. 2002). Although perforation of the esophagus is easily determined with contrast

6   Peptic Stricture

Focal narrowing of the esophagus results from a variety of inflammatory and neoplastic processes, but peptic stricture of the lower esophagus is one of the most common causes (Ferguson 2005; Pregun et al. 2009). Gastro-esophageal reflux disease can cause

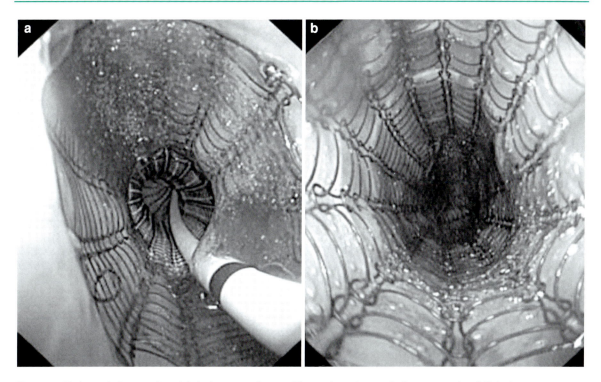

Fig. 14 **a** Endoscopic image of partial deployment of a metallic esophageal stent. **b** Same stent after full deployment

morphologic changes of reflux esophagitis that may progress to fibrotic narrowing and stricture formation (Luedtke et al. 2003; Johnston and Wong 2004; Ott 1994). The typical peptic stricture is located at the esophagogastric junction and is usually found in the presence of hiatus hernia (Fig. 10). Differential considerations for focal narrowings in the lower esophagus include mucosal ring, malignant strictures, and intrinsic strictures due to other factors, such as sclerotherapy, radiation, or caustic ingestion; in addition, extrinsic processes or those arising from the stomach may involve or invade the esophagus and mimic peptic stricture. Thus, in patients with dysphagia and focal esophageal narrowing, radiographic and endoscopic examination is warranted in assessing these differential causes before therapy is initiated.

Once the diagnosis of peptic stricture is established and malignancy (and Barrett's esophagus) has been excluded, therapeutic options can be considered. The clinical course of peptic stricture is usually chronic and progressive, and the importance of controlling the underlying causes of this disease (i.e., anti-reflux therapy) must be understood. More aggressive treatment of peptic stricture includes intralesional steroid injections, peroral esophageal dilatations, and

surgery (Ferguson 2005; Johnston and Wong 2004). Steroid injections into the site of stricture have been controversial, but may reduce inflammation and delay or possibly prevent fibrosis; however, patients receiving this form of therapy often require dilatations or even anti-reflux surgery.

Esophageal dilatation is usually the initial method of choice for treatment of benign strictures and has proven safe and effective in relieving associated dysphagia (Johnston and Wong 2004). Esophageal dilatation involves repetitive passage of increasingly larger dilators across a stricture, usually on a frequent basis, until a lumen size of 14–15 mm or larger is obtained. The three main types of dilators used in the United States are: (1) mercury-filled rubber types (Maloney or Hurst), (2) wire-guided Savary-Gilliard dilators (Fig. 11), and (3) balloon dilators that can be passed endoscopically or over a guide wire. These procedures may be performed using fluoroscopic guidance, but may be done in an outpatient setting, or performed by the patient at home. Esophageal perforation is the most serious complication of stricture dilation, although a variety of lesser problems, such as placement in the trachea or curling in the esophagus, may occur (Johnston and Wong 2004; Ferguson 2005).

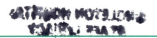

Fig. 15 a Radiographic appearance of partial deployment of an esophageal metallic stent for palliative treatment of esophageal carcinoma. **b** Water-soluble contrast examination of the esophagus the next day shows full deployment of the stent and patency of the lumen without complications, such as perforation

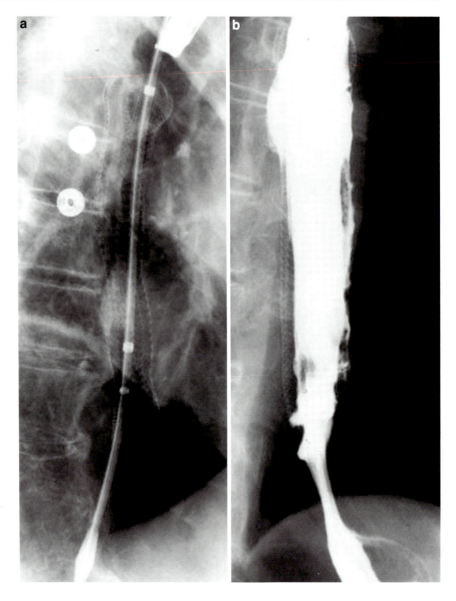

The esophageal perforation rate with the more modern dilators is extremely low, and is about 0.1–0.4 % per procedure; however, the risk is higher in more complex and narrower strictures (Ferguson 2005). Radiographic evaluation of patients following stricture dilation with suspected esophageal injury is similar to evaluating any individual with suspected esophageal perforation.

Surgical therapy for peptic stricture is indicated in those who have failed repeated esophageal dilatations or are not suitable for aggressive medical therapy (Johnston and Wong 2004). Anti-reflux operations available to patients with reflux disease and often refractory complications have evolved in recent years from open thoracic or abdominal procedures to those performed using laparoscopic techniques (Klingler et al. 1999). The standard open Nissen fundoplication was the most commonly used procedure, and whether partial or complete fundic wraps were used depended on factors such as the effectiveness of esophageal peristalsis and potential avoidance of post-operative dysphagia or "gas-bloat" syndrome. These procedures have been modified for laparoscopic use; however, post-operative complications, both acute and late in origin, can occur, which may warrant radiographic evaluation (Fig. 12) (Baker et al. 2007).

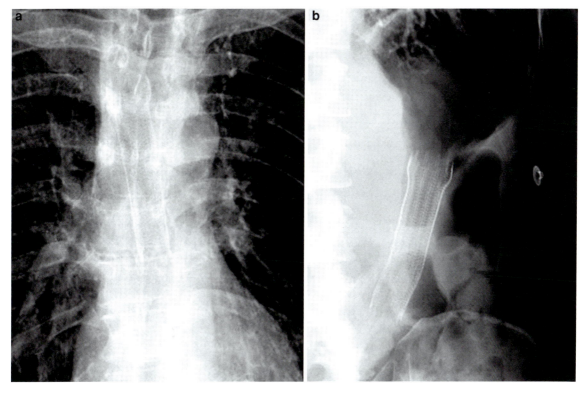

Fig. 16 **a** Fully deployed metallic stent in the mid-esophagus at the level of the aortic arch and carina on a plain chest radiograph. **b** Patient developed dysphagia and the stent was no longer seen in its previous location on the chest film. An abdominal radiograph showed that the stent had dislodged and migrated into the stomach

7 Esophageal Malignancy

Squamous cell carcinoma and adenocarcinoma are the most common primary esophageal malignancies (Chen et al. 1999; Lagergren and Lagergren 2010). Early diagnosis of esophageal carcinoma portends a better prognosis because the size of the lesion and extent of invasion into the esophageal wall are related; however, in the absence of effective screening programs, esophageal malignancy is usually diagnosed as a more advanced tumor, that has invaded adjacent organs and is associated with a poor survival (Fig. 13). Adenocarcinoma has increased dramatically in prevalence; this malignancy typically originates in the lower esophagus and may arise from the esophageal glands, heterotopic gastric mucosal, or metaplastic columnar epithelium, a so-called Barrett's carcinoma (Dent 2011). Indeed, the most common origin is believed to be dysplastic Barrett's epithelium. Surgery for esophageal malignancy may be performed for curative intent, but endoscopic procedures and the use of a variety of endoluminal stents can be used to manage these patients.

Malignant obstruction of the esophagus and palliation of dysphagia or associated complications (e.g., mediastinal sinus tract or airway fistula) are commonly treated with endoscopic methods (Sharma and Kozarek 2010). Mucosal ablation or resection techniques for possible curative treatment of early esophageal malignancy or management of Barrett's esophagus were discussed previously. A tissue diagnosis is important initially because esophageal stricture or obstruction may be due to a benign or malignant cause, and early treatment may be similar. Tumor ablation combined with serial dilatations can destroy and reduce malignant tissue bulk and also increase the luminal diameter of the esophagus to relieve dysphagia and improve nutrition of the patient. If the various tumor ablation techniques and standard dilatations are not successful or need to be repeated frequently, endoscopic stent placement offers another option.

Endoscopic stent placement for malignant obstruction of the esophagus has evolved in recent years, from the use of plastic stents to the deployment of expandable metallic stents (Bethge and Vakil 2001; van Heel et al. 2010; Qureshi et al. 2009). Large-diameter plastic stents were successful in relieving dysphagia in selected patients, but have been replaced by the metallic stents; complications included migration, tumor overgrowth, and obstruction, which were evaluated with radiographic filming and contrast examinations. Expandable metallic stents provide a newer approach to palliative treatment of malignant strictures that offers several advantages (Fig. 14). The stent introducers are smaller in diameter (some pass through the endoscopic channels), which limits the need for extensive dilatation of the area of malignant narrowing and thus avoidings potential complications, such as perforation of the esophagus (Fig. 15). The expandable stents are also designed to slowly create radial forces that enlarge the luminal diameter until the stent is fully expanded. Coated stents are available that help to prevent tumor in-growth through the metallic mesh and permit the closure of sinus tracts, fistulas, and perforations. Disadvantages of metallic stents include their cost, difficulties with migration, and the continued problem of tumor growth and occlusion. As with plastic stents, radiographic imaging is helpful in evaluation of the position of the stents in the esophagus and associated complications (Fig. 16) (Battersby et al. 2012; Vleggaar and Siersema 2011).

8   Conclusion

In conclusion, management of esophageal diseases in the past consisted primarily of diagnosis and possibly surgical or radiation treatment. Major advancements in esophageal intervention have occurred in recent years, especially with the use of endoscopic techniques. The endoscopist typically performs many of these interventional procedures, but imaging may be required before, during, or after the endoscopic intervention is performed. In this chapter we have discussed a variety of esophageal problems amenable to endoscopic intervention and reviewed the role of imaging in assisting in the management of these disorders and their potential complications.

References

Albillos A, Peñas B, Zamora J (2010) Role of endoscopy in primary prophylaxis for esophageal variceal bleeding. Clin Liver Dis 14:231–250

Ackroyd R, Watson DI, Devitt PG, Jamieson GG (2001) Laparoscopic cardiomyotomy and anterior partial fundoplication for achalasia. Surg Endosc 15:683–686

Ayantunde AA, Oke T (2006) A review of gastrointestinal foreign bodies. Int J Clin Pract 60:735–739

Baker ME, Einstein DM, Herts BR, Remer EM, Motta-Ramirez GA, Ehrenwald E, Rice TW, Richter JE (2007) Gastroesophageal reflux disease: integrating the barium esophagram before and after antireflux surgery. Radiology 243:329–339

Bethge N, Vakil N (2001) A prospective trial of a new self-expanding plastic stent for malignant esophageal obstruction. Am J Gastroenterol 96:1350–1354

Battersby NJ, Bonney GK, Subar D, Talbot L, Decadt B, Lynch N (2012) Outcomes following oesophageal stent insertion for palliation of malignant strictures: A large single centre series. J Surg Oncol 105:60–65

Chen LQ, Hu CY, Ghadirian P, Duranceau A (1999) Early detection of esophageal squamous cell carcinoma and its effects on therapy: an overview. Dis Esophagus 12:161–167

Colon V, Grade A, Pulliam G, Johnson C, Fass R (1999) Effect of doses of glucagon used to treat food impaction on esophageal motor function of normal subjects. Dysphagia 14:27–30

Dent J (2011) Barrett's esophagus: A historical perspective, an update on core practicalities and predictions on future evolutions of management. J Gastroenterol Hepatol 26: 11–30 (suppl 1)

Emami MH, Raisi M, Amini J, Tabatabai A, Haghighi M, Tavakoli H, Hashemi M, Fude M, Farajzadegan Z, Goharian V (2008) Pneumatic balloon dilation therapy is as effective as esophagomyotomy for achalasia. Dysphagia 23:155–160

Ferguson DD (2005) Evaluation and management of benign esophageal strictures. Dis Esophagus 18:359–364

Francis DL, Katzka DA (2010) Achalasia: update on the disease and its treatment. Gastroenterology 139:369–374

Garman KS, Shaheen NJ (2011) Ablative therapies for Barrett's esophagus. Curr Gastroenterol Rep 13:226–239

Garza JM, Kaul A (2010) Gastroesophageal reflux, eosinophilic esophagitis, and foreign body. Pediatr Clin North Am 57:1331–1345

Ginsberg GG, Pfau PR (2010) Foreign bodies, bezoars, and caustic ingestions. In: Feldman M, Friedman LS, Brandt LJ (eds) Sleisenger and fordtran: gastrointestinal and liver disease, 9th edn. WB Saunders, Philadelphia

Imperiale TF, O'Connor B, Vaezi MF, Richter JE (2000) A cost-minimization analysis of alternative treatment strategies for achalasia. Am J Gastroenterol 95:2737–2745

Johnston MH, Wong R (2004) Esophageal strictures. In: Castell DO, Richter JE (eds) The esophagus, 4th edn. Lippincott, Williams & Wilkins, Philadelphia

Kaszar-Seibert DJ, Korn WT, Bindman DJ, Shortsleeve MJ (1990) Treatment of acute esophageal food impaction with a combination of glucagon, effervescent agent, and water. AJR 154:533–534

Katilius M, Velanovich V (2001) Heller myotomy for achalasia: quality of life comparison of laparoscopic and open approaches. JSLS 5:227–231

Katz PO, Gilbert J, Castell DO (1998) Pneumatic dilatation is effective long-term treatment for achalasia. Dig Dis Sci 43:1973–1977

Klingler PJ, Bammer T, Wetscher GJ, Glaser KS, Seelig MH, Floch NR, Branton SA, Hinder RA (1999) Minimally invasive surgical techniques for the treatment of gastroesophageal reflux disease. Dig Dis 17:23–36

Kochhar R, Goenka MK, Mehta SK (1992) Esophageal strictures following endoscopic variceal sclerotherapy. Dig Dis Sci 37:347–352

Lagergren J, Lagergren P (2010) Oesophageal cancer. BMJ 341:1207–1212

Larghi A, Lightdale CJ, Memeo L, Bhagat G, Okpara N, Rotterdam H (2005) EUS followed by EMR for staging of high-grade dysplasia and early cancer in Barrett's esophagus. Gastrointest Endosc 62:16–23

Levine MS (2005) Barrett esophagus: update for radiologists. Abdom Imaging 30:133–141

Luedtke P, Levine MS, Rubesin SE, Weinstein DS, Laufer I (2003) Radiologic diagnosis of benign esophageal strictures: a pattern approach. Radiographics 23:897–909

Narra S, Al-Kawas FH (2010) The importance of preparation and innovation in the endoscopic management of esophageal foreign bodies. Gastroenterol Hepatol 6:795–797

Ott DJ (1994) Gastroesophageal reflux disease. Radiol Clinics North Am 32:1147–1166

Ott DJ, Chen MYM (1998) What is the value of the radiological diameter of the esophagogastric junction following dilation? In: Giuli R, Galmiche JP, Jamieson GG, Scarpignato C (eds) The esophagogastric junction. John Libbey, Paris, pp 1356–1359

Ott DJ, Donati D, Wu WC, Chen MYM, Gelfand DW (1991) Radiographic evaluation of achalasia immediately after pneumatic dilatation with the Rigiflex dilator. Gastrointest Radiol 16:279–282

Patti MG, Herbella FA (2010) Fundoplication after laparoscopic Heller myotomy for esophageal achalasia: what type? J Gastrointest Surg. 14:1453–1458

Pregun I, Hritz I, Tulassay Z, Herszényi L (2009) Peptic esophageal stricture: medical treatment. Dig Dis 27:31–37

Qureshi I, Shende M, Luketich JD (2009) Surgical palliation for Barrett's esophagus cancer. Surg Oncol Clin N Am 18:547–560

Richter JE (2008) Update on the management of achalasia: balloons, surgery and drugs Expert Rev. Gastroenterol Hepatol 2:435–445

Richter JE, Boeckxstaens GE (2011) Management of achalasia: surgery or pneumatic dilation. Gut 60:869–876

Seewald S, Ang TL, Omar S, Groth S, Dy F, Zhong Y, Seitz U, Thonke F, Yekebas E, Izbicki J, Soehendra N (2006) Endoscopic mucosal resection of early esophageal squamous cell cancer using the Duette mucosectomy kit. Endoscopy 38:1029–1031

Shah VH, Kamath PS (2010) Portal hypertension and gastrointestinal bleeding. In: Feldman M, Friedman LS, Brandt LJ (eds) Sleisenger & Fordtran: gastrointestinal and liver disease, 9th edn. WB Saunders, Philadelphia

Shaheen NJ, Sharma P, Overholt BF et al. (2009) Radiofrequency ablation in Barrett's esophagus with dysplasia. N Engl J Med 360:2277–2288

haheen NJ, Greenwald BD, Peery AF et al. (2010) Safety and efficacy of endoscopic spray cryotherapy for Barrett's esophagus with high-grade dysplasia. Gastrointest Endosc 71:680–685

Sharara AI, Rockey DC (2001) Gastroesophageal variceal bleeding. N Engl J Med 345:669–681

Sharma P, Kozarek R (2010) Role of esophageal stents in benign and malignant diseases. Am J Gastroenterol 105:258–273

Vaezi MF, Baker ME, Achkar E, Richter JE (2002) Timed barium oesophagram: better predictor of long term success after pneumatic dilation in achalasia than symptom assessment. Gut 50:765–770

van Heel NC, Haringsma J, Spaander MC, Bruno MJ, Kuipers EJ (2010) Esophageal stents for the relief of malignant dysphagia due to extrinsic compression. Endoscopy 42:536–540

Vleggaar FP, Siersema PD (2011) Expandable stents for malignant esophageal disease. Gastrointest Endosc Clin N Am 21:377–388

Wallace MB (2004) Special endoscopic imaging and optical techniques. In: Castell DO, Richter JE (eds) The esophagus, 4th edn. Lippincott, Williams & Wilkins, Philadelphia

Wu WT, Chiu CT, Kuo CJ, Lin CJ, Chu YY, Tsou YK, Su MY (2011) Endoscopic management of suspected esophageal foreign body in adults. Dis Esophagus 24:131–137

Wiseman EF, Ang YS (2011) Risk factors for neoplastic progression in Barrett's esophagus. World J Gastroenterol 17:3672–3683

Yamamoto AJ, Levine MS, Katzka DA, Furth EE, Rubesin SE, Laufer I (2001) Short-segment Barrett's esophagus: findings on double-contrast esophagography in 20 patients. AJR Am J Roentgenol 176:1173–1178

The Importance of Enteral Nutrition

Christina Stene and Bengt Jeppsson

Contents

C. Stene (✉)
Department of Surgery, Ängelholm Hospital,Institute
of Clinical Sciences, Lund University,
Malmö, Sweden
e-mail: christina.stene@med.lu.se

B. Jeppsson
Department of Surgery,
University Hospital of Skane-Malmö,
Institute of Clinical Sciences, Lund University,
Malmö, Sweden

Abstract

Many neurological diseases are followed by a disturbance of nutritional intake to some extent and thus constitute the most common indication for nutritional support and enteral access. Several studies have shown that malnutrition is a common condition, with as many as 40% of admitted patients being identified as undernourished and 78% of these further found to be deteriorated in their nutritional status during hospital stay (McWirtrer and Pennington in BMJ 308:945–948, 1994). Malnutrition being a preventable disorder, it is thus of great importance to identify patients at risk of malnutrition and prevent impairment of nutritional status (Johansen et al. in Clin Nutr 23:539–550, 2004). With adequate nutritional care, improved healing is augmented, resulting in better care and quality of life, lowered costs due to reduced length of hospital stay, fewer complications, and decreased mortality. Gut starvation hampers the immunological response. Even small amounts of enteral nutrition maintain gastrointestinal mucosal integrity and improve barrier function, thus minimizing immunological complications and enhancing clinical recovery.

O. Ekberg (ed.), *Dysphagia*, Medical Radiology. Diagnostic Imaging, DOI: 10.1007/174_2012_578,
© Springer-Verlag Berlin Heidelberg 2012

1 The Importance of Enteral Nutrition

The value of nutritional support and the risks and implications of malnutrition of sick patients who are to undergo elective surgical intervention have been well documented in the literature in recent decades. Neurological diseases constitute the most common indication for nutritional support and enteral access since a wide variety of neurological conditions result in dysphagia, aspiration, swallowing disorders, or a combination of these symptoms (Phillips and Ponsky 2011).

Malnutrition is common prior to or after stroke, with dysphagia—a frequent manifestation of stroke—adding to nutrition risk (Corrigan et al. 2011). Malnutrition is a preventable disorder. During the acute and rehabilitation phases of stroke, nutritional intervention is the mainstay of the interdisciplinary approach to the care and treatment of these patients.

When cognitive functions are affected, such as visual neglect, or there is a concomitant depressive state where the patient is reluctant to eat, or there is a neurological deficit, e.g., paresis of the upper extremities or apraxia, the patient's ability to ingest food will be hampered, thus influencing nutritional intake and increasing the risk of malnutrition (Corrigan et al. 2011).

In elderly multimorbid patients, nutritional and fluid intake is often compromised and preventive nutritional support has to be considered at an early stage as restoration of body cell mass here is more difficult than in younger persons. Further, difficulties in performing assisted feeding are more pronounced in the elderly (Volkert et al. 2006).

For patients with a normal-functioning gastrointestinal tract who require nutritional support, enteral access is the preferred mode through which to administer nourishment. Enteral nutrition has been proven to be safe and possesses a clear cost advantage as well as giving metabolic and immunity-linked benefits. Enteral access encompasses local nasogastric or nasoenteric tubes, endoscopic options comprising percutaneous endoscopic gastrostomy (PEG) and percutaneous endoscopic jejunostomy, and a surgical approach (gastrostomy, e.g., Witzel technique, or jejunostomy), the later confined to patients who opted for or were chosen for abdominal surgery or in cases where the endoscopic procedure is deemed not feasible.

Parenteral nutrition should be restricted to patients with contraindications for the use of the enteral pathway, e.g., with a nonfunctioning gastrointestinal tract due to ileus/mechanical obstruction, fistulas of the upper gastrointestinal tract, or a reduced visceral blood flow.

To evaluate or assess the nutritional status of a patient, the specific demands of that individual must be reflected upon to form a basis for selection of the optimal treatment strategy for the patient on his or her journey through the disease (Howard et al. 2006). Knowledge of the various treatment methods, risks, and advantages associated with the different options is a prerequisite for being able to lead the patient through the most effective and tailored nutritional support.

Satisfactory supply of nutrients is important for the many tasks of the gastrointestinal tract. In addition to its role in digestion of food and the absorption of nutrients, it also constitutes a barrier between the luminal content and the blood circulation and lymphatics, and also houses a large proportion of the immune system of the body. This explains the importance of maintaining the gut in as good a condition as possible during periods of disease and reduced ability in providing the body with a normal dietary intake.

Technical progress concerning access to the gastrointestinal tract as well as the diverse formulae suitable for upgrading a variety of states of impaired nutritional needs has now made it unacceptable to allow patients who are unable to maintain nutritional support in a normal way or other ways to become malnourished and for this to result in any complications, distress, or even death by starvation (Dudrick and Palesty 2011).

If 7 days has elapsed without the patient being able to achieve a sufficient oral intake of aliments or if the patient has been unable to take in at least 60% of the estimated daily nutrient demands, nutritional support should be initiated without delay, in the first instance by the enteral route (Arends et al. 2006; Jayarajan and Daly 2011). Nutritional support is indispensable for patients who cannot achieve full supply of energy and substrate demands.

Early enteral feeding has largely shown positive results compared with the parenteral feeding, resulting in a better outcome, with a reduction in the complication rate, lower incidence of infections and

Intestinal lumen

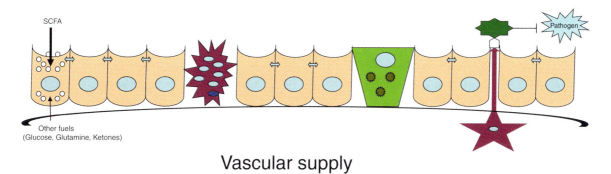

Vascular supply

Fig. 1 Immunocompetent cells of different characters are located between the intestinal mucosal cells. The main part of nourishment for enterocytes and colonocytes is received from the intestinal lumen and only a minor part is received from the circulation

sepsis, improved wound healing, and a decreased length of hospital stay. Immunological benefits are also seen in enteral feeding. The European Society for Clinical Nutrition and Metabolism (ESPEN) and the American Society for Parenteral and Enteral Nutrition (ASPEN) have recommended gut feeding as the method of choice when the gastrointestinal tract is able to tolerate enteral supply.

It has been shown that it is not necessary to remove an orogastric feeding tube in order to assess the state of dysphagia since an objective swallowing evaluation can be performed with such a tube in place (Leder et al. 2011).

The cells of the intestinal mucosa (the enterocytes and colonocytes) receive around 70% of their nourishment from the intestinal lumen and only a minor part, around 20–30%, from the circulation (Fig. 1). The inner epithelial cell layer has a high cell turnover, the cells being exchanged every 2–3 days, thus requiring sufficient nutritional supply for this high metabolism. The presence of nutrients in the intestinal lumen is the most potent stimulus for proliferation of mucosal cells as well as for other functions such as hormonal release and production of intestinal juices involved in the absorption of nutritional components. The daily endogenous gastrointestinal fluid production is about 8,000–9,000 ml, of which the small intestine itself accounts for around 3,500 ml.

Dietary fibers are fermented by bacteria in the colon to short chain fatty acids (SCFAs) that are absorbed by the liver and included in the energy metabolism. SCFAs have been shown to have a beneficial effect on the microcirculation of the intestinal mucosa, as well as a trophic effect since they constitute energy substrates for the colonic mucosa, stimulating fluid and electrolyte absorption (Schneider et al. 2006). The amino acid glutamine is the preferred source of fuel for the enterocytes.

Intake of nutrients per se may be at any rate as essential as body mass and structure to preserve normal function and its effects on the intestinal structure are closely linked to loss of luminal nutrition rather than to the metabolic consequences itself. In healthy volunteers it has been observed that if the gastrointestinal tract is not used or there is a short-term loss of nutrients in the intestinal lumen, the absorptive capacity of the small intestine is reduced within 36 h. A sustained total parenteral nutrition leads to atrophy of enterocytes of the small intestine as well as changes in the enteric nerve system, which may explain difficulties encountered during transition from total parenteral nutrition to oral feeding.

Many studies have shown that the concept of "minimal enteral nutrition," meaning a supply of small amounts of enteral nutrition to provide the intestinal mucosa with necessary nutrients and then completing the rest of the patient's nutritional demands by the intravenous route, is an useful way of preserving gut integrity.

The gut absorptive function is dependent on gut motility, and therefore stimulation of gastrointestinal motility is an important part of nutritional support. Enteral nutrition also enhances biliary and pancreatic secretions, which are important for maintenance of gut integrity and reduction of the risk of gallbladder sludge or gallstone formation.

Many factors seem to be of great importance with regard to wound healing, but nutritional status and especially lately nutritional intake seem to be a crucial aspect to bear in mind when dealing with patients.

2 The Importance of Gut Function

2.1 Surface

The intestinal mucosa, constituting the innermost layer of the intestinal wall, is made up of three layers (epithelium, connective tissue, and smooth muscle) and is responsible for the important functions of the gastrointestinal tract: absorption, digestion, and secretion. The structure of the mucosa is very specialized depending on in which part of the gastrointestinal tract it is exerting its function. It is folded (constituting villi), resulting in an increased surface area.

The intestinal surface is considered to cover a very large area; the exact size is difficult to establish and differs between individuals, extending to around 250 m^2 (equivalent to a doubles tennis court). It is in fact the body's largest surface area, considering all the food that is passing through it. Its main function is absorption of nutrients. The small intestine has a length of about 3.5 m. The minimal length required to ensure significant absorption of nutrients is about 1 m.

When blood flow to the gastrointestinal mucosa ceases, the absorptive surface area is reduced, a fact attributed to changes within villi comprising among other changes decreased villus height, reduction of cell proliferation and cell migration, and augmented apoptosis and cell death. Restoration of blood circulation providing nutritional supply leads to restored absorptive cell mass and the rates of nutrient absorption may be enhanced.

2.2 Bacteria

The gut microbiota fulfills several tasks, among which the most important are protective, immunoregulatory, and metabolic functions. All humans are intimately associated with an extensive population of microbial organisms existing in a symbiotic relationship (Fukatsu and Kudsk 2011). We host at least ten bacterial cells for every human cell. The gut constitutes a reservoir of bacteria, considering that every healthy human harbors 1–2 kg of bacteria, made up of up to 1,000 different species. This is beneficial as long as the balance between health-enhancing bacteria and potential pathogens is maintained. However, when the balance between commensal bacteria and the potentially pathogenic bacteria is altered, the situation may rapidly become detrimental. Since the intestinal microbiota contributes considerably to the production of amino acids and the gut microbes are also involved in the production of fatty acids and in the synthesis of vitamins, e.g., the essential nutrient vitamin B_{12}, alterations in gut function will have wide implications.

Bacteria are, as previously mentioned, highly involved in the process of degrading dietary fibers, thus contributing to a large extent to the intestinal mucosal cells' nourishment and the energy metabolism. Critically ill patients often have a pathologic colonization of the gastrointestinal tract, which is a key factor in the development of multiple-organ failure. The colonization may cause infection by the patient's endogenous flora. This development is the result of a combination of an impaired local defense, the lack of enteral stimulation, and the presence of invasive measures, e.g., the use of broad-spectrum antibiotics that causes a change in the endogenous flora. An alteration of the intestinal microbiota caused by even short-term antibiotic treatment may persist for several years (Jernberg et al. 2007).

Potential pathogens are prevented from colonizing and interacting with epithelial and immunological cells by the microbiota occupying intestinal surfaces (Fig. 2).

2.3 Barrier Function: Translocation

Besides its task to absorb nutrients, the gut constitutes a barrier between the outer surface and the internal milieu of the body.

Fig. 2 A balanced intestinal microbial flora under normal conditions and during disorder (e.g., in patients undergoing antibiotic therapy, total parenteral nutrition, starvation, or any other condition leading to altered composition of the luminal microbial content resulting in increased susceptibility to pathogenic attacks)

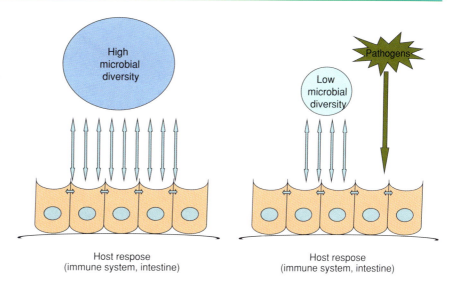

Under normal circumstances, several barriers, in collaboration with the adaptive immune system, effectively prevent the entry of bacteria into the systemic circulation (Fukatsu and Kudsk 2011). An impaired mucosal barrier may lead to passage of bacteria and/or endotoxins through the mucosal wall to the blood and further to other organs, a process termed "translocation." A subsequent activation of the immune response may enhance a septic reaction in a critically ill patient.

The absence of nutrients in the intestinal lumen, as well as total parenteral nutrition, leads to gut starvation with mucosal atrophy and risk of translocation. The presence of food in the gut lumen stimulates the mucosa mechanically as well as increasing blood flow. There is always an advantage in trying to nourish the patient through the gastrointestinal tract to achieve a normal barrier function.

2.4 Immune Function

The gastrointestinal tract constitutes one of the body's largest immunocompetent organs and is considered to harbor around 40% of the immune defense. Between the mucosal cells, various types of immunocompetent cells with different purposes are located, some capable of producing secretory antibodies, mucins, and macrophages, thus keeping the symbiotic microflora alert.

Enteral nutrition has positive effects on intestinal immunity and a local trophic effect on the gastrointestinal mucosa. A connection between the intestinal immune system in gut mucosa and the airway system has been described, with positive effects when enteral nutrition is provided.

Changes in immune function result in a reduced ability to prevent, fight, and recover from infection. Increased immune system activity increases the need for amino acids such as glutamine and alanine to facilitate protein synthesis in muscles and liver in order to prevent breakdown of endogenous proteins.

3 Metabolism

3.1 Starvation

The body is well prepared to withstand starvation (Fig. 3).

During a short period of starvation (12–24 h) glucose is released from breakdown of glycogen through glycogenolysis (giving around 4,000 kJ) to maintain blood glucose levels relatively invariable and to provide vital organs with a substrate. Degradation of fat occurs to a small extent as does degradation of amino acids. When starving is prolonged, the situation will be altered, as in Fig. 4.

The glycogenolysis is now modest since the glycogen supply is ended after 24 h fasting. The large energy store is the fat depot (210,000–250,000 kJ) and a continuous degradation of triglycerides to free fatty acids (FFAs) and glycerol takes place. FFAs and glycerol form ketone bodies in the liver and are used

Fig. 3 Metabolic changes during short-term fasting. *AA* amino acid, *FFA* free fatty acid

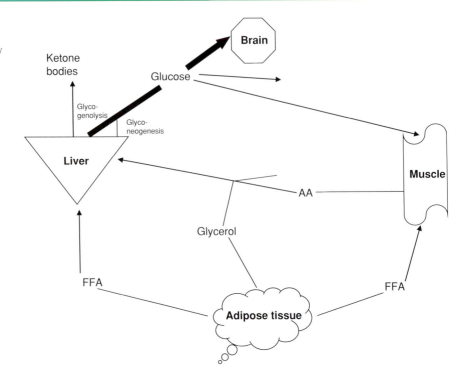

Fig. 4 Metabolic changes during long-term fasting

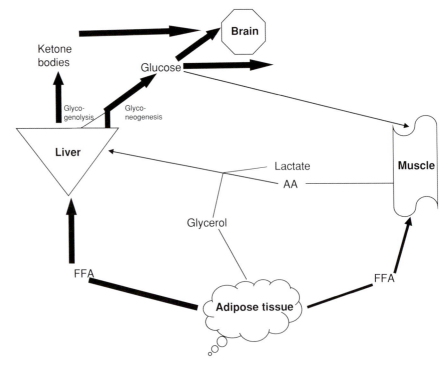

in the glyconeogenesis. FFAs may also be used directly by muscles as an energy source. The vital organs of the body, i.e., the brain, heart, red blood cells, etc., have now adapted their energy consumption in a way to use mainly ketone bodies and much less glucose. In this situation, the body avoids degradation of endogenous protein to save the muscles and other parts of body protein.

Fig. 5 Metabolic changes in trauma, sepsis, etc

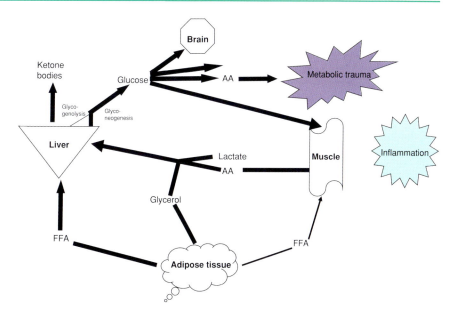

3.2   Starvation and Trauma/Sepsis

The situation is completely altered if during fasting the body is exposed to a metabolic trauma, e.g., either a planned or an acute operation, an accident, or a complication such as septicemia. Degradation of fat continues, but fat utilization in muscles and also in the liver with production of ketone bodies is strongly reduced. The body thereafter again uses glucose as an energy source, mainly obtaining glucose through glyconeogenesis from amino acids. A considerable degradation of muscle protein and release of amino acids occurs, and these are converted to glucose in the liver. At the same time, the amount of circulating amino acids increases and they are used as material for wound healing as well as for the production of acute-phase reactant proteins. The most important difference from the condition of long-term fasting is the imperfect fat use and the increasing proteolysis. These changes are to a great extent ruled by the neuroendocrine response with an increased release of stress hormones such as cathecholamines, cortisol, and glucagon. Simultaneously, this is also induced by some cytokines, released from activated macrophages and lymphocytes. Among these interleukin-1 is considered to play a crucial role.

On condition that adequate fluid supply is provided, a human may survive a long-term fasting period of up to 2 months.

The pathophysiological processes behind the body's response to trauma as described above are not fully known, but inflammation seems to play a vital role.

Starving in combination with trauma reduces the survival time to 20–30 days (Fig. 5).

3.3   Starvation and Cancer

The same pattern of reaction is seen in a patient with a malignant disease. The presence of a tumor involves some metabolic changes similar to those occurring in trauma. Around 50% of all cancer patients are expected to die of starvation. The tumor cells have an imperative need for glucose, and by incomplete combustion of glucose a huge amount of lactate is produced. Lactate is converted into glucose in the liver, and there is an exchange of glucose and lactate between the liver and tumor cells. In this process the body loses a great amount of energy when converting lactate to glucose. The degradation of fat depots continues unaltered as the production of ketone bodies seems to be normal. Simultaneously, a potent proteolysis occurs to keep the glyconeogenesis ongoing as well as to synthesize acute-phase proteins and also to meet the tumor cells' need for amino acids. It seems this proteolytic effect of the tumor is also mediated by cytokines, especially interleukin-1 and tumor necrosis factor. These substances also have

Fig. 6 Metabolic changes in cancer

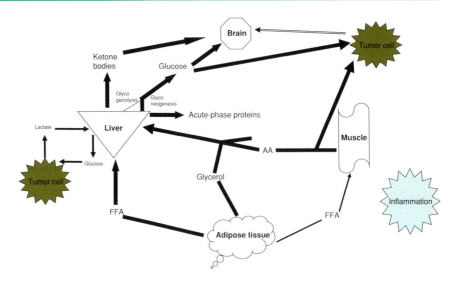

a direct effect on the saturation center in the brain, resulting in loss of appetite (anorexia), which further deteriorates the nutritional status of the patient.

In tumor patients, inflammation also plays an important role and thus decreasing inflammation is of value in the short term to reduce metabolic complications of starvation and in the long term in playing a role in cancer survival.

The patient is put into a catabolic condition not only by the tumor but also by the surgical/metabolic trauma. The stores of glucose in the liver and muscles as glycogen contain approximately 1,000 kcal (4,186 kJ) of energy. The total energy in fat in the form of triglycerides is approximately 50,000–60,000 kcal (209,340–251,208 kJ). If the body's muscle mass is converted into energy, this will result in about 10,000 kcal (41,868 kJ). Thus, it is evident that if these processes with strongly increased proteolysis cannot be broken down, the body's muscle mass will decrease rapidly, and since this will affect the respiratory muscles, the patient will be ruined (Fig. 6).

What can be done to cease this course of events? We know that adequate pain relief is important to reduce the stress response contributing to the inflammatory state. Epidural anesthesia is especially effective in this aspect. Providing anabolic hormones (androgens, growth hormone) reduces the proteolysis in muscle. It will also be hampered by muscular activity. Energy consumption may be reduced to a certain extent by increasing the indoor temperature. The most important thing is to ensure that the patient has an adequate nutritional supply.

4   Malnutrition

Malnutrition, described more specifically in the chapter "Complications of Oropharyngeal Dysphagia: Malnutrition and Aspiration Pneumonia" by Carrión et al. in this volume, is a condition arising as a result of too little, too much, or unbalanced intake of energy, protein, or other nutrients leading to measurable unfavorable effects on tissue, organs, body constitution, and body functions that will affect the outcome of clinical treatment. "Malnutrition" means "wrong alimentation" but is commonly used to describe insufficient nutrition, a state where intake during a long period is lower than the need of nutrients. Preexisting malnutrition occurs frequently, and is often seen upon admission to hospital in a variety of disease states, but malnutrition may also develop during the hospital stay. It has been estimated that over 50 million Europeans are at risk of disease-related malnutrition and up to 40% of hospital inpatients are expected to suffer from malnutrition.

The Council of Europe issued a resolution in November 2003 (Council of Europe, Committee of Ministers 2003) stating that screening for nutritional status must be performed on all admitted patients, that a plan for nutritional care must be made upon diagnosis of malnutrition, and that nutritional support must be an integral part of all therapies.

Nutritional screening is a rapid and simple process conducted by admission staff or community health care teams, whereas *nutritional assessment* is a detailed examination of metabolic, nutritional, or functional variables by an expert clinician, dietician, or nutrition nurse (Howard et al. 2006).

4.1 Consequences

Malnutrition is a risk factor for complications to hospital care and leads to an unfavorable outcome of treatment comprising infections, extended bed rest resulting in prolonged length of hospital stay, increased costs, and a delayed recovery, as well as a higher (up to eight times higher) mortality rate.

4.2 Diagnostics

All patients should undergo nutritional screening, and in the case of malnutrition, an assessment should be conducted regularly during the hospital stay. A patient at risk of malnutrition is defined as fulfilling one or more of the following criteria:

Involuntary weight loss.

Eating difficulties (e.g., loss of appetite, swallowing or chewing disabilities, problems of getting food into the mouth, problems concerning the oral cavity or teeth, nausea/vomiting).

Underweight (body mass index below 20 kg/m^{-2} if under 70 years and below 22 kg/m^{-2} if over 70 years). The presence of concomitant diseases/infections should also be taken into consideration.

5 Treatment of Insufficient Nutritional Intake

Oral nutrition is the first choice. Hospital food in adequate amounts should be energy-dense, contain balanced nutriments, and be palatable. If food intake is not sufficient, oral nutritional supplements (ONS; also denominated "sip feeds") as nutritional drinks and/or protein drinks are to be given. Mechanical alteration of food, as well as altered consistency of beverages, to achieve various textures might be one way of retaining some degree of oral intake. The possibility of fortification of food, or enriching food, should also be taken into consideration.

Mortality, morbidity, and complication rates are significantly reduced by using ONS compared with routine clinical care in patients at risk of disease-

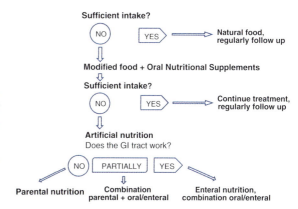

Nutritional treatment

Fig. 7 Stepwise decision tree

related malnutrition. Reduction of hospital length of stay has also been observed (Stratton et al. 2003).

ONS can:

- Improve energy and nutrient intake
- Improve body weight or attenuate weight loss
- Improve functional outcomes
- Improve clinical outcomes

The next step, if the above measures are not successful, is enteral nutrition by a feeding tube. The needs for each patient concerning energy and protein are determined by age, weight, activity, and degree of illness parameters. The nutritional plan as well as all other medical treatment should be documented in the medical record. If needed, e.g., in conditions of dysphagia, ENT tumors, or radiation injuries of the mouth, throat, or upper gastrointestinal tract, a feeding tube may be placed in the duodenum or in the jejunum. A percutaneous gastrostomy can also be considered.

If most of the patient's nutritional needs cannot be supplied by the above-mentioned measures, parental nutrition must be undertaken as a supplement to enteral nutrition, or exclusively if enteral nutrition fails or if one expects that gastrointestinal function may not allow enteral nutrition.

Nutrition is not a question of whether or not/all or nothing, but is a question of both feeding pathways:

Supplementation with enteral nutrition if complete oral nutrition cannot be achieved.

Supplementation with parenteral nutrition if total oral and enteral nutrition cannot be achieved.

Specialized nutritional teams trained and organized to provide nutritional support and working to standard protocols produce the best results, with

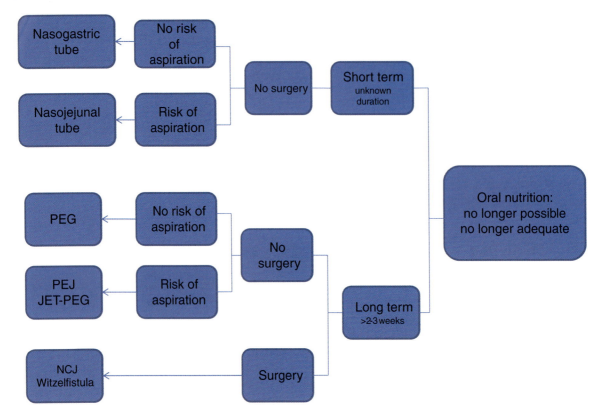

Fig. 8 Tube systems for enteral nutrition. *PEJ* percutaneous endoscopic jejunostomy, *JET-PEG* jejunal tube percutaneous endoscopic gastrostomy (a jejunal catheter placed through the percutaneous endoscopic gastrostomy to the jejunum beyond the ligament of Treitz when there are gastroduodenal motility problems), *NCJ* needle catheter jejunostomy

fewer complications and better outcomes than those who provide occasional or ad hoc treatment (Howard et al. 2006) (Fig. 7).

The patient's medical/surgical history and actual condition will be decisive for which feeding pathway should be used. This decision ought to be made shortly after hospital admission, to increase the opportunity for the patient to recover without complications. Enteral feeding is the preferred method if the gastrointestinal tract is functioning and no other contraindications exist. Assessing whether assisted feeding will be required short term or long term is the first step in this pathway, as depicted in Fig. 8.

Since successful nutritional care is built upon multidisciplinary cooperation, a nutritional support team including representatives of different professional groups working together to meet the patient's nutritional demands is fundamental.

Nutritional intervention can prevent or at least ameliorate any deterioration in nutritional status when normal eating is still possible but is inadequate to meet nutritional needs.

5.1 Calculation of Nutritional Needs

At the most, 7–10 days of inadequate oral intake is an indication for considering nutritional support (Arends et al. 2006) (Fig. 9).

To be able to start nutritional support early, it is useful to have some simplified rules to begin with as are outlined here in general terms. To start with, the energy need for most patients is about 25–30 kcal/kg per day, corrected if needed as shown in Fig. 10, especially during recovery and rehabilitation.

Energy and fluid needs should be assessed individually, taking into consideration the actual diagnosis and situation, in that metabolic needs may increase dramatically depending on the medical situation as illustrated in Fig. 11.

Nutritional treatment - different combinations

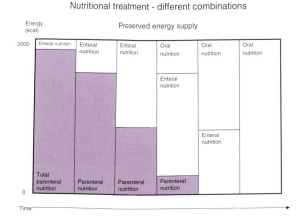

Calculation of nutritional needs

Fig. 9 Oral, enteral, and parenteral nutrition should complement each other to maintain adequate energy supply

The need for fluid should be estimated to around 30 ml/kg per day. The minimal need for protein is 0.8 g/kg per day although it may be 1.0–1.5 g/kg per day for sick patients. Vitamins and trace elements are given if required. If the patient is severely undernourished, a refeeding syndrome has to be avoided (i.e., when more nutrients are given than the tissue can metabolize, a condition that is more common when the supply is provided intravenously).

5.2 Enteral Solutions

Essentially two different kinds of enteral solutions are available. Most prevalent are so-called polymeric solutions, composed of whole protein, triglycerides, and glucose polymers along with electrolytes, trace elements, and vitamins. These solutions are available either in standard mode or as solutions with high energy and protein content. As a rule, the standard diet contains 6 g of nitrogen per liter and provides 1 kcal/ml, whereas the concentrated solution comprises 8–10 g of nitrogen per liter and an energy content of 1.5 kcal/ml. More than 90% of all patients needing enteral nutrition can satisfactorily be given these solutions. The second type of enteral solution is referred to as "elementary diet," meaning a split product where the components consist of amino acids, monosaccharides, essential fatty acids, minerals, and vitamins. The advantage of this solution is that it is more easily absorbed than the traditional enteral solution.

The characteristics of some commonly used enteral solutions shown listed in Fig. 12.

More than 100 "solutions" including homogenates, emulsions, suspensions, and powders mixed with water for enteral feeding are commercially available. Furthermore, ordinary foods can be modified for use as enteral feedings for infusion into the stomach. Some of these solutions are designed for general nutrition, whereas others are formulated for specific metabolic or clinical conditions and the contents thus differ greatly.

Solutions for enteral feeding can be classified as follows (Dudrick and Palesty 2011):

1. Natural foods—modified for providing complete nutrition by various routes.
2. Polymeric solutions—macronutrients in the form of isolates of intact protein, triglycerides, and carbohydrate polymers designed to provide complete nutrition by various routes.
3. Monomeric solutions—mixtures of proteins as peptides and/or amino acids; fat as long-chain triglycerides or a combination of long-chain triglycerides and medium-chain triglycerides; and carbohydrates as partially hydrolyzed starch maltodextrins and glucose oligosaccharides; for patients with disturbances of absorption or digestion.
4. Special metabolic solutions—for patients with unique metabolic requirements, e.g., failure of liver/lungs/kidneys/heart; including immune-modulating solutions (containing, e.g., ω-3 polyunsaturated fat, RNA, arginine, glutamine, taurine, carnitine, N-acetylcysteine, antioxidants, vitamins, and trace elements).
5. Modular solutions—nutritional components that may be given individually or mixed together to meet special needs of a patient (e.g., increased number of calories/amount of nitrogen, various minerals).
6. Hydration solutions—provide water, minerals, and small quantities of carbohydrates and/or amino acids as supplementation or as minimal humane support primarily for dehydrated and/or cachectic patients.
7. Medical foods—designed for special dietary purposes or as foods for which health claims have been made and which must be used under medical supervision.

Fig. 10 Estimation of energy demands

Average of energy demands per kg/daily

Basic metabolism (BMB)	= 90 kJ = 22 kcal
Confinement in bed: BMB + 30%	= 120 kJ = 29 kcal
Walking: BMB + 50%	= 140 kJ = 33 kcal
Convalescence: BMB + 80%	= 170 kJ = 40 kcal

Corrections

Thin patient	+ 10%
Obese patient	- 10%
Age between 18 - 30 years	+ 10%
Age 70+ years	- 10%
For each degree of temperature rise	+ 10%

Procentual energy increase in different clinical conditions

Increase (%)	Conditions
→ 100	Burn injury
40	Deep infections, sepsis
20	Trauma, multiple fractures
10	Elective surgery
10	Resting condition
0	Basic metabolism

Enteral solutions

Fig. 11 Increased energy needs in different clinical states

8. Nutritional supplements—intended to supplement/fortify the diet with one or more nutrients otherwise consumed in less than recommended amounts, e.g., vitamins, minerals, amino acids, proteins, enzymes, and metabolites.

Use of the 1–1.5 kcal/ml polymeric high-protein enteral formula is appropriate in most cases. Elemental or semielemental formulae are rarely needed. Fiber-containing formulations can be used in the rehabilitation setting and in patients requiring long-term enteral feeding. Nutritional support includes food fortification, ONS, tube feeding, and parenteral nutrition and aims for increased intake of macronutrients and/or micronutrients.

Positive biological actions of both fibers and their fermentation products (e.g., SCFAs) and the possibility of incorporating different fibers into enteral formulae without increased risk of tube obstruction have changed the enteral feeding approach. Different types of fibers with different biological effects are known. Specific types of fiber are used according to the underlying disease. A formula enriched with a mixture of six fibers has been shown to increase fecal SCFA levels in patients undergoing long-term total enteral nutrition (Schneider et al. 2006).

A high fiber content helps the gut maintain gut physiological function, improve gastrointestinal tolerance (e.g., prevention of diarrhea and constipation), and ameliorate glycemic and lipid control. The recommended fiber intake is 15–30 g/day (Lochs et al. 2006). A high fiber content also stimulates gut microbes.

Since many patients who are in need of nutritional support may also have an imbalance of their gut flora, often secondary to antibiotic use, starvation, and medication, it has been suggested that the addition of "healthy" bacteria such as lactobacilli or bifidobacteria (probiotics) may be of some use. Interesting data are available for this use in intensive care patients and in patients prior to surgery. However, more studies are needed to elucidate the main clinical role of probiotics and prebiotics in improving gut barrier function in this group of patients.

5.3 Immunonutrition

Several different substances have been tested as adjuncts to postoperative nutritional treatment regarding their pharmacological effects in animal

Type	Content	Application/disadvantages
Caloric content (kcal/ml)	1 1,5 2	Risk for dehydration
Protein content (energy%)	<20% standard >20% high	Trauma/septichemia
Osmolality (mOsm/kg)	isotonic < 350 slightly hypertonic 350-550 strongly hypertonic >550	Diarrhoea, espec at intrajejunal admin
Fat content (energy%)	Standard >20% Low 5-20% Fat free <5%	Fat free solutions should be used for insufficiency of the pancreas, hyperlipidemia
Type of fat	LCT LCT/MCT ω-3/ω-6	At malabsorption and trauma With anti-inflam activity
Fiber content	With fiber "Lowresidue"	Prevents constipation Ameliorate colonic mucosa
Electrolyte content Mineral content	Sodium 400-900 mg/1000 kcal Potassium 16-40 Eq/1000 kcal	NB! Sodium intake at renal failure and malabsorption
Pharmaconutrients	Glutamine, anti-oxidants, arginine, omega-3-fatty acids	Immune enhancing, critically ill
Elementar diets	oligopeptides a/o amino acids	For malabsorption

Fig. 12 Characteristics of enteral solutions

models and in vitro experiments. Arginine (improved wound healing), glutamine (improved resistance to infections and a preferred nutrient for enterocytes), ω-3 fatty acids (restraining several inflammatory mediators and cytokines), and nucleotides are among the most used constitutionally essential substrates recommended for patients undergoing major abdominal surgery procedures and have also been shown to improve postoperative outcomes for patients undergoing tumor surgery of the head and neck area (Felekis et al. 2010). These substrates have been shown to upregulate host immune response, to control inflammatory response, and to modulate nitrogen balance and protein synthesis after metabolic trauma. The substitutes should be given 5–7 days before and after the intervention.

Perioperative immunonutrition aims at modulating altered immunological and metabolic functions in the context of major surgery, which is the most studied setting in this field. Perioperative administration of immunonutrition-supplemented enteral formula significantly reduced postoperative infections, morbidity, costs, and length of hospital stay in patients undergoing surgery for cancer (Braga et al. 1999; Cerantola et al. 2010; Jayarajan and Daly 2011).

5.4 Technique

Improved clinical outcome and a reduction in complication and mortality rates are observed when enteral tube feeding (ETF) is provided, as shown in a systematic review and meta-analysis (Stratton et al. 2003). In this way, an increased total energy supply can be provided as well as a higher volume of nutrient intake, and a more complete nutrient supply is possible at the critical time of recovery.

In cases where oral nutritional support is either unable to increase total nutrient intake sufficiently (e.g., in a patient with poor appetite) or is contraindicated (e.g., cerebrovascular accident, patient with dysphagia and risk of aspiration, or with an upper gastrointestinal tract condition that prevents enteral supply), ETF is the most appropriate way to increase nutritional intake. ETF is clearly indicated in patients with neurological dysphagia and should be initiated as soon as possible (Volkert et al. 2006).

It is important to use the gastrointestinal tract to achieve a trophic effect and activity in the small intestine mucosa, something that probably could be achieved only by a small amount of enteral nutrition. Some studies (Elia et al. 1987) assert that as little as 300 ml/day is required to prevent changes of intestinal permeability caused by total starvation. This implies that two to three teaspoons of the contents to the gastrointestinal lumen per hour may be sufficient to maintain the activity and barrier function of the gut.

Most patients with enteral nutritional supply will receive this via a nasogastric tube. It is important to know where the tube tip is located to avoid the risk of aspiration. If the stomach is atonic or if there is an increased risk of regurgitation, the tip should be placed in the duodenal or jejunal part of the small intestine. Tubes carrying a load, a balloon, or a helical tip are more prone to pass through the pylorus and remain in the duodenum or jejunum. Administration of pharmaceuticals, e.g., metoclopramide, may facilitate passage.

A gastrostomy may be established without an open surgical procedure by using the percutaneous technique for a PEG. The technique to achieve this is outlined in Fig. 13. Compared with nasogastric tube feeding, PEG feeding is well tolerated subjectively by the patient as well as socially, by being less stigmatizing, gives less esophageal reflux and aspiration pneumonia problems, and is superior regarding nutritional efficacy (Löser et al. 2005).

A gastroscope is introduced into the stomach, which is then insufflated. The source of light is identified from the outside and a cannula is introduced through the stomach wall into the insufflated stomach, through which a thread is conducted (Fig. 13a). The thread is captured by the instrument, which then is

removed (Fig. 13b). Thereafter, a polyurethane or silicon rubber catheter, with a "disk" at the end, is inserted with help of the thread (Fig. 13c) and is taken out through the abdominal wall (Fig. 13d). For long-term or permanent use, the catheter may be replaced after approximately 4 weeks when a stable stoma is formed by a so-called gastric button/gastroport (Fig. 13e). This procedure has considerably facilitated the establishment of a gastrostomy in a less invasive way.

PEG feeding is easy to establish and to use, with its low risk of complications making it routine practice worldwide and the method of choice for medium-term and long-term enteral feeding, for maintenance and improvement of nutritional status, and for maintenance and improvement of quality of life. Feeding via a PEG is preferred if it is expected that the patient's nutritional intake is likely to be inadequate and supplementary enteral nutrition will be necessary for a period exceeding 2–3 weeks (Löser et al. 2005).

It is important to try supplementary oral nutrition by special drinks and individual nutritional and swallowing advice first; but if this does not stabilize or improve the patient's situation, additional enteral nutrition via a PEG should be considered early in ongoing disease in order to stop the deterioration of the nutritional status and consecutively to stabilize and even improve the patient's quality of life (Löser et al. 2005).

A meta-analysis (Lipp and Lusardi 2009) has shown that prophylactic antibiotics should be routinely administered when establishing a PEG to reduce the incidence of postoperative infections. One single dose given orally is preferable.

The primary aim of ETF is:
- To avoid further loss of body weight
- To correct significant nutritional deficiencies
- To rehydrate the patient
- To stop the related deterioration of the quality of life of the patient owing to inadequate oral nutritional intake

There are many indications for using a PEG tube. In an oncological setting, a PEG tube may be used either in a palliative situation in patients with inoperable stenosing tumors in the ENT area or in the upper gastrointestinal tract, or prior to treatment such as surgery, chemotherapy, or radiotherapy as a temporary measure to be removed after completion of

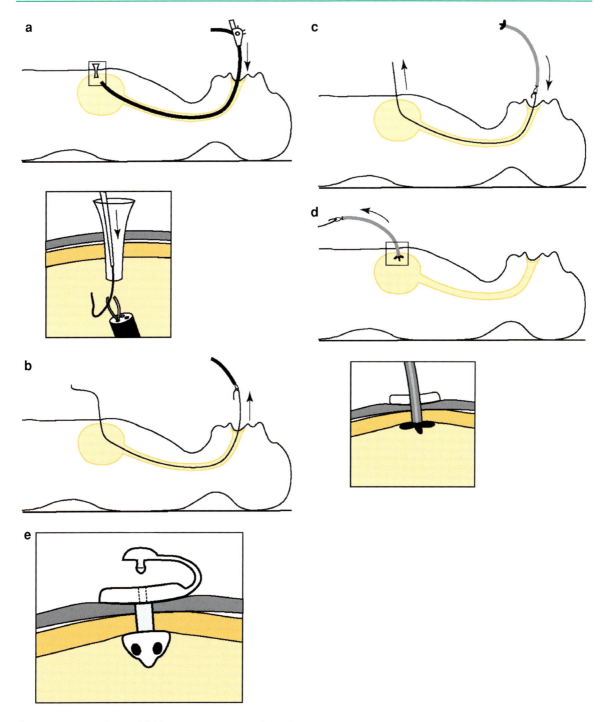

Fig. 13 Principles for establishing a percutaneous endoscopic gastrostomy

treatment when the patient has recaptured an adequate and lasting oral nutritional intake.

A PEG tube my be used in patients with neurological conditions such as dysphagia after cerebrovascular stroke or craniocerebral trauma, and in patients with, e.g., cerebral tumors, bulbar paralysis, Parkinson's disease, amyotrophic lateral sclerosis, or cerebral palsy. In fact, dysphagic conditions in neurological disorders are the most common and established indications for a PEG. The assessment of safe swallow and adequacy of nutritional supply is crucial in determining which patients with neurological dysphagia should be referred for a PEG. As in stroke patients with dysphagia and inadequate oral food intake, early feeding via a PEG is helpful and highly effective, and in contrast to nasogastric tube feeding allows in parallel adequate training to reenable swallowing. Most the patients with amyotrophic lateral sclerosis will receive a PEG, and the decision for this should be made early in the course of the disease.

In elderly demented patients, all published data support an individualized but critical and restrictive approach to PEG feeding.

A PEG tube may be used in a variety of other clinical conditions, such as wasting in AIDS, short bowel syndrome, reconstructive facial surgery, prolonged coma, polytrauma, Crohn's disease, cystic fibrosis, chronic renal failure, and congenital abnormalities, e.g., tracheoesophageal fistula, as well as for palliative drainage of gastric juices and secretions in the small intestine in the presence of a chronic gastrointestinal stenosis or ileus.

In a nonselected patient population, less than 40% of patients with a PEG tube have a malignant underlying disorder. The main therapeutic indications are benign neurological disorders (approximately 50% of cases) and ENT disorders, which are usually malignant (approximately 30% of cases).

PEG tubes can be used liberally. Appropriate supplementary enteral nutrition via a PEG system is more effective than oral nutrition alone in those cases in which the patients undergo several weeks of chemotherapy/radiotherapy. PEG should be considered early in order to ensure adequate nutritional support and to prevent the well-known drawbacks of prolonged nasogastric tube feeding. PEG feeding can prevent ongoing weight loss and maintain nutritional status, but full reversal of weight loss is rare even in benign diseases.

Since 1980 when PEG was first introduced, a variety of systems for ETF have been developed especially by endoscopic insertions, making enteral feeding today an efficient and highly effective means of ensuring nutrition when the patient is not able to achieve a sufficient intake orally. The low complication rates for this easy-to-use technique and the high degree of acceptance by patients leads to a pronounced amelioration of nutritional status, general well-being, and quality of life. For ETF purposes, it is recommended to use PEG early in the course of disease.

5.5   Complications

The complication rate is low, and only 1–4% of cases result in serious complications requiring treatment (Löser et al. 2005).

Next to local wound infection, aspiration of gastric content is the most common complication of ETF. This risk may be reduced by placing the tip of the tube quite distant in the small intestine, i.e., in the duodenal or jejunal part. It is also favorable to raise the head and the upper part of the body by approximately 30° with respect to the bed.

Blockage of the tube is not unusual, and it is recommended to flush the tube every 24 h. Diarrhea occurs in one third of patients, and is caused by several factors, one of which could be the simultaneous administration of antibiotics. Administration of prebiotics and/or probiotics through the tube may improve this condition. In some cases when the patient was earlier receiving long-term total parenteral nutrition, mucosal atrophy and hypoalbuminemia may be noted. Nausea and vomiting is found in 10–20% of patients but may be treated successfully with antiemetic or prokinetic drugs, or with a reduced rate of nutrient supply/infusion. Interactions with simultaneously provided pharmacological treatment may sometimes be a problem, especially when theophylline, warfarin, or digoxin is administered.

Infections may sometimes occur in connection with the PEG wound or be related to contamination of the device. It is recommended that the device be changed every 24 h and that an opened bag of enteral solution not be kept at room temperature for more than 4 h.

5.6   Contraindications

A nonfunctioning gastrointestinal tract is a contraindication to enteral nutrition. In the case of ileus, mechanical obstruction of the gastrointestinal tract, fistulas in the upper part of the gut, or a reduced splanchnic blood flow, nutrition should be provided parenterally.

Contraindications to the establishment of a PEG comprise serious coagulation disorders, interposed organs, marked peritoneal carcinomatosis, severe asci-tes, peritonitis, anorexia nervosa, severe psychosis, advanced dementia, and a clearly limited life expectancy.

6 Evaluation of the Effect of Nutritional Treatment

ONS and ETF have been shown to improve clinically relevant outcomes such as body weight, mortality, complication rates, length of hospital stay, quality of life, and a number of functional measures, e.g., muscle strength and immune function.

A patient with good nutritional status is better prepared with regard to the outcome of surgery, including rate and degree of complications, morbidity, and survival.

Nourishment per os or via a nasogastric tube leads to:
- Significantly fewer infectious complications and shorter length of hospital stay
- A lower rate of anastomotic leakages
- A lower cost per day
- A more physiologic manner for the body to gather nutriments
- A positive influence concerning immune function and gut barrier function

An adequate nutritional supply is achieved when common parameters are followed over time, such as stabilized/gained body weight, reduction of edemas, decreased inflammation with a declining C-reactive protein level, improved muscle function measured by grip strength or gait ability, a higher degree of mobilization/physical activities, and reduced problems related to constipation.

7 Ethical Aspects

Enteral feeding has a 500-year history in Europe, but findings concerning efforts to provide nutrition enterally have been dated to as early as 3500–1500 BC in Egypt (Dudrick and Palesty 2011). The legislative attitude in Europe differs to some extent between countries and is mainly influenced by ancient Greco-Roman views, religious opinions, and more modern society apprehensions. The Hippocratic tradition is based on beneficence (do good) and nonmaleficence (do no harm) (Körner et al. 2006).

The "four principles" approach to medical ethics, from a "nutritional view" are a follows:
1. Autonomy—the principal of self-determination. Wishes of the patient must be respected.
2. Nonmaleficence—the deliberate avoidance of harm. The expected benefit of nutritional support must outweigh the risks.
3. Beneficence—the providing of "good." Nutritional support therapy in most circumstances will provide benefit.
4. Justice—protection of a patient who is incompetent in understanding or making a decision. Fair and equitable resources for all. Provide cost-effective nutritional support.

Artificial nutrition and hydration constitute medical treatments. Decisions to withhold or withdraw nutritional support are subject to the same ethical considerations as any other therapeutic intervention.

Judgments concerning quality of life are of increasing importance in assessing the efficacy of the treatment. Clinicians must act in the best interests of the patient. It may sometimes be a delicate balance between the patient's legal rights and professional judgment, and medical decisions should be made after consultation with those close to the patient.

8 Conclusions

A malnourished patient is a high-risk patient and has a higher rate of complications, a prolonged length of hospital stay, and an increased mortality. A good nutritional condition is a prerequisite for avoiding complications and to regain health. Food is part of the medical treatment. An accurate diet is a prerequisite if every other medical treatment is to be effective or enhanced. The sick individual's nutrition should be taken into consideration in the same way as all other medical treatments and should thus be subject to the same requests for investigation, diagnosis, planning of treatment, and investigation/documentation.

The principle of nutritional treatment in hospitals should always be that food or nourishment ought to be provided the natural way if possible. If 7–10 days of care has elapsed without sufficient oral nutritional intake, nutritional support should be considered.

Even if the enteral supply is as low as a volume of 10–15 ml/h, it is of importance for maintaining the integrity and barrier function of the gut. "To nourish the gut enterally—and the rest of the body intravenously…!" If oral and/or enteral nutrition is not satisfactory to complete the patient's nutritional demands, enteral and parenteral nutrition should be used in combination to cover the nutritional needs and to minimize the adverse effects and complications of both regimens when not used in combination. If there is doubt as to whether tube feeding/enteral nutrition will be beneficial or when the prognosis of the underlying condition is uncertain, a trial treatment should be given for a defined period and the goals and criteria for continuing or discontinuing the feeding should be defined in advance.

For patients with neurological diseases, nutritional support should be given at an early stage to prevent malnutrition developing and thereby impairing recovery in those whose neurological condition improves.

References

Arends J, Bodoky G, Bozetti F, Fearon K et al (2006) ESPEN guidelines on enteral nutrition: non-surgical oncology. Clin Nutr 25:245–259

Braga M, Gianotti L, Radaelli G (1999) Perioperative immunonutrition in patients undergoing cancer surgery: results of a randomized double-blind phase 3 trial. Arch Surg 134:428–433

Cerantola Y, Hübner M, Grass F, Demartines N, Schäfer M (2010) Immunonutrition in gastrointestinal surgery. Br J Surg 98:37–48

Corrigan ML, Escuro AA, Celestin J, Kirby DF (2011) Nutrition in the stroke patient. Nutr Clin Pract 26:242–252

Council of Europe, Committee of Ministers (2003) Resolution ResAP (2003)3 on food and nutritional care in hospitals. https://wcd.coe.int/ViewDoc.jsp?id=85747

Dudrick SJ, Palesty AJ (2011) Historical highlights of the development of enteral nutrition. Surg Clin N Am 91: 945–964

Elia M, Goren A, Behrens R, Barber RW, Neale G (1987) Effect of total starvation and very low calorie diets on intestinal permeability in man. Clin Sci 73:205–210

Felekis D, Eleftheriadou A, Papadakos G, Bosinakou I, Ferekidou E, Kandiloros D, Katsaragakis S, Charalabopoulos K, Manolopoulos L (2010) Effect of perioperative immuno-enhanced enteral nutrition on inflammatory response, nutritional status, and outcomes in head and neck cancer patients undergoing major surgery. Nutr Cancer 62(8):1105–1112

Fukatsu K, Kudsk K (2011) Nutrition and gut immunity. Surg Clin N Am 91:755–770

Howard P, Jonkers-Schuitema C, Furniss L, Kyle U, Muehlebach S, Ödlind-Olin A, Page M, Wheatley C (2006) Managing the patient journey through enteral nutritional care. Clin Nutr 25:187–195

Jayarajan S, Daly JM (2011) The relationships of nutrients, routes of delivery, and immunocompetence. Surg Clin N Am 91:737–753

Jernberg C, Löfmark S, Edlund C, Jansson JK (2007) Long-term ecological impacts of antibiotic administration on the human intestinal microbiota. ISME J 1:56–66

Johansen N, Kondrup J, Munk Plum L, Bak L et al (2004) Effect of nutritional support on clinical outcome in patients at nutritional risk. Clin Nutr 23:539–550

Körner U, Bondolfi A, Bühler E, MacFie J, Meguid MM, Messing B, Oehmichen F, Valentini L, Allison SP (2006) Ethical and legal aspects of enteral nutrition. Clin Nutr 25:196–202

Leder SB, Lazarus CL, Suiter DM, Acton LM (2011) Effects of orogastric tubes on aspiration status and recommendations for oral feeding. Otolaryngol Head Neck Surgery 144(3): 372–375

Lipp A, Lusardi G (2009) A systemic review of prophylactic antimicrobials in PEG placement. J Clin Nurs 18(7): 938–948

Lochs H, Picard C, Allison SP (2006) Evidence supports nutritional support. Clin Nutr 25:177–179

Löser C, Aschl G, Hébuterne X, Mathus-Vliegen EMH, Muscaritoli M, Niv Y, Rollins H, Singer P, Skelly RH (2005) ESPEN guidelines on artificial enteral nutrition—percutaneous endoscopic gastrostomy (PEG). Clin Nutr 24:848–861

McWirtrer JP, Pennington CR (1994) Incidence and recognition of malnutrition in hospital. BMJ 308:945–948

Phillips MS, Ponsky J (2011) Overview of enteral and parenteral feeding access techniques: principles and practice. Surg Clin N Am 91:897–911

Schneider S, Girard-Pipau F, Anty R, van der Linde E, Philipsen-Geerling B (2006) Effects of total enteral nutrition supplemented with a multi-fibre mix on faecal short-chain fatty acids and microbiota. Clin Nutr 25:82–90

Stratton RJ, Green CJ, Elia M (2003) Disease-related malnutrition: an evidence-based approach to treatment. CAB International, Wallingford

Volkert D, Berner YN, Berry E, Cederholm T et al (2006) ESPEN guidelines on enteral nutrition: geriatrics. Clin Nutr 25:330–360

Part V
Complications

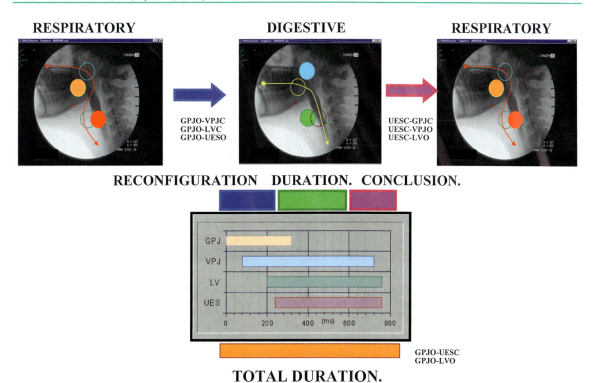

RESPIRATORY   DIGESTIVE   RESPIRATORY

GPJO-VPJC   UESC-GPJC
GPJO-LVC   UESC-VPJO
GPJO-UESO   UESC-LVO

RECONFIGURATION   DURATION.   CONCLUSION.

GPJO-UESC
GPJO-LVO

TOTAL DURATION.

Fig. 1 Configuration of the oropharynx during swallow response. Each phase of the response (reconfiguration, duration, and conclusion) is defined by opening or closure events occurring at the glossopalatal junction (*GPJ*), velopharyngeal junction closure (*VPJC*), laryngeal vestibule (*LV*), and upper esophageal sphincter (*UES*). *GPJC* glossopalatal junction closure, *GPJO* glossopalatal junction opening, *LVC* laryngeal vestibule closure, *LVO* laryngeal vestibule opening, *UESC* upper esophageal sphincter closure, *UESO* upper esophageal sphincter opening, *VPJO* velopharyngeal junction opening

patient (Finestone et al. 1995). Dysphagia, rate of 47% on admission, was associated with malnutrition ($P = 0.032$) and significantly declined over time (Finestone et al. 1995) in patients with stroke.

Neurodegenerative diseases such as multiple sclerosis and Parkinson's disease may also be characterized by oropharyngeal dysphagia as a secondary complication and therefore their clinical course is influenced by its consequences. In a Japanese study published in 1999, the authors investigated the relationship between weight loss and dysphagia in Parkinson's disease. The dysphagic subjects accounted for 31% of the Parkinson's disease patients and for 7% of control subjects ($P < 0.005$), although half of the dysphagic Parkinson's disease patients was not aware of the swallowing impairment. The body mass index (BMI; weight in kilograms divided by/height in meters squared) in the dysphagic group (19.1 ± 3.6 kg/m^2) was significantly lower than in the nondysphagic group (21.6 ± 3.0 kg/m^2) ($P < 0.005$). Patients in the dysphagic group showed significantly lower carbohydrate intake (186 ± 49 g) than those in

the nondysphagic group (215 ± 52 g) ($P < 0.05$). Finally, the biochemical indices of nutritional status were lower in the dysphagic group than in the nondysphagic group (Nozaki et al. 1999).

2   Pathophysiology and Diagnosis

2.1   Pathophysiology of Dysphagia

Oropharyngeal dysphagia may result from a wide range of *structural alterations* that may impair bolus progression. The most common structural abnormalities include esophageal and ear–neck–throat tumors, neck osteophytes, postsurgical esophageal stenosis, and Zenker's diverticulum (Clavé et al. 2004). Dysphagia may also be a side effect in patients with head and neck cancer undergoing radiotherapy (García-Peris et al. 2007). However, oropharyngeal dysphagia is more frequently a functional disorder of deglutition affecting oropharyngeal swallow response caused by

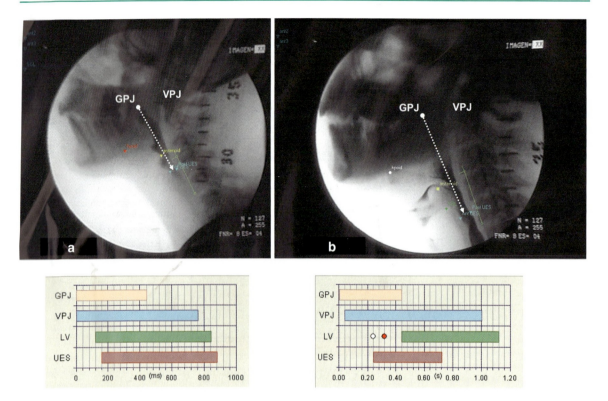

Fig. 2 Videofluoroscopic pictures and oropharyngeal swallow response during the ingestion of a 5-mL nectar bolus in **a** a healthy individual and **b** an older patient with neurogenic dysphagia and aspiration associated with stroke. An increased total duration of the swallow response may be seen, as well as a delayed closure of the laryngeal vestibule and delayed opening of the upper sphincter. The *white dot* indicates the time when contrast material penetrates the laryngeal vestibule, and the *red dot* indicates passage into the tracheobronchial tree (aspiration). *GPJ* glossopalatal junction, *VPJ* velopalatal junction, *LV* laryngeal vestibule, *UES* upper esophageal sphincter

ageing or stroke or associated with systemic or neurological diseases. In biomechanical terms, the oropharyngeal swallow response consists of the temporal arrangement of oropharyngeal structures from a respiratory to a digestive pathway, the transfer of the bolus from the mouth to the esophagus, and the recuperation of the respiratory configuration (Kahrilas et al. 1996; Jean 2001) (Fig. 1). Sensory input by physicochemical properties of the bolus is required during bolus preparation, triggering and modulating the swallow response. Taste, pressure, temperature, nociceptive, and general somatic stimuli from the oropharynx and larynx are transported through cranial nerves V, VII, IX, and X to the central pattern generator, within the nucleus tractus solitarius (NTS), where they are integrated and organized with information originating from the cortex. Swallowing has a multiregional and asymmetrical cerebral representation in caudal sensorimotor and lateral premotor cortex,

insula, temporopolar cortex, amygdala, and cerebellum. This observation explains why 30–50% of unilateral hemispheric stroke patients will develop dysphagia (Hamdy et al. 1999). Once activated, the central pattern generator triggers a swallow motor response involving motor neurons in the brainstem and axons traveling through the cervical spinal cord (C1–C2) and cranial nerves (V, VII, IX–XII) (Jean 2001). The duration of the swallow response in healthy humans is in the range 0.6–1 s (Jean 2001). Healthy subjects presented a short reaction time in the submental muscles (Nagaya and Sumi 2002), short swallow response (glossopalatal junction opening–laryngeal vestibule opening less than 740 ms), fast laryngeal vestibule closure (LVC; less than 160 ms), and fast upper esophageal sphincter (UES) opening (less than 220 ms) (Clavé et al. 2006). In contrast, the swallow response is impaired in older people, especially in patients with neurogenic dysphagia (Clavé et al. 2006; Nagaya and Sumi 2002; Kahrilas et al. 1997). Older patients have prolonged reaction time in the submental muscles (Nagaya and Sumi 2002), and the overall duration of oropharyngeal swallow response in these subjects is significantly longer than in healthy volunteers owing to delay in the early phase of oropharyngeal reconfiguration from a respiratory to a digestive pathway (Clavé et al. 2006). We found that prolonged intervals to LVC and UES opening were the key abnormalities of swallow response, double those of healthy subjects and leading to unsafe deglutition and aspiration in neurological older patients (Fig. 2) (Clavé et al. 2006; Kahrilas et al. 1997). This delayed swallow response in the elderly and in patients with neurogenic dysphagia can be attributed to an impairment of sensations (Teismann et al. 2007, 2009), a decrease in the number of neurons in the brain, and a delay in the synaptic conduction of the afferent inputs to the central nervous system (CNS) caused by ageing (Nagaya and Sumi 2002) and by other risk factors for dysphagia such as neurodegenerative diseases and stroke (Clavé et al. 2005a; Turley and Cohen 2009). Other conditions such as delirium, confusion, and dementia, and the effects of sedative, neuroleptic, or antidepressant drugs can also contribute to impaired swallow response in frail older patients (Turley and Cohen 2009). Transfer of the bolus from the mouth through the pharynx is mainly caused by the squeezing action of the tongue (Nicosia and Robbins 2001). Older adults present with lingual weakness, a finding that has been related to sarcopenia of the head and neck musculature and frailty (Robbins et al. 2005). Tongue propulsion is assessed by direct measurements with oral sensors (Robbins et al. 2005) or by videofluoroscopic studies which measure the bolus velocity and kinetic energy during swallow (Clavé et al. 2006). Older adults generate lower maximum isometric pressures than younger adults (Robbins et al. 2005). We showed that young healthy adults have high bolus velocity (more than 35 cm/s) and strong bolus propulsion forces (more than 0.33 mJ) (Clavé et al. 2006). In contrast, older people with oropharyngeal dysphagia have impaired tongue propulsion forces (less than 0.14 mJ) and slower bolus velocity (less than 10 cm/s) (Clavé et al. 2006). Therefore, functional oropharyngeal dysphagia in the elderly and in neurological patients is associated with impairment of efficacy and safety of swallow caused by weak tongue propulsion and prolonged and delayed swallow response. Pathogenesis of impaired safety is related to a delay in several physiologic protective reflexes in oropharyngeal reconfiguration (mainly LVC) caused by a slow neural swallow response and is associated with several risk factors such as ageing, neurodegenerative diseases, confusion, dementia, and drugs. Pathogenesis of impaired efficacy is related to alterations in bolus propulsion caused by a weak muscular tongue squeeze associated with sarcopenia and weakness (Clavé et al. 2005a).

2.2 Screening, Assessment, and Diagnosis of Dysphagia

The goal of the diagnostic program for dysphagia is to evaluate two deglutition-defining characteristics: (1) *efficacy*, the patient's ability to ingest all the calories and water he or she needs to remain adequately nourished and hydrated; and (2) *safety*, the patient's ability to ingest all needed calories and water with no respiratory complications (Clavé et al. 2004, 2005a, b 2006). To assess both characteristics of deglutition, two groups of diagnostic methods are available (1) clinical methods such as deglutition-specific medical history and clinical examination, usually used as screening methods; and (2) the exploration of deglutition using specific complementary studies such as videofluoroscopy (VFS).

2.2.1 Clinical Screening

Clinical screening for oropharyngeal dysphagia should be low risk, quick, and low cost and aim at selecting the highest risk patients who require further assessment. In involves:

1. *Deglutition-specific questionnaires.* The ten-item Eating Assessment Tool (EAT-10) is a self-administered, symptom-specific outcome instrument for dysphagia. The EAT-10 has displayed excellent internal consistency, test–retest reproducibility, and criterion-based validity. The normative data suggest that an EAT-10 score of 3 or higher is abnormal. The instrument may be utilized to document the initial dysphagia severity in persons with swallowing disorders. (Belafsky et al. 2008). There is also a validated specific symptom inventory to assess the severity of oropharyngeal dysphagia in patients with neuromyogenic dysphagia (Wallace et al. 2000). The inventory consists of 17 questions each answered on a 100-mm visual

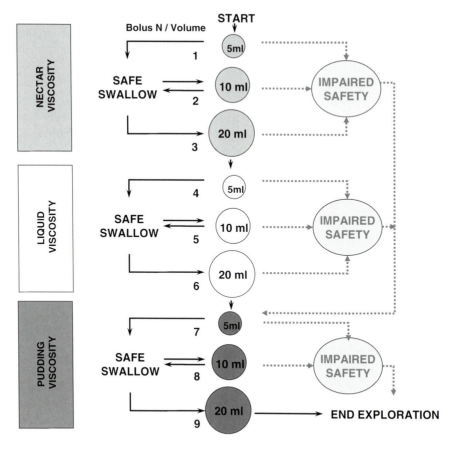

Fig. 3 Algorithms for bolus volume and viscosity administration during the volume–viscosity swallow test (V-VST). The strategy of the V-VST aims at protecting patients from aspiration by starting with nectar viscosity and the volumes are increased from 5- to 10- and 20-mL boluses in a progression of increasing difficulty. When patients have completed the nectar series without major symptoms of aspiration (cough and/ or fall in oxygen saturation of 3% or greater), a less "safe" liquid viscosity series is assessed also with boluses of increasing difficulty (5–20 mL). Finally, a "safer" pudding viscosity series (5–20 mL) is assessed using similar rules. If the patient shows a sign of impaired safety at nectar viscosity, the series is interrupted, the liquid series is omitted, and a safer pudding viscosity series is assessed. If the patient shows a sign of impaired safety at liquid viscosity, the liquid series is interrupted and the pudding series is assessed

analogue scale. Applied to patients with neuromyogenic dysphagia, the 17-question inventory shows strong test–retest reliability over 2 weeks. Also, face, content, construct validity, and score correlated highly with an independent global assessment severity score (Wallace et al. 2000).

2. *Clinical examination.* Current methods for clinical screening of dysphagia are, for example, the water swallow test (Gordon et al. 1987), the 3-oz water test developed in the Burke Rehabilitation Center (DePippo et al. 1992), the timed swallow test (Nathadwarawala et al. 1992), and the standardized bedside swallow assessment (Westergren 2006; Smithard et al. 1998). Patients are asked to drink 50 mL (Palmer et al. 2001), 3 oz (DePippo et al. 1992), 150 mL (Nathadwarawala et al. 1992), or 60 mL (Westergren 2006; Smithard et al. 1998) of water from a glass without interruption. Coughing during or after completion or the presence of a postswallow wet-hoarse voice quality, or a swallow speed of less than 10 mL/s is scored as abnormal. These clinical bedside methods can detect dysphagia, although with differing diagnostic accuracy. Burke's 3-oz water swallow test identified 80% of patients aspirating during subsequent VFS examination (sensitivity 76%, specificity 59%) (DePippo et al. 1992). The standardized bedside swallow assessment showed a variable sensitivity (47–68%) and specificity (67–86%) in detecting aspiration when used by speech–swallow therapists or

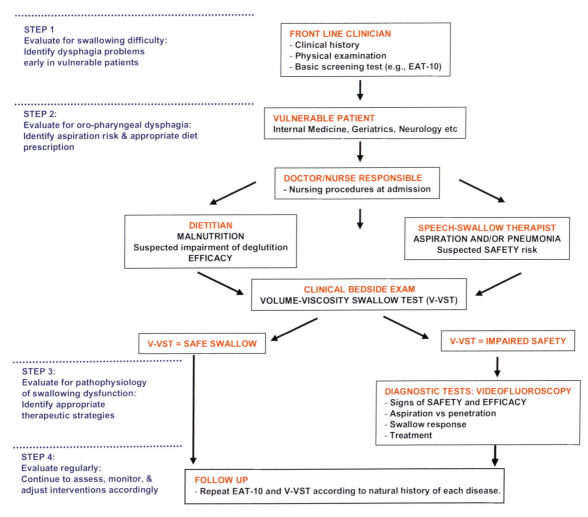

STEP 1
Evaluate for swallowing difficulty:
Identify dysphagia problems
early in vulnerable patients

FRONT LINE CLINICIAN
- Clinical history
- Physical examination
- Basic screening test (e.g., EAT-10)

STEP 2
Evaluate for oro-pharyngeal dysphagia:
Identify aspiration risk & appropriate diet
prescription

VULNERABLE PATIENT
Internal Medicine, Geriatrics, Neurology etc

DOCTOR/NURSE RESPONSIBLE
- Nursing procedures at admission

DIETITIAN
MALNUTRITION
Suspected impairment of deglutition
EFFICACY

SPEECH-SWALLOW THERAPIST
ASPIRATION AND/OR PNEUMONIA
Suspected SAFETY risk

CLINICAL BEDSIDE EXAM
VOLUME-VISCOSITY SWALLOW TEST (V-VST)

V-VST = SAFE SWALLOW

V-VST = IMPAIRED SAFETY

STEP 3:
Evaluate for pathophysiology
of swallowing dysfunction:
Identify appropriate
therapeutic strategies

DIAGNOSTIC TESTS: VIDEOFLUOROSCOPY
- Signs of SAFETY and EFFICACY
- Aspiration vs penetration
- Swallow response
- Treatment

STEP 4:
Evaluate regularly:
Continue to assess, monitor, &
adjust interventions accordingly

FOLLOW UP
- Repeat EAT-10 and V-VST according to natural history of each disease.

Adapted from Clavé P, Arreola V, Romea M, Medina L, Palomera E, Serra-Prat M. Accuracy of the volume-viscosity swallow test for clinical screening of oropharyngeal dysphagia and aspiration. Clinical Nutrition. 2008;27(6):806-15.

Fig. 4 Algorithm for screening, diagnosis, and treatment of oropharyngeal functional dysphagia at the Hospital de Mataró, Barcelona, Spain. Note the involvement of several professional domains of the multidisciplinary dysphagia team and the vertical and horizontal flows of information. The *boxes* indicate the diagnostic screening strategy of patients at risk; the *arrows* indicate flow of information on patient status, and the *dotted lines* indicate therapeutic interventions. *EAT-10* ten-item Eating Assessment Tool

physicians (Westergren 2006; Smithard et al. 1998). These screening procedures involve continuous swallowing of quite large amounts of liquid and may place the patient at high risk of aspiration. Furthermore, many of these studies on bedside screening lack methodological quality and, therefore, the psychometric properties of the screening procedure being studied cannot be determined accurately (Bours et al. 2009). Clavé et al. developed a safer clinical method (the V-VST) using a series of 5–20-mL nectar, liquid, and pudding boluses sequentially administered in a progression of increasing difficulty (Fig. 3). Cough, fall in oxygen saturation of 3% or greater, and changes in quality of voice were considered clinical signs of impaired safety, whereas piecemeal deglutition and oropharyngeal residue were considered signs of impaired efficacy. The V-VST is a safe, quick, and accurate clinical method with 88.2% sensitivity for impaired safety, 100% sensitivity for aspiration, and up to 88.4% sensitivity for impaired efficacy of swallows (Clavé et al. 2004). Figure 4 shows the algorithm for management (screening, diagnosis, and treatment) of oropharyngeal dysphagia at the Hospital de Mataró, Barcelona, Spain (Clavé et al. 2005b). The V-VST is considered to be a highly adequate instrument for screening for dysphagia and agrees with the recommendations stated in the systematic review on bedside screening for dysphagia by Bours et al. (2009), which combine a water test and pulse oximetry and use coughing, choking, and voice alteration as end points. The use of different viscosities in the V-VST can be considered to be an improvement compared with a simple water test using only liquid.

2.2.2 Videofluoroscopy

VFS is the gold standard to study the oral and pharyngeal mechanisms of dysphagia (Clavé et al. 2004; Cook and Kahrilas 1999). If VFS is not available, fiber-optic endoscopic evaluation of swallowing may be used as a valuable diagnostic instrument instead (Langmore et al. 1991). VFS is a dynamic exploration that evaluates the safety and efficacy of deglutition, characterizes the alterations of deglutition in terms of videofluoroscopic symptoms, and helps to select and assess specific therapeutic strategies. The technical requirements for clinical VFS are an X-ray tube with fluoroscopy and a videotape recorder; additionally, there are computed-assisted methods of analysis of images allowing quantitative temporal and spatial measurements (Clavé et al. 2006). The main observations during VFS are done in the lateral plane while the patient is swallowing 5–20-mL boluses of at least three consistencies: liquid, nectar, and pudding. We keep the patient at a minimal risk of aspiration by starting the study with low volumes and thick consistencies, introducing liquids and high volumes as tolerated (Clavé et al. 2006). Major signs of impaired efficacy during the oral stage include apraxia and decreased control and bolus propulsion by the tongue. Many older patients have deglutitional apraxia (difficulty, delay, or inability to initiate the oral stage) following a stroke. This symptom is also seen in patients with Alzheimer's disease, with dementia, and with diminished oral sensitivity. Impaired lingual control (inability to form the bolus) or propulsion results in oral or vallecular residue when alterations occur at the base of the tongue. The main sign regarding safety during the oral stage is glossopalatal (tongue–soft palate) seal insufficiency, a serious

dysfunction that results in the bolus falling into the hypopharynx before the triggering of the oropharyngeal swallow response and while the airway is still open, which causes predeglutitive aspiration (Clavé et al. 2004; Logemann 1993). Videofluoroscopic signs of safety during the pharyngeal stage include penetrations and/or aspirations. Penetration refers to the entering of contrast material into the laryngeal vestibule within the boundaries of the vocal cords. When aspiration occurs, contrast material goes beyond the vocal cords into the tracheobronchial tree (Fig. 2b). The potential of VFS regarding image digitalization and quantitative analysis currently allows accurate swallow response measurements in patients with dysphagia (Fig. 2). A slow closure of the laryngeal vestibule and a slow opening of the UES (as seen in Fig. 2b) are the most characteristic aspiration-related parameters (Clavé et al. 2006; Kahrilas et al. 1997). Penetration and aspiration may also result from an insufficient or delayed hyoid and laryngeal elevation, which fails to protect the airway. A high, permanent postswallow residue may lead to postswallow aspiration, since the hypopharynx is full of contrast material when the patient inhales after swallowing, and then contrast material passes directly into the airway (Clavé et al. 2004; Logemann 1993). Thereafter, VFS can determine whether aspiration is associated with impaired glossopalatal seal (predeglutitive aspiration), a delay in triggering the pharyngeal swallow or impaired deglutitive airway protection (laryngeal elevation, epiglottic descent, and closure of vocal folds during swallow response), or an ineffective pharyngeal clearance (postswallow aspiration) (Clavé et al. 2004).

2.3 Pathophysiology of Malnutrition in Patients with Dysphagia

2.3.1 Screening and Assessment of Malnutrition

The assessment of the nutritional status is a complex and time-consuming procedure which requires trained personnel. The procedure and thus the diagnosis of malnutrition is based on a combination of data extracted from the patient's history, physical examination, and specific laboratory parameters.

The patient's history will focus on finding out possible changes in diet and body weight and will explore the socioeconomic aspects and symptoms that may influence the nutritional status in the context of the disease in the patient. The patient will be asked about his or her usual weight, to assess weight changes over time, recorded toxic habits, medication, gastrointestinal symptoms, and the presence of known diseases. It is important to ask the patient about his or her usual diet and performed in recent weeks to estimate intake. The physical examination should be directed to detect the loss of muscle and fat and the presence of edema and ascites. Body weight, as an absolute value, has its limitations; however, combined with the individual's height, i.e., the BMI, it can be used to diagnose a situation of malnutrition. One of the best indicators of malnutrition or risk of malnutrition is the assessment of weight changes over time. It is considered that unintentional weight loss of 5% of previous weight in 1 month or 10% in 3 months is highly suggestive of malnutrition. The skinfold measurement by a precision caliper provides an estimate of fat mass, triceps skinfold being the most used. In contrast, the measurement of body circumferences can estimate the individual's muscle mass, arm circumference being the most used. As for the triceps skinfold, measurements should then be compared with reference values. It is important to note that skinfolds and circumferences have significant interobserver variability, which limits the reproducibility of the data. Among the markers, there is no ideal single biochemical marker for malnutrition, as most laboratory parameters are limited by being insensitive and not very specific or being affected by nonnutritional factors. Of these, the most commonly used is serum albumin, a protein with liver synthesis and relatively long half-life, which is a good marker of nutritional status and prognosis in the absence of overt inflammation. The dosage of proteins synthesized by the liver but having a shorter half-life than albumin, i.e., prealbumin, could be of help to monitor changes of the nutritional status during a short period of time (Gil).

Considering the complexity of the assessment of the nutritional status, it is important that simpler tools are used by untrained personnel to detect the patients at risk of malnutrition, in order to request a more detailed evaluation by specialized personnel, and for a timely start of nutritional intervention. To this end, a number of screening tools for nutritional risk have been developed. The validated nutritional screening method for the hospitalized patient is the nutritional risk screening 2002 developed by the European Society for Clinical Nutrition and Metabolism (ESPEN) and built on the retrospective analysis of 128 controlled trials focusing on nutritional assessment, nutritional support, and patient outcomes. Very simple and fast to complete, it has a low variability between observers, the most subjective assessment being the severity of the disease (Kondrup 2003). The Malnutrition Universal Screening Tool developed by the British Society for Parenteral and Enteral Nutrition in 2003 has been validated to identify adult patients who are malnourished or at risk of malnourishment (both default and excess). ESPEN recommends its use in the community, but it can also be utilized in institutionalized patients or patients admitted to the hospital. The Malnutrition Universal Screening Tool has been shown to predict the duration of hospital stay and mortality. The method is simple and reproducible between different observers and it is linked to specific protocols and recommendations for treatment (Malnutrition Advisory Group 2000). The Subjective Global Assessment (SGA), validated in the majority of the population, designed by Baker in 1982, is a dynamic process of nutritional assessment that is structured and simple with high predictive power and a high rate of interobserver agreement. However, it requires training and is more appropriate for the detection of established malnutrition rather than acute changes in nutritional status or nutritional risk (Detsky et al. 1987). The method validated for the geriatric population is the MNA, with a high positive predictive value and high specificity and sensitivity, recommended by the ESPEN for the screening of elderly patients. The MNA identifies patients at risk before any other visible changes occur. The first part consists of a screening (MNA Short Form) and the second considers food habits, social status, functional ability, and physical examination (Vellas et al. 1999).

2.4 Types and Mechansims of Malnutriton in Dysphagia

There is a strong relationship between the prevalence and severity of dysphagia and the incidence of malnutrition (Clavé et al. 2005a, 2006). Up to 50% of nursing home residents and up to 70 % of geriatric patients in hospital show signs of malnutrition. However, the true prevalence of malnutrition among patients with dysphagia, the pathophysiological aspects of malnutrition associated with oropharyngeal dyspagia, the relevance of oropharyngeal dyspagia as a cause of malnutrition, and the type of malnutrition associated with diseases also causing oropharyngeal dysphagia are not fully settled.

Three types of malnutrition have been described: starvation-related malnutrition, chronic-disease-related malnutrition, and acute-disease-related or injury-related malnutrition (Jensen et al. 2010). Starvation-related malnutrition develops in situations of chronic energy and protein deficiency but where the ratio between the amount of energy and protein is maintained. It is characterized by absence of inflammation, and loss of the body's muscle mass and subcutaneous fat, eventually leading to emaciation. Chronic-disease-related malnutrition is characterized by the presence of chronic inflammation of mild to moderate degree, and by a variable degree of reduced food intake because of disease-associated anorexia. Cancer, liver cirrhosis, chronic obstructive pulmonary disease, and chronic renal failure are clinical conditions frequently characterized by this type of malnutrition. Acute-disease-related or injury-related malnutrition is characterized by acute and severe inflammation, which impairs the ability to use nutrients introduced by the diet or infused by artificial nutrition. Critically ill patients frequently develop this type of malnutrition. Chronic-disease-related malnutrition is the most common form of malnutrition in hospital (Jensen et al. 2010). The existence of disease-associated malnutrition is very common and the prevalence may range between 20 and 50% of patients, depending on the variability of the diagnostic criteria used (Norman et al. 2008). In developed countries the main cause of malnutrition is disease. Any disorder, whether chronic or acute, has the potential to result in or aggravate malnutrition in more than one way: response to trauma, infection, or inflammation may alter metabolism, appetite, absorption, or assimilation of nutrients. (Campbell 1999). The catabolic effects of several mediators such as cytokines (interleukin-1, interleukin-6, and tumor necrosis factor alpha), glucocorticoids, and catecholamines, and the lack of insulin-like growth factor 1 have been extensively studied in recent years; their relevance is, however, not yet entirely understood (Tisdale 2005). Drug-related side effects: (e.g., chemotherapy, morphine derivatives, antibiotics, sedatives, neuroleptics, digoxin,

antihistamines, and captopril) can cause anorexia or interfere with the ingestion of food. In geriatric patients further factors such as dementia, immobilization, anorexia, and poor dentition can further worsen the situation.(Markson 1997; Morley 1997). The cause and prevalence of malnutrition in different diseases and settings are extensively discussed in the recently published ESPEN guidelines on enteral nutrition (Anker et al. 2006; Arends et al. 2006; Cano et al. 2006; Kreymann et al. 2006; Lochs et al. 2006; Meier et al. 2006; Ockenga et al. 2006; Plauth et al. 2006; Volkert et al. 2006). Apart from the pathological causes of malnutrition, socioeconomic factors such as low income and isolation may also contribute to the development of malnutrition (Pirlich et al. 2005). The situation can be further aggravated in hospital owing to adverse hospital routines that lead to insufficient nutrient intake (Dupertuis et al. 2003). Several studies have found evidence to suggest that hospitalized patients often receive less than an optimal level of nutritional care owing to lack of training and awareness of hospital staff (Kondrup et al. 2002). Patients are frequently ordered to have nil by mouth without being fed by another route or are called for an investigation immediately prior to the food being served, multiple episodes of fasting before an investigation occur, and meals are often considered unpalatable. Depression, dementia, and lack of feeding assistance lead to further decreased nutrient intake (Incalzi et al. 1996; Sullivan et al. 1999).

We studied the prevalence of malnutrition among patients with chronic dysphagia caused by nonprogressive brain disorders (e.g., stroke, brain injury) or by neurodegenerative diseases (e.g., ALS, multiple sclerosis). The prevalence and the type of malnutrition were studied using the SGA (Vellas et al. 1999). Anthropometric measures (triceps skinfold thickness, arm circumference, and arm muscle circumference), BMI, percentage weight loss, plasma albumin level, and lymphocyte count were also recorded. The prevalence and the type of malnutrition were similar between nonprogressive brain disorder and neurodegenerative disease patients with neurogenic dysphagia. Malnutrition was found in 16% of nonprogressive brain disorder patients according to the SGA (SGA B or C), in 24.1% according to BMI, and in 20% according to weight loss greater than 10%. In neurodegenerative disease patients, malnutrition was found in 22% of patients according to the SGA, in 21.9% according to BMI, and in 23.5% according to weight loss greater than 10%. The study found a strong correlation between dysphagia and malnutrition as the clinical severity (Wallace et al. 2000) of dysphagia scored 325.6 ± 12.3 points in patients with normal nutritional status and 529 ± 34.5 points in patients with or at risk of malnutrition ($P < 0.05$). The type of malnutrition in both groups of patients with neurogenic dysphagia was uniformly of the chronic type. Significant differences were found in relation to anthropometric parameters between well-nourished patients and malnourished patients in (1) skeletal muscle measured as upper arm muscle circumference of 28.4 ± 0.4 versus 24.8 ± 0.5 cm ($P < 0.05$), and (2) fat mass measured as triceps skinfold of 15.5 ± 0.6 versus 10.9 ± 1.0 mm ($P < 0.05$). In contrast, measurements of visceral protein level were found to be within the normal range in most patients with neurogenic dysphagia and malnutrition as plasma albumin level was 40.2 ± 0.7 versus 40.9 ± 1.9 g/L and the lymphocyte counts were similar among patients with SGA A and patients with SGA B or C (Clavé et al. 2006).

2.4.1 Sarcopenia and Dysphagia

The tongue plays a key role in bolus propulsion. We and others found elderly patients with dysphagia showed impaired tongue propulsion (Rofes et al. 2010) and decreased tongue volume due to sarcopenia (Robbins et al. 2002; Robbins et al. 2005). Older adults show lingual weakness, a finding that has been related to sarcopenia of the head and neck musculature and frailty (Robbins et al. 2005) and one of the major causes for dysphagia in the elderly, associated with impairment in efficacy and safety of swallow (Rofes et al. 2011).

Depending on the literature definition used for sarcopenia, the prevalence in 60–70 years old is reported as 5–13%, whereas the prevalence ranges from 11 to 50% in people over 80 years old (Morley 2008). Even with a conservative estimate of prevalence, sarcopenia affects more than 50 million people today and will affect more than 200 million in the next 40 years. The impact of sarcopenia on older people is far-reaching; its substantial tolls are measured in terms of morbidity (Sayer et al. 2005), disability (Janssen et al. 2002), high costs of health care (Janssen et al. 2004a), and mortality (Gale et al. 2007). The European Working Group on Sarcopenia in Older People (EWGSOP) has recently developed a

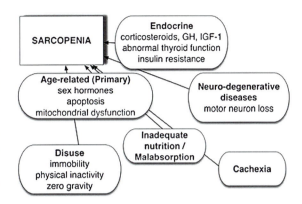

Fig. 5 Mechanisms of sarcopenia. *GH* growth hormone, *IGF-1* insulin-like growth factor 1. (Cruz-Jentoft et al. 2010)

practical clinical definition and consensus diagnostic criteria for age-related sarcopenia (Cruz-Jentoft et al. 2010) It defined sarcopenia as a syndrome characterized by progressive and generalized loss of skeletal muscle mass and strength with a risk of adverse outcomes such as physical disability, poor quality of life, and death (Delmonico et al. 2007; Goodpaster et al. 2006). It recommends using the presence of both low muscle mass and low muscle function (strength or performance) for the diagnosis of sarcopenia. The rationale for use of two criteria is that muscle strength does not depend solely on muscle mass, and the relationship between strength and mass is not linear (Goodpaster et al. 2006; Janssen et al. 2004b). There are several mechanisms that may be involved in the onset and progression of sarcopenia. These mechanisms involve, among others, protein synthesis, proteolysis, neuromuscular integrity, and muscle fat content. (Fig. 5). Sarcopenia can be considered "primary" (or age-related) when no other cause is evident but ageing itself, whereas sarcopenia can be considered "secondary" when one or more other causes are evident. Sarcopenia staging, which reflects the severity of the condition, is a concept that can help guide clinical management of the condition. EWGSOP suggests a conceptual staging as "presarcopenia," "sarcopenia," and "severe sarcopenia" (Cruz-Jentoft et al. 2010). The parameters of sarcopenia are the amount of muscle and its function. The measurable variables are mass, strength, and physical performance. The following sections briefly review measurement techniques that can be used and discuss their suitability for research and clinical practice settings. A wide range of techniques can be used to assess muscle mass (Lukasi 2005). We present here the proposals of EWGSOP:

1. *Body imaging techniques.* Three imaging techniques have been used for estimating muscle mass or lean body mass—computed tomography, magnetic resonance imaging (MRI), and dual-energy X-ray absorptiometry (DXA). Computed tomography and MRI are considered to be very precise imaging systems that can separate fat from other soft tissues of the body, making these methods gold standards for estimating muscle mass in research. High cost, limited access to equipment at some sites, and concerns about radiation exposure limit the use of these whole-body imaging methods in routine clinical practice (Chien et al. 2008). DXA is an attractive alternative method both for research and for clinical use to distinguish fat, bone mineral, and lean tissues. This whole-body scan exposes the patient to minimal radiation. The main drawback is that the equipment is not portable, which may preclude its use in large-scale epidemiology studies (Chien et al. 2008).

2. *Bioimpedance analysis (BIA).* BIA estimates the volume of fat and lean body mass. The test itself is inexpensive, easy to use, readily reproducible, and appropriate for both ambulatory and bedridden patients. BIA measurement techniques, used under standard conditions, have been studied for more than 10 years (NIH 1996), and BIA results under standard conditions have been found to correlate well with MRI predictions (Janssen 2000). Prediction equations have been validated for multiethnic adults (Sullivan et al. 1999) and reference values have been established for adult white men and women, including older subjects (Roubenoff et al. 1997; Kyle et al. 2001a, b). Thus, BIA might be a good portable alternative to DXA.

3. *Total body potassium (TBK) or partial body potassium (PBK) per fat-free soft tissue.* As skeletal muscle contains more than 50% of the TBK pool, TBK is the classic method for estimation of skeletal muscle. More recently, PBK of the arm has been proposed as a simpler alternative (Wielopolski et al. 2006). PBK of the arm is safe and inexpensive. TBK is the classic method for the estimation of skeletal muscle, but this method is not used routinely.

4. *Anthropometric measurements.* Calculations based on mid-upper arm circumference and skinfold thickness have been used to estimate muscle mass in ambulatory settings. However, age-related changes in fat deposits and loss of skin elasticity contribute to estimation errors in older people. There are relatively few studies validating anthropometric measures in older and obese people; these and other confounders make anthropometric measures vulnerable to error and questionable for individual use (Rolland et al. 2008).

5. *Muscle strength.* There are fewer well-validated techniques to measure muscle strength. Although lower limbs are more relevant than upper limbs for gait and physical function, handgrip strength has been widely used and is well correlated with most relevant outcomes. Again, cost, availability, and ease of use can determine whether the techniques are better suited to clinical practice or are useful for research. It must be remembered that factors unrelated to muscle, e.g., motivation or cognition, may hamper the correct assessment of muscle strength (Cruz-Jentoft et al. 2010).

6. *Physical performance.* A wide range of tests of physical performance are available, including the Short Physical Performance Battery, which includes usual gait speed, 6-min walk test, and the stair climb power test (Working Group on Functional Outcome Measures 2008). Tongue strength can be assessed by several standardized instruments for lingual pressure measurements, air-filled bulbs between the tongue and hard palate, and manometric devices or by assessing the bolus velocity and kinetic energy during videofluoroscopic studies (Clavé et al. 2006).

3   Complications of Dysphagia: Aspiration Pneumonia and Malnutrition

The severity of oropharyngeal dysphagia ranges from moderate difficulty to complete inability to swallow. Oropharyngeal dysphagia may give rise to two groups of clinically relevant complications: (1) malnutrition and/or dehydration caused by a decrease in the efficacy of deglutition, present in up to 25–75% of patients with dysphagia; (2) choking and tracheobronchial aspiration caused by the decrease in deglutition safety and which results in pneumonia in 50% of cases, with an associated mortality of up to 50% (Clavé et al. 2004, 2005a). Figure 6 summarizes

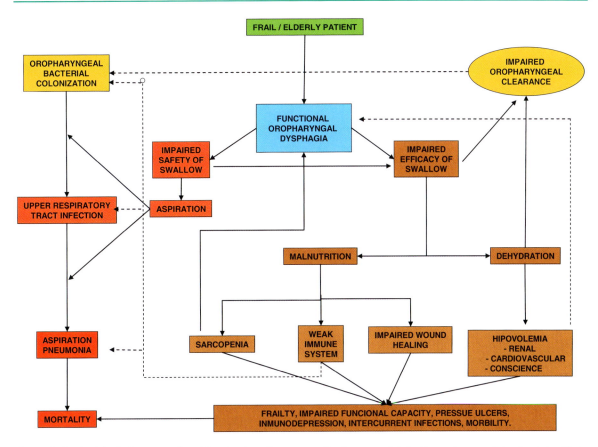

Fig. 6 Pathophysiological aspects of nutritional and respiratory complications associated with oropharyngeal dysphagia in elderly patients

the pathophysiological aspects of complications related to oropharyngeal dysphagia in the elderly and in neurological patients.

3.1 Respiratory Complications: Aspiration Pneumonia

The incidence and the prevalence of aspiration pneumonia in the community are poorly defined. They increase in direct relation with age and underlying diseases. The risk of aspiration pneumonia is higher in older patients because of the high incidence of dysphagia (Loeb et al. 2003). In elderly nursing home residents with oropharyngeal dysphagia, aspiration pneumonia occurs in 43–50% during the first year, with a mortality of up to 45% (Cook and Kahrilas 1999). We recently studied 134 older patients (over 70 years) consecutively admitted with pneumonia in an acute geriatric unit in a general hospital. Of the 134 patients,

53% were over 84 years old and 55% showed clinical signs of oropharyngeal dysphagia; the mean Barthel score was 61 points, indicating a frail population. Patients with dysphagia were older and showed lower functional status, higher prevalence of malnutrition and comorbidities, and higher Fine's pneumonia severity scores. Patients with dysphagia had higher mortality at 30 days (22.9 vs. 8.3%, $P = 0.033$) and at 1 year of follow-up (55.4 vs. 26.7%, $P = 0.001$) (Fig. 7). Therefore, oropharyngeal dysphagia is a highly prevalent clinical finding and an indicator of disease severity in older patients with pneumonia (Cabre et al. 2010).

The pathogenesis of aspiration pneumonia has been revised recently (Marik and Kaplan 2003; Almirall et al. 2007) and presumes the contribution of risk factors that alter swallowing function, cause aspiration, and predispose the oropharynx to bacterial colonization. Aspiration observed during VFS is associated with a 5.6-fold to sevenfold increase in the

Fig. 7 Accumulated survival at 1 year according to the presence of clinical signs of oropharyngeal dysphagia and the functional status (preadmission Barthel score) (Cabre et al. 2010)

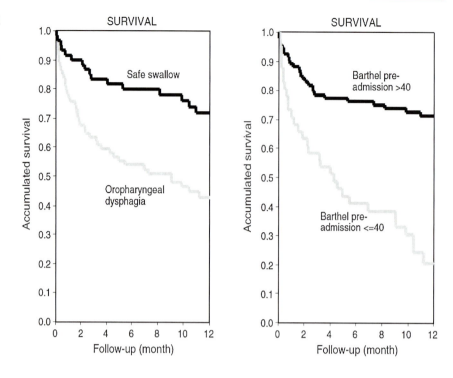

risk of pneumonia (Schmidt et al. 1994). Up to 45% of older patients with dysphagia had penetration into the laryngeal vestibule, 30% had aspiration, half of them without cough (silent aspiration), and 45% had oropharyngeal residue (Clavé et al. 2005a). It is accepted that detection of aspiration by VFS is a predictor of pneumonia risk and/or probability of rehospitalization (Cook and Kahrilas 1999). It is also well known that not all patients who aspirated during VFS develop pneumonia. Impairment in host defenses such as abnormal cough reflex (Addington et al. 1999; Marik and Kaplan 2003), impaired pharyngeal clearance (Palmer et al. 2001), amount and bacterial concentration of aspirate, and weakened immune system also strongly contributed to the development of aspiration pneumonia (Almirall et al. 2007). Impairment of cough reflex increases the risk of aspiration pneumonia in stroke patients (Addington et al. 1999). Several risks factors contribute to oropharyngeal colonization, such as:

1. Older age. Swallow response, cough reflex, and breathing coordination are impaired in older people.
2. Malnutrition. Poor nutritional status is a marker of a population highly susceptible to acquiring pneumonia as in the elderly as malnutrition depresses the immune system.

3. Smoking status, number of cigarettes smoked per day, and lifetime smoking.
4. Poor oral hygiene. This is probably the most common infectious sequela of poor oral health in the elderly, particularly those who reside in nursing homes, is aspiration pneumonia. The oral environment in people who still have their teeth is quite different from the flora that thrive in the toothless person but all of them result in oropharyngeal colonization by potential respiratory tract pathogens.
5. Antibiotics. It has been suggested that inappropriate antibiotic treatment could be a risk factor for pneumonia. In some patients who are smokers or who have chronic bronchitis, the use of antibiotics in the previous 3 months may provoke a variety of respiratory flora, predisposing the patient to opportunistic infection with colonization of more aggressive organisms, which could be causative pathogens of aspiration pneumonia.
6. Dry mouth. Many medications reduce salivary flow or create xerostomia as a side effect. This creates a favorable environment for growth of bacteria that are pathogenic to the lungs if they are aspirated.
7. Immunity. Older adults can have reduced oropharyngeal clearance, reduced numbers of T cells,

Pathophysiological aspects of aspiration pneumonia and oropharyngeal dysphagia

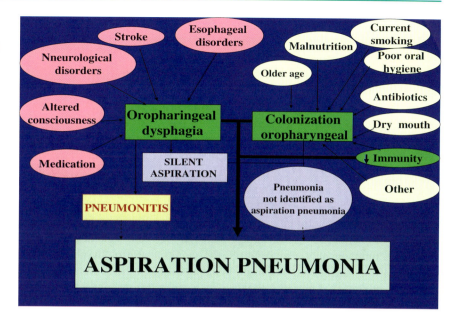

reduced helper T-cell activity and response to antigens, reduced numbers of B cells and B-cell response to antigens, reduced antibody response, reduced phagocytosis, and reduced numbers of Toll-like receptors on phagocytic cells.

8. Feeding tubes. These reduce salivary flow and subsequently alter oropharyngeal colonization in tube-fed patients, but the prevalence of gastroesophageal reflux disease has also been shown to be increased in tube-fed patients and to predispose them to pneumonia (Fig. 8). Increased incidence of oropharyngeal colonization with respiratory pathogens is also caused by impairment of salivary clearance (Palmer et al. 2001). The microbial cause of aspiration pneumonia involves *Staphylococcus aureus*, *Haemophilus influenzae*, and *Streptococcus pneumoniae* for community-acquired aspiration pneumonia and Gram-negative aerobic bacilli in nosocomial pneumonia (Almirall et al. 2007). It is worth bearing in mind the relative unimportance of anaerobic bacteria in aspiration pneumonia (Almirall et al. 2007). Surprisingly, in the clinical setting, oropharyngeal dysphagia and aspiration are usually not considered etiologic factors in older patients with pneumonia (Marik and Kaplan 2003; Almirall et al. 2007).

There are many unanswered questions about the monitoring and treatment of aspiration pneumonia. In a recent editorial, Connolly (2010) raised the following points: (1) Should we be instituting a policy of universal screening for dysphagia in elderly people presenting with pneumonia (or indeed in the frail, hospitalized elderly in general)? (2) Should we modify our treatment of pneumonia in older people to "cover" Gram-negative bacteria and staphylococci? (3) What evidence is there that mouth colonization by potentially unpleasant bacteria is of any clinical significance? (4) Should we screen for mouth colonization? (5) Can we eradicate such colonization, and if so does this affect the incidence or prevalence of morbidity and/or mortality from lower respiratory tract infection? (6) If eradication attempts are deemed useful and feasible, what methods should we use? (7) What are the possible side effects of such policies and what will be the costs? These and other questions must be answered in the next few years if we want to reduce the incidence of this important complication.

3.2 Complications of Malnutrition

The consequences of malnutrition for patients with oropharyngeal dysphagia can be very serious. Impaired ventilatory drive and immune function, delayed wound healing and convalescence from illness, and decreased functional status are the main contributors for the enhanced morbidity in malnutrition (Norman et al. 2008).

Impaired nutritional status results in impaired ventilatory drive and decreased respiratory muscle function. Malnutrition and protein depletion reduces muscle mass and impairs the strength of the respiratory muscles. This leads to decreased vital capacity, increase in airflow resistance and residual volume (Arora and Rochester 1982), and lower strength of cough (Finestone et al. 1995). The weight of the diaphragm is related directly and significantly to body weight, and lung function tests were correlated with BMI and lean mass in different patient groups, including those with chronic obstructive pulmonary disease or cystic fibrosis (Dureuil and Matuszczak 1998). The reduction of contractile force present in starvation-related malnutrition can be reversed completely with nutritional replenishment (Elia et al. 2005). Malnutrition may also influence the clinical outcome of the patient with dysphagia by depressing immune response. Epidemiological observations confirmed that infection and malnutrition aggravate each other. However, nutrition does not influence all infections equally (Scrimshaw et al. 1968; Chandra 1990, 1996; Keusch et al. 1983). For some infections (e.g., pneumonia, bacterial and viral diarrhea, measles, tuberculosis), there is overwhelming evidence that the clinical course and final outcome are negatively affected by nutritional deficiency. For other infections (e.g., viral encephalitis, tetanus), the permissive role of impaired nutritional status is limited. It is now established that nutritional deficiency is commonly associated with impaired immune responses, particularly cell-mediated immunity, phagocyte function, cytokine production, secretory antibody response, antibody affinity, and the complement system (Chandra and Newberne et al. 1977; Gershwin et al. 1984; Bendich and Chandra 1990; Chandra 1992). In fact, malnutrition is the most common cause of immunodeficiency worldwide. Another important fact is age: it is recognized that in many older subjects the immune system is not capable of providing defense against microorganisms, malignant cells, and other "foreign" agents. Ageing is associated with a reduction in the levels of many immune responses in most but not all elderly individuals. Changes in immunity associated with ageing include decreased delayed hypersensitivity, reduced interleukin-2 production, decreased lymphocyte response to mitogens and antigens, low rate of seroconversion, and decreased antibody titer after vaccination. Immune dysfunction as assessed by the prevalence of autoantibodies also increases in the elderly (Chandra 2002).

4   Treatment

Treatment of dysphagia and malnutrition in older patients differs greatly among centers. This variability can contribute to some controversy on the effect of swallowing therapy in preventing malnutrition and aspiration pneumonia. In addition, there are a limited number of studies addressing these—unresolved—questions. A recent review found that there are insufficient data to determine the effectiveness of treatments for dysphagia prevention in older adults (Loeb et al. 2003). In contrast, other authors found that treatment of dysphagia is cost-effective and the use of dysphagia-preventive programs is correlated with a reduction in aspiration pneumonia rates (Logemann 1995).

4.1   Treatment of Oropharyngeal Dysphagia

Management strategies for oropharyngeal dysphagia in older patients may be grouped into six major categories and simultaneously applied to the treatment of each patient (Logemann 1995). During VFS, a combination of strategies may be selected to compensate each patient's specific deficiency, and the usefulness of VFS in treating the patient's symptoms is thus explored. Swallow therapy aims at improving the speed, strength, and range of movement of muscles involved in the swallow response and at modifying the mechanics of swallow to improve bolus transfer and avoid or minimize aspiration. It should be remarked that the largest body of literature concerns swallow therapy in older patients after strokes (Cook and Kahrilas 1999). Furthermore, a recent systematic review on the effects of therapy in oropharyngeal dysphagia by speech and language therapists indicated that many questions remain about the actual therapeutic effects, even though some positive significant outcome studies have been published (Speyer et al. 2010). Nutritional and respiratory status should always be monitored in dysphagic patients in order to assess the efficacy of treatments.

1. *Postural strategies, body and head positions.* Verticality and symmetry should be sought during the patient's ingestion. Attention must be paid to controlling breathing and muscle tone. Postural

strategies are easy to adopt—they cause no fatigue—and allow modification of oropharyngeal and bolus path dimensions. Anterior neck flexion (chin tuck) protects the airway (Bulow et al. 2001; Logemann et al. 1989; Lewin et al. 2001), posterior flexion (head extension or chin raise) facilitates gravitational pharyngeal drainage and improves oral transit velocity, head rotation (head turn maneuver) toward the paralyzed pharyngeal side directs food to the healthy side, increases pharyngeal transit efficacy, and facilitates UES opening (Turley and Cohen 2009; Robbins et al. 2005), whereas head tilt to the stronger side prior to the swallow directs the bolus down to the stronger side by utilizing the effects of gravity; deglutition in the lateral or supine decubitus protects against aspirating hypopharyngeal residues.

2. *Change in bolus volume and viscosity.* Reductions in bolus volume and enhancement of bolus viscosity significantly improve safety signs, particularly regarding penetration and aspiration (Clavé et al. 2006). Viscosity is a physical property that can be measured and expressed in SI units (Pa s). The prevalence of penetrations and aspirations is maximal with water and thin fluids (20 mPa s) and decreases with nectar (270 mPa s) and pudding (3,900 mPa s) viscosity boluses (Clavé et al. 2006). In addition, clinical studies also found dietary modifications can reduce the risk of aspiration pneumonia (Cook and Kahrilas 1999). Patients with decreased efficiency of deglutition need dietary adjustments to concentrate their caloric and protein requirements in the low volume of food they can swallow. Modifying the texture of liquids is particularly important to ensure that patients with neurogenic or ageing-associated dysphagia remain adequately hydrated and aspiration-free (Clavé et al. 2004). This may be easily achieved by using appropriate thickening agents (Clavé et al. 2006).

3. *Neuromuscular praxis.* The goal is to improve the physiology of deglutition (the tonicity, sensitivity, and motility of oral structures, particularly the lips and tongue, and pharyngeal structures). Lingual control and propulsion may be improved by using rehabilitation and biofeedback techniques (Robbins et al. 2005). Improved isometric strength after 2 months of progressive resistance lingual exercises has proved to correspond with

spontaneous increased pressure generation during swallowing in stroke patients, thus showing significant improvement in swallowing function and dietary intake (Robbins et al. 2005). Of late, the rehabilitation of hyoid muscles with cervical flexion exercises (Shaker exercise) has been shown to improve hyoid and laryngeal elevation, to increase UES opening, to reduce pharyngeal residue, and to improve dysphagia symptoms in patients with neurogenic dysphagia (Shaker et al. 2002). The management of patients with impaired UES opening as a consequence of propulsive deficiencies should be basically oriented to increase bolus propulsion force and to rehabilitate the extrinsic mechanisms of UES opening, particularly the activity of hyoid muscles (Shaker et al. 2002). The tongue-holding or Masako maneuver is presumed to compensate for the reduction in tongue base–pharyngeal wall contact in swallowing, thus contributing to an increased anterior movement of the posterior pharyngeal wall during swallowing. However, the use of the maneuver per se, which inhibits posterior retraction of the base of the tongue, results in increasing the amount of pharyngeal residue after the swallow. Another motor treatment for improving muscles strength is *neuromuscular electrostimulation* (NMES). The first study using NMES in dysphagic patients was performed by Freed et al.(2001). Since then, several studies have been published with controversial therapy outcome (Leelamanit et al. 2002; Burnett et al. 2003; Blumenfeld et al. 2006; Kiger et al. 2006), probably owing to the diversity in treatment parameters (frequency, pulse duration, or treatment intensity) and lack of a standard protocol for the use of NMES. However, although NMES as an adjunct to standard treatment is still controversial, a meta-analysis showed a small but significant treatment effect for transcutaneous NMES on patients with dysphagia (Bogaardt et al. 2009).

4. *Specific swallowing maneuvers.* These are maneuvers the patient must be able to learn and perform in an automated way. Each maneuver is specifically directed to compensate for specific biomechanical alterations (Clavé et al. 2005a; Logemann 1995).

   – *Supraglottic and super supraglottic swallow.* Its aim is to close the vocal folds before and during deglutition in order to protect the airway from aspiration, and by coughing immediately after the swallow to clear any residue. The difference between these related maneuvers is the degree of effort in the preswallow breath-hold. The super supraglottic swallow requires an effortful breath-hold, whereas the supraglottic swallow requires a breath-hold with no extra effort. It is useful in patients with penetrations or aspirations during the pharyngeal stage or slow pharyngeal motor pattern.

– *Effortful, forceful, or hard swallow.* Its aim is to increase the posterior motion of the tongue base during deglutition in order to improve bolus propulsion. It is useful in patients with low bolus propulsion (Clavé et al. 2005a; Logemann 1995).

– *Double deglutition.* Its aim is to minimize the amount of postswallow residue before a new inspiration. It is useful in patients with post-swallow residue (Logemann 1995).

– *Mendelsohn maneuver.* It allows for increased extent and duration of laryngeal elevation and therefore increased duration and amplitude of UES opening (Logemann 1995).

5. *Surgical/drug-based management of UES disorders.* Identifying an obstructive pattern at the UES allows patient treatment using a surgical cricopharyngeal section (Shaw et al. 1996) or an injection of botulinum toxin (Ravich 2001). Impaired neural UES relaxation observed in spastic neurological diseases such as Parkinson's disease and brain injury is characterized by delayed or absent swallow response, short hyoid motion, weak bolus propulsion, and reduced or even absent neuromuscular relaxation and reduced sphincter compliance on manometry (Williams et al. 2002). Treatment must combine treatment of neurogenic dysphagia and improvement of neuromuscular relaxation of the sphincter. The efficacy of cricopharyngeal myotomy in patients with impaired swallow response is fair to poor and injection of botulinum toxin in the sphincter could be a therapeutic alternative for these patients. Patients with impaired UES opening associated with Zenker's diverticulum or isolated cricopharyngeal bars show normal swallow response, wide hyoid motion, and strong bolus propulsion and reduced sphincter compliance caused by sphincter fibrosis (Clavé et al. 2007). Treatment of this group of patients is surgical and combines cricopharyngeal myotomy and resection of the diverticulum. Surgical results in older patients with Zenker's diverticulum and preserved swallow response are excellent (Clavé et al. 2007).

6. *Sensorial enhancement strategies.* Oral sensorial enhancement strategies are particularly useful in patients with apraxia or impaired oral sensitivity (very common in older patients) (Logemann 1995). The aim these strategies is the initiation or acceleration of the oropharyngeal swallow response. Most sensorial enhancement strategies include a mechanical stimulation of the tongue, bolus modifications (volume, temperature, and taste), or a mechanical stimulation of the pharyngeal pillars. Acid flavors such as lemon and lime (Hamdy et al. 2003; Logemann et al. 1995) and cold substances such as ice cream and ice (Rosenbek et al. 1996) trigger the mechanism of deglutition, but may not reach clinical or statistical significance even after intense training.

7. *Pharmacology of swallow response.* Several drugs, most centrally acting, can elicit oropharyngeal dysphagia in older people. Neural activity in the NTS is inhibited by γ-aminobutyric acid (GABA) (Wang and Bieger 1991; Hockman et al. 1996), and benzodiazepine administration can potentiate the GABA system in the CNS and cause dysphagia (Dantas and Nobre Souza 1997). Ethanol also acts in the CNS, binding to the $GABA_A$ receptor, and alcohol ingestion can predispose to oropharyngeal aspiration (Dua et al. 2009). Neuroleptics are widely used in the older demented population for control of aggressive or disruptive behavior, and dopamine antagonists such as phenothiazines and haloperidol can impair swallow function. Moreover, extrapyramidal signs and xerostomia are common adverse effects of these drugs clearly associated with dysphagia (Sokoloff and Pavlakovic 1997; Dziewas et al. 2007). Use of neuroleptics is also associated with a 60% greater risk of pneumonia (Knol et al. 2008). Studies using pharmacological stimulant agents have also shown some promising positive effects (Loeb et al. 2003). Several types of pharmacological and mechanical stimulation increase the concentration of substance P (SP) in saliva and improve the swallowing reflex and cough-reflex sensitivity. The increase in the serum SP concentration with volatile black pepper oil or capsaicin might be closely related to improvement of the swallow response

Fig. 9 Algorithm for indication of percutaneous endoscopic gastrostomy (*PEG*) in patients with oropharyngeal dysphagia and impaired safety of swallow. *VFS* videofluoroscopy

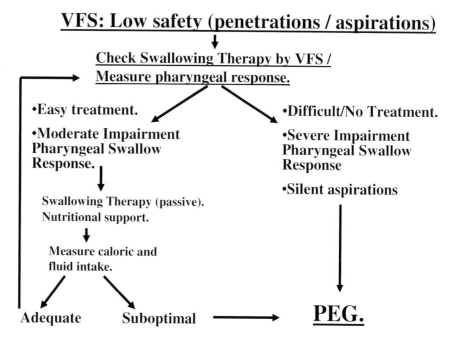

(Ebihara et al. 1993, 2005, 2006). Capsaicin and piperine (active substance from black pepper) act as transient receptor potential channel vanilloid 1 (TRPV1) agonists. TRPV1 is widely expressed on sensory neurons innervating the pharynx and larynx, projecting to NTS, and colocalizes with SP (Hamamoto et al. 2009). Other stimulants of TRPV1, such as heat and acid, have also been reported to improve swallowing (Hamdy et al. 2003; Logemann et al. 1995; Watando et al. 2004). Moreover, intervention with an angiotensin-converting enzyme inhibitor also resulted in an increase in the serum SP concentration, and reduced the incidence of aspiration pneumonia (Nakayama et al. 1998; Sekizawa et al. 1998). Use of a dopamine agonist such as amantadine and a folic acid supplement known to activate dopaminergic neurons also prevented aspiration pneumonia (Nakagawa et al. 1999) Higher doses of L-dopa may reduce swallowing abnormalities (Sueli 2005). The development of physical or drug-based strategies to accelerate the swallow response is a relevant field of research for the management of neurogenic dysphagia and ageing-associated dysphagia (Clavé et al. 2005a).

8. *Percutaneous endoscopic gastrostomy (PEG).* VFS will help in *treatment selection* depending upon the severity of efficacy or safety impairment in each patient: (1) patients with mild efficacy alterations

and correct safety may have a family-supervised restriction-free diet; (2) in patients with moderate alterations, dietary changes will be introduced aiming at decreasing the volume and increasing the viscosity of the alimentary bolus; (3) patients with severe alterations will require additional strategies based upon increased viscosity and the introduction of postural techniques, active maneuvers, and oral sensorial enhancement; and (4) there is a group of patients with alterations so severe that they cannot be treated despite using rehabilitation techniques— in these patients, VFS objectively demonstrates the inability of the oral route and the need to perform a PEG (Fig. 9) (Clavé et al. 2004). However, there is little evidence that nonoral feeding reduces the risk of aspiration (Cook and Kahrilas 1999). Even though no absolute criteria exist, a number of dysphagia teams have indicated gastrostomy in (1) patients with severe alterations of efficacy during the oral or pharyngeal stages, or with malnutrition; (2) patients with safety alterations during the pharyngeal stage who do not respond to rehabilitation; and (3) patients with significant silent aspirations, particularly in neurodegenerative conditions. For long-term nutritional support, PEG should be preferred to nasogastric tubes since it is associated with less treatment failure, better nutritional status, and may also be more convenient for the patient

(Addington et al. 1999). In patients with severe neurological dysphagia, tube feeding has to be initiated as early as possible (Robbins et al. 2005) For most patients requiring gastrostomy, a small amount of food may still be safely administered through the oral route (Clavé et al. 2004).

4.2 Treatment of Malnutritition

A recent resolution of the Council of Europe on food and nutritional care in hospitals claimed that undernutrition among hospital patients leads to extended hospital stays, prolonged rehabilitation, diminished quality of life, and unnecessary health care costs, and identified functional oropharyngeal dysphagia as a major contributor to malnutrition (Milne et al. 2006). Robinson et al. (1987) showed that patients with an impaired nutritional status on hospital admission experienced a 30% increase of hospital stay and this was associated with a doubling of the costs, even though the patients belonged to the same disease-related group and therefore had the same reimbursement. A recent study from South America even reported an increase of treatment costs by 300% (Correia and Waitzberg 2003) This is in contrast with the results of trials that showed that the prevalence of malnutrition can be reduced by proper nutritional care (O'Flynn et al. 2005) and that nutritional therapy in malnourished patients resulted in a significant reduction of the length of stay by an average of approximately 2.5 days and in treatment costs (Tucker and Miguel 1996; Kruizenga et al. 2005). Recommendations from this resolution (Milne et al. 2006) which are related to dysphagia include (1) the development of dietary management at national levels as well as national descriptors for texture modification, (2) documentation and assessment of food intake, (3) detailed food service contracts to include texture-modified menus, (4) a meal serving system adjusted to patients, and (5) informing and involving patients/families in the process by giving them help and guidance in ordering and consuming food. If a patient is at nutritional risk or is malnourished, nutritional counseling will be given to improve the oral feeding. This is the first nutritional intervention previous to any nutritional support. In some circumstances, nutritional counseling is not enough to maintain or recover proper nutritional status, and oral nutritional supplements (ONS) are indicated. Milne et al. (2006) reviewed 55 randomized controlled trials that studied the clinical and nutritional benefits of ONS in older patients on hospital admission, at home, and in nursing homes. They concluded that ONS can improve nutritional status and reduce morbidity and mortality in malnourished patients during hospital admission. The scientific evidence does not support ordinary supplementation in older people at home or in older well-nourished patients in any clinical setting (hospital, home, or nursing home). However, in patients with stroke and dysphagia, the FOOD study (Dennis et al. 2005) evaluated the effect of systematically adding an oral supplement to the hospital diet. These data did not support indiscriminate use of ONS in patients with stroke and ONS must be prescribed only for malnourished patients on admission or for those in whom nutritional status is impaired.

5 Conclusions

Identification of functional oropharyngeal dysphagia as a major neurological and geriatric syndrome will soon cause many changes in the provision of medical and social services. Education of health professionals on diagnosis and treatment of dysphagia and its complications, early diagnosis, development of specific complementary explorations in the clinical setting, improvement in therapeutic strategies to avoid aspirations and malnutrition, and research into its pathophysiological aspects are the cornerstones to allow maximal recovery potential for older patients with functional oropharyngeal dysphagia. In many hospitals there is a big discrepancy between the high prevalence, morbidity, mortality, and costs caused by nutritional and respiratory complications of functional oropharyngeal dysphagia and the restricted availability of human and material resources dedicated to dysphagic patients. Dysphagia with oropharyngeal aspiration is not usually considered an etiologic factor in older patients with community-acquired pneumonia (Marik and Kaplan 2003; Almirall et al. 2007) or with malnutrition (Clavé et al. 2005b).

Therefore, diagnosis and management of oropharyngeal dysphagia needs a *multidisciplinary approach*. A *multidisciplinary dysphagia team* should include several professional domains: nurses, speech–swallow therapists, gastroenterologists, ENT specialists, neurologists, surgeons, rehabilitation physicians, dietitians, radiologists, geriatricians, etc. The goals of a multidisciplinary dysphagia team include: (1) early identification of older patients with dysphagia; (2) diagnosis of any medical or surgical cause of dysphagia that may respond to specific treatment; (3) characterization of specific biomechanical events responsible for functional dysphagia in each patient; and (4) the design of a set of therapeutic strategies to provide patients with safe and effective deglutition, or the provision of an alternative route to oral feeding based on objective and reproducible data (Clavé et al. 2004, 2005b). The involvement of the patient's family in the diagnostic and therapeutic process is of capital importance.

References

Addington WR, Stephens RE, Gilliland KA (1999) Assessing the laryngeal cough reflex and the risk of developing pneumonia after stroke: an interhospital comparison. Stroke 30:1203–1207

Almirall J, Cabre M, Clavé P (2007) Aspiration pneumonia. Med Clin (Barc) 129:424–432

Anker SD, John M, Pedersen PU, Raguso C, Cicoira M, Dardai E, Laviano A, Ponikowski P, Schols AM, Becker HF, Böhm M, Brunkhorst FM, Vogelmeier C (2006) ESPEN guidelines on enteral nutrition: cardiology and pulmonology. Clin Nutr 25:311–318

Arends J, Bodoky G, Bozzetti F, Fearon K, Muscaritoli M, Selga G, van Bokhorst-de van der Schueren MA, von Meyenfeldt M, DGEM (German Society for Nutritional Medicine), Zürcher G, Fietkau R, Aulbert E, Frick B, Holm M, Kneba M, Mestrom HJ, Zander A (2006) ESPEN guidelines on enteral nutrition: non-surgical oncology. Clin Nutr 25:245–259

Arora NS, Rochester DF (1982) Respiratory muscle strength and maximal ventilatory ventilation in undernourished patients. Am Rev Respir Dis 126:5–8

Belafsky PC, Mouadeb DA, Rees CJ, Pryor JC, Postma GN, Allen J, Leonard RJ (2008) Validity and reliability of the Eating Assessment Tool (EAT-10). Ann Otol Rhinol Laryngol 117:919–924

Bendich A, Chandra RK (1990) Micronutrients and immune functions. New York Academy of Sciences, New York

Blumenfeld L, Hahn Y, Lepage A, Leonard R, Belafsky PC (2006) Transcutaneous electrical stimulation versus traditional dysphagia therapy: a nonconcurrent cohort study. Otolaryngol Head Neck Surg 135:754–757

Bogaardt H, Van Dam D, Wever NM, Bruggeman CE, Koops J, Fokkens WJ (2009) Use of neuromuscular electrostimulation in the treatment of dysphagia in patients with multiple sclerosis. Ann Otol Rhinol Laryngol 118:241–246

Bours GJ, Speyer R, Lemmens J, Limburg M, de Wit R (2009) Bedside screening tests vs videofluoroscopy or fibreoptic endoscopic evaluation of swallowing to detect dysphagia in patients with neurological disorders: systematic review. J Adv Nurs 65:477–493

Bulow M, Olsson R, Ekberg O (2001) Videomanometric analysis of supraglottic swallow, effortful swallow, and chin tuck in patients with pharyngeal dysfunction. Dysphagia 16:190–195

Burnett TA, Mann EA, Cornell SA, Ludlow CL (2003) Laryngeal elevation achieved by neuromuscular stimulation at rest. J Appl Physiol 94:128–134

Cabre M, Serra-Prat M, Palomera E, Almirall J, Pallares R, Clavé P (2010) Prevalence and prognostic implications of dysphagia in elderly patients with pneumonia. Age Ageing 39:39–45

Cabré M, Monteis R, Roca M, Palomera E, Serra M, Clavé P (2010) Association between oropharyngeal dysphagia and malnutrition in hospitalized patients in acute geriatric unit. Rev Esp Geriatr Gerontol 45:17

Campbell IT (1999) Limitations of nutrient intake. The effect of stressors: trauma, sepsis and multiple organ failure. Eur J Clin Nutr 53:S143–S147

Cano N, Fiaccadori E, Tesinsky P, Toigo G, Druml W, Kuhlmann M, Mann H, Hörl WH (2006) ESPEN guidelines on enteral nutrition: adult renal failure. Clin Nutr 25: 295–310

Chai J, Chu FC, Chow TW, Shum NC (2008) Prevalence of malnutrition and its risk factors in stroke patients residing in an infirmary. Singapore Med J 49:290–296

Chandra RK, 1990 McCollum Award Lecture (1990) Nutrition and immunity: lessons from the past and new insights into the future. Am J Clin Nutr 53:1087–1101

Chandra RK (1992) Nutrition and Immunology. ARTS Biomedical, St John's

Chandra RK (1996) Nutrition, immunity and infection: from basic knowledge of dietary manipulation of immune responses to practical application of ameliorating suffering and improving survival. Proc Natl Acad Sci 93:14304–14307

Chandra RK (2002) Nutrition and the immune system from birth to old age. Eur J Clin Nutr 56:S73–S76

Chandra RK, Newberne PM (1977) Nutrition, immunity and infection. Mechanisms of interactions. Plenum, New York

Chien MY, Huang TY, Wu YT (2008) Prevalence of sarcopenia estimated using a bioelectrical impedance analysis prediction equation in community-dwelling elderly people in Taiwan. J Am Geriatr Soc 56:1710–1715

Clavé P, Terre R, de Kraa M, Serra M (2004) Approaching oropharyngeal dysphagia. Rev Esp Enferm Dig 96: 119–131

Clavé P, Verdaguer A, Arreola V (2005a) Oral-pharyngeal dysphagia in the elderly. Med Clin (Barc) 124:742–748

Clavé P, Almirall J, Esteve A, Verdaguer A, Berenguer M, Serra-Prat M (2005b) Dysphagia—a team approach to prevent and treat complications. Hosp Healthc Eur N5–N8

Clavé P, de Kraa M, Arreola V, Girvent M, Farre R, Palomera E, Serra-Prat M (2006) The effect of bolus viscosity on swallowing function in neurogenic dysphagia. Aliment Pharmacol Ther 24:1385–1394

Clavé P, Arreola V, Velasco M, Quer M, Castellvi JM, Almirall J, Garcia Peris P, Carrau R (2007) Diagnosis and treatment of functional oropharyngeal dysphagia. Features of interest to the digestive surgeon. Cir Esp 82:62–76

Connolly MJ (2010) Of proverbs and prevention: aspiration and its consequences in older patients. Age Ageing 39:2–4

Cook IJ, Kahrilas PJ (1999) AGA technical review on management of oropharyngeal dysphagia. Gastroenterology 116:455–478

Correia MI, Waitzberg DL (2003) The impact of malnutrition on morbidity, mortality, length of hospital stay and costs evaluated through a multivariate model analysis. Clin Nutr 22:235–239

Cruz-Jentoft AJ, Baeyens JP, Bauer JM, Boirie Y, Cederholm T, Landi F, Martin FC, Michel JP, Rolland Y, Schneider SM, Topinková E, Vandewoude M, Zamboni M (2010) European working group on sarcopenia in older people. Sarcopenia: European consensus on definition and diagnosis: report of the European working group on sarcopenia in older people. Age Ageing 39:412–423

Dantas RO, Nobre Souza MA (1997) Dysphagia induced by chronic ingestion of benzodiazepine. Am J Gastroenterol 92:1194–1196

Delmonico MJ, Harris TB, Lee JS, Visser M, Nevitt M, Kritchevsky SB, Tylavsky FA, Newman AB (2007) Alternative definitions of sarcopenia, lower extremity performance, and functional impairment with aging in older men and women. J Am Geriatr Soc 55:769–774

Dennis MS, Lewis SC, Warlow C (2005) FOOD trial collaboration. Routine oral nutritional supplementation for stroke patients in hospital (FOOD): a multicentre randomised controlled trial. Lancet 365:755–763

DePippo KL, Holas MA, Reding MJ (1992) Validation of the 3-oz water swallow test for aspiration following stroke. Arch Neurol 49:1259–1261

Detsky AS, McLaughlin JR, Baker JP, Johnston N, Whittaker S, Mendelson RA, Jeejeebhoy KN (1987) What is subjective global assessment of nutritional status? J Parenter Enteral Nutr 11:8–13

Dua KS, Surapaneni SN, Santharam R, Knuff D, Hofmann C, Shaker R (2009) Effect of systemic alcohol and nicotine on airway protective reflexes. Am J Gastroenterol 104:2431–2438

Dupertuis YM, Kossovsky MP, Kyle UG, Raguso CA, Genton L, Pichard C (2003) Food intake in 1707 hospitalised patients: a prospective comprehensive hospital survey. Clin Nutr 22:115–123

Dureuil B, Matuszczak Y (1998) Alteration in nutritional status and diaphragm muscle function. Reprod Nutr Dev 38:175–180

Dziewas R, Warnecke T, Schnabel M, Ritter M, Nabavi DG, Schilling M, Ringelstein EB, Reker T (2007) Neuroleptic-induced dysphagia: case report and literature review 1. Dysphagia 22:63–67

Ebihara T, Sekizawa K, Nakazawa H, Sasaki H (1993) Capsaicin and swallowing reflex. Lancet 341:432

Ebihara T, Takahashi H, Ebihara S, Okazaki T, Sasaki T, Watando A, Nemoto M, Sasaki H (2005) Capsaicin troche for swallowing dysfunction in older people. J Am Geriatr Soc 53:824–828

Ebihara T, Ebihara S, Maruyama M, Kobayashi M, Itou A, Arai H, Sasaki HA (2006) Randomized trial of olfactory stimulation using black pepper oil in older people with swallowing dysfunction. J Am Geriatr Soc 54:1401–1406

Ekberg O, Hamdy S, Woisard V, Wuttge-Hannig A, Ortega P (2002) Social and psychological burden of dysphagia: its impact on diagnosis and treatment. Dysphagia 17:139–146

Elia M, Stratton R, Russell C, Green C, Pang F (2005) The cost of disease-related malnutrition in the UK and economic considerations for the use of oral nutritional supplements (ONS) in adults: executive summary. British Association for Parenteral and Enteral Nutrition, Redditch

Finestone HM, Greene-Finestone LS, Wilson ES, Teasell RW (1995) Malnutrition in stroke patients on the rehabilitation service and at follow-up: prevalence and predictors. Arch Phys Med Rehabil 76:310–316

Foley NC, Martin RE, Salter KL, Teasell RW (2009) A review of the relationship between dysphagia and malnutrition following stroke. J Rehabil Med 41:707–713

Freed ML, Freed L, Chatburn RL, Christian M (2001) Electrical stimulation for swallowing disorders caused by stroke. Respir Care 46:466–474

Gale CR, Martyn CN, Cooper C, Sayer AA (2007) Grip strength, body composition, and mortality. Int J Epidemiol 36:228–235

García-Peris P, Parón L, Velasco C, de la Cuerda C, Camblor M, Bretón I, Herencia H, Verdaguer J, Navarro C, Clavé P (2007) Long-term prevalence of oropharyngeal dysphagia in head and neck cancer patients: Impact on quality of life. Clin Nutr 26:710–717

Gershwin ME, Beach RS, Hurley LS (1984) Nutrition and Immunity. Academic Press, New York

Gil A Tratado de nutrición. Ángel Gil Hernández, vol IV, 2nd edn. chap 1

Goodpaster BH, Park SW, Harris TB, Kritchevsky SB, Nevitt M, Schwartz AV, Simonsick EM, Tylavsky FA, Visser M, Newman AB (2006) The loss of skeletal muscle strength, mass, and quality in older adults: the health, aging and body composition study. J Gerontol A Biol Sci Med Sci 61:1059–1064

Gordon C, Hewer RL, Wade DT (1987) Dysphagia in acute stroke. Br Med J (Clin Res Edu) 295:411–414

Hamamoto T, Takumida M, Hirakawa A, Tatsukawa T, Ishibashi T (2009) Localization of transient receptor potential vanilloid (TRPV) in the human larynx. Acta Otolaryngol 129:560–568

Hamdy S, Rothwell JC, Brooks DJ, Bailey D, Aziz Q, Thompson DG (1999) Identification of the cerebral loci processing human swallowing with H2(15)O PET activation1. J Neurophysiol 81:1917–1926

Hamdy S, Jilani S, Price V, Parker C, Hall N, Power M (2003) Modulation of human swallowing behaviour by thermal and chemical stimulation in health and after brain injury. Neurogastroenterol Motil 15:69–77

Hockman CH, Weerasuriya A, Bieger D (1996) GABA receptor-mediated inhibition of reflex deglutition in the cat. Dysphagia 11:209–215

Incalzi RA, Gemma A, Capparella O, Cipriani L, Landi F, Carbonin P (1996) Energy intake and in-hospital starvation. A clinically relevant relationship. Arch Intern Med 156:425–429

Janssen I, Heymsfield SB, Baumgartner RN, Ross R (2000) Estimation of skeletal muscle mass by bioelectrical impedance analysis. J Appl Physiol 89:465–471

Janssen I Heymsfield SB, Ross R (2002) Low relative skeletal muscle mass (sarcopenia) in older persons is associated with functional impairment and physical disability. J Am Geriatr Soc 50:889–896

Janssen I, Shepard DS, Katzmarzyk PT, Roubenoff R (2004a) The healthcare costs of sarcopenia in the United States. J Am Geriatr Soc 52:80–85

Janssen I, Baumgartner R, Ross R, Rosenberg IH, Roubenoff R (2004b) Skeletal muscle cutpoints associated with elevated physical disability risk in older men and women. Am J Epidemiol 159:413–421

Jean A (2001) Brain stem control of swallowing: neuronal network and cellular mechanisms. Physiol Rev 81:929–969

Jensen GL, Mirtallo J, Compher C, Dhaliwal R, Forbes A, Grijalba RF, Hardy G, Kondrup J, Labadarios D, Nyulasi I, Castillo Pineda JC, Waitzberg D (2010) Adult starvation and disease-related malnutrition: a proposal for etiology-based diagnosis in the clinical practice setting from the International Consensus Guideline Committee. Clin Nutr 29:151–153

Kahrilas PJ, Lin S, Chen J, Logemann JA (1996) Oropharyngeal accommodation to swallow volume. Gastroenterology 111:297–306

Kahrilas PJ, Lin S, Rademaker AW, Logemann JA (1997) Impaired deglutitive airway protection: a videofluoroscopic analysis of severity and mechanism. Gastroenterology 113:1457–1464

Keusch GT, Wilson CS, Waksal SD (1983) Nutrition, host defenses, and the lymphoid system. Arch Host Defense Mech 2:275–359

Kiger M, Brown CS, Watkins L (2006) Dysphagia management: an analysis of patient outcomes using VitalStim therapy compared to traditional swallow therapy. Dysphagia 21:243–253

Knol W, van Marum R, Jansen PA, Souverein PC, Schobben AF, Egberts AC (2008) Antipsychotic drug use and risk of pneumonia in elderly people. J Am Geriatr Soc 56:661–666

Kondrup J, Johansen N, Plum LM, Bak L, Larsen IH, Martinsen A, Andersen JR, Baernthsen H, Bunch E, Lauesen N (2002) Incidence of nutritional risk and causes of inadequate nutritional care in hospitals. Clin Nutr 21:461–468

Kondrup J, Rasmussen HH, Hamberg O, Stanga Z (2003) Nutritional risk screening (NRS 2002): a new method based on an analysis of controlled clinical trials. Clin Nutr 22:321–336

Kreymann KG, Berger MM, Deutz NE, Hiesmayr M, Jolliet P, Kazandjiev G, Nitenberg G, van den Berghe G, Wernerman J, DGEM (German Society for Nutritional Medicine), Ebner C, Hartl W, Heymann C, Spies C (2006) ESPEN guidelines on enteral nutrition: intensive care. Clin Nutr 25:210–223

Kruizenga HM, Van Tulder MW, Seidell JC, Thijs A, Ader HJ, Van Bokhorst-de van der Schueren MA (2005) Effectiveness and cost-effectiveness of early screening and treatment of malnourished patients. Am J Clin Nutr 82:1082–1089

Kyle UG, Genton L, Slosman DO, Pichard C (2001a) Fat-free and fat mass percentiles in 5225 healthy subjects aged 15 to 98 years. Nutrition 17:534–541

Kyle UG, Genton L, Karsegard L, Slosman DO, Pichard C (2001b) Single prediction equation for bioelectrical impedance analysis in adults aged 20–94 years. Nutrition 17:248–253

Langmore SE, Schatz K, Olson N (1991) Endoscopic and videofluoroscopic evaluations of swallowing and aspiration. Ann Otol Rhinol Laryngol 100:678–681

Leelamanit V, Limsakul C, Geater A (2002) Synchronized electrical stimulation in treating pharyngeal dysphagia. Laryngoscope 112:2204–2210

Lewin JS, Hebert TM, Putnam JB, DuBrow RA (2001) Experience with the chin tuck maneuver in postesophagectomy aspirators. Dysphagia 16:216–219

Lochs H, Dejong C, Hammarqvist F, Hebuterne X, Leon-Sanz M, Schutz T, van Gemert W, van Gossum A, Valentini L, DGEM (German Society for Nutritional Medicine), Lübke H, Bischoff S, Engelmann N, Thul P (2006) ESPEN guidelines on enteral nutrition:gastroenterology. Clin Nutr 25:260–274

Loeb MB, Becker M, Eady A, Walker-Dilks C (2003) Interventions to prevent aspiration pneumonia in older adults: a systematic review. J Am Geriatr Soc 51:1018–1022

Logemann JA (1993) Manual for the videofluorographic study of swallowing, 2nd edn. Pro-Ed, Austin

Logemann JA (1995) Dysphagia: evaluation and treatment. Folia Phoniatr Logop 47:140–164

Logemann JA, Kahrilas PJ, Kobara M, Vakil NB (1989) The benefit of head rotation on pharyngoesophageal dysphagia. Arch Phys Med Rehabil 70:767–771

Logemann JA, Pauloski BR, Colangelo L, Lazarus C, Fujiu M, Kahrilas PJ (1995) Effects of a sour bolus on oropharyngeal swallowing measures in patients with neurogenic dysphagia. J Speech Hear Res 38:556–563

Lukasi H (ed), Heymsfield M (2005) Assessing muscle mass. Human body composition. Human Kinetics, Champaign

Malnutrition Advisory Group (MAG) (2000) MAG—guidelines for detection and management of malnutrition. British Association for Parenteral and Enteral Nutrition, Redditch

Marik PE, Kaplan D (2003) Aspiration pneumonia and dysphagia in the elderly. Chest 124:328–336

Markson EW (1997) Functional, social, and psychological disability as causes of loss of weight and independence in older community living people. Clin Geriatr Med 13:639–652

Meier R, Ockenga J, Pertkiewicz M, Pap A, Milinic N, Macfie J, DGEM (German Society for Nutritional Medicine), Löser C, Keim V (2006) ESPEN guidelines on enteral nutrition: pancreas. Clin Nutr 25:275–284

Milne A, Avenell A, Potter J (2006) Meta-analysis: protein and energy supplementation in elderly people at risk from malnutrition. Ann Intern Med 144:37–48

Morley JE (1997) Anorexia of aging: physiologic and pathologic. Am J Clin Nutr 66:760–773

Morley JE (2008) Sarcopenia: diagnosis and treatment. J Nutr Health Aging 12:452–456

Nagaya M, Sumi Y (2002) Reaction time in the submental muscles of normal older people. J Am Geriatr Soc 50:975–976

Nakagawa T, Wada H, Sekizawa K, Arai H, Sasaki H (1999) Amantadine and pneumonia. Lancet 353:1157

Nakayama K, Sekizawa K, Sasaki H (1998) ACE inhibitor and swallowing reflex. Chest 113:1425

Nathadwarawala KM, Nicklin J, Wiles CM (1992) A timed test of swallowing capacity for neurological patients. J Neurol Neurosurg Psychiatry 55:822–825

Nicosia M, Robbins J (2001) The fluid mechanics of bolus ejection from the oral cavity. J Biomech 34:1537–1544

NIH (1996) Bioelectrical impedance analysis in body composition measurement: national institutes of health technology assessment conference statement. Am J Clin Nutr 64: 524S–532S

Norman K, Richard C, Lochs H, Pirlich M (2008) Prognostic impact of disease-related malnutrition. Clin Nutr 27:5–15

Nozaki S, Saito T, Matsumura T, Miyai I, Kang J (1999) Relationship between weight loss and dysphagia in patients with Parkinson's disease. Rinsho Shinkeigaku 39: 1010–1014

O'Flynn J, Peake H, Hickson M, Foster D, Frost G (2005) The prevalence of malnutrition in hospitals can be reduced: results from three consecutive cross-sectional studies. Clin Nutr 24:1078–1088

Ockenga J, Grimble R, Jonkers-Schuitema C, Macallan D, Melchior J.C, Sauerwein H.P, Schwenk A, DGEM (German Society for Nutritional Medicine), Süttmann U (2006) ESPEN guidelines on enteral nutrition: wasting in HIV and other chronic infectious diseases. Clin Nutr 25:319–329

Palmer LB, Albulak K, Fields S, Filkin AM, Simon S, Smaldone GC (2001) Oral clearance and pathogenic oropharyngeal colonization in the elderly. Am J Respir Crit Care Med 164:464–468

Pirlich M, Schutz T, Kemps M, Luhman N, Minko N, Lubke HJ, Rossnagel K, Willich SN, Lochs H (2005) Social risk factors for hospital malnutrition. Nutrition 21:295–300

Plauth M, Cabre E, Riggio O, Assis-Camilo M, Pirlich M, Kondrup J, DGEM (German Society for Nutritional Medicine), Ferenci P, Holm E, Vom Dahl S, Müller M.J, Nolte W (2006) ESPEN guidelines on enteral nutrition: liver disease. Clin Nutr 25:285–294

Ravich WJ (2001) Botulinum toxin for UES dysfunction: therapy or poison? Dysphagia 16:168–170

Robbins J, Langmore S, Hind JA, Erlichman M (2002) Dysphagia research in the 21st century and beyond: proceedings from dysphagia experts meeting, August 21, 2001. J Rehabil Res Dev 39:543–548

Robbins J, Gangnon RE, Theis SM, Kays SA, Hewitt AL, Hind JA (2005) The effects of lingual exercise on swallowing in older adults. J Am Geriatr Soc 53:1483–1489

Robinson G, Goldstein M, Levine GM (1987) Impact of nutritional status on DRG length of stay. J Parenter Enteral Nutr 11:49–51

Rofes L, Arreola V, Romea M, Palomera E, Almirall J, Cabré M, Serra-Prat M, Clavé P (2010) Pathophysiology of oropharyngeal dysphagia in the frail elderly. Neurogastroenterol Motil 22:851–858. Epub 2010 Jun 7

Rofes L, Arreola V, Almirall J, Cabré M, Campins L, García-Peris P, Speyer R, Clavé P (2011) Diagnosis and management of oropharyngeal dysphagia and its nutritional and respiratory complications in the elderly. Gastroenterol Res Pract 201:818979

Rolland Y, Czerwinski S, Abellan Van Kan G, Morley JE, Cesari M, Onder G, Woo J, Woo J, Baumgartner R, Pillard F, Boirie Y, Chumlea WM, Vellas B (2008) Sarcopenia: its assessment, etiology, pathogenesis, consequences and future perspectives. J Nutr Health Aging 12:433–450

Rosenbek JC, Robbins J, Roecker EB (1996) A penetration-aspiration scale. Dysphagia 11:93–98

Roubenoff R, Baumgartner RN, Harris TB, Dallal GE, Hannan MT, Economos CD, Stauber PM, Wilson PW, Kiel DP (1997) Application of bioelectrical impedance

analysis to elderly populations. J Gerontol A Biol Sci Med Sci 52:129–136

Sayer AA, Dennison EM, Syddall HE, Gilbody HJ, Phillips DI, Cooper C (2005) Type 2 diabetes, muscle strength, and impaired physical function: the tip of the iceberg? Diabetes Care 28:2541–2542

Schmidt J, Holas M, Halvorson K, Reding M (1994) Videofluoroscopic evidence of aspiration predicts pneumonia and death but not dehydration following stroke. Dysphagia 9:7–11

Scrimshaw NS, Taylor CE, Gordon JE (1968) Interactions of nutrition and infection. World Health Organization, Geneva

Sekizawa K, Matsui T, Nakagawa T, Nakayama K, Sasaki H (1998) ACE inhibitors and pneumonia. Lancet 352:1069

Serra-Prat M, Hinojosa G, López D, Juan M, Fabré E, Voss DS, Calvo M, Marta V, Ribó L, Palomera E, Arreola V, Clavé P (2011) Prevalence of oropharyngeal dysphagia and impaired safety and efficacy of swallow in independently living older persons. J Am Geriatr Soc 59:186–187

Shaker R, Easterling C, Kern M, Nitschke T, Massey B, Daniels S, Grande B, Kazandjian M, Dikeman K (2002) Rehabilitation of swallowing by exercise in tube-fed patients with pharyngeal dysphagia secondary to abnormal UES opening. Gastroenterology 122:1314–1321

Shaw DW, Cook IJ, Jamieson GG, Gabb M, Simula ME, Dent J (1996) Influence of surgery on deglutitive upper oesophageal sphincter mechanics in Zenker's diverticulum. Gut 38:806–811

Smithard DG, O'Neill PA, Park C, England R, Renwick DS, Wyatt R, Morris J, Martin DF (1998) Can bedside assessment reliably exclude aspiration following acute stroke? Age Ageing 27:99–106

Sokoloff LG, Pavlakovic R (1997) Neuroleptic-induced dysphagia. Dysphagia 12:177–179

Speyer R, Baijens L, Heijnen M, Zwijnenberg I (2010) Effects of therapy in oropharyngeal dysphagia by speech and language therapists: a systematic review. Dysphagia 25: 40–65

Sullivan DH, Sun S, Walls RC (1999) Protein-energy undernutrition among elderly hospitalized patients: a prospective study. JAMA 281:2013–2019

Teismann IK, Steinstraeter O, Stoeckigt K, Suntrup S, Wollbrink A, Pantev C, Dziewas R (2007) Functional oropharyngeal sensory disruption interferes with the cortical control of swallowing. BMC Neurosci 8:62

Teismann IK, Steinstrater O, Warnecke T, Suntrup S, Ringelstein EB, Pantev C, Dziewas R (2009) Tactile thermal oral stimulation increases the cortical representation of swallowing. BMC Neurosci 10:71

Tisdale MJ (2005) Molecular pathways leading to cancer cachexia. Physiology (Bethesda) 20:340–348

Tucker HN, Miguel SG (1996) Cost containment through nutritional intervention. Nutr Rev 54:111–121

Turley R, Cohen S (2009) Impact of voice and swallowing problems in the elderly. Otolaryngol Head Neck Surg 140:33–36

Vellas B, Guigoz Y, Garry PJ, Nourhashemi F, Bennahum D, Lauque S, Albarede JL (1999) The Mini Nutritional Assessment (MNA) and its use in grading the nutritional state of elderly patients. Nutrition 15:116–122

Volkert D, Berner Y.N, Berry E, Cederholm T, Coti B.P, Milne A, Palmblad J, Schneider S, Sobotka L, Stanga Z, DGEM

(German Society for Nutritional Medicine), Lenzen-Grossim-linghaus R, Krys U, Pirlich M, Herbst B, Schütz T, Schröer W, Weinrebe W, Ockenga J, Lochs H (2006) ESPEN guidelines on enteral nutrition: geriatrics. Clin Nutr 25:330–360

Wallace KL, Middleton S, Cook IJ (2000) Development and validation of a self-report symptom inventory to assess the severity of oral-pharyngeal dysphagia. Gastroenterology 118:678–687

Wang YT, Bieger D (1991) Role of solitarial GABAergic mechanisms in control of swallowing. Am J Physiol 261:639–646

Watando A, Ebihara S, Ebihara T, Okazaki T, Takahashi H, Asada M, Sasaki H (2004) Effect of temperature on swallowing reflex in elderly patients with aspiration pneumonia. J Am Geriatr Soc 52:2143–2144

Westergren A (2006) Detection of eating difficulties after stroke: a systematic review. Int Nurs Rev 53:143–149

Wielopolski L, Ramirez LM, Gallagher D, Sarkar SR, Zhu F, Kaysen GA, Levin NW, Heymsfield SB, Wang ZM (2006) Measuring partial body potassium in the arm versus total body potassium. J Appl Physiol 101:945–949

Williams RB, Wallace KL, Ali GN, Cook IJ (2002) Biomechanics of failed deglutitive upper esophageal sphincter relaxation in neurogenic dysphagia. Am J Physiol Gastrointest Liver Physiol 283:16–26

Working group on functional outcome measures (2008) Working group on functional outcome measures for clinical trials functional outcomes for clinical trials in frail older persons: time to be moving. J Gerontol A Biol Sci Med Sci 63:160–164

Dehydration in Dysphagia

Zeno Stanga, Samuel Hannes Baldinger, and Pere Clavé

Contents

Abstract

Dehydration–increased depletion of bodily fluids–is a major problem in the elderly. In patients with dysphagia, this imbalance of body fluids is often accelerated due to restricted fluid intake, leading to increased mortality in hospitalized older adults. As a result, the hydration status of patients with a swallowing disorder must be closely monitored and rapidly corrected. In the following, dehydration and fluid balance, as well as their pathophysiology and disorders, will be discussed in detail. Furthermore, risk factors for and signs and symptoms of dehydration in the elderly in general and in dysphagic patients in particular will be outlined. In addition, management of dehydration with oral, enteral and parenteral replacement of fluids will be explained. Parenteral hypodermoclysis, for example, has been shown to be as safe and effective as intravenous replacement, with a similar or better adverse event profile in a number of systematic reviews.

1 Learning Points

- To be aware of dysphagia-related dehydration.
- To be familiar with the pathophysiology of dehydration.
- To recognize the signs and symptoms of dehydration.
- To know the treatment strategies for dehydration.

Z. Stanga (✉) · S. H. Baldinger
University Polyclinic for Endocrinology,
Diabetes and Clinical Nutrition,
University Clinic for General Medicine,
University Hospital, Bern, Switzerland
e-mail: zeno.stanga@insel.ch

P. Clavé
Universitat Autònoma de Barcelona,
Hospital de Mataró, Barcelona, Spain

O. Ekberg (ed.), *Dysphagia*, Medical Radiology. Diagnostic Imaging, DOI: 10.1007/174_2011_349,
© Springer-Verlag Berlin Heidelberg 2012

2 Introduction

Fluid balance and electrolytes are vital to all life and are involved in countless regulatory mechanisms, such as cell shape, body temperature, signal transduction, and transportation systems. Dehydration is a large problem among elderly persons in long-term-care facilities, in acute care hospitals, as well as in the community. Dysphagia— a frequent consequence of neuromuscular or obstructive disease—is directly related to dehydration (Vivanti et al. 2009). An assessment of total water intake from food, beverages and enteral and parenteral sources among dysphagic adult patients receiving thickened fluids showed that no patients achieved their calculated fluid requirements unless enteral or parenteral fluids were given (Vivanti et al. 2009). Therefore, it is important to be aware of the risk of dehydration especially in patients with dysphagia. Special attention should be paid to signs and symptoms of dehydration in such patients. Treatment should be initialized promptly because the consequences of dehydration can be severe and has been associated with increased mortality among hospitalized older adults (Warren et al. 1994).

3 Definition of Dehydration

Different suggestions for the definition of dehydration exist. From a clinical point of view, rapid weight loss of greater than 3% of body weight has been proposed (Weinberg and Minaker 1995). From a pathophysiological point of view however, dehydration is a state of water depletion which results in a relative deficit of body water in relation to sodium with consequently increased sodium values, increased plasma osmolality, and a resulting loss of intracellular volume, often referred to as hypertonic dehydration or hypovolemic hypernatremia. Although the terms "hypotonic dehydration" and "isotonic dehydration" are widely used, pathophysiologically they characterize a condition of volume depletion rather than dehydration.

4 Prevalence of Dehydration

The true prevalence of dehydration is difficult to assess. It depends on the indicators used to define dehydration. Among community-dwelling adults it can be as high as 60% when defined as plasma sodium level of 145 mmol/l or greater, blood urea nitrogen (BUN) to creatinine ratio greater than 20, osmolarity greater than 295 mOsm/l, or hypotonic hypovolemia (Stookey et al. 2005). Another study found that 48% of older adults visiting an emergency department had laboratory values indicating dehydration; only in 26% of them did physicians document assessment for signs of dehydration (Bennett et al. 2004). In older adults, dehydration is one of the ten most frequent diagnoses for hospitalization (Xiao et al. 2004), and dehydration has been reported to be the most common fluid and electrolyte imbalance in older adults (Martin and Larsen 1994).

5 Risk Factors

5.1 Impact of Dysphagia

Dysphagia has been shown to be directly related to dehydration (Vivanti et al. 2009). In one study, daily fluid intake of thickened liquids was only 22% of the recommended amount of 1,500 ml/day (Whelan 2001).

5.2 Other Risk Factors

Although decreased sensitivity to antidiuretic hormone (ADH) has been shown in older adults and the sense of thirst appears to diminish (Phillips et al. 1993), even in otherwise healthy persons, several studies showed that, under normal conditions, older adults maintain adequate hydration. However, physical or emotional illness, surgery, trauma, or higher physiologic demands increase the risk of dehydration (Luckey and Parsa 2003).

A study following nursing home residents for 6 months found that 31% were dehydrated during that period and one third of those had had prior episodes of dehydration (Mentes et al. 2006). Dehydration in nursing homes has been linked to inadequately trained nurses. Residents with moderate to severe dysphagia, severe cognitive and functional impairment, aphasia or inability to speak the official language of the country, and a lack of family or friends to assist them at mealtimes are at great risk of dehydration (Kayser-Jones et al. 1999).

Female gender and polypharmacy have also been shown to increase the risk of dehydration in nursing

Fig. 1 Fluids compartments

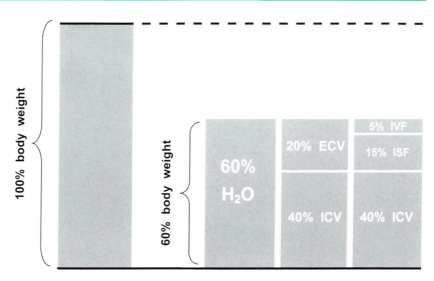

H₂O = water; ECV = extracellular volume; ICV = intracellular volume;
IVF = intravascular fluid; ISF = interstitial fluid

home residents (Lavizzo-Mourey et al. 1988). Dehydration occurs more frequently in older adults with diabetes, cancer, cardiac disease, or acute infections (Xiao et al. 2004; Warren et al. 1994) or especially in patients having multiple comorbidities (Bennett et al. 2004; Lavizzo-Mourey et al. 1988).

6   Pathophysiology of Dehydration

6.1   Fluid Compartments

Figure 1 illustrates water distribution in the body. Depending on age and gender, about 50–60% of body weight is from water. Since women generally have a higher percentage of body fat and a smaller muscle mass than men, they have somewhat less body fluid. Two different compartments are functionally separated by cell membranes. About two thirds of body water or 40% of total body weight is found in the intracellular space; the remaining one third of body water, accounting for 20% of total body weight, is found in the extracellular space (i.e., for an adult weighing 70 kg, about 60%, approximately 42 l, is water; the extracellular volume is about 14 l and the intracellular volume is about 28 l).

Extracellular water can further be subdivided into extravascular and intravascular fluid, functionally separated by the capillary wall. Extravascular fluid

counts for approximately 3/4 of extracellular fluid or 15% of total body weight. Only 1/12 of total body water is found intravascular, counting 5% of total body weight.

The extravascular component again can be subdivided into the interstitial fluids, the transcellular fluids, such as water in the gastrointestinal tract, and fluids in cartilages, connective tissues and bones.

6.2   External Fluid Balance

The skin, the respiratory tract, the endocrine system, the kidneys, and the gastrointestinal tract are involved in fluid balance. The average total fluid intake and output is about 2,600 ml/day (30–40 ml/kg body weight). Liquids account for about 1,500 ml of daily input; 800 ml comes from liquids within solid food and the remaining 300 ml comes from oxidation water (Fig. 2).

The main water output of 1,500 ml/day passes via the kidneys. A considerable amount is lost via the skin (600 ml) and the lungs (400 ml); together also referred to as insensible perspiration (Fig. 2). Only 100–150 ml/day is lost with the feces.

To understand the mechanisms of fluid balance, it is important to understand that maintenance of effective arterial blood volume is primarily related to the regulation of sodium balance. In contrast, maintenance of

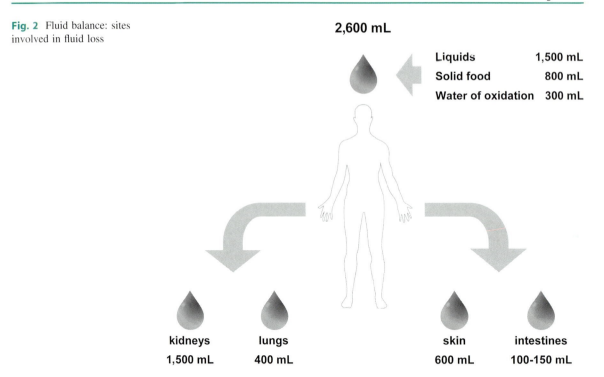

Fig. 2 Fluid balance: sites involved in fluid loss

Table 1 Electrolyte balance (mmol/l)

	ECV	ICV
Na$^+$	143	12
K$^+$	4	155
Cl$^-$	103	3.8
HCO$_3^-$	25	8

ECV extracellular volume, *ICV* intracellular volume

osmolality is related to the regulation of water balance. Maintenance of volume always overrides maintenance of osmolality. The ability of the kidney to excrete urine with an osmolality different from that of plasma plays a central role in the regulation of water balance. The kidney can conserve sodium very efficiently, but the capacity to excrete excess sodium is limited.

6.3   Internal Fluid Balance

The distribution of fluid between the different compartments is kept constant within close limits. The membranes separating the two main compartments, the intracellular and the extracellular space, are semipermeable, meaning that they allow only selected solutes to pass through. Water, however, can pass freely. The membranes with their Na-K-ATPase pump therefore maintain the different solute compositions within each compartment.

Osmolality is defined as the amount of solute particles per kilogram of solution. Plasma osmolality can be directly measured or calculated as 2 × serum sodium (mmol/l) + BUN (mg/dl)/2.8 + plasma glucose (mg/dl)/18. It normally ranges from 275 to 290 mOsm/kg.

Tonicity is determined by those solutes which determine the transcellular distribution of water, called effective osmoles. Urea for example is an inactive osmole since it can pass freely through the membrane and an elevation of serum urea level does not lead to movement of water out of the cell. Still it contributes to plasma osmolality.

Sodium, with normal serum concentrations of 135–145 mmol/l, is the major extracellular cation determining plasma osmolality, whereas potassium is the key determinant for intracellular osmolality (Table 1). Only 2% of the body's potassium is found in the extracellular fluid; the normal serum concentration range is from 3.5 to 5.0 mmol/l. The intracellular concentration is much higher, approximately 140 mmol/l (Table 1). Electroneutrality is granted by chloride and bicarbonate anions as well as proteins.

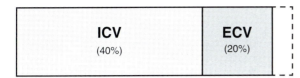

Fig. 3 Disorders of water balance: isotonic dehydration

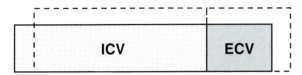

Fig. 4 Disorders of water balance: hypotonic dehydration

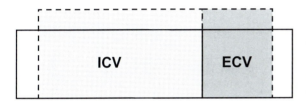

Fig. 5 Disorders of water balance: hypertonic dehydration

Osmotic forces are the primary determinant of water distribution in the body. A change in osmolality in one compartment makes the fluid hypertonic compared with the other compartments and triggers water movement across the cell membrane from lower to higher osmolality. Since water can freely cross cell membranes, the osmolality of the intracellular and the extracellular space is the same.

6.4   Disorders of Fluid Balance

6.4.1   Isotonic and Hypotonic Dehydration

"Isotonic dehydration" is a somewhat confusing term, in fact referring to a state of volume depletion rather than dehydration. It occurs when there is a balanced loss of solutes and water. The extracellular fluid volume decreases when severe isotonic dehydration occurs, leading to tissue hypoperfusion, whereas the plasma osmolality and consequently the intracellular fluid volume remain normal (Fig. 3).

Isotonic dehydration happens during vomiting, diarrhea, fistulae, use of diuretics, third space sequestration, burns, sedative and carbon monoxide intoxication, sunstroke, blood loss, or complete fast.

Volume depletion results in a decreased blood flow to the kidneys and triggers the renin–angiotensin–aldosterone system, which results in increased sodium and water reabsorption. ADH secretion triggers water retention in order to correct volume depletion.

Hypotonic dehydration occurs when sodium is lost at a greater rate than water, resulting in serum osmolality less than 270 mmol/l and serum sodium concentrations of less than 135 mmol/l. The low serum osmolality results in a reduction of the extracellular space (Fig. 4). It can occur when lost salt and fluid are partly replaced by hypotonic fluids.

These forms of dehydration should be treated with isotonic fluids.

6.4.2   Hypertonic Dehydration

Pathophysiologically, hypertonic dehydration is the literal form of dehydration. It results when water losses exceed those of sodium. Serum sodium concentrations exceed 145 mmol/l and the BUN to creatinine ratio is greater than or equal to 25. The elevation of the serum sodium concentration and therefore osmolality causes water to be pulled out of the cells into the extracellular fluid (Fig. 5).

Acute hypernatremia causes movement of water out of the brain. The decrease in brain volume can cause rupture of veins, causing intracerebral or subarachnoidal hemorrhage. As a compensatory mechanism, the cells of the brain begin to accumulate solutes, initially sodium and potassium, in order to pull water back to the cell and restore cell volume. Later, the accumulation of osmolytes occurs. These consist primarily of myoinositol and the amino acids glutamine and glutamate (Heilig et al. 1989; Lien et al. 1990).

Hypertonic dehydration occurs, as in dysphagia, owing to decreased water intake or during either renal or extrarenal excessive water losses. Renal water losses occur with use of loop diuretics or osmotic diuretics, in postobstructive disease, in the polyuric phase of acute renal failure, or in renal or central diabetes insipidus. Extrarenal water losses occur transcutaneously by sweating, as in the condition of fever, or burns or via the respiratory tract in hyperventilation. The increasing plasma osmolality triggers ADH release and thirst (Fig. 6). But also nonosmolar, volume-dependent receptors exist which trigger ADH secretion. Secretion of ADH from the supraoptic and

Fig. 6 Compensatory
mechanism of the regulation
of sodium and water. *ADH*
antidiuretic hormone

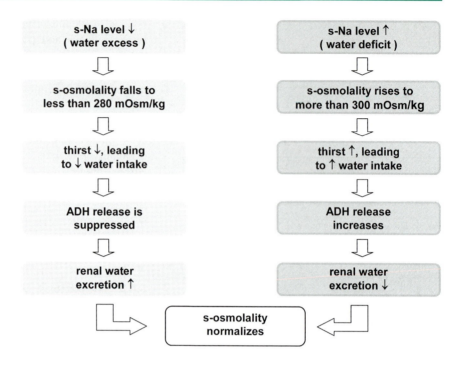

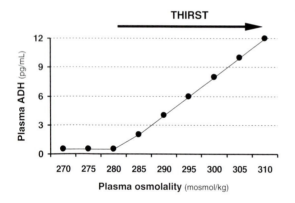

Fig. 7 Osmotic regulation of ADH release and thirst (Robertson et al. 1982)

paraventricular nuclei of the thalamus results in decreased excretion of free water. In humans the threshold for ADH secretion is 280–285 mOsm/kg. Above this threshold there is a relatively linear rise of ADH secretion with rising plasma osmolality (Fig. 7). The trigger value for the sense of thirst, which is the major protective mechanism against hypernatremia, is somewhat higher than for ADH secretion (Robertson 1987). This form of dehydration must be treated with hypotonic fluids (see Chap. 8).

7 Symptoms and Signs

Symptoms of dehydration can be very subtle (Table 2). They include lethargy, weakness, irritability, dizziness, and thirst, although in elderly patients the sense of thirst seems to be diminished. With rising sodium levels, especially in the setting of acute development, vomiting can occur and consciousness levels can become distinctively depressed up to delirium and coma. Also, seizures can occur and, as mentioned already, so can hemorrhage due to decreased brain volume. In general, central nervous system symptoms occur when dehydration results in a 1% loss of body weight and are very prominent for 5% loss (Lieberman 2007; Thomas et al. 2008). Chronic hypernatremia is less likely to cause neurologic effects than is acute hypernatremia, defined as development in less than 48 h.

Common clinical findings in dehydrated patients are dry skin and mucous membranes, fever, confusion, sunken eyeballs, poor skin turgor, decreased jugular venous pressure, oliguria, orthostatic hypotension with a greater risk of collapse, and tachycardia (Table 2). Although physical examination may suggest the presence of dehydration, physicians

Table 2 Signs, symptoms, and laboratory findings related to dehydration

Common symptoms

  Thirst

  Lethargy

  Weakness

  Dizziness

  Irritability

  Delirium

  Seizures

  Coma

  Fever

  Orthostatic hypotention

Common clinical signs

  Dry mucous membranes,

  Sunken eyes

  Muscle weakness

  Decreased skin turgor

  Rapid weight loss (3–5% of body weight)

  Decreased venous filling pressure

  Tachycardia

  Dark urine color and decreasing urine output

Laboratory findings

  Serum BUN to creatinine ratio >25

  Serum osmolality >300 mmol/kg

  Serum sodium concentration >150 mmol/l

  Urine osmolality >700 mmol/kg in a patient with hypernatremia (but not in diabetes insipidus or with use of diuretics)

  Urine specific gravity >1,029

should not rely only on clinical signs and symptoms to indicate that dehydration is present. In the final analysis, the diagnosis of dehydration can be confirmed biochemically.

Laboratory finding are increased hematocrit, increased serum sodium, BUN, and creatinine levels, and increased BUN to creatinine ratio (above 20), compared with previous values. In a patient with hypernatremia, a urine sodium concentration of less than 25 mmol/l indicates an inadequately low fluid replacement (Table 2).

The resulting prerenal kidney failure can lead to accumulation of active metabolites of certain drugs. In particular, patients receiving opioids should be closely monitored for adverse effects of opioid intoxication.

8 Management of Dehydration

8.1 General Management

Symptoms and vital signs of patients with dehydration should be carefully monitored and fluid intake and output should be accurately recorded. Skin and mouth care must be provided to maintain the integrity of the skin surface and oral mucous membranes.

As study showed that an effective standard to calculate fluid requirement for normal weight, underweight, and overweight patients is as follows: 100 ml/kg for the first 10 kg of body weight, 50 ml/kg for the next 10 kg of body weight, and 15 ml/kg for the remaining body weight (Chidester and Spangler 1997). In the case of fever, an additional 100–150 ml per degree Celsius higher than 37°C is needed. Caution should be paid to signs of overhydration, especially in patients with congestive heart failure.

8.2 Oral/Enteral Replacement

Whenever possible, oral rehydration should be favored. To replace missing fluids in a patient with dysphagia, thickened liquids, frozen juice bars, or food with high fluids (e.g., pureed fruits and vegetables) should be offered first. Sodium-containing solutions and food should be avoided (Mentes 2006). Water boluses given via a feeding tube (e.g., percutaneous endoscopic gastrostomy) may be necessary if hydration cannot be maintained.

8.3 Parenteral Replacement

8.3.1 Hypodermoclysis

With hypodermoclysis (HDC), fluid is infused into the subcutaneous space through a fine cannula. Several studies and reviews found that HDC is a safe and effective alternative to intravenous fluid administration in order to rehydrate older adults with mild to moderate dehydration who are unable to take adequate fluids orally (Remington and Hultman 2007; Slesak et al. 2003; Dasgupta et al. 2000). Favored sites for HDC are the thighs, abdomen, back, and arms, and are shown in Fig. 8.

Fluid can be infused using gravity at a rate of 20–80 ml/h. Over 24 h, up to 1.5 l can be delivered at

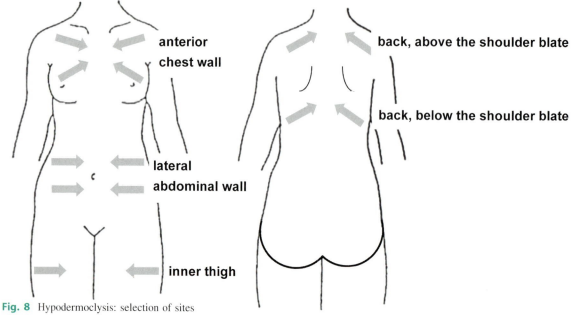

Fig. 8 Hypodermoclysis: selection of sites

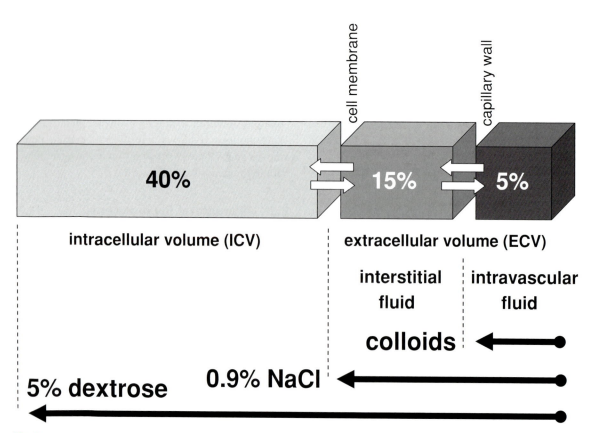

Fig. 9 Distribution of infused fluids

one site or 3 l can be delivered using two sites (Walsh 2005; Sasson and Shvartzman 2001; Jain et al. 1999). Other authors recommend an infusion rate of 82–148 ml/h (Thomas et al. 2008). Our experience in the outpatient clinic shows that the infusion of 1 l solution within 2 h is safe. Commonly, normal saline, isotonic dextrose–saline, 5% dextrose, and Ringer's solutions are used accordingly to the clinical situation. The achievable volume has been variously reported to be 1,500 ml/day, or up to 3,000 ml/day using two sites (Thomas et al. 2008). In a study of 60 residents in a long-term-care facility with dementia and mild to moderate dehydration, more subjects receiving intravenous fluids were agitated (80%) compared with subjects receiving subcutaneous fluids (37%). No difference was found in the amount of fluid administered or in improvement of dehydration parameters (O'Keefe and Lavan 1996). Lipshitz et al. (1991) demonstrated that radioactive technetium injected at the site of the infusion is absorbed into the blood supply within 60 min.

Subcutaneous infusions with hyaluronidase (an enzyme that degrade hyaluronan, resulting in an opening of the interstitial space) usually allow a faster infusion rate, a lower rate of moderate edema, and less discomfort.

The administration of up to 20 mmol potassium chloride per liter seems to be uncomplicated, but there have been no systematic studies. Local adverse effects occurred rarely and were similar in the HDC and intravenous groups. They included edema, erythema, and cellulitis. There was also no difference in the incidence of systemic adverse effects such as cardiac failure and hyponatremia (Slesak et al. 2003). Both methods showed the same effectiveness. HDC requires less nursing time and the cost of intravenous supplies was reported to be approximately 4 times greater than that of HDC supplies (O'Keefe and Lavan 1996). HDC seem to be particularly well suited for use in the nursing home, because the cannula can be sited out of the reach of the patient, making it less likely for it to become dislodged (Remington and Hultman 2007). Patients or their caretakers may also easily be taught to manage this technique at home. It is appropriate for treatment of mild to moderate dehydration or for the prevention of dehydration but is not an alternative for intravenous hydration in the condition of severe dehydration or hypovolemic shock.

8.3.2 Intravenous Rehydration

Severe dehydration usually requires the application of intravenous fluids. Although there is no exact definition of severe dehydration, a serum sodium concentration greater than 150 mmol/l, serum osmolality greater than 300 mOsm/kg, or a BUN to creatinine ratio greater than 25 indicates a distinctive lack of water. The free water deficit in patients with hypernatremia can be calculated as

$$\text{free water deficit (l)} = 0.6 \times \text{body weight (kg)} \times [(\text{plasma sodium}/140) - 1]$$

As an example, for a patient with a body weight of 60 kg and a serum sodium concentration of 150 mmol/l, the free water deficit is $0.6 \times 60 \times [(150/140)-1] = 2.5$ l. The deficit can be replaced with use of an isotonic dextrose solution. In the case of hypovolemia, dextrose–saline (2.5% glucose, 0.45% sodium chloride) should be preferred. Approximately, the doubled total volume is needed to achieve the same serum sodium level as with isotonic dextrose solution. One should be aware that the addition of potassium chloride or bicarbonate reduces the amount of free water in the same proportion as the addition of sodium chloride. Figure 9 demonstrates the distribution of infused fluids in the different compartments of the body (Allison and Lobo 2004).

In the setting of acute hypernatremia, lasting less than 48 h, the free water deficit should be replaced rapidly. However, rapid application of hypotonic solutions will cause fluids to move quickly from the intravascular space to the extravascular space and then into the cells. Especially in the brain, where osmolytes have accumulated in the cells in order to maintain normal cell volume (see Sect. 6.4.2), the rapid application of hypotonic solutes can cause brain edema. A slow correction is therefore mandatory for patients with hypernatremia lasting longer than 48 h. In the first 24 h, maximally 50% of the replacement should be completed and special attention should be paid to signs of cerebral edema such as headache and seizures. The remaining deficit can be corrected in the next 48–72 h. Ongoing water and sodium losses through the urine and insensible perspiration should be taken into account.

Take Home Messages

- Dehydration is a large, probably underestimated problem in dysphagic patients.
- Special attention must be paid to signs and symptoms of dehydration in this population.
- It is important to distinguish between dehydration and volume depletion, since the treatment approaches are different.
- Dehydration should be treated with hypotonic fluids according to the calculated water deficit.
- Volume depletion should be treated with isotonic fluids.
- Whenever possible, oral rehydration should be favored to treat mild dehydration.
- HDC is a safe and effective alternative to intravenous fluid administration to treat mild to moderate dehydration in patients with contraindications for oral rehydration, particularly in dysphagic patients.

References

Allison SP, Lobo DN (2004) Fluid and electrolytes in the elderly. Curr Opin Clin Nutr Metab Care 7(1):27–33

Bennett JA, Thomas V, Riegel B (2004) Unrecognized chronic dehydration in older adults: examining prevalence rate and risk factors. J Gerontol Nurs 30(11):22–28

Chidester JC, Spangler AA (1997) Fluid intake in the institutionalized elderly. J Am Diet Assoc 97(1):23–28

Dasgupta M, Binns MA, Rochon PA (2000) Subcutaneous fluid infusion in a long-term care setting. J Am Geriatr Soc 48(7):795–799

Heilig CW, Stromski ME, Blumenfeld JD, Lee JP, Gullans SR (1989) Characterization of the major brain osmolytes that accumulate in salt-loaded rats. Am J Physiol 257(6):F1108–F1116

Jain S, Mansfield B, Wilcox MH (1999) Subcutaneous fluid administration–better than the intravenous approach? J Hosp Infect 41(4):269–272

Kayser-Jones J, Schell ES, Porter C, Barbaccia JC, Shaw H (1999) Factors contributing to dehydration in nursing homes: inadequate staffing and lack of professional supervision. J Am Geriatr Soc 47(10):1187–1194

Lavizzo-Mourey R, Johnson J, Stolley P (1988) Risk factors for dehydration among elderly nursing home residents. J Am Geriatr Soc 36(3):213–218

Lieberman HR (2007) Hydration and cognition: a critical review and recommendations for future research. J Am Coll Nutr 26(5):555S–561S

Lien YH, Shapiro JI, Chan L (1990) Effects of hypernatremia on organic brain osmoles. J Clin Invest 85(5):1427–1435

Lipschitz S, Campbell AJ, Roberts MS, Wanwimolruk S, McQueen EG, McQueen M, Firth LA (1991) Subcutaneous

fluid administration in elderly subjects: validation of an under-used technique. J Am Geriatr Soc 39:6–9

Luckey AE, Parsa CJ (2003) Fluid and electrolytes in the aged. Arch Surg 138(10):1055–1060

Martin JH, Larsen PD (1994) Dehydration in the elderly surgical patient. Assoc Operat Rm Nurs J 60(4):666–671

Mentes JC (2006) Oral hydration in older adults: greater awareness is needed in preventing, recognizing, and treating dehydration. Am J Nurs 106(6):40–49

Mentes JC, Wakefield B, Culp K (2006) Use of a urine color chart to monitor hydration status in nursing home residents. Biol Res Nurs 7(3):197–203

O'Keefe ST, Lavan JN (1996) Subcutaneous fluids in elderly hospital patients with cognitive impairment. Gerontology 42(1):36–39

Phillips PA, Johnston CI, Gray L (1993) Disturbed fluid and electrolyte homoeostasis following dehydration in elderly people. Age Ageing 22(1):S26–S33

Remington R, Hultman T (2007) Hypodermoclysis to treat dehydration: a review of the evidence. J Am Geriatr Soc 55(12):2051–2055

Robertson GL (1987) Physiology of ADH secretion. Kidney Int 21:S20–S26

Robertson GL, Aycinena P, Zerbe RL (1982) Neurogenic disorders of osmoregulation. Am J Med 72:339–353

Sasson M, Shvartzman P (2001) Hypodermoclysis: an alternative infusion technique. Am Fam Physician 64(9):1575–1578

Slesak G, Schnürle JW, Kinzel E, Jakob J, Dietz PK (2003) Comparison of subcutaneous and intravenous rehydration in geriatric patients: a randomized trial. J Am Geriatr Soc 51(2):155–160

Stookey JD, Pieper CF, Cohen HJ (2005) Is the prevalence of dehydration among community-dwelling older adults really low? Informing current debate over the fluid recommendation for adults aged 70+ years. Public Health Nutr 8(8):1275–1285

Thomas DR, Cote TR, Lawhome L, Levenson SA, Rubenstein LZ, Smith DA, Stefanacci RG, Tangalos EG, Morley JE, Council Dehydration (2008) Understanding clinical dehydration and its treatment. J Am Med Dir Assoc 9:292–301

Vivanti AP, Campbell KL, Suter MS, Hannan-Jones MT, Hulcombe JA (2009) Contribution of thickened drinks, food and enteral and parenteral fluids to fluid intake in hospitalised patients with dysphagia. J Hum Nutr Diet 22(2):148–155

Walsh G (2005) Hypodermoclysis: an alternate method for rehydration in long-term care. J Infus Nurs 28(2):123–129

Warren JL, Bacon WE, Harris T, McBean AM, Foley DJ, Phillips C (1994) The burden, outcomes associated with dehydration among US elderly, 1991. Am J Public Health 84(8):1265–1269

Weinberg AD, Minaker KL (1995) Dehydration. Evaluation and management in older adults. Council on Scientific Affairs, American Medical Association. JAMA 15 274(19):1552–1556

Whelan K (2001) Inadequate fluid intakes in dysphagic acute stroke. Clin Nutr 20(5):423–428

Xiao H, Barber J, Campbell ES (2004) Economic burden of dehydration among hospitalized elderly patients. Am J Health Syst Pharm 61(23):2534–2540

Index

O. Ekberg (ed.), *Dysphagia*, Medical Radiology. Diagnostic Imaging, DOI: 10.1007/978-3-642-17887-0,
© Springer-Verlag Berlin Heidelberg 2012

Printing and Binding: Stürtz GmbH, Würzburg